Membrane Transport
in Red Cells

Membrane Transport in Red Cells

Edited by

J. CLIVE ELLORY

*Fellow of Queens' College Cambridge
and Lecturer in Physiology
The Physiological Laboratory
Cambridge University, England*

and

VIRGILIO L. LEW

*Fellow of King's College Cambridge
and Assistant Director of Research
The Physiological Laboratory
Cambridge University, England*

1977

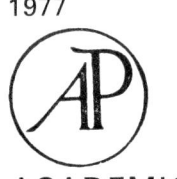

ACADEMIC PRESS
London   New York   San Francisco
A Subsidiary of Harcourt Brace Jovanovich, Publishers

ACADEMIC PRESS INC. (LONDON) LTD.
24/28 Oval Road, London NW1 7DX

United States Edition published by
ACADEMIC PRESS INC.
111 Fifth Avenue, New York, New York 1003

Copyright © 1977 by
ACADEMIC PRESS INC. (LONDON LTD.
All rights reserved. No part of this book may be reproduced in any form by photostat, microfilm, or any other means, without written permission from the publishers

Library of Congress Catalog Card Number: 77 74365
ISBN: 0 12 237150 X

Printed in Great Britain by
THE GARDEN CITY PRESS LIMITED
LETCHWORTH, HERTFORDSHIRE SG6 1JS

List of contributors

L. Beaugé, *Department of Biophysics, University of Maryland School of Medicine, Baltimore, Maryland, U.S.A.*
J. D. Cavieres, *The Physiological Laboratory, University of Cambridge, U.K.*
J. C. Ellory, *The Physiological Laboratory, University of Cambridge, U.K.*
H. G. Ferreira, *Laboratorio de Fisologia, Institutio Gulbenkian de Ciencia, Oeiras, Portugal.*
P. A. G. Fortes, *Department of Biology, University of California, San Diego, La Jolla, California, U.S.A.*
S. B. Hladky, *The Physiological Laboratory, University of Cambridge, U.K.*
G. D. Holman, *Department of Physiology, King's College, University of London, London, U.K.*
U. V. Lassen, *Zoophysiological Laboratory B., August Krogh Institute, University of Copenhagen, Denmark.*
V. L. Lew, *The Physiological Laboratory, University of Cambridge, U.K.*
F. M. Kregenow, *Laboratory of Kidney and Electrolyte Metabolism, National Heart and Lung Institute, N.I.H., Bethesda, Maryland, U.S.A.*
K. Martin, *Pharmacology Department, University of Cambridge, U.K.*
R. Motais, *Laboratory of Comparative Physiology, University of Nice, France.*
R. J. Naftalin, *Department of Physiology, King's College, University of London, London, U.K.*
J. C. Parker, *Division of Hematology, Department of Medicine, University of North Carolina, Chapel Hill, North Carolina, U.S.A.*
T. J. Rink, *The Physiological Laboratory, University of Cambridge, U.K.*
R. I. Sha'afi, *Department of Physiology, University of Connecticut Health Center, Farmington, Connecticut, U.S.A.*
S. K. Srivastava, *Department of Human Biological Chemistry and Genetics, University of Texas Medical Branch, Galveston, Texas, U.S.A.*
J. S. Wiley, *Austin Hospital, Department of Medicine, University of Melbourne, Heidelberg, Victoria, Australia 3084.*
J. D. Young, *A.R.C. Institute of Animal Physiology, Babraham, Cambridge, U.K.*

Preface

Cell biologists and scientists interested in membranes tend to regard the red cell ambivalently. On the one hand it is often considered a dead cell. Mammalian red cells lack nuclei and the various intracellular organelles. They are biochemically limited, and atypical in the sense of being highly specialized for a particular respiratory function. On the other hand, the red cell presents an excellent model for membrane transport studies. Although it lacks electrically-excitable channels, it does possess a suprising variety of transport systems, both active and passive, some of which are also widely distributed amongst other animal cells. Unlike the plasma membrane of giant cell systems like the squid axon, the red cell membrane is directly exposed to the bulk solution in which it is suspended. Furthermore, reversible haemolysis and selective ionophore treatments allow the composition of the internal medium of red cells to be controlled better than in any other cell.

It is the main purpose of this book to present the reader interested in membrane physiology with an overall picture of the transport systems peculiar to red cells, and of the use of the red cell membrane as an experimental model for the study of more general transport mechanisms. Such a project has to reflect the variety and versatility of transport systems currently being investigated in red cells from various species.

Original contributions were requested from active workers in each of the different fields covered. The organisation of these contributions into an appropriate sequence was simply done by grouping the different chapters into four sections: cation transport; anion transport and the related problems of pH and potential; non-electrolyte transport and finally comparative and clinical studies. Inevitably there are differences both in style and in scientific interpretation, but no editorial attempts have been made to avoid overlapping or conflicting views, since we feel that these can be fruitful and positive components of a multiauthor work like this. Allowing the contributors literary freedom necessarily leads to differences in terminology. In the discussion of membrane potential, where semantic confusion might have arisen we requested a clarifying comment from S. B. Hladky.

We hope that the collection of articles presented here bring to the attention not only of the specialist but also of scientists and clinicians working in related fields the range and sophistication of the transport processes that exist in the red cell membrane.

Cambridge, May 1977

J. CLIVE ELLORY
VIRGILIO L. LEW

Contents

List of contributors	v
Preface	vii
The sodium pump in human red cells J. D. Cavieres	1
Passive fluxes of sodium and potassium across red cell membranes L. Beaugé and V. L. Lew	39
Passive Ca transport and cytoplasmic Ca buffering in intact red cells H. G. Ferreira and V. L. Lew	53
The effect of Ca on the K permeability of red cells V. L. Lew and H. G. Ferreira	93
Choline transport in red cells K. Martin	101
pH equilibrium across the red cell membrane S. B. Hladky and T. J. Rink	115
Electrical potential and conductance of the red cell membrane U. V. Lassen	137
A comment on the semantics of the "determination" of membrane potential S. B. Hladky	173
Anion movements in red blood cells P. A. George Fortes	175
Organic anion transport in red blood cells R. Motais	197
Water and small nonelectrolyte permeation in red cells R. I. Sha'afi	221
Transport of sugars in human red cells R. J. Naftalin and G. D. Holman	257
Red cell amino acid transport J. D. Young and J. C. Ellory	301
Glutathione movements S. K. Srivastava	327

Genetic abnormalities of cation transport in the human erythrocyte 337
J. S. Wiley

The sodium pump in ruminant red cells 363
J. C. Ellory

Transport in avian red cells 383
F. W. Kregenow

Solute and water transport in dog and cat red blood cells 427
J. C. Parker

Index 467

The sodium pump in human red cells

J. D. CAVIERES
Physiological Laboratory, Cambridge University, UK

1 Introduction	1
2 Cation fluxes and adenosine triphosphatase activity	2
3 Enzymic properties of the sodium pump	8
3.1 Phosphorylation, dephosphorylation and ATP–ADP exchange	9
3.2 K-phosphatase activity	15
3.3 Ouabain inhibition and binding	17
4 Kinetic properties and models	22
4.1 ATPase reaction and inactivation studies	22
4.2 External and internal cation sites	23
4.3 Models	27
Acknowledgement	32
References	33

1 Introduction

Knowledge of the characteristics of sodium and potassium fluxes across the cell membrane has arisen in a great proportion from studies conducted with human red cells. The experimental system presents some clear advantages, like the homogeneity of the cell type, the absence of anatomical compartments, the possibility to distribute in aliquots, as well as the convenient handling of the intracellular composition which can be achieved by lysis and reconstitution of the resulting ghosts. Despite all these merits, red cells present a remarkably low density of sodium pumps (about 1/170 that of brain membranes or 1/400 that of kidney membranes (Bader *et al.*, 1968)) and hence they are not a suitable source for studies involving isolation and purification of the enzyme. However, just as little understanding of the pump mechanisms can be achieved by studying broken membrane preparations without due regard to the ionic fluxes, the same is true of the reciprocal situation. Accordingly, I will also consider enzymatic and other studies made with membrane preparations from tissues rich in the pump enzyme, and which can be extended in large measure to human erythrocytes.

Several other reviews on the sodium pump have been recently published, including those of Dahl and Hokin (1974), Glynn and Karlish (1975a), Jørgensen (1975a), Schwartz et al. (1975), Skou (1975), and Whittam and Chipperfield (1975).

2 Cation fluxes and adenosine triphosphatase activity

Shortly after the advent of radioactive isotopes, human and other erythrocytes were found to display a measurable permeability to potassium ions under physiological conditions (Mullins et al., 1941). Since the concentrations of Na and K in human red cells were far from those corresponding to electrochemical equilibrium, maintenance of a steady state presupposed the existence of an active process (at the expense of metabolic energy) for the transport of Na outwards and K inwards, or both (a Na–K pump), and which prevented the colloid-osmotic lysis of the cells. Danowski (1941) and Harris (1941) showed that while storage of erythrocytes at 4°C led to K loss and Na gain in the cells, rewarming of the suspensions to 37°C, in the presence of metabolic substrates, reversed these changes; glucose (Maizels, 1951) and inosine (Harris and Prankerd, 1955) were the best substrates for this purpose.

Shaw (1954, 1955) demonstrated that the influx of ^{42}K in washed horse red cells had a dependence on external K (K_o) which could be described in terms of one saturable and one linear component. The saturable portion of the influx implied dependence on a limited number of K-binding sites on the outside of the cell membrane, and this was consistent with a proposal (Shaw, 1954) of carrier molecules for the translocation of K inwards and Na outwards across the lipid barrier. Glynn (1956) studied Na and K fluxes in human erythrocytes and showed that starvation of the cells reduced the size of the saturable component of K influx. He also demonstrated that part of the Na efflux in media containing physiological Na concentrations depended on the presence of external K. The external K concentration for half-maximal activation ($K_{\frac{1}{2}}$) of K influx, about 2 mM, was very similar to $K_{\frac{1}{2}}$ for the activation of Na efflux by external K. Thus the proposal of a linkage of K influx and Na efflux through the Na pump was substantiated. The stoichiometry of the linkage was studied by Post and Jolly (1957) by measuring net Na and K fluxes in human red cells whose cation composition had been altered by cold storage: they found that 1·5 Na ions were pumped outwards per K pumped inwards.

In 1953, Schatzmann discovered that the cardiac glycoside strophanthin prevented the reversal of the changes of cell cation concentrations elicited by cold storage of the erythrocytes. Strophanthin seemed by then not to have any metabolic effects and it was rightly thought that it should interfere with the cation-transport machinery directly. Cardiac glycosides were shown to inhibit part of the K influx and of the Na efflux in human red cells and, in addition, part of the Na influx (Glynn, 1957). The last effect pointed at the existence of a pump-mediated exchange diffusion of Na, in addition to the exchange of Na for K.

A method then became available for resealing erythrocyte ghosts prepared by osmotic lysis (Hoffman et al., 1960; Hoffman, 1962a), making it possible to control the composition of the solutions bathing both sides of the cell membrane. The aglycone strophanthidin was found to inhibit Na efflux when present in the incubation medium, but not when incorporated inside ghosts at the lysing stage (Hoffman, 1966), thus confirming ouabain microinjection experiments with squid giant axons (Caldwell and Keynes, 1959). The dependence of the Na pump on adenosine triphosphate (ATP) was demonstrated by Gárdos (1954) by resealing the nucleotide into partially lysed red cells and in the presence of arsenate (to inhibit glycolytic phosphorylation), and by Hoffman (1960, 1962b) by using resealed ghosts prepared from metabolically depleted human red cells.

Working with crab nerve membranes, Skou (1957) described an adenosine triphosphatase (ATPase) activity that, besides Mg^{2+}, required Na and K ions as activators. His results implied separate sites for Na and K and cross-inhibition at high concentration ratios; these properties were consistent with the involvement of this (Na + K)-ATPase in Na and K transport. Post et al. (1960) and Dunham and Glynn (1961) described a similar enzymic activity in human erythrocyte ghosts and showed that cardiac glycosides inhibited a fraction of the ATPase activity. The Na and K concentrations for half-maximal activation of the ATPase coincided with those for the activation of the fluxes by internal Na and external K. At high Na concentrations, therefore, there was a decrease of the apparent affinity for K; similarly, the activation of K influx in intact erythrocytes by external K occurred with a lower affinity in high Na than in choline medium (Post et al., 1960).

Skou (1960) extended his studies with crab nerve ATPase and showed the existence of an ATP–AD^{32}P exchange reaction (no adenylate kinase was present), but no $^{32}P_i$–ATP exchange could be demonstrated. Several monovalent cations could replace for K in coactivating the ATPase in the presence of high Na, with affinities Rb,K > NH_4 > Cs > Li; potassium at high concentrations behaved as a competitive inhibitor towards Na. However, it is also apparent from Skou's (1960) results that monovalent cations other than Na, notably Li, can also activate his ATPase in the absence of Na, although to a much lesser extent. What this may mean is unclear, for the possibility of active Li efflux seems ruled out (in human red cells, at any rate) by experiments of McConaghey and Maizels (1962), who examined net fluxes of several alkali metal cations in cells loaded by lactose treatment. They demonstrated that while Rb, Cs and Li would replace for K at the external sites (with affinities K,Rb > Cs > Li) in supporting active Na efflux, none would replace for Na in being actively extruded from the cells. In particular, in Na-free systems (inside and out) the cells failed to extrude any Li into K + Li or into Cs + Li media; in these conditions, Li at both sides of the membrane simply followed the reciprocal chloride distribution ratio (McConaghey and Maizels, 1962).

Using yet another method for controlling the intracellular composition, Sen and Post (1961, 1964) subjected red cells to half-isotonic conditions which would lyse part of them (which were discarded) and induce a "pre-haemolytic" increase of permeability in the others. Working with high ATP, high Na "reconstituted red cells", they found that, provided that glycolysis was inhibited, there was a ratio of $1 \cdot 16 \times (3 \text{ Na} + 2 \text{ K})$ net transport cycles per high-energy phosphate bond spared by ouabain. They also showed that ADP and P_i were released intracellularly, and that ADP would not replace for ATP in the ATPase of broken ghosts if the membranes were properly ridden of adenylate kinase activity. Using Hoffman's ghosts instead, Glynn (1962) showed that the ouabain-sensitive ATPase activity was stimulated by internal Na and external K, and not vice versa. Laris and Letchworth (1962), Whittam (1962) and later Garrahan and Glynn (1967d) confirmed this finding.

Whittam and Ager (1965) measured ATPase activity as the sum of P_i release and lactate production (because of glycolytic reutilization of P_i). Loading human red cells by the lactose treatment of McConaghey and Maizels (1962), they found that ATPase activity and active K influx correlated linearly upon variation of the external K concentration, with a K : ∼ P ratio of 2·2 and in agreement with the findings of Sen and Post (1961); the ratio did not depend on the internal Na concentration and, hence, on the pump turnover rate. A linear correlation between ATPase and K influx was also obtained when the plot was done for varying ouabain concentrations, thus showing identical ouabain affinities for both processes in a simultaneous measurement. Parker and Hoffman (1967) observed that ouabain could inhibit lactate production in human red cells if they were loaded to contain a high Na concentration. Coupling of ATP hydrolysis by the pump to glycolytic phosphorylation of ADP was found to occur at the level of the phosphoglycerokinase reaction.

In a series of papers, Garrahan and Glynn (1967a,b,c,d,e) examined the behaviour of the sodium pump in human red cells and its dependence on several external and internal variables. Using fresh cells, they confirmed that the stoichiometry for Na–K exchange was different from 1 : 1; measuring tracer fluxes, the quotient ouabain-sensitive (O.S.) Na efflux to

O.S. K influx was nearly 1·3, but it could have been as high as 1·8 if part of the O.S. K influx represented K–K exchange through the pump. The O.S. Na : $\sim$ P ratio was in turn found close to 2·9 (Garrahan and Glynn, 1967d). Thus 3 Na were pumped out and 2 K pumped in per ATP hydrolysed, as found by Post and Jolly (1957) and Sen and Post (1964) measuring net fluxes. When the O.S. Na efflux of red cells was measured in K-free media (Garrahan and Glynn, 1967a), the rather surprising observation was made that there was a substantial O.S. Na efflux into Na-free solutions (see Fig. 1) and that as the external Na concentration was raised the O.S. Na efflux passed through a minimum at about 5 mM Na_o, to increase again almost linearly up to 140 mM Na_o (see also Sachs,

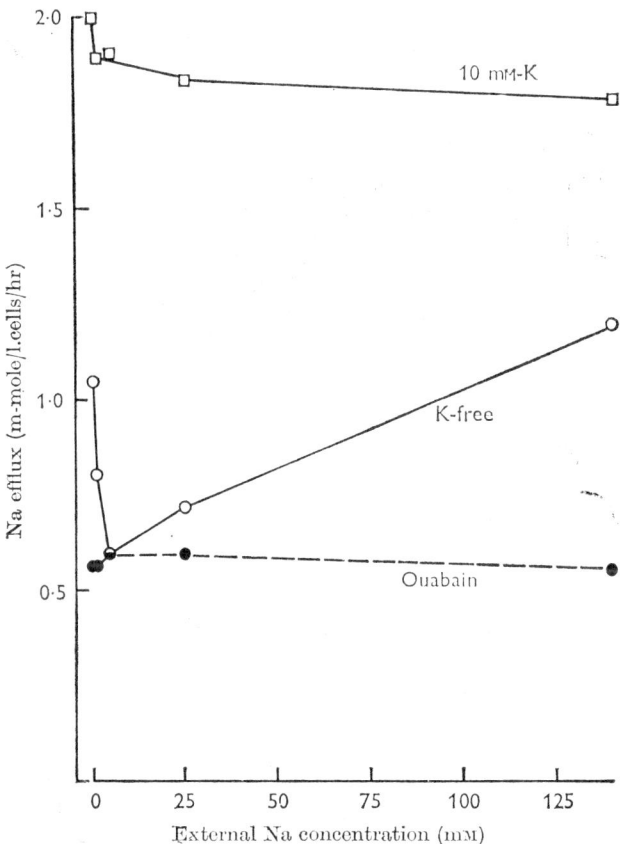

FIG. 1. The effect of external Na concentration on the Na efflux from fresh red cells, with and without external potassium or 7×10^{-5} M ouabain. Choline replacement. Reproduced from Garrahan and Glynn (1967a).

1970). The linear portion of the efflux was matched by an almost equal O.S. Na influx, and thus constituted a 1–1 exchange of internal for external Na ions through the pump (Garrahan and Glynn, 1967a).

External K ions activated the O.S. K influx following a sigmoid curve at high external Na and a quasi-hyperbola in choline medium (Fig. 2) (Garrahan and Glynn, 1967b; Sachs and Welt, 1967). In high Na medium, external K ions inhibited the O.S. Na influx following a curve which was the "mirror image" of the activation of O.S. K influx (Garrahan and Glynn, 1967c). Thus the appearance of Na–K exchange as the external K concentration increases occurs at the expense of Na–Na exchange through

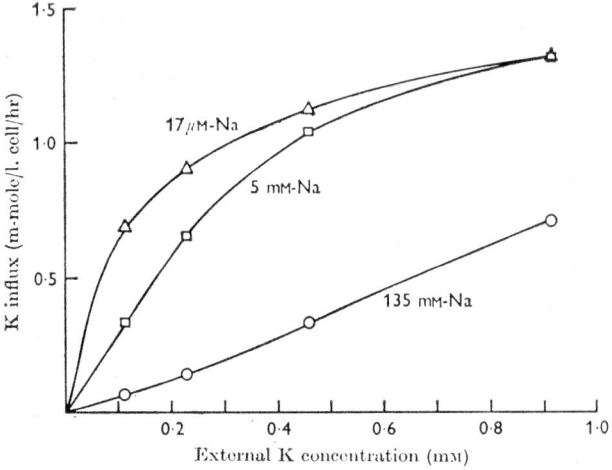

FIG. 2. The activation of K influx by external K in fresh red cells and the effect of external Na. Choline replaces Na. Reproduced from Garrahan and Glynn (1967b).

the pump. Although ATP seemed necessary for Na–Na exchange in resealed ghosts, this mode of operation of the pump was favoured by either low ATP or high P_i concentrations, or low internal Na and high internal K; in fact, at a low intracellular [ATP] : [ADP][P_i] ratio, external K ions inhibited the O.S. Na efflux (Garrahan and Glynn, 1967c). Finally, resealed ghosts with a low [ATP] : [ADP][P_i] ratio were shown to incorporate $^{32}P_i$ into ATP if the cation gradients were steeper than normal. The incorporation suggested that in these conditions the pump could run backwards, leading to ATP synthesis (Garrahan and Glynn, 1967e; Lant and Whittam, 1968).

The reversal of the pump was later demonstrated by Glynn et al. (1970)

and Lant et al. (1970), who showed the existence of an O.S. K efflux in red cells. In the absence of external K ions, the O.S. K efflux varied linearly with the external Na concentration (Glynn et al., 1970). In the presence or absence of external Na, the O.S. K efflux was activated by external K ions with $K_{\frac{1}{2}}$ values which were similar to those for the activation of Na–K exchange in comparable conditions. Since in these circumstances O.S. K influx greatly exceeded the O.S. K efflux, K–K exchange through the pump should occur only once every four or more Na–K exchange cycles. In the absence of external K, however, the O.S. K efflux was associated with an O.S. influx of Na superimposed on to the component of Na–Na exchange, i.e. with reversal of the entire pump cycle (Glynn et al., 1970). Using starved, phosphate-loaded erythrocytes, Glynn and Lew (1970) found an O.S. $^{32}P_i$ incorporation into ATP, which was activated by external Na with a low affinity (just as O.S. K efflux or O.S. Na efflux into K-free media are activated) and inhibited by external K (as the O.S. Na influx is). The pump reversal yielded a ratio of O.S. K efflux to O.S. ATP synthesis not very different from 3 (Glynn and Lew, 1970).

The effect of various nucleotides on Na–Na and Na–K exchanges in resealed ghosts was examined by Glynn and Hoffman (1971), who found that only ATP would sustain Na–K exchange significantly and Na–Na exchange in some measure; Na–Na exchange varied linearly with ADP concentration, but no relationship between ADP and Na–K exchange was found. The ADP requirement and the negligible ATP hydrolysis concomitant with it (Garrahan and Glynn, 1967c,d) suggested that Na–Na exchange could be associated to the ATP–ADP exchange reaction originally described by Skou (1960), just as Na–K exchange is to the overall (Na + K)-ATPase reaction. That Na–Na exchange through the pump has an absolute requirement for ATP could be shown after extensive inhibition and dilution of red cell adenylate kinase, and since the β,γ-imido analogue of ATP was found ineffective, the ATP activation should be mediated by phosphorylation of the pump (Cavieres and Glynn, 1976).

The characteristics of the O.S. K–K exchange have been further studied by Simons (1974, 1975) using resealed ghosts. The exchange is activated by internal K with $K_{\frac{1}{2}}$ of about 10 mM, and is strongly inhibited by internal Na ions. Since the O.S. K–K exchange is, in fact, activated by internal P_i (Glynn et al., 1970; Simons, 1974), it should represent the reversal of the dephosphorylation step of the pump cycle, probably associated with the P_i–H_2O exchange that Dahms and Boyer (1973) have demonstrated with a purified electroplax (Na + K)-ATPase preparation. Surprisingly though, K–K exchange also requires ATP (with a low affinity), although it is not hydrolysed and can be replaced by nonphosphorylating analogues (Simons, 1974, 1975). This and other similar findings clearly show that ATP is needed by the pump in a capacity different from that in the phosphorylation reaction or in Na–Na exchange (see below).

The O.S. Na efflux in (Na + K)-free medium (Garrahan and Glynn, 1967a) was further characterized by Lew et al. (1973), who found that the efflux did not represent an exchange for K leaking from the cells, and was then uncoupled. However, it needed ATP. They proposed that the uncoupled Na efflux could have its counterpart in the spontaneous dephosphorylation which occurs in the absence of potassium ions. Experiments studying the uncoupled Na efflux and the Na-ATPase activity at low ATP concentrations (Karlish and Glynn, 1974; Glynn and Karlish, 1976) will be considered, for convenience, in the next section.

The Na pump, in human erythrocytes at any rate, can then work in five different "modes", namely Na–K, Na–Na and K–K exchanges, K–Na exchange (reversal) and Na–0 (uncoupled Na efflux) (Glynn and Karlish, 1975b). Of them, Na–K, Na–Na and Na–0 have been identified in nerve (Keynes and Swan, 1959; Caldwell et al., 1960; Baker, 1964; Baker et al., 1969).

The results on pump-mediated fluxes and ATPase activity rest, especially in the case of kinetic analysis, on the assumption that the observed ouabain-sensitive fractions occur as a result of the activity of the pump. The identification of pump and ouabain-sensitive properties has benefited from inhibition experiments using an anti-pump antibody. Antisera raised in rabbits against a highly purified pig kidney (Na + K)-ATPase preparation, inhibited the O.S. (Na + K)-ATPase of broken ghosts from human erythrocytes as well as that from other sources; and also the O.S. Na–K and Na–Na exchanges exactly when incorporated into resealed ghosts (Jørgensen et al., 1973): the antiserum also inhibited the O.S. K–K exchange and the O.S. uncoupled Na efflux (Glynn et al., 1974).

3 Enzymic properties of the sodium pump

A number of enzymic reactions which appear associated to the activity of the pump-ATPase have been described in crude membrane extracts and microsomal preparations from kidney, brain and electric organ amongst other tissues, including red cells. The attribution of phosphorylation and dephosphorylation, ATP–ADP exchange, K-phosphatase activity and ouabain binding to (Na + K)-ATPase, rested in their sensitivity to Na and K or in their susceptibility to ouabain inhibition. Identification has been possible now that (Na + K)-ATPase has been obtained in a high degree of purity (for review see Jørgensen, 1975). I will examine each of these properties as they occur in different preparations and will attempt to connect them with the translocating properties of the enzyme, as they emerge from the studies conducted with human erythrocytes.

3.1 PHOSPHORYLATION, DEPHOSPHORYLATION AND ATP–ADP EXCHANGE

That membrane preparations could be phosphorylated by [γ^{32}P]ATP at 0°C was demonstrated by Charnock and Post (1963) and Post et al. (1965) using guinea-pig kidney microsomes and by Albers et al. (1963) with eel electric organ ATPase. The TCA*-stable labelling was accelerated by Na, inhibited by the addition of K and stabilized by ouabain, which relieved the K inhibition (Charnock and Post, 1963). The $K_{\frac{1}{2}}$ for Na stimulation in the absence of K was 1·6 mM, similar to that for the Na-activation of (Na + K)-ATPase at low K levels (Post et al., 1960). The phosphorylation rate was half-maximal at about 1 μM [γ^{32}P]ATP, i.e. 1/100 or less the value of $K_{\frac{1}{2}}$ for ATP in the overall (Na + K)-ATPase reaction. Addition of an excess unlabelled ATP exposed a spontaneous dephosphorylation whose rate was increased by low concentrations of K (Post et al., 1965). The phosphorylated protein met the minimal requirement to be the intermediate in the (Na + K)-ATPase reaction, for its formation was catalysed by Na ions and its breakdown by K ions (Post and Sen, 1965).

Oligomycin, a well-known inhibitor of oxidative phosphorylation, decreases the rate of (Na + K)-ATPase in resealed ghosts at the same pace as Na–K exchange (Whittam et al., 1964). In kidney microsomes, oligomycin also slows down the hydrolysis of the phosphorylated intermediate, but not its formation (Whittam et al., 1964). At concentrations which maximally inhibit the (Na + K)-ATPase of electric organ microsomes, oligomycin does not inhibit an ATP-[^{14}C]ADP exchange reaction; the exchange can instead be inhibited by K, ouabain and high Mg concentrations (Fahn et al., 1966). This finding led Albers and his colleagues to propose the scheme

$$E_1 + \text{ATP} \xrightleftharpoons{\text{Na}^+,\ \text{low Mg}^{++}} E_1 \sim \text{P} + \text{ADP}$$

$$E_1 \sim \text{P} \xrightarrow[\text{oligomycin}]{\text{high Mg}^{++}} E_2 - \text{P}$$

$$E_2 - \text{P} \xrightarrow{\text{K}^+} E_2 + \text{P}_i$$

where the phosphorylated intermediate would exist in at least two forms: a

* TCA = trichloroacetic acid.

first one ($E_1 \sim P$) which is sensitive to ADP and not to K, and a second ($E_2 - P$) which is K-sensitive and ADP-insensitive. The conversion of $E_1 \sim P$ into $E_2 - P$ would then be accelerated by Mg ions and inhibited by oligomycin.

Similar phosphorylation, dephosphorylation and ATP-ADP exchange reactions have been found by Blostein (1968, 1970) in membranes of human erythrocytes. But in this case, oligomycin increases the rate of ATP-ADP exchange (Blostein, 1970), an observation also made by Stahl (1968) for rat brain ATPase. Since, on the other hand, the O.S. Na-Na exchange in red cells is inhibited by oligomycin (Garrahan and Glynn, 1967d), then Na-Na exchange must involve at least one step beyond the point of release of ADP (Glynn et al., 1971), possibly $E_1 \sim P \rightarrow E_2 - P$.

Post et al. (1969) allowed kidney membranes to equilibrate with [γ^{32}P]ATP plus Na, with and without K, so as to allow the nucleotide to bind without phosphorylating. Then Mg ions and a chase of nonradioactive ATP were added so that only bound [γ^{32}P]ATP could phosphorylate. The result showed that K did not affect the phosphorylation capacity of the enzyme, though it increased the dephosphorylation rate (see Fig. 3). In a complementary experiment, the enzyme was equilibrated with [γ^{32}P]ATP plus Mg ions and without Na or K and then chased with nonradioactive ATP plus Na plus varying concentrations of ADP. It was found that ADP

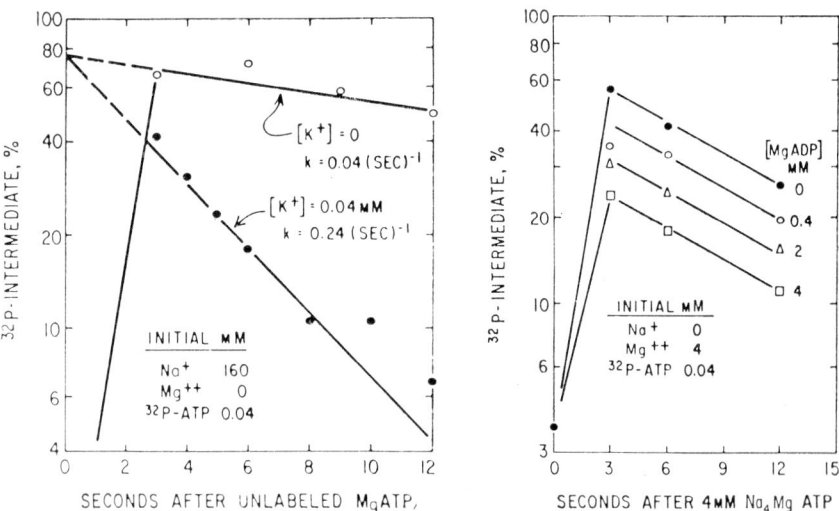

FIG. 3. K-sensitive and ADP-sensitive phosphoenzymes. Phosphorylation started *and* chased at zero-time. Reaction mixture completed at the *left* with Mg $\pm$ K ions and at the *right* with Na ions $\pm$ variable MgADP concentrations. Excess cold ATP included at zero-time as chasing agent. Reproduced from Post et al. (1969).

did not affect the dephosphorylation rate, but decreased the initial amount of phosphorylated enzyme. Since ADP was not present during the initial equilibration with [γ^{32}P]ATP, its effect should be attributed to rapid reversal of phosphorylation. As ADP, on the other hand, does not increase the dephosphorylation rate, it follows that the remaining phosphoenzyme must represent an ADP-insensitive form arising from that which was ADP-sensitive (Post et al., 1969).

Blostein (1970) found that when membranes of human erythrocytes are phosphorylated by $2\,\mu$M [γ^{32}P]ATP at 37°C and the reaction is then chased by K or nonradioactive ATP, rapid dephosphorylation occurs. Membranes treated with ouabain or oligomycin will lose K sensitivity, but the bound ^{32}P will still experience turnover on addition of excess nonradioactive ATP (since the spontaneous dephosphorylation should have also been blocked by the inhibitors, the observed turnover must arise *either* from ADP contamination in the excess ATP *or* from ADP still bound to the enzyme, see Blostein (1975)).

Departing from the scheme of Fahn et al. (1966) and Post et al. (1969), Fukushima and Tonomura (1973) have proposed that after starting the phosphorylation by [γ^{32}P]ATP, the K-sensitive phosphoenzyme appears first and the ADP-sensitive phosphoenzyme later. They support this claim in their Fig. 6 which shows that when ADP is added at 0·1 and 0·2 sec after [γ^{32}P]ATP, there is no decrease in the level of ^{32}P-phosphoenzyme formed until then, but that decrements which are progressively larger are obtained when ADP is added after longer intervals. However, the evidence is blurred by the fact that at the shortest times dephosphorylation was not observed after EDTA* either; this implies that at the beginning of the reaction they are observing a rapid labelling of a small extent and which has slow or no turnover (cf. Skou and Hilberg, 1969). If this initial labelling is deducted as a baseline, the ADP-induced decays are grossly exponential at all times and with comparable time-courses. Using also a rapid-mixing technique, Mårdh (1975) has provided a clear demonstration of transient accumulation of an ADP-sensitive phosphoenzyme when bovine brain ATPase is phosphorylated by [γ^{32}P]ATP *in the presence* of K.

Evidence for the role of the phosphoenzyme as intermediate in the ATPase reaction has been provided by Neufeld and Levy (1970) for the steady state, by Kanazawa et al. (1970) during the transient state of phosphorylation by [γ^{32}P]ATP and by Mårdh and Zetterqvist (1972, 1974) measuring phosphorylation and dephosphorylation rates with observations in the millisecond range. On this basis, a catalytic centre activity of 6000 min^{-1} was calculated for the Na pump in native erythrocyte membranes at

* EDTA = ethylenediaminotetraacetic acid. It blocks phosphorylation by chelation of Mg ions.

2 mM ATP and 37°C (Blostein, 1970). A value of 12 000 min^{-1} had been reported by Bader et al. (1968) in similar conditions. In (Na + K)-ATPase preparations from various tissues and species it ranged between 4000 and 13 000 min^{-1} (Bader et al., 1968).

When the ATPase activity of erythrocyte membranes is measured in the presence of Mg and Na ions, the addition of K ions inhibits the activity at 0·1 μM ATP and activates it at higher ATP concentrations (Blostein, 1970). Similar observations have been made with other preparations (Czerwinski et al., 1967; Neufeld and Levy, 1969). Na-ATPase and (Na + K)-ATPase behaved kinetically as if they were separate enzymes, but Post et al. (1972) have pointed out that the Na-ATPase activity of kidney membranes can be accounted for by the spontaneous splitting of the phosphorylated intermediate. They also found that during the normal dephosphorylation of $E_2 - P$ as stimulated by K and its congeners, an "occluded form" of the dephosphoenzyme ensued whose release, as assessed by rephosphorylation by [γ^{32}P]ATP, could be accelerated by high Na and by increasing the total ATP concentration. Consequently, a second, low-affinity ATP effect was postulated, as characteristic of the (Na + K)-activated hydrolysis (see Fig. 4). Occlusion of the dephosphoenzyme in the presence of K and its congeners would explain the inhibition of the Na-ATPase activity by K at low ATP concentrations; a membrane Na-UTPase activity, which presents a low affinity for the substrate, is always inhibited by K ions (Siegel and Goodwin, 1972).

A high-affinity binding of ATP to (Na + K)-ATPase preparations in the absence of Mg ions has been studied by Hegyvary and Post (1971) and Nørby and Jensen (1971), who have found a low dissociation constant (0·12–0·22 μM), of the order of $K_{\frac{1}{2}}$ for the phosphorylation reaction (Post et al., 1965). The reversible binding is not affected by Na, but K inhibits it, and this can be reversed by Na (Hegyvary and Post, 1971). This behaviour has been explained by proposing two forms of the dephosphoenzyme before turnover: E_1, with high ATP affinity and low affinity for K, and E_2, with the inverse properties. Then the native enzyme would mainly be in the E_1 form. Similar conclusions have been reached by Post et al (1973) who have observed that the onset of the phosphorylation by [γ^{32}P]ATP plus Mg and Na ions at 0°C shows a delay when the dephosphoenzyme has been in previous contact with K, but not when with Na and no K; and by Karlish et al (1976) who have found that the rate of binding of a fluorescent ATP analogue is considerably decreased when the enzyme has been in previous contact with K and no Na. Independent evidence comes from NEM-inactivation experiments of Skou (1974a) and a trypsin-inactivation study by Jørgensen (1975b).

A two-component decay of ^{32}P-phosphoenzyme, not fully accounted by

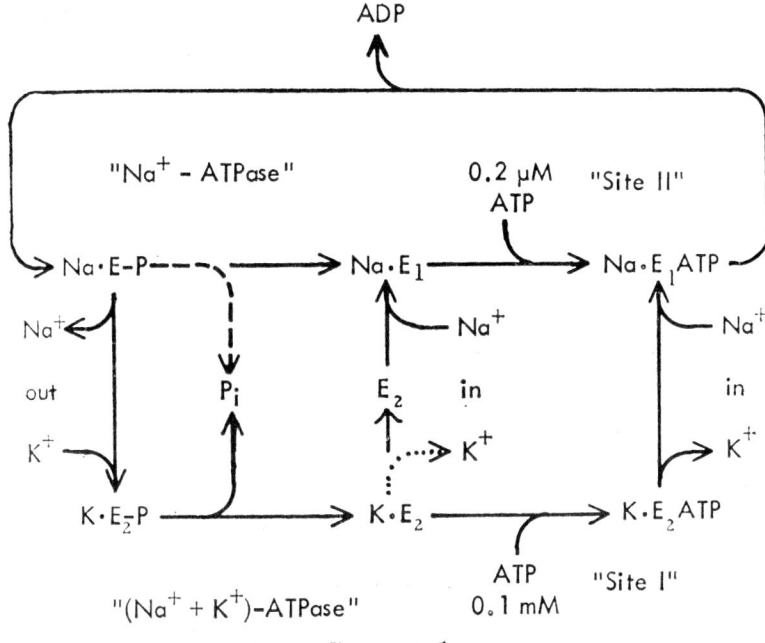

SCHEME 1

FIG. 4. Relationships amongst (Na + K)-ATPase and Na-ATPase activities and the occluded dephosphoenzyme form (KE_2). Reproduced from Post et al. (1972).

$^{32}P_i$ liberation, has been found for (Na + K)-ATPase preparations from bovine brain (Kanazawa et al., 1970; Tonomura and Fukushima, 1974) and human red cell membranes (Blostein, 1975). In these cases, the phosphorylation being conducted at very low [γ^{32}P]ATP concentrations, the fast initial dephosphorylation seems associated with ATP resynthesis, possibly from ADP still bound to the enzyme. These results are consistent with the ability of K ions to release bound ATP (Hegyvary and Post, 1971; Nørby and Jensen, 1971) and with the finding that EDTA blocks the conversion of $E_1 \sim P$ to $E_2 - P$ (Klodos and Skou, 1975).

When the uncoupled Na efflux of resealed ghosts is compared with their O.S. Na–K exchange, ATP or CTP activate the former with higher affinities than the latter (Karlish and Glynn, 1974), suggesting that the uncoupled Na efflux is associated to the Na-ATPase activity of the membranes, as Na-K exchange is to the (Na + K)-ATPase. Making use of a regenerating system incorporated into resealed ghosts, Glynn and Karlish (1976) could measure a small O.S. Na$_i$-ATPase activity at [γ^{32}P]ATP concentrations as low as 1 μM, and in media lacking Na and K. The simultaneous measurement of O.S. efflux of ^{24}Na gave a Na : $\sim$ P ratio between 2 and 3 whether in the absence or in the presence of external K ions. When the O.S. Na-ATPase of resealed ghosts was measured in K-free media and as a function of external Na concentration, the hydrolysis reached a minimum at about 5 mM Na$_o$, to increase again linearly towards higher external Na concentrations. This reactivation matches the observation by Post et al. (1972) that with kidney membranes high Na concentrations increased the (spontaneous) dephosphorylation rate of the ^{32}P-phosphoenzyme as they gave way to a second phase of activation of the Na-ATPase activity. The Na-ATPase activity of resealed ghosts was, in addition, inhibited by external K, both in the presence and in the absence of external Na (Glynn and Karlish, 1976), and this was explained by occlusion of the enzyme as KE_2 (see Fig. 4) occurring after the dephosphorylation catalysed by external K. The effect of external Na on the O.S. Na-ATPase was strikingly similar to that on the O.S. Na efflux in K-free media (Garrahan and Glynn, 1967b; Lew et al., 1973) where the uncoupled Na efflux decreased towards 5 mM Na$_o$, to give way to a 1-1 exchange of internal for external Na ions (see Fig. 1). But in the Na-ATPase experiment, intracellular ADP is virtually absent due to the action of the creatine phosphate/phosphokinase regenerating system, and hence there should not be a proper Na–Na exchange through the pump. It might be that in these conditions, high external Na leads to a 3–2 Na–Na exchange, or else that uncoupled Na efflux occurs again while Na ions sit on external sites without being translocated inwards (Glynn and Karlish, 1976). At any rate, Na binding at one external pump site seems not to lead to O.S. Na influx in conditions of Na–K exchange (Cavieres and Ellory, 1975).

These findings, as well as the nonphosphorylating ATP requirement of K–K exchange (Simons, 1974, 1975) reaffirm the need to postulate a "low-affinity ATP site". This seemed not necessary for the uncoupled Na efflux or associated Na-ATPase activity, and may not be for Na–Na exchange (Glynn and Hoffman, 1971) or the ATP–ADP exchange probably associated with it.

Phosphorylation of the ATPase by ^{32}P$_i$ (in the absence of ouabain) has also been demonstrated (Post et al., 1975). ^{32}P$_i$ can phosphorylate in exchange with phosphoenzyme formed from ATP, or else directly on to the native dephosphoenzyme; it can also label the occluded dephosphoenzyme formed by phosphorylation from nonradioactive ATP and dephosphorylation in the presence of Rb or Li. The ^{32}P-enzyme formed can be either K-sensitive or K-insensitive, depending on the conditions for its formation and the concentration of Mg ions. But it is in no case ADP-sensitive, and hence these should be envisaged as forms of $E_2 - $ P. However, AT^{32}P can be formed from ^{32}P-enzymes thus obtained (Post et al., 1974; Taniguchi and Post, 1975) by treatment with very high concentrations of Na and

CDTA* (to spare the AT^{32}P from hydrolysis). Since the system is apparently devoid of compartmentalization that allows gradients to be formed (or limits the access of Na to its "reversal site"), the energy for the ATP synthesis must arise from a conformational change of the enzyme ($E_2 - P \rightarrow E_1 \sim P$?) brought about by the high Na concentration. This stepwise route to ATP synthesis is indeed one of the strongest evidences for the existence of two phosphorylated intermediates in sequence. A reversible phosphorylation by P_i is probably associated to the O.S. K–K exchange, considering its requirement for inorganic phosphate (Glynn et al., 1970; Simons, 1974). ATP synthesis from P_i plus ADP (Garrahan and Glynn, 1967e; Lant and Whittam, 1968; Glynn and Lew, 1970; Post et al., 1974; Taniguchi and Post, 1975) would in turn imply coupled reversal of Na and K fluxes through the Na pump (Glynn et al., 1970).

These examples of association of ion-translocating and biochemical events amount to substantial evidence for the involvement of the phosphorylated enzyme as intermediate in the pump cycle, and for the connection of some "partial reactions" of the enzyme with Na and K movements catalysed by the sodium pump.

3.2 K-PHOSPHATASE ACTIVITY

Judah et al. (1962) observed that K ions stimulated the hydrolysis of p-nitrophenylphosphate (PNPP) by a preparation of human erythrocyte ghosts; Na ions inhibited the K-stimulated hydrolysis. A similar enzymic activity was then found in membranes of several other tissues (Albers and Koval, 1966; Fujita et al., 1966; Nagai et al., 1966), varying in parallel with (Na + K)-ATPase activities and correlating with various inactivating treatments. The $K_{\frac{1}{2}}$ for the K activation is about 3 mM, and the affinities for cation replacement in the activation are Rb > K > NH$_4$ > Cs > Na > Li (series III of Eisenman, 1960) (Albers and Koval, 1966; Nagai et al., 1966). In the absence of K, sodium ions stimulate at low concentrations ($K_{\frac{1}{2}}$ about 10 mM) but high concentrations are inhibitory (Fujita et al., 1966; Nagai et al., 1966). Lineweaver-Burk plots for the K-activation in the presence of Na bend downwards (Nagai et al., 1966; Robinson, 1969a). This suggests that Na displays both activatory and inhibitory effects also in the presence of K. Interestingly enough, Na seems to change the kinetics of substrate interaction: the double-reciprocal plots shown by Nagai et al. (1966) for the dependence on PNPP concentration are linear in the absence of Na but bend upwards in its presence, as if Na disclosed the existence of a second PNPP site (which in its absence might be swamped by a large difference of affinities). This recalls suggestions regarding the

* CDTA = 1,2-diaminocyclohexanetetracetic acid, a divalent cation chelating agent.

ATPase and its substrate (Glynn and Lew, 1969; Post et al., 1972; Glynn and Karlish, 1976), although the kinetics in this case are different (Neufeld and Levy, 1969). K-phosphatase also hydrolyses carbamyl-phosphate and acetyl-phosphate (Bond et al., 1966; Yoshida et al., 1966); the latter can also substitute for ATP as a substrate for (Na + K)-ATPase, phosphorylating the enzyme by the Na-dependent route (Bond et al., 1971).

Fujita et al. (1966) and Nagai et al. (1966) also observed that K-phosphatase was inhibited by ATP, ADP and P_i, although they did not agree on the inhibition pattern. Ouabain inhibited rabbit brain (Na + K)-ATPase with $K_\frac{1}{2} = 1$ μM and the associated K-phosphatase with $K_\frac{1}{2} = 30$ μM (Fujita et al., 1966). This difference, however, may have merely reflected different ouabain-binding conditions, since ATP reduced $K_\frac{1}{2}$ for ouabain inhibition of K-phosphatase. Yet more conflicting evidence came from experiments of Bader and Sen (1966) who found that Na would not activate the phosphatase reaction in kidney membranes in the absence of K, that ATP would behave as a competitive inhibitor towards acetyl-phosphate even in the absence of Na and that ouabain affinities of both enzyme activities were identical. The low affinity for ATP as inhibitor ($K_i = 2$ mM, Bader and Sen, 1966) suggests that even in the presence of Na it is binding of ATP at a nonphosphorylating site that elicits the inhibition.

The idea of close association between (Na + K)-ATPase and the K-phosphatase activity was strengthened further by the finding that Na plus ATP (or other nucleotide triphosphates) stimulated the K-phosphatase of membrane preparations, although they both inhibited when used separately (Nagai and Yoshida, 1966; Robinson, 1969a; Yoshida et al., 1969). A similar observation has been made with human red cells (Rega et al., 1968; Garrahan et al., 1970). The combination of Na plus ATP (or CTP) increases the apparent affinity for K (Rega et al., 1968; Yoshida et al., 1969; Garrahan et al., 1970), for ouabain, and also for Na as an activator at low K concentrations (Yoshida et al., 1969). In these conditions, Na ions do not increase the maximal phosphatase activity, but no other cation will replace for Na in these effects.

Using intact human erythrocytes and their resealed ghosts, Garrahan et al., (1969) and Rega et al., (1970) studied the "sidedness" of the phosphatase reaction. Using acetylphosphate as the substrate (since PNPP and p-nitrophenol move readily across the red cell membrane, Garrahan and Rega, 1972), the hydrolysis was found to occur at the internal side of the membrane (Garrahan et al., 1969). When present in the outside medium, K activated and Na inhibited the phosphatase, whereas the activation by ATP, Mg and Na were found to be intracellular (Rega et al., 1970). The activation by K in broken ghosts is due mainly to an increase in the substrate affinity (Garrahan et al., 1969). On the other hand, the effect of Na plus ATP must involve phosphorylation of the enzyme: in brain microsomes, oligomycin inhibits (Na + K)-ATPase but not the K-phosphatase activity (Israel and Titus, 1967), yet oligomycin has been found to abolish completely the stimulatory effect of Na plus ATP (Askari and Koyal, 1968). Besides, there must be a phosphorylated-enzyme stage in the phosphatase reaction, since p-nitrophenol has been reported to release first and P_i later in the reaction sequence (Robinson, 1970).

The above considerations are consistent with the current view that the K-phosphatase represents the terminal step of the (Na + K)-ATPase reaction, where the synthetic substate is replacing for the phosphorylated intermediate at the hydrolytic stage. There are agents which can decrease the (Na + K)-ATPase activity and stimulate the K-phosphatase concomitantly (Fujita et al., 1966; Robinson, 1969b; Albers and Koval, 1972). PNPP cannot replace ATP in supporting O.S. Na and K fluxes in human red cells (Garrahan and Rega, 1972), but PNPP inhibits Na–K and Na–Na exchanges with the same affinity as shown as a substrate of the K-phosphatase reaction; ATP can partially reverse the inhibition. Finally, it seems that the K-phosphatase activity is only loosely coupled to the overall ATPase cycle, since antibodies against (Na + K)-ATPase preparations fail to inhibit K-phosphatase (Askari and Rao, 1972), or inhibit it partially (Glynn et al., 1974), at antiserum concentrations fully inhibitory for (Na + K)-ATPase.

3.3 OUABAIN INHIBITION AND BINDING

Binding of tritiated digoxin to cardiac muscle membranes (Matsui and Schwartz, 1968; Schwartz et al., 1968) and to electric organ ATPase (Albers et al., 1968) was found in the presence of ATP plus Na and Mg ions or in the presence of Mg ions and inorganic phosphate. Binding in the first set of conditions was inhibited by K ions and that in the second set by Na ions. The labelling occurred with a high affinity for the glycoside and was practically irreversible at 0°C. The fact that it could follow the "Na-activated route" suggested that digoxin was binding to the phosphoenzyme, although other nucleoside triphosphates which did not appear to be substrates for the (Na + K)-ATPase nor support the active fluxes would replace for ATP in supporting the binding. It was later recognized that ITP, UTP and CTP could also phosphorylate the enzyme, albeit with lower affinity than ATP, and that adenylate kinase contamination in the preparations could be held responsible for ADP effects also observed (Schoner et al., 1968; Skou and Hilberg, 1969; Siegel and Goodwin, 1972; Tobin et al., 1972). As a counterpart to the "Na-inhibited route" of binding, Mg ions plus ouabain could activate an incorporation of $^{32}P_i$ to the enzyme, to an extent comparable to that obtained with $[\gamma^{32}P]ATP$ + Mg + Na (Albers et al., 1968; Lindenmayer et al., 1968).

Based on phosphorylation experiments, Sen et al., (1969) postulated that ouabain combined to the P-intermediate to form an ouabain-phosphoenzyme insensitive to K ions and which slowly released P_i:

$$E_2 - P \xrightarrow{\text{ouabain}} E_2 - P\,Ou \underset{+ P_i}{\overset{- P_i}{\rightleftharpoons}} E_2\,Ou \underset{+ \text{ouabain}}{\overset{- \text{ouabain}}{\rightleftharpoons}} E_2$$

to produce an ouabain-inhibited dephosphoenzyme which, in the case of guinea-pig kidney membranes, happened to dissociate readily at 37°C (cf. Erdmann and Schoner, 1973). This ouabain-inhibited dephosphoenzyme (E_2Ou) would be the form arising by incubating the enzyme with ouabain in the absence of Na ions; in this case, P_i incorporation on to the enzyme-ouabain complex would stabilize and accelerate the "Na-inhibited route". The protective effect of Na had a concentration dependence which was identical to that for the formation of the phosphorylated intermediate with ATP + Mg (Sen et al., 1969). The β,γ-methylene analogue of ATP inhibits ouabain binding in the presence of Na + Mg + P_i (the conditions chosen so that ATP would activate, Tobin et al., 1973) and this lends support to the hypothesis of Sen et al., (1969). Hansen et al., (1971) have reported that in Mg-free conditions, the binding of ouabain, ATP and ADP is mutually exclusive.

By counting the tritiated glycoside bound to human red cell ghosts at 100 per cent inhibition of the (Na + K)-ATPase activity (Ellory and Keynes, 1969) and to intact erythrocytes, measuring inhibition of K influx (Hoffman and Ingram, 1968; Hoffman, 1969), 200 sites per cell and a turnover number of 10 500 min^{-1} were obtained (assuming one glycoside site per ATPase molecule). An upper limit of about 1000 sites per red cell has been estimated by Glynn (1957), using the biological assay method. Glynn also observed that in red cells, the inhibition of K influx caused by a small concentration of scillaren-A could be prevented by increasing the external K concentration. Similarly, Schatzmann (1965) observed that, besides decreasing the rate of the ATPase activity of resealed ghosts, ouabain seemed to decrease the affinity of the pump for external K, and to increase the affinity of external Na as an inhibitor, Undoubtedly, the glycoside was attacking the ATPase at a locus which interacted strongly with the external cation binding sites.

At low concentrations of ouabain and Mg ions (with no other ligands present), K inhibits the binding of ouabain to guinea-pig kidney membranes with $K_{\frac{1}{2}}$ of about 0·1 mM. The K affinity decreases at higher ligand concentrations or in the presence of P_i (Tobin and Sen, 1970). This is quite interesting, for phosphorylation of the enzyme would then not be necessary for the existence of high-affinity K sites (cf. Nørby and Jensen, 1971), as opposite to the results obtained with K-phosphatase and in beryllium-inactivation experiments (see below).

Cation effects are better defined when both sides of the membrane are under control, as occurs with red cells (Hoffman and Ingram, 1968; Hoffman, 1969; Beaugé and Adragna, 1971; Gardner and Conlon, 1972; Gardner and Frantz, 1974; Sachs, 1974; Bodemann and Hoffman, 1976a, b, c). With human erythrocytes, the binding follows a hyperbola (Gardner and Conlon, 1972) as happens with other preparations (Hansen, 1971; Erdmann and Schoner, 1973; Hansen and Skou, 1973; but see Taniguchi and Iida, 1972). The time-course of the binding has been found either to level off when 100 per cent inhibition of the maximally inhibitable K influx is attained (Gardner and Conlon, 1972), or to continue into a region of "unspecific binding" (Glynn, 1957; Hoffman and Ingram, 1968; Hoffman, 1969). When the apparent dissociation constant of the ouabain binding was plotted against the concentration of monovalent cation in the medium, hyperbolae were obtained, upright for K ions and inverted for Na ions (Gardner and Frantz, 1974). These patterns were interpreted in terms of partially-competitive cation interaction, implying that there existed one glycoside binding site and one monovalent-cation binding site. Sodium binding at the latter would then lead to a discrete increase of glycoside affinity, while potassium binding, to a decrease (Gardner and Conlon, 1972). The calculated values for the ouabain dissociation constants were 1.4×10^{-7} M in the (nominal) absence of Na or K, 5×10^{-10} M at saturating Na concentrations and 2.6×10^{-7} M at saturating K concentration. Gardner and Frantz (1974) then found that while external K and Rb increased the ouabain dissociation constant, external Cs and Li aligned with Na in decreasing it. Then, external monovalent cation sites modulating ouabain binding might not necessarily equate with those activating the fluxes, for Cs and Li can support active Na efflux, admittedly with lower affinities than K and Rb (McConaghey and Maizels, 1962). Caesium ions had earlier been found not to affect the *rate* of ouabain binding (Hoffman and Ingram, 1968; Hoffman, 1969), although leading to reduced levels of bound ouabain at maximal inhibition of K influx. Sachs (1974) altered the internal cation composition of human red cells (by using the *p*-chloromercuribenzenesulphonate (PCMBS) method of Garrahan and Rega, 1967) and found that external Na *did not* affect the rate of ouabain binding to cells with a reduced K content (cf. Bodemann and Hoffman, 1976a). This suggested that the effect of external Na in nominally K-free media would result from competition with K leaking from normal, high K cells. Perhaps this is also the basis for the activating effect of external Cs on the binding rate (cf. Hoffman and Ingram, 1968). Sachs (1974) also proposed a model for glycoside-cation interactions, based on direct competition between K and ouabain or K and Na at one of two external potassium sites. This seems, however, unlikely, for although it is conceivable that K and ouabain can exclude each other from a domain of binding, it is difficult to understand how Na binding at the same site could not be equally deleterious towards ouabain.

Using rat brain and guinea-pig kidney (Na + K)-ATPase, Han et al., (1976) have observed that K, Rb and Li present higher affinities for catalysing dephosphorylation than for inhibiting ouabain binding, and have postulated that different external cation sites are involved in each process. However, this seems uncertain since the phosphoenzyme levels were observed in the absence of ouabain, and cardiac glycosides reduce the apparent affinity at the "K-loading sites" (Schatzmann, 1965; Sachs, 1974).

A comprehensive examination of internal and external variables governing ouabain binding has been made by Bodemann and Hoffman (1976a, b, c) by making use of resealed ghosts from human erythrocytes. When the binding is supported by internal ATP, external Na ions do not affect the rate of binding in the absence of external K or at saturating external K concentrations; internal Na, however, *inhibits* the binding provided extracellular K is present (see Fig. 5). In addition, internal K ions also inhibit when in the presence of external K (Bodemann and Hoffman, 1976a). The authors propose that any set of conditions leading to Na–K or K–K exchange will be unfavourable for the binding of ouabain, but not those leading to Na–Na exchange. The binding supported by internal Mg and P_i is inhibited by internal Na even in the absence of external K. Extracellular K also inhibits the (Mg + P_i)-promoted binding, but now independently from the level of internal Na, and subject to competition by external Na. Independent inhibition by internal Na or external K is also observed when UTP promotes ouabain binding (Bodemann and Hoffman, 1976b). Finally, when internal Mg_{free} concentrations are very much reduced by resealing EDTA into ghosts, both ATP- and P_i-supported binding is diminished. In these circumstances, the remaining ATP-promoted binding loses its sensitivity to inhibition by internal Na, gains sensitivity to stimulation by external Na (in the presence of external K) and the inhibitory effect of external K loses its Na_i requirement (Bodemann and Hoffman, 1976c). Considering the loss of sensitivity to internal Na in low Mg_{free} conditions, and since blockage of the $E_1 \sim P \rightarrow E_2 - P$ transition should occur (Post et al., 1969), the authors are inclined to think that the ATP-supported ouabain binding may not involve phosphorylation but just ATP

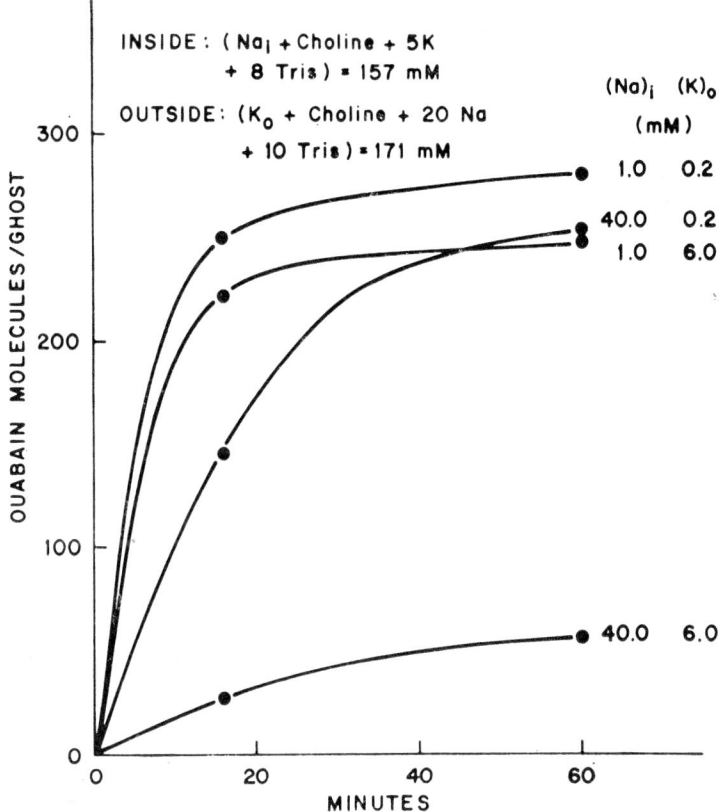

FIG. 5. The effect of internal Na and external K on the rate of ouabain binding to reconstituted red cell ghosts. Reproduced from Bodemann and Hoffman (1976a).

binding to the enzyme. The effects of external Na and K (as well as those on the UTP-supported binding) would then be explained by a decrease in the ATP binding affinity, brought about by *external* K.

Although it is not certain that the K effect on ATP binding is intracellular rather than extracellular (Hegyvary and Post, 1971; Nørby and Jensen 1971), some of these experiments admit alternative interpretations which are compatible with the need of phosphorylation for ouabain to bind. For instance, at very low Mg_{free} concentrations, the O.S. Na–K exchange was reduced by only half (Bodemann and Hoffman, 1976c), and hence the level of K-sensitive phosphoenzyme must have been high enough for it to qualify as the form at which ouabain binds (Sen *et al.*, 1969), subject to the inhibitory effect of external K ions by virtue of catalysis of dephosphorylation. This would be so if, even at very low Mg_{free} concentrations, the rate-limiting step for the overall pump cycle lied elsewhere, possibly at the release of the K-inhibited dephosphoenzyme or occluded form (KE_2, Post et al., 1972; see Fig. 4 in this chapter). The combined requirement for internal Na and external K in order to inhibit the ATP-supported binding coincides with the need for simultaneous binding of Na_i and K_o to effect Na–K exchange (Garay and Garrahan, 1973) and, conceivably, hydrolysis of the K-sensitive phosphoenzyme.

4 Kinetic properties and models

4.1 ATPase reaction and inactivation studies

The interactions of ATP, Mg, Na, K and inhibitors with rat brain ATPase give parabolic Lineweaver-Burk plots in most cases (Squires, 1965; Ahmed et al., 1966) and this implies multi-site interactions of the ligands with the enzyme. Potassium has been found to behave as uncompetitive activator at high Na concentrations (Robinson, 1967) which is consistent with the formation of a phosphorylated intermediate and K attack beyond the point of ADP liberation (Glynn and Lew, 1969). Peter and Wolf (1972), on the other hand, have obtained kinetic patterns which can be interpreted assuming that the enzyme must combine K first, and then Na and ATP randomly before P_i can be released. This implies, amongst other things, that the "circular carrier" model of Shaw (1954) could not, in its original form, describe the interactions of Na and K with the ATPase.

An alternative approach has been to analyse the effects of different ligands on the rate at which some agents inactivate (Na + K)-ATPase. For instance, the inactivation caused by beryllium ions is accelerated by K and inhibited by Na (Toda, 1968). The cation site in question presents moderate affinity for K ($K_{\frac{1}{2}} = 1\cdot 4$ mM) and K-analogues (Robinson, 1973, 1975) similar to those for the K-phosphatase activity. Coincidentally, Na decreases the K affinity at the "inactivation sites", but Na plus CTP increase it to values close to those observed in the K-activation of (Na + K)-ATPase and Na–K exchange. Sodium ions, in turn, protect (Na + K)-ATPase from inactivation by dicyclohexylcarbodiimide (Robinson, 1974), with $K_{\frac{1}{2}} = 2\cdot 3$ mM; 1 mM ATP decreases $K_{\frac{1}{2}}$, but not ATP plus Mg, and this makes it necessary to postulate the existence of Na sites round the cycle of the ATPase reaction. Skou (1974a, b) has found curves for the Na and K effects on NEM-inactivation of the enzyme which are identical to those obtained by activating the native ATPase with these ions. Increasing the ATP concentration causes a reduction of $K_{\frac{1}{2}}$ for the Na-protective effect on the inactivation and, conversely, a high Na:K ratio greatly increases the ATP affinity for the process. Similar results are obtained by studying the effect of ATP on the activation of the native enzyme by Na and K (Skou, 1974b). The reciprocal effects of ATP and Na have been interpreted by Skou in terms of two forms of the internal configuration: i_s, with high Na and ATP affinities, and i_p with high K and low ATP and Na affinities (cf. E_1 and E_2 of Hegyvary and Post, 1971). Skou also found that both ATP and ATPMg would be effective in promoting the increase in relative Na affinity, and this conflicts with the observations by Robinson (1974) on the dicyclohexylcarbodiimide inactivation.

4.2 EXTERNAL AND INTERNAL CATION SITES

When either the total or the O.S. K influx in human red cells are measured in high Na media, the dependence on external K concentration follows a sigmoid curve (Garrahan and Glynn, 1967b; Sachs and Welt, 1967) (see Fig. 2); similar behaviour can be observed with rat red cells (Beaugé and Ortiz, 1971) and high K or low K sheep erythrocytes (Hoffman and Tosteson, 1971; see Chapter 15 in this book). Sachs and Welt (1967) fitted the curve of activation of ATP-dependent K influx by external K in high Na media, to an equation derived after assuming that K must bind at two external pump sites (K_K about 0·5 mM at each site) before translocation occurs. They also found that at high Na_o and low K_o concentrations, external Rb, Cs and Li ions had a biphasic effect on the active K influx: at low concentrations, these K analogues activated K influx, at higher concentrations they inhibited it (Sachs and Welt, 1967). Similar situations arise when Li influx in lactose-treated red cells is measured at variable external K concentrations (McConaghey and Maizels, 1962) and the O.S. K influx is measured at varying concentrations of thallous ions (Cavieres and Ellory, 1974). This effect of substrate-analogues is characteristic of systems presenting multi-site binding for the substrate (Monod et al., 1965). Thallous ions activate the O.S. Na efflux with a high Tl^+ affinity (Lishko et al., 1973; Cavieres and Ellory, 1974), substituting for K stoichiometrically at the external pump sites (Cavieres and Ellory, 1974). When the external Na concentration is reduced to nearly zero, the activation of the K influx in red cells is apparently hyperbolic, but even at Na_o concentrations as low as 15 μM, an inflexion of the curve can be found (Garrahan and Glynn, 1967b). In these conditions, the curve of activation of the O.S. Na efflux of resealed ghosts by external K can be fitted with dissociation constants 4 and 100 μM at the external K sites (Lew et al., 1973).

At high external K, the O.S. K influx (or Rb influx) does not seem to change with the external Na concentration and hence the inhibition by Na_o should be of a competitive type (Garrahan and Glynn, 1967b; Beaugé and Ortiz, 1971). If the O.S. K influx in human red cells is measured at variable Na_o concentrations and at fixed K concentrations above c. 0·1 mM, Dixon plots (1/v v. Na_o concentration) are linear, both in the case of fresh, low Na cells (Sachs, 1967; Priestland and Whittam, 1968), or of cells loaded by PCMBS or nystatin treatment, to contain high Na (Sachs, 1974; Cavieres and Ellory, 1975). This implies that Na ions need binding at only one external site to enact the competitive inhibition and Sachs (1974) has proposed that this is one of the external K sites. However, when the K concentration in the medium is very low, the Dixon plots become hyperbolic (Cavieres and Ellory, 1975), the kinetic pattern corresponding to partially-competitive inhibition (Dixon and Webb, 1964). This means that external Na exerts its effect on the K affinity by binding at a site different from the two K sites (a "third external (Na) site"), and that KXK and $K\overset{Na}{X}K$ forms are equally effective in promoting K translocation inwards. The dissociation constant for external Na with the KXK form was estimated as 40–50 mM (Cavieres and Ellory, 1975), but it must lie between 0·14 and 0·24 mM for the combination with the unliganded form (Cavieres and Ellory, 1977). The latter estimate makes it very likely that this is the same as the "high affinity Na site" involved in the inhibition of the O.S. Na efflux in (Na+ K)-free media (Garrahan and Glynn, 1967b; Sachs, 1970; Lew et al., 1973) and its associated Na-ATPase activity (Glynn and Karlish, 1976). However, at saturating external K and high external Na, occupation of the allosteric site by Na ions cannot lead to any significant O.S. Na influx (cf. Garrahan and Glynn, 1967c). Conversely, it may be proposed that in the presence of external K, in a given pump unit external Na ions would bind most times at the allosteric site and thus inhibit K influx; raising the Na_o concentration, and if the K_o concentration is low enough, would achieve binding of Na at the two external K sites to promote Na–Na exchange. Simultaneous measurements of O.S. K influx and O.S. Na influx as a function of external Na concentration should help to decide about this scheme (but see Garay and Garrahan, 1973).

The interaction of Na ions with the internal sites of the sodium pump in human red cells is subject to inhibition by internal K ions (Garay and Garrahan, 1973; Knight and Welt, 1974). An equation describing three equivalent Na sites at which internal K inhibits by direct competition has been fitted by Garay and Garrahan (1973) to their flux data. The dissociation constant for Na at each site (K_{Na}) lies between 0·2 and 0·5 mM, while the inhibition constant for K (K_{iK}) is close to 9 mM (Garay and Garrahan, 1973, 1975). In addition to their competitive effect, internal K ions appear to increase the maximal rate of exchanges above a basal level.* The fitted V^{max} value for the Na–K exchange curve was an apparently hyperbolic function of the internal K concentration, suggesting the pres-

* See Fig. 5b, Ellory (this volume) for illustration on this point.

ence of a single activatory internal K site with $K_{\frac{1}{2}}$ of about 9 mM (Garay and Garrahan, 1973), a value closely similar to K_{iK} at each internal Na site, and to $K_{\frac{1}{2}}$ for the activation of O.S. K–K exchange by internal K in resealed ghosts (Simons, 1974). This effect might perhaps be related to the inhibition of ATP-promoted ouabain binding to resealed ghosts by internal K (Bodemann and Hoffman, 1976a). The maximal Na–Na exchange rate, however, varied linearly with the internal K concentration (Garay and Garrahan, 1973), as if the K affinity at one internal stimulatory site were very low in this case. The observed effects of internal K are not due to an increase of the glycolytic rate of the cells (Garay and Garrahan, 1975). These K effects are not well understood, but there are independent indications of their occurrence in human red cells (Knight and Welt, 1974) and in both low K and high K type sheep erythrocytes (Sachs et al., 1974).

A rather crucial point concerning the overall kinetics of the pump has been the experimental observation that independence obtains between internal and external cation sites in their activiation of Na–K and Na–Na exchanges, both in human erythrocytes (Garay and Garrahan, 1973) and sheep red cells (Hoffman and Tosteson, 1971). In the analysis of Baker and Stone (1966) for viable kinetic models of the Na pump, the apparent dissociation constants for one action at one side does not depend on the cation concentrations at the other side when internal and external sites must be loaded before the rate-limiting step. The pump turnover, then, depends on the probability (or saturation function) of having internal and external cation sites loaded simultaneously with their respective activators or

$$v = \frac{V^{max}}{\left(1 + \frac{K'_{Na}}{[Na_i]}\right)^3 \left(1 + \frac{K'_{K}}{[K_o]}\right)^2}$$

where K'_{Na} and K'_{K} represent the apparent dissociation constants for Na_i and K_o, respectively (subject to the respective inhibitions by K_i and Na_o), having omitted, for simplicity, the activation by internal K. Increasing intracellular P_i and decreasing intracellular ATP concentrations have been found to inhibit Na–K exchange in such way that neither internal ATP, P_i or Na or external K affect the affinities of each other at their respective sites (Garay and Garrahan, 1975). These experiments have been interpreted as indicating that internal Na and external K sites must exist during the whole transport cycle, and that at least one of the two sets must keep constant affinity throughout (Garrahan and Garay, 1974; Garay and Garrahan, 1975). Considering that in human red cells, 3 Na ions are transported outwards and 2 K ions inwards per pump cycle (Sen and Post, 1964; Whittam and Ager, 1965; Garrahan and Glynn, 1967d), the number of internal Na and external K sites which seem to best fit the results, coincides with the stoichiometry and is consistent with the possibility that activation and translocation sites are the same.

As was mentioned earlier, K congeners in the external medium can activate O.S. Na efflux. The sequence of affinities at the external K sites is Rb > K > Cs > Li, as assessed from the activation of Na efflux (McConaghey and Maizels, 1962) or from the effectiveness in coactivating and inhibiting active K influx (Sachs and Welt, 1967). This corresponds to series III of Eisenman, omitting Na (Eisenman, 1960; Diamond and Wright 1969). No explicit data are available concerning the selectivity sequence of the internal pump sites but the information, however, seems contained in the article of Maizels (1968). His Fig. 1 shows the Na efflux from red cells loaded by lactose treatment, to contain Na + B (where B stands for K, Rb, Cs or Li) and exchanging with a Na-free medium containing 150 mM BCl. The Na efflux follows in all cases a sigmoid dependence on internal Na, while the apparent Na affinity and V^{max} depend on which B was used. His Fig. 2 replots the same experiments as Na efflux rate constant against log Na$_i$: all curves are bell-shaped, presenting maxima (cf. Sachs, 1970) at Na$_i$ values which are characteristic of B. Now, for any system requiring the concurrent occupation of n equivalent sites before the rate-limiting step $v = V^{max}/(1 + K'/C)^n$, where K' is the apparent dissociation constant for the activator (Na in this case) at each site and C its concentration. The rate constant for the efflux is v/C, so by putting $d[v/C]/dC = 0$, one obtains

$$K' = \frac{C_{peak}}{n - 1}$$

where C_{peak} is the activator concentration corresponding to the maximum in the rate-constant plots. Then, if $n = 3$, from the data in Fig. 2 of Maizels (1968), $K'_{Na} = 5.8$ mmol (l cell water)$^{-1}$ at 140 mmol K (or Rb) per litre cell water. This agrees very well with the value of 5.81 mmol (l cell water)$^{-1}$ given in Figs. 1 and 5 of Garay and Garrahan (1975). Since for competitive inhibition, $K'_{Na} = K_{Na}(1 + [K]/K_{iK})$ and if $K_{iK} = 9$ mmol (l cell water)$^{-1}$ at each Na site (Garay and Garrahan, 1973), the K_{Na} (in the absence of inhibitor) is 0.34 mM. Using this value and the same plot in the article of Maizels (1968), one obtains $K_{iCs} = 31$ and $K_{iLi} = 35$ mmol (l cell water)$^{-1}$. Thus, the affinity sequence at the "Na-loading sites" of human red cells is

$$Na > K, Rb > Cs > Li$$

which can only be compatible with sequence VII of Eisenman (where K > Rb) (Diamond and Wright, 1969).

It is also apparent from Fig. 1 of Maizels (1968) that the Na_i-activation curves tend to different V^{max} values in the order K ⩾ Rb, Cs > Li. The lower V^{max} of Li should not be due to incomplete saturation at the external "K sites" because of a low Li affinity, for at 5 mM Na_o external Li activates the O.S. Na efflux in red cells with $K_{\frac{1}{2}}$ about 13 mM (Beaugé and del Campillo, 1976), and yet in those experiments the maximal Li_o-activation of O.S. efflux is about half that attained by external K. It is conceivable that the lower Li activation could be due to an intracellular action; however, when the O.S. K influx human erythrocytes (loaded by nystatin treatment to contain high sodium and low potassium) is measured in Na-free medium with and without 50 mM Li, all K influx time-courses are linear up to at least 1 h and hence any Li build-up in the cells does not lead to inhibition of the sodium pump (unpublished experiment of J. C. Ellory and J. D. Cavieres). It is possible, although not very likely, that the pump shuttles more slowly or with a lower Na : ∼ P ratio when performing Na–Li exchange. Or it may also be that Li ions have some Na-like action at the "third external (Na) site", thus occupying all three external pump sites at high external Li concentration and self-inflicting inhibition of its activation of Na–Li exchange through the pump (Cavieres and Ellory, 1977).

4.3 MODELS

Since it seems that internal and external cation sites should exist simultaneously at some stage before the rate-limiting step of Na–K or Na–Na exchange, the "circular model" of the carrier (Shaw, 1954), though consistent with the phosphorylation-dephosphorylation cycle, cannot as such account for the translocation kinetics. Nor can the P-intermediate cycle. Similarly, the mechanical models of Opit and Charnock (1965), Jardetzky (1968) and Lowe (1968) cannot accommodate the simultaneity of external and internal binding (Caldwell, 1970). A kinetic model, differing from that of Shaw (1954) in that the energy for the cyclical change of affinity of the cation sites is fed to the external form of the carrier and in that cation binding is not subject to saturation, has been proposed by Caldwell (1968). The model can fit a number of observations on the O.S. Na efflux in red cells and muscle and can be consistent with the independence of internal and external sites; however, it cannot easily account for the conditions for K–K exchange through the pump (Glynn and Lew, 1969). Garrahan and Garay (1974) have pointed out that additional requirements for the observed independence are that, on a time-average basis, the fraction of the pump held in an occluded conformation must be small and (as mentioned in section 4.2) that either the external K sites or the internal Na sites must not change their affinity appreciably round the cycle.

Simultaneous models (external and internal units) for Na and K translocation have been proposed by Skou (1971), Repke and Schön (1973), Stein et al. (1973) and Repke et al. (1974), as well as by Hoffman and Tosteson (1971) and Garrahan and Garay (1974). The question of the actual mechanism has been tackled by Stein et al. (1973) by suggesting that external and internal sub-units rotate their cation sites by 180° to make them face each other while simultaneously changing to the converse affinities. Exchange of Na for K is then effected at the central cavity ("internal transfer"). Kyte (1974) has cast doubt on the feasibility of models implying rotational movement of sub-units or large macromolecular entities. Antibodies against the large polypeptide (mol wt = 85 000–100 000, see Jørgensen, 1975, for references) of the purified (Na + K)-ATPase can bind at the inner side of membrane-bound enzyme (Kyte, 1974), as it occurs with the anti-pump antibody and human red cells (Jørgensen et al., 1973). But unlike Jørgensen's antibodies, the anti-large chain antibody binds without inhibiting (Na + K)-ATPase activity. It follows that it is very difficult that the large polypeptide, say, can experience any important rotational movement with a large immunoglobulin attached to it (Kyte, 1974).

Repke and Schön (1973) proposed a flip-flop model of the sodium pump, which, taking the half-of-the-sites-reactivity concept of Lazdunski (1972), incorporates the sequence of steps of the phosphorylation-dephosphorylation cycle, considering spatial separation of a "carrier moiety" from a "catalytic moiety". Although the tightly coupled model of Repke and Schön (1973) cannot easily explain the Na-ATPase activity or why non-phosphorylating analogues of ATP can activate O.S. K-K exchange (Simons, 1975), schemes like theirs, involving two sub-units working at least part of the time 180° out of phase, allow for the simultaneity of internal and external cation sites and provide a means of graded free-energy transfer from the chemical bond to the electrochemical system, without quasi-irreversible steps of high dissipation. Reciprocating models benefit, besides, from the fact that the molecular weight of membrane-bound (Na + K)-ATPase is around 300 000, as determined from its target size to radiation inactivation (Kepner and Macey, 1968), and this can be accounted for by two large and two small polypeptides (Kyte, 1971; Jørgensen, 1975). However, there are reasons why (Na + K)-ATPase cannot be a strictly half-of-the-sites enzyme (see Glynn and Karlish, 1975a,b).

Based on Eisenman's (1960) hypothesis for the occurrence of cation selectivity series, Skou (1964) has proposed a model for translocation, consisting of a channel with three negative charges in a row, whose negative field-strength, and hence their alkali cation selectivity, would undergo cyclical changes upon phosphorylation and dephosphorylation of a neighbouring site. Unfortunately, this otherwise ingenious array cannot account for an overall Na–K exchange different from 1 Na for 1 K per cycle.

If external and internal sites are different entities, Eisenman's theory readily explains their different selectivities for monovalent cations in terms of their anionic radii: the external K sites (sequence III), preferring cations of small hydration-free energy, should be weak sites, that is, of large anionic radius. The internal Na sites (sequence VII) should present smaller radius. But if internal and external sites occur cyclically in some sort of reciprocating array, their change of selectivity should happen while they are not available for exchange with the internal or external media (cf. Garrahan and Garay, 1974).

Regarding factors that may change the selectivity series of a site, Eisenman (1960) has pointed out that inter-site spacing is the only factor that will change the sequence, and markedly. For instance, for a negative site 1·4 Å in radius, its sequence will be IIIa for infinitely separated (d > 4 Å) sites in a matrix, while it will shift to sequence X for the case of the closest (crystal lattice) packing (Fig. 3 of Eisenman, 1960). Considering then the existence of three internal Na sites and two external K sites plus the external Na site, a simple assumption is that a set of three sites experiences a cyclical change of affinities in each of two sub-units 180° out of phase. A schematic array for the change of affinity is proposed in Fig. 6. The model assumes proximity of the monovalent cation sites, two of which are pictured as similar while the third is thought different in nature. When they face the internal side of the pump, the macromolecular structure restricts them to be closely packed together: they then present a high Na selectivity (sequence VII). When they face the external aspect, in turn, they separate and while two sites change their selectivity to sequence III, a third pump site (supposedly of higher intrinsic field-strength) maintains its high Na selectivity. The change of sequence by change of the inter-site spacing could conceivably be also achieved if the net density of negative charges in the neighbourhood of the "pores" is higher on the inside than on the outside.

In red cells, at any rate, the stoichiometry of 3 Na transported out for 2 K transported in will lead in this as in any "circular carrier" model to returning one empty site to the inside; it follows that in any sequential model attempting to represent the normal stoichiometry, it must be assumed that one of the external sites is "different". Looking at the problem in this way, the proposal of an allosteric external Na site (Cavieres and

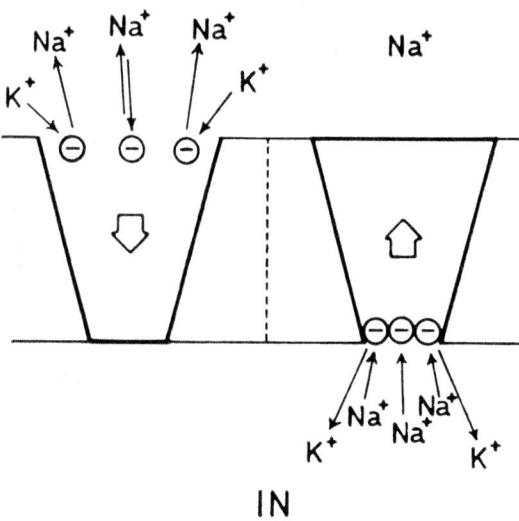

FIG. 6. Proposed change of selectivity of a multi-site carrier with reciprocation, by change of the inter-site spacing upon translocation. For details see text.

Ellory, 1975, 1977), fits in well. Since, as discussed before, $_K^{Na}X_K^{}$ could not lead to translocation of Na inwards, one of the difficulties with the scheme of Fig. 6 is disposing of Na bound at the "third external site" *after* K has bound *and* become unavailable for exchange with the external medium (for, otherwise, allosteric inhibition by Na_o would not occur). Examination of the possibility of having at this very stage any events which could explain the loss of bound Na towards the external medium points at just one candidate: the hydrolysis of the phosphoenzyme. Thus, if the active centre of the enzyme was directly involved in the translocating process, it might be that Na is released because the "third external site" consists of one of the phosphoryl oxygens of the phosphorylated intermediate.

EPR and PRR studies on Mn^{2+} binding to (Na + K)-ATPase have revealed a high-affinity binding site ($K_{\frac{1}{2}} + 0.88\ \mu M$) similar to that disclosed kinetically from (Na + K)-ATPase measurements, and at which Mg ions competed (Grisham and Mildvan, 1974). Inorganic phosphate can bind to the enzyme-Mn^{2+} complex in the presence of Na and K in a way that implies, in addition, the formation of a covalent bond between phosphate and the enzyme. $K_{\frac{1}{2}}$ for the K effect was 2 mM and for the Na effect 40 mM. Grisham and Mildvan (1974) proposed a model of the active centre, combining "biochemical" and "translocating" events, where a phosphoryl oxygen constitutes the only carrier for pumping Na out and K inwards. They assumed that stoichiometries higher than 1 (Na + K)/ATP could be obtained by multiple shuttling of the phosphorylated moiety across the barrier. This is, however, not viable, for such an action could only achieve facilitated diffusion and not active transport. Considering that the phosphorylation of (Na + K)-ATPase by $^{32}P_i$ is not activated but inhibited by "internal" Na ions (Post et al., 1975), and that the value of 40 mM reported by Grisham and Mildvan for $K_{\frac{1}{2}(Na)}$ is quite consistent with *external* (rather than internal) binding to the $P_i - Mn^{2+}$-enzyme complex (Cavieres and Ellory, 1975), it is more likely that this low-affinity Na effect rather consists in stabilization of the complex by Na binding at the "third external site".

In Fig. 7, a hypothetical arrangement is proposed where the phosphoryl at the active centre is again assumed directly involved in ion translocation, with one of its oxygen atoms acting as the "third site" of the pump. In step A, representing the K-sensitive phosphoenzyme in its pre-hydrolytic stage, three negative charges are available to the external medium through

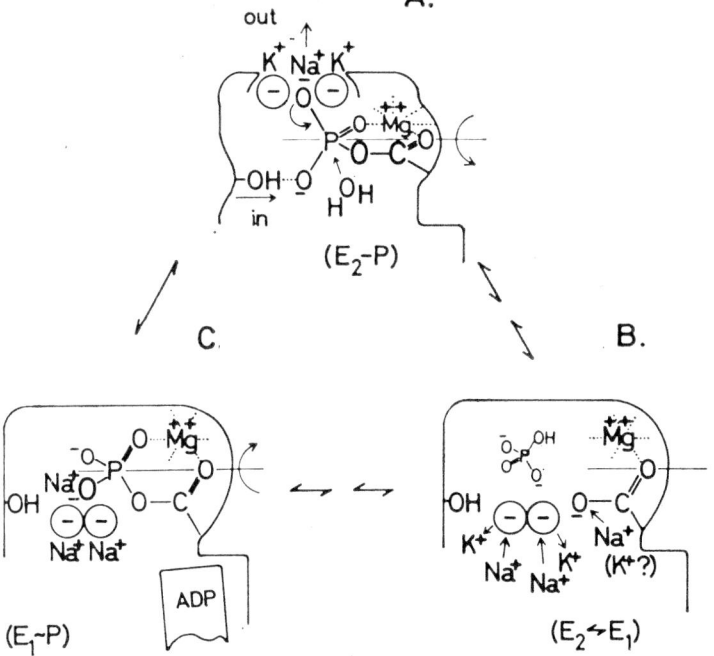

FIG. 7. Hypothetical relationships between monovalent cation sites and the active centre of (Na + K)-ATPase. One of the phosphoryl oxygens would constitute one of the cation sites. For discussion see text.

a narrow gate or pore: they consist of two related negative groups plus the phosphoryl oxygen. The phosphoryl is assumed held in orientated position by co-ordination of a third oxygen atom by Mg^{2+} which, in turn, binds to the carbonyl oxygen of the acyl moiety combining phosphate (probably an aspartyl residue, Post and Kume, 1973) and to the enzyme elsewhere. Binding of Na at the phosphoryl oxygen contributes to stabilize the phosphoenzyme, and thus explain its action as a "brake" for the pump. Binding of K at the two "external" K sites facilitates the attack of the phosphoryl by some group in the enzyme (here symbolized as the —OH of a serine or threonine residue) so as to labilize the P—O bond with aspartyl and allow nucleophilic attack by water. The labilization reaction (K-phosphatase) has to be by electron withdrawal, since there exists a K-stimulated, ouabain-inhibited P_i–$H_2^{18}O$ exchange in (Na + K)-ATPase (Dahms and Boyer, 1973) and this implies that it is the P—O bond and not the O—C bond that is split. The redistribution of electronic density amongst the different atoms will lead to Na loss to the external medium, as indicated. In step B ($E_2 \leftrightarrow E_1$), the hydrolysis of the phosphoryl group has produced the indirect translocation of one negative charge inwards, on to the carboxyl oxygen; the polypeptide chain has experienced a conformational change that has allowed the C—O···Mg plane to rotate by 90° as indicated in A, with simultaneous shuttling of the two loaded K sites inwards. The carboxyl oxygen (? the activatory internal K site of Garay and Garrahan, 1973) plus the other two sites now constitute three internal sites, closely packed together. In step C ($E_1 \sim P$), and ensuing phosphorylation by ATP, the phosphoryl oxygen has taken over as third (internal) Na site. Following redistribution of the energy between the "high-energy" acyl-phosphate and the protein structure, the six-member ring, the polypeptide chain and its two additional Na sites rotate back 90° and all three sites become available, with their sodiums, to the external medium by opening of the "pore".

In a kinetic model of the Na pump, Stone (1968) has proposed a separation of functional units within the machinery, so that the three outgoing Na sites originate differently. The interactions at the external aspect were somehow similar to those described by Cavieres and Ellory (1975, 1977). Calculations made by Stone (1968) in order to fit his model to the current data in the literature gave for Na binding at an external site which did not bind K, a $K_{\frac{1}{2}} = 150$ mM when the two K sites were occupied, and 0·5 mM when they were empty.

ACKNOWLEDGEMENT

I wish to thank Professor I. M. Glynn for his critical reading of the manuscript.

References

ALBERS, R. W., FAHN, S. and KOVAL, G. J. (1963). *Proc. Nat. Acad. Sci. U.S.A.* **50**, 474–481.
ALBERS, R. W. and KOVAL, G. J. (1966). *J. Biol. Chem.* **241**, 1896–1898.
ALBERS, R. W. and KOVAL, G. J. (1972). *J. Biol. Chem.* **247**, 3088–3092.
ALBERS, R. W., KOVAL, G. J. and SIEGEL, G. J. (1968). *Molec. Pharmacol.* **4**, 324–336.
ASKARI, A. and KOYAL, D. (1968). *Biochem. Biophys. Res. Commun.* **32**, 227–232.
ASKARI, A. and RAO, S. N. (1972). *Biochem. Biophys. Res. Commun.* **49**, 1323–1328.
BADER, H., POST, R. L. and BOND, G. H. (1968). *Biochim. Biophys. Acta*, **150**, 41–46.
BADER, H. and SEN, A. K. (1966). *Biochim. Biophys. Acta*, **118**, 116–123.
BAKER, P. F. (1964). *Biochim. Biophys. Acta*, **88**, 458–460.
BAKER, P. F., BLAUSTEIN, M. P., KEYNES, R. D., MANIL, J., SHAW, T. I. and STEINHARDT, R. A. (1969). *J. Physiol.* **200**, 459–496.
BAKER, P. F. and STONE, A. J. (1966). *Biochim Biophys. Acta*, **126**, 321–329.
BEAUGÉ, L. A. and ADRAGNA, N. (1971). *J. Gen. Physiol.* **57**, 576–592.
BEAUGÉ, L. A. and DEL CAMPILLO, E. (1976). *Biochim Biophys. Acta*, **433**, 547–554.
BEAUGÉ, L. A. and ORTIZ, O. (1971). *J. Physiol.* **218**, 533–549.
BLOSTEIN, R. (1968). *J. Biol. Chem.* **243**, 1957–1965.
BLOSTEIN, R. (1970). *J. Biol. Chem.* **245**, 270–275.
BLOSTEIN, R. (1975). *J. Biol. Chem.* **250**, 6118–6124.
BODEMANN, H. H. and HOFFMAN, J. F. (1976a). *J. Gen. Physiol.* **67**, 497–525.
BODEMANN, H. H. and HOFFMAN, J. F. (1976b). *J. Gen. Physiol.* **67**, 527–545.
BODEMANN, H. H. and HOFFMAN, J. F. (1976c). *J. Gen. Physiol.* **67**, 547–561.
BOND, G. H., BADER, H. and POST, R. L. (1966). *Fed. Proc.* **25**, 567.
BOND, G. H., BADER, H. and POST, R. L. (1971). *Biochim. Biophys. Acta*, **241**, 57–67.
CALDWELL, P. C. (1968). *Physiol. Rev.* **48**, 1–64.
CALDWELL, P. C. (1970). *In* "Membranes and Ion Transport" (E. E. Bittar, ed), vol. I, pp. 433–461. Wiley, London.
CALDWELL, P. C., HODGKIN, A. L., KEYNES, R. D. and SHAW, T. I. (1960). *J. Physiol.* **152**, 591–600.
CALDWELL, P. C. and KEYNES, R. D. (1959). *J. Physiol.* **148**, 8–9P.
CAVIERES, J. D. and ELLORY, J. C. (1974). *J. Physiol.* **243**, 243–266.
CAVIERES, J. D. and ELLORY, J. C. (1975). *Nature*, **255**, 338–340.
CAVIERES, J. D. and ELLORY, J. C. (1977). In preparation.
CAVIERES, J. D. and GLYNN, I. M. (1976). *J. Physiol.* **263**, 214–215P.
CHARNOCK, J. S. and POST, R. L. (1963). *Nature*, **199**, 910–911.
CZERWINSKI, A., GITELMAN, H. J. and WELT, L. G. (1967). *Amer. J. Physiol.* **213**, 786–792.
DAHL, J. L. and HOKIN, L. E. (1974). *A Rev. Biochem.* **43**, 327–356.
DAHMS, A. S. and BOYER, P. D. (1973). *J. Biol. Chem.* **248**, 3155–3162.
DANOWSKI, T. S. (1941). *J. Biol. Chem.* **139**, 693–705.
DIAMOND, J. M. and WRIGHT, E. M. (1969). *A. Rev. Physiol.* **31**, 581–646.
DIXON, M. and WEBB, E. C. (1964). "Enzymes," ch. VIII. Longmans, London.
DUNHAM, E. T. and GLYNN, I. M. (1961). *J. Physiol.* **156**, 274–293.
EISENMAN, G. (1960). *In* "Membrane Transport and Metabolism" (A. Kleinzeller and A. Kotyk, eds), pp. 163–179. Academic Press, New York and London. (Published 1961.)

ELLORY, J. C. and KEYNES, R. D. (1969). *Nature*, **221**, 776.
ERDMANN, E. and SCHONER, W. (1973). *Biochim. Biophys. Acta*, **307**, 386–398.
FAHN, S., KOVAL, G. J. and ALBERS, R. W. (1966). *J. Biol. Chem.* **241**, 1882–1889.
FUJITA, M., NAKAO, T., TASHIMA, Y., MIZUNO, N., NAGANO, K. and NAKAO, M. (1966). *Biochim. Biophys. Acta*, **117**, 42–53.
FUKUSHIMA, Y. and TONOMURA, Y. (1973). *J. Biochem., Tokyo*, **74**, 135–142.
GARAY, R. P. and GARRAHAN, P. J. (1973). *J. Physiol.* **231**, 297–325.
GARAY, R. P. and GARRAHAN, P. J. (1975). *J. Physiol.* **249**, 51–67.
GARDNER, J. D. and CONLON, T. H. (1972). *J. Gen. Physiol.* **60**, 609–629.
GARDNER, J. D. and FRANTZ, C. (1974). *J. Membrane Biol.* **16**, 43–64.
GÁRDOS, G. (1954). *Acta Physiol. Hung.* **6**, 191–199.
GARRAHAN, P. J. and GARAY, R. P. (1974). *Ann. N.Y. Acad. Sci.* **242**, 445–457.
GARRAHAN, P. J. and GLYNN, I. M. (1967a). *J. Physiol.* **192**, 159–174.
GARRAHAN, P. J. and GLYNN, I. M. (1967b). *J. Physiol.* **192**, 175–188.
GARRAHAN, P. J. and GLYNN, I. M. (1967c). *J. Physiol.* **192**, 189–216.
GARRAHAN, P. J. and GLYNN, I. M. (1967d). *J. Physiol.* **192**, 217–235.
GARRAHAN, P. J. and GLYNN, I. M. (1967e). *J. Physiol.* **192**, 237–256.
GARRAHAN, P. J., POUCHAN, M. I. and REGA, A. F. (1969). *J. Physiol.* **202**, 305–327.
GARRAHAN, P. J., POUCHAN, M. I. and REGA, A. F. (1970). *J. Membrane Boil.* **3**, 26–42.
GARRAHAN, P. J. and REGA, A. F. (1967). *J. Physiol.* **193**, 459–466.
GARRAHAN, P. J. and REGA, A. F. (1972). *J. Physiol.* **223**, 595–617.
GLYNN, I. M. (1956). *J. Physiol.* **134**, 278–310.
GLYNN, I. M. (1957). *J. Physiol.* **136**, 148–173.
GLYNN, I. M. (1962). *J. Physiol.* **160**, 18–19P.
GLYNN, I. M. and HOFFMAN, J. F. (1971). *J. Physiol.* **218**, 239–256.
GLYNN, I. M., HOFFMAN, J. F. and LEW, V. L. (1971). *Phil. Trans. Roy. Soc. B*, **262**, 91–102.
GLYNN, I. M. and KARLISH, S. J. D. (1975a). *A. Rev. Physiol.* **37**, 13–55.
GLYNN, I. M. and KARLISH, S. J. D. (1975b). *In* "Energy Transformation in Biological Systems" (Ciba Found. Symp. 31), pp. 205–223. North-Holland, Amsterdam.
GLYNN, I. M. and KARLISH, S. J. D. (1976). *J. Physiol.* **256**, 465–496.
GLYNN, I. M., KARLISH, S. J. D., CAVIERES, J. D., ELLORY, J. C., LEW, V. L. and JØRGENSEN, P. L. (1974). *Ann. N.Y. Acad. Sci.* **242**, 357–371.
GLYNN, I. M. and LEW, V. L. (1969). *J. Gen. Physiol.* **54**, 289s–305s.
GLYNN, I. M. and LEW, V. L. (1970). *J. Physiol.* **207**, 393–402.
GLYNN, I. M., LEW, V. L. and LÜTHI, U. (1970). *J. Physiol.* **207**, 371–391.
GRISHAM, C. M. and MILDVAN, A. S. (1974). *J. Biol. Chem.* **249**, 3187–3197.
HAN, C. S., TOBIN, T., AKERA, T. and BRODY, T. M. (1976). *Biochim. Biophys. Acta*, **429**, 993–1005.
HANSEN, O. (1971). *Biochim. Biophys. Acta*, **233**, 122–132.
HANSEN, O., JENSEN, J. and NØRBY, J. G. (1971). *Nature, New Biol.* **234**, 122–124.
HANSEN, O. and SKOU, J. C. (1973). *Biochim. Biophys. Acta*, **311**, 51–66.
HARRIS, J. E. (1941). *J. Biol. Chem.* **141**, 579–595.
HARRIS, E. J. and PRANKERD, T. A. J. (1955). *Biochem. J.* **61**, xix.
HEGYVARY, C. and POST, R. L. (1971). *J. Biol. Chem.* **246**, 5234–5240.
HOFFMAN, J. F. (1960). *Fed. Proc.* **19**, 127.
HOFFMAN, J. F. (1962a). *J. Gen. Physiol.* **45**, 837–859.
HOFFMAN, J. F. (1962b). *Circulation*, **26**, 1201–1213.

HOFFMAN, J. F. (1966). *Amer. J. Med.* **41**, 666–680.
HOFFMAN, J. F. (1969). *J. Gen. Physiol.* **54**, 343s–350s.
HOFFMAN, J. F. and INGRAM, C. J. (1968). In "Metabolism and Membrane Permeability of Erythrocytes and Trombocytes" (E. Deutsch, E. Gerlach and K. Moser eds), pp. 420–424. G. Thieme Verlag, Stuttgart.
HOFFMAN, J. F., TOSTESON, D. C. and WHITTAM, R. (1960). *Nature*, **185**, 186–187.
HOFFMAN, P. G. and TOSTESON, D. C. (1971). *J. Gen. Physiol.* **58**, 438–466.
ISRAEL, Y. and TITUS, E. (1967). *Biochim. Biophys. Acta*, **139**, 450–459.
JARDETSKY, O. (1966). *Nature*, **211**, 969–970.
JØRGENSEN, P. L. (1975a). *Quart. Rev. Biophys.* **7**, 239–274.
JØRGENSEN, P. L. (1975b). *Biochim. Biophys. Acta*, **401**, 399–415.
JØRGENSEN, P. L., HANSEN, O., GLYNN, I. M. and CAVIERES, J. D. (1973). *Biochim. Biophys. Acta*, **291**, 795–800.
JUDAH, J. D., AHMED, K. and McLEAN, A. E. M. (1962). *Biochim. Biophys. Acta*, **65**, 472–480.
KANAZAWA, T., SAITO, M. and TONOMURA, Y. (1970). *J. Biochem., Tokyo*, **67**, 693–711.
KARLISH, S. J. D. and GLYNN, I. M. (1974). *Ann. N.Y. Acad. Sci.* **242**, 461–470.
KARLISH, S. J. D., YATES, D. W. and GLYNN, I. M. (1976). *Nature*, **263**, 251–253.
KEPNER, G. R. and MACEY, R. I. (1968). *Biochim. Biophys. Acta*, **163**, 188–203.
KEYNES, R. D. and SWAN, R. C. (1959). *J. Physiol.* **147**, 591–625.
KLODOS, I. and SKOU, J. C. (1975). *Biochim. Biophys. Acta*, **391**, 474–485.
KNIGHT, A. B. and WELT, L. G. (1974). *J. Gen. Physiol.* **63**, 351-373.
KYTE, J. (1971). *Biochem. Biophys. Res. Commun.* **43**, 1259–1265.
KYTE, J. (1974). *J. Biol. Chem.* **249**, 3652–3660.
LANT, A. F., PRIESTLAND, R. N. and WHITTAM, R. (1970). *J. Physiol.* **207**, 291–301.
LANT, A. F. and WHITTAM, R. (1968). *J. Physiol.* **199**, 457–484.
LARIS, P. C. and LETCHWORTH, P. E. (1962). *J. Cell. Comp. Physiol.* **60**, 229–234.
LAZDUNSKI, M. (1972). In "Current Topics in Cellular Regulation" (B. I. Horecker and E. R. Stadtman, eds), vol. 6, pp. 267–310. Academic Press, New York and London.
LEW, V. L., HARDY, M. A. and ELLORY, J. C. (1973). *Biochim. Biophys. Acta*, **323**, 251–266.
LINDENMAYER, G. E., LAUGHTER, A. H. and SCHWARTZ, A. (1968). *Arch. Biochem. Biophys.* **127**, 187–192.
LISHKO, V. K., KOLCHYNSKA, L. I. and PARKHOMENKO, M. T. (1973). *Ukr. Biokhem. Zh.* No. 1, 42-46.
LOWE, A. G. (1968). *Nature*, **219**, 934–936.
MAIZELS, M. (1951). *J. Physiol.* **112**, 59–83.
MAIZELS, M. (1968). *J. Physiol.* **195**, 657–679.
MÅRDH, S. (1975). *Biochim. Biophys. Acta*, **391**, 464–473.
MÅRDH, S. and ZETTERQVIST, Ö. (1972). *Biochim. Biophys. Acta*, **255**, 231–238.
MÅRDH, S. and ZETTERQVIST, Ö. (1974). *Biochim. Biophys. Acta*, **350**, 473–483.
MATSUI, H. and SCHWARTZ (1968). *Biochim. Biophys. Acta*, **151**, 655–663.
McCONAGHEY, P. D. and MAIZELS, M. (1962). *J. Physiol.* **162**, 485–509.
MONOD, J., WYMAN, J. and CHANGEUX, J-P. (1965). *J. Molec. Biol.* **12**, 88–118.
MULLINS, L. J., FENN, W. O., NOONAN, T. R. and HAEGE, L. (1941). *Amer. J. Physiol.* **135**, 93–101.
NAGAI, K., IZUMI, F. and YOSHIDA, H. (1966). *J. Biochem., Tokyo*, **59**, 295–303.
NAGAI, K. and YOSHIDA, H. (1966). *Biochim. Biophys. Acta*, **128**, 410–412.

NEUFELD, A. H. and LEVY, H. M. (1969). *J. Biol. Chem.* **244**, 6493–6497.
NEUFELD, A. H. and LEVY, H. M. (1970). *J. Biol. Chem.* **245**, 4962–4967.
NØRBY, J. G. and JENSEN, J. (1971). *Biochim. Biophys. Acta*, **233**, 104–116.
OPIT, L. J. and CHARNOCK, J. S. (1965). *Nature*, **208**, 471–474.
PETER, H. W. and WOLF, H. U. (1972). *Biochim. Biophys. Acta*, **290**, 300–309.
POST, R. L., HEGYVARY, C. and KUME, S. (1972). *J. Biol. Chem.* **247**, 6530–6540.
POST, R. L. and JOLLY, P. (1957). *Biochim. Biophys. Acta*, **25**, 118–128.
POST, R. L. and KUME, S. (1973). *J. Biol. Chem.* **248**, 6993–7000.
POST, R. L., KUME, S. and ROGERS, F. N. (1973). *In* "Mechanisms in Bioenergetics" (G. F. Azzone, L. Ernster, S. Papa, E. Quagliariello and N. Siliprandi, eds), pp. 203–218. Academic Press, New York and London.
POST, R. L., KUME, S., TOBIN, T., ORCUTT, B. and SEN, A. K. (1969). *J. Gen. Physiol.* **54**, 306s–326s.
POST, R. L., MERRITT, C. R., KINGSOLVING, C. R. and ALBRIGHT, C. D. (1960). *J. Biol. Chem.* **235**, 1796–1802.
POST, R. L. and SEN, A. K. (1965). *J. Histochem. Cytochem.* **13**, 105–112.
POST, R. L., SEN, A. K. and ROSENTHAL, A. S. (1965). *J. Biol. Chem.* **240**, 1437–1445.
POST, R. L., TANIGUCHI, K. and TODA, G. (1974). *Ann. N.Y. Acad. Sci.* **242**, 80–91.
POST, R. L., TODA, G. and ROGERS, F. N. (1975). *J. Biol. Chem.* **250**, 691–701.
PRIESTLAND, R. N. and WHITTAM, R. (1968). *Biochem. J.* **109**, 369–374.
REGA, A. F., GARRAHAN, P. J. and POUCHAN, M. I. (1968). *Biochim. Biophys. Acta*, **150**, 742–744.
REGA, A. F., GARRAHAN, P. J. and POUCHAN, M. I. (1970). *J. Membrane Biol.* **3**, 14–25.
REPKE, K. R. H. and SCHÖN, R. (1973). *Acta Biol. Med. Germ.* **31**, K19–K30.
REPKE, K. R. H., SCHÖN, R., HENKE, W., SCHÖNFELD, W., STRECKENBACH, B. and DITTRICH, F. (1974). *Ann. N.Y. Acad. Sci.* **242**, 203–219.
ROBINSON, J. D. (1967). *Biochemistry*, **6**, 3250–3258.
ROBINSON, J. D. (1969a). *Biochemistry*, **8**, 3348–3355.
ROBINSON, J. D. (1969b). *Molec. Pharmacol.* **5**, 584–592.
ROBINSON, J. D. (1970). *Biochim. Biophys. Acta*, **212**, 509–511SC.
ROBINSON, J. D. (1973). *Arch. Biochem. Biophys.* **156**, 232–243.
ROBINSON, J. D. (1974). *FEBS Lett.* **38**, 325–328.
ROBINSON, J. D. (1975). *Biochim. Biophys. Acta*, **384**, 250–264.
SACHS, J. R. (1967). *J. Clin. Invest.* **46**, 1433–1441.
SACHS, J. R. (1970). *J. Gen. Physiol.* **56**, 322–341.
SACHS, J. R. (1974). *J. Gen. Physiol.* **63**, 123–143.
SACHS, J. R., ELLORY, J. C., KROPP, D. L., DUNHAM, P. B. and HOFFMAN, J. F. (1974). *J. Gen. Physiol.* **63**, 389–414.
SACHS, J. R. and WELT, L. G. (1967). *J. Clin. Invest.* **46**, 65–76.
SCHATZMANN, H. J. (1953). *Helv. Physiol. Pharmac. Acta*, **11**, 346–354.
SCHATZMANN, H. J. (1965). *Biochim. Biophys. Acta*, **94**, 89–96.
SCHONER, W., BEUSCH, R. and KRAMER, R. (1968). *Eur. J. Biochem.* **7**, 102–110.
SCHWARTZ, A., LINDENMAYER, G. E. and ALLEN, J. C. (1975). *Pharmacol. Rev.* **27**, 3–134.
SCHWARTZ, A., MATSUI, H. and LAUGHTER, A. H. (1968). *Science*, **160**, 323–325.
SEN, A. K. and POST, R. L. (1961). *Fed. Proc.* **20**, 138.
SEN, A. K. and POST, R. L. (1964). *J. Biol. Chem.* **239**, 345–352.
SEN, A. K., TOBIN, T. and POST, R. L. (1969). *J. Biol. Chem.* **244**, 6596–6604.

Shaw, T. I. (1954). Ph.D. Thesis, University of Cambridge.
Shaw, T. I. (1955). *J. Physiol.* **129**, 464–475.
Siegel, G. J. and Goodwin, B. (1972). *J. Biol. Chem.* **247**, 3630–3637.
Simons, T. J. B. (1974). *J. Physiol.* **237**, 123–155.
Simons, T. J. B. (1975). *J. Physiol.* **244**, 731–739.
Skou, J. C. (1957). *Biochim. Biophys. Acta*, **23**, 394–401.
Skou, J. C. (1960). *Biochim. Biophys. Acta*, **42**, 6–23.
Skou, J. C. (1964). *Prog. Biophys. Mol. Biol.* **14**, 131–166.
Skou, J. C. (1971). *Current Topics in Bioenergetics*, **4**, 357–389.
Skou, J. C. (1974a). *Biochim. Biophys. Acta*, **339**, 234–245.
Skou, J. C. (1974b). *Biochim. Biophys. Acta*, **339**, 246–257.
Skou, J. C. (1975). *Quart. Rev. Biophys.* **7**, 401–434.
Skou, J. C. and Hilberg, C. (1969). *Biochim. Biophys. Acta*, **185**, 198–219.
Stahl, W. L. (1968). *J. Neurochem.* **15**, 511–518.
Stein, W. D., Lieb, W. R., Karlish, S. J. D. and Eilam, Y. (1973). *Proc. Nat. Acad. Sci. U.S.A.* **70**, 275–278.
Stone, A. J. (1968). *Biochim. Biophys. Acta*, **150**, 578–586.
Taniguchi, K. and Iida, S. (1972). *Biochim. Biophys. Acta*, **288**, 98–102.
Taniguchi, K. and Post, R. L. (1975). *J. Biol. Chem.* **250**, 3010–3018.
Tobin, T., Akera, T., Hogg, R. E. and Brody, Th. M. (1973). *Molec. Pharmacol.* **6**, 278–281SC.
Tobin, T., Baskin, S. I., Akera, T. and Brody, Th. M. (1972). *Molec. Pharmacol.* **8**, 256–263.
Tobin, T. and Sen, A. K. (1970). *Biochim. Biophys. Acta*, **198**, 120–131.
Toda, G. (1968). *J. Biochem., Tokyo*, **64**, 457–464.
Tonomura, Y. and Fukushima, Y. (1974). *Ann. N.Y. Acad. Sci.* **242**, 92–105.
Whittam, R. (1962). *Biochem. J.* **84**, 110–118.
Whittam, R. and Ager, M. E. (1965). *Biochem. J.* **97**, 214–227.
Whittam, R. and Chipperfield, A. R. (1975). *Biochim. Biophys. Acta*, **415**, 149–171.
Whittam, R., Wheeler, K. P. and Blake, A. (1964). *Nature*, **203**, 720–724.
Yoshida, H., Izumi, F. and Nagai, K. (1966). *Biochim. Biophys. Acta*, **120**, 183–186PN.
Yoshida, H., Nagai, K., Ohashi, T. and Nakagawa, Y. (1969). *Biochim. Biophys. Acta*, **171**, 178–185.

Passive fluxes of sodium and potassium across red cell membranes

L. BEAUGÉ and V. L. LEW

Physiological Laboratory, Cambridge University, UK

1 Introduction	39
2 The passive fluxes of potassium	40
2.1 Ouabain-sensitive components	40
2.2 K fluxes in the presence of ouabain	42
3 The passive fluxes of sodium	45
3.1 Ouabain-sensitive components	45
3.2 Na fluxes in the presence of ouabain	46
4 Can the ouabain-poisoned Na pump perform cation translocation?	48
References	50

1 Introduction

The human red blood cell membrane is a choice model for studies on active Na and K transport. Many workers in this field often felt a curious attraction for a group of fluxes usually described as ouabain-resistant or ouabain-insensitive. This interest may seem difficult to explain. To anybody only marginally concerned with this field these fluxes look a complex mixture of "left over" leaks with the only interesting and rather disturbing property of not being diffusional. In 1966, Hoffman and Kregenow suggested the existence of a second active Na extrusion mechanism in human red blood cells which could operate in the presence of ouabain, when the Na pump was presumed to be fully inhibited. A few years earlier Kleinzeller and Knotkova (1954) had observed that kidney cells incubated *in vitro* can regulate their volume in the presence of ouabain. This was confirmed by Whittembury (1968), who also suggested the existence of a link between Hoffman and Kregenow's pump II and the osmoregulatory mechanism found in kidney slices in the presence of ouabain. The ouabain-insensitive Na flux component became thus associated with an important physiological function and this stimulated and inspired much of the subsequent work done in this field.

More than a comprehensive review, this chapter will provide a critical analysis of the passive components of the Na and K fluxes in red blood cells. The possible nature of the mechanisms which mediate these fluxes will be discussed.

Under physiological conditions, the Na pump is only about 75 per cent saturated with external K and because of the different ion translocating modes of this mechanism (see Glynn and Karlish, 1975) a number of passive Na and K flux components are also known to occur through it. Thus, the Na pump normally mediates a substantial K–K exchange and also a small measure of Na–Na exchange and K–Na reversal.

It is usually assumed that ouabain is a specific inhibitor of the Na pump and that it blocks all the biochemical reactions mediated by the (Na + K)-ATPase as well as all the ion movements occurring through the translocating part of the pump apparatus. It may therefore seem safe to analyse, as it is often done, the Na and K flux components in red cells, in terms of their ouabain sensitivity or insensitivity, the ouabain-sensitive fluxes representing pump-mediated transport and the ouabain-insensitive fluxes representing leaks or transport across unidentified mechanisms. However, although there is good evidence suggesting that ouabain inhibits the uphill Na and K transport together with the associated hydrolysis of ATP, the evidence that it blocks all other transport and enzymic activities of the Na pump is less convincing. This has led a number of workers to suggest that altered forms of the Na pump machinery may also perform cation translocation (Brinley and Mullins, 1968; Sachs, 1971; Beaugé and Ortiz, 1973; Beaugé and Adragna, 1974), and also Ca-activated or Ca-induced substrate hydrolysis or ion transport (Blum and Hoffman, 1971; Rega *et al.*, 1973; Lew, 1974; see also Lew and Beaugé, 1977).

In the following section we will briefly review the available information about the passive components of the Na and K movements in red blood cells and will consider the possibility that some of these fluxes represent biochemically silent transport through the intact or ouabain-altered pump.

2 The passive fluxes of potassium

2.1 OUABAIN-SENSITIVE COMPONENTS

2.1.1 *K–K exchange*

The Na pump is able to catalyze a 1–1 exchange of potassium ions without the simultaneous hydrolysis of ATP (although the presence of ATP is required) (Glynn *et al.*, 1970; Glynn *et al.*, 1971). This passive K exchange has not been considered a normal mode of operation of the Na pump (see Glynn and Karlish, 1975). This is not really justified since under physiological conditions the K–K exchange is much nearer to its maximum value than the "normal" Na–K exchange which is only about 20–30 per cent saturated with internal Na. The K–K exchange is activated by K and inhibited by Na, on both membrane surfaces. The K_m for external K is about 1·5 mM in the presence of Na in the medium. Internally, 4 mM Na inhibited 90 per cent of the exchange in the presence of 9 mM K (Simons, 1974). Under physiological conditions, therefore, the K–K exchange will not be significantly inhibited by internal Na and will be about 75 per cent saturated with external K. This amounts to a flux of about 0·2–0·4 mmol (l cells)$^{-1}$ h^{-1} (Glynn et al., 1970) which represents about 15–30 per cent of the total K influx.

2.1.2 Na–K "reversal" exchange

The large electrochemical gradients of Na and K which exist across the human red cell membrane under normal conditions ought to be able to drive the pump backwards to some extent. External K inhibits this reversal (Glynn and Lew, 1970) with the same apparent affinity as it stimulates or inhibits all other pump-mediated fluxes. It is therefore reasonable to conclude, although very difficult to measure, that a small reversal rate occurs under physiological conditions. This could represent a K efflux and a Na influx of about 30–60 μmol (l cells)$^{-1}$ h^{-1}.

2.1.3 Nucleotide and P_i requirements of the K–K exchange and K–Na reversal

The ouabain-sensitive K–K exchange requires ATP and P_i, but it is not affected by ADP (Glynn et al., 1970; Glynn et al., 1971; Simons, 1974). The apparent K_m for ATP is about 100 μM. Since ATP hydrolysis was not associated with these fluxes and since nonhydrolysable ATP analogues were also able to sustain some degree of exchange, it was assumed that the nucleotide acted without phosphorylation of the pump (Simons, 1975). P_i-free resealed ghosts showed no ouabain-sensitive K–K exchange (Simons, 1974) and inosine, which reduces the level of P_i in intact cells, also inhibited the ouabain-sensitive K efflux (Glynn et al., 1970) into Na-containing media with or without K. It is not yet clear whether P_i is required for the K–K exchange in order to provide a phosphorylated intermediate which allows K to shuttle backwards and forwards, or whether P_i has to go on and off the enzyme with each translocation cycle. In the case of the K–Na exchange, the P_i requirement seems to represent the reversal of the final biochemical step of the forward ATPase reaction. The nucleotide dependence of this flux has not yet been measured although ADP must be an obvious requirement.

2.2 K FLUXES IN THE PRESENCE OF OUABIN

2.2.1 *The electrodiffusional "leak"*

A fraction of the K influx varies linearly with the external K concentration up to 150 mM. This has been found originally in the absence of ouabain (Shaw, 1955; Glynn, 1956) but it is also present in ouabain-poisoned cells (Beaugé and Adragna, 1974). It is independent of the metabolic state of the cells (Glynn, 1956) and it is strongly influenced by pH. A change of pH from 6·0 to 8·7 increases its value six- to eightfold (Beaugé and Adragna, 1974). At physiological pH its rate-constant has a value of 0·006 h^{-1} (Glynn, 1956) which is equivalent to a P_K of the order of 10^{-10} cm sec^{-1}. This P_K is close to that found for lipid bilayers (Hladky et al., 1974) and it seems reasonable to assume that it represents the membrane ground permeability to potassium. If this is so, Ussing's flux-ratio equation predicts a K efflux of about 0·4 mmol (l cells)$^{-1}$ under physiological conditions.

2.2.2 *The saturable components of the K fluxes*

In the presence of ouabain and external Na there is a large component of the K influx which shows saturation (Glynn, 1957; Garrahan and Glynn, 1967; Beaugé and Adragna, 1971; Wiley and Cooper, 1974). The half-maximum is attained at a K concentration between 4 and 7 mM. Under the same experimental conditions, external K stimulates a K efflux. The kinetic characteristics of the K-activated K efflux, however, are quite different from those of the K influx; the apparent K_m is lower, about 1·5 mM, and the maximum efflux is about one-half that of the K influx (Glynn et al., 1970). These differences suggest a complex relationship or no relation at all between these two fluxes. In the absence of external Na the absolute magnitude of the K influx is reduced by 40–50 per cent; in addition, in the presence of only 5 mM Na, external K does not stimulate the K efflux (Glynn et al., 1970). The Na dependence of the K influx has an apparent K_m for Na of about 16 mM at 1 mM external K (Beaugé and Adragna, 1971). The Na dependence of the K-stimulated K efflux has not been investigated. If one considers the kinetic properties of the Na-dependent K influx and compares them with those of the K-stimulated K efflux in Na media the similarities are quite striking. This can be seen in Fig. 1 where the values of individual experiments have been normalized to allow comparison with other fluxes through the Na pump.

The findings discussed above strongly suggest that in ouabain-poisoned cells external Na is required to catalyze a K–K exchange with a 1–1 stoichiometry. However, as it will be seen later, the effects of external Na

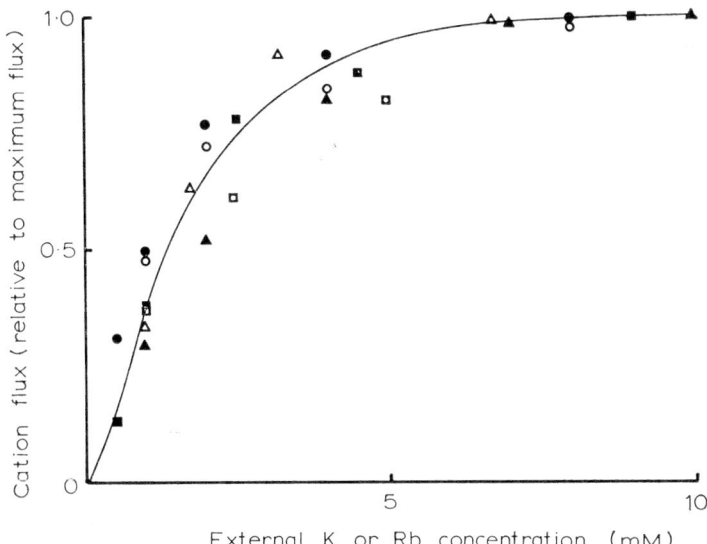

FIG. 1. Saturable components of the K or Rb influx, the K efflux and the K-stimulated active Na efflux as a function of the external K or Rb concentration. All values were normalized relative to the maximum flux. The correspondence between symbols, fluxes and sources is indicated below.

Symbol	Flux	Reference
○	ouabain-sensitive K-stimulated K efflux in Na media	Glynn et al., 1970
●	K-stimulated K efflux in Na media with ouabain	Glynn et al., 1970
▲	Na-dependent K influx in the presence of ouabain	Wiley and Cooper, 1974
■	Na-dependent Rb influx in the presence of ouabain	Beaugé and Adragna, 1971
△	saturable total K influx in Na media	Garrahan and Glynn, 1967a
□	K-activated Na efflux in Na media	Glynn, 1956

on the influx of K have their counterpart on a stimulatory effect of external K on the influx of Na. This has led Wiley and Cooper (1974) to suggest that at least part of the Na and K influx occurs through a cotransport mechanism. In some avian red cells the influx of Na and K is accompanied by an increase in cell volume (Kregenow, 1971; Schmidt andMcManus, 1974); this would indeed suggest some kind of cotransport or at least that the K–K exchange is not 1–1. In human red cells the evidence for such a cotransport mechanism is not at all convincing. Although there is a K-dependent net Na gain, a net K gain stimulated by external Na has only been seen in K-depleted, Li-loaded cells (Wiley and Cooper, 1974). This makes it difficult to distinguish between a K–Li exchange and a net gain of KCl.

Figure 2, constructed with data from Garrahan and Glynn (1967b), and Glynn et al. (1970) shows that, in the absence of K, increasing external Na from 0 to 5 mM largely stimulates the K efflux; from 5 mM upwards the K efflux is steadily reduced to the levels found in the absence of Na, or even further. This suggests the interesting possibility that the failure of K to stimulate the K efflux in 5 mM Na media results from the fact that this flux is already fully activated. If this were true, then one should expect K to activate the K efflux both in full-Na and in Na-free media, although not necessarily in the same way. This has not been tested yet but evidence from measurements of K influx in Na-free media (Beaugé and Adragna, 1971) suggest that there is a smaller saturable component with a lower affinity for external K.

In the presence of ouabain the K-activated K efflux into Na-media also requires ATP (Glynn et al., 1971). A similar dependence was found for the Na-dependent component of the K influx (Beaugé and Adragna,

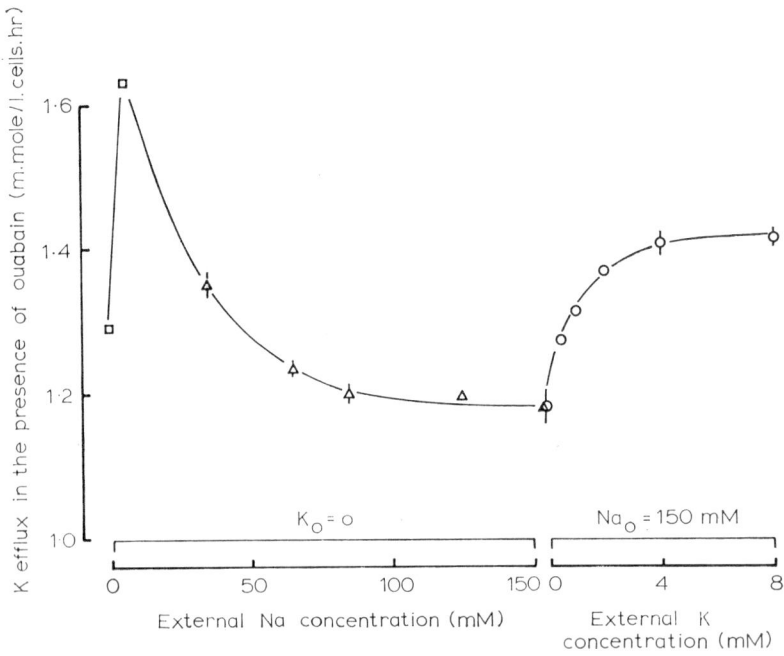

FIG. 2. The effects of external Na and K on the efflux of K in the presence of ouabain. The points correspond to absolute values taken from different experiments of Garrahan and Glynn (1967b) (□) and Glynn et al. (1970) (△, ○).

1971). There is no evidence of ATP hydrolysis associated with these fluxes and it is not known whether P_i is required as well.

2.3.3 *A comparison between the ouabain-sensitive K fluxes and the K fluxes in the presence of ouabain*

All the K fluxes considered above, together with the active Na and K fluxes, have a number of features in common:

a. The apparent affinity for external K seems to be the same for all these fluxes in high Na media (Fig. 1).
b. ATP or ADP are always required.
c. External pH affects both the ouabain-sensitive K influx and the saturable components of the K influx in the presence of ouabain in the same way (Beaugé and Adragna, 1974). This indicates either that groups with similar ionization properties are involved or that K binds to the same sites for both fluxes.
d. Inhibitory-type interactions between Na and K are transformed into stimulatory interactions by ouabain. This may merely reflect the reactivity of two different mechanisms which interact with the same ligands, but a more interesting alternative is that of a single system, the Na pump, with a multiplicity of reactive modalities.

3 The passive fluxes of sodium

3.1 OUABAIN-SENSITIVE COMPONENTS

3.1.1 *The efflux of Na as part of a Na–Na exchange*

The ouabain-sensitive Na–Na exchange is one of the passive transport modes mediated by the Na pump. Its biochemical counterpart is the ATP–ADP exchange reaction (see chapter by Cavieres). It is now established that it requires both ATP and ADP, but there is no associated hydrolysis of ATP (Garrahan and Glynn, 1967b; Cavieres and Glynn, 1976). External K inhibits the Na–Na exchange with the same K_m as it activates and inhibits all other fluxes through the pump in high Na media ($K_m =$ 1·5–2 mM). This means that under physiological conditions, with a plasma K concentration of about 4 mM, 25–30 per cent of the ouabain-sensitive Na efflux represents Na–Na exchange. This is equivalent to a flux of about 0·5 mmol (l cells)$^{-1}$ h^{-1}.

3.1.2 *The influx of Na as part of a Na–Na exchange and a K–Na reversal*

The Na–Na exchange and the K–Na reversal present under physiological conditions will account for all the ouabain-sensitive passive Na influx.

The reversal rate of the Na pump in these conditions is about a fortieth of the forward rate. This means that under physiological conditions about 0·5 per cent of the pumps contribute to dissipate the Na and K gradients which are maintained by the fraction of actively transporting pumps.

3.2 Na fluxes in the presence of ouabain

3.2.1 *Electrodiffusional "leak"*

As with the K influx of Na as a function of the external Na concentration can be divided into a linear and a saturable component. The rate-constant of the linear component estimated from results by Garrahan and Glynn (1967b) and Wiley and Cooper (1974) is about $0·008$ h^{-1}. This corresponds to a maximum value of P_{Na} of about $1·1 \times 10^{-10}$ cm sec^{-1}, which is of the same order as that of the P_K, indicating that the ground permeability of the human red blood cell membrane does not discriminate between these two alkali metal ions in analogy with the properties of lipid bilayers (Hladky et al., 1974).

3.2.2 *Saturable components of the Na fluxes*

A nonlinear component of Na influx has been found in ouabain-poisoned cells in the presence of external K (Glynn, 1957; Wieth, 1970) as well as free solutions (Garrahan and Glynn, 1967; Wiley and Cooper, 1974). In the absence of ouabain, a saturable component of the Na influx was also found when there was enough K in the medium to inhibit completely the Na–Na exchange through the Na pump (Solomon, 1952; Sachs, 1970). This indicates that we are not in the presence of an ouabain-induced flux.

The Na efflux in the presence of ouabain also shows saturation kinetics (Fig. 3). This has been seen in red cells from a variety of species such as man (Sachs, 1971; Dunn, 1973; Garay and Garrahan, 1973; Beaugé, 1975), rat (Beaugé and Oritiz, 1973) and beef (Motais, 1973) irrespective of the procedure used for loading cells with different internal Na concentrations.

Lubowitz and Whittam (1969) found that internal Na stimulates Na influx and suggested that the saturable components of the Na fluxes in the presence of ouabain result from the operation of an exchange diffusion mechanism (see also Dunn, 1970). These findings were never confirmed and there is now good evidence from a number of other laboratories which indicates that the Na influx is independent of the internal Na concentration (Beaugé and Ortiz, 1973; Dunn, 1973; Garay and Garrahan, 1973; Beaugé, 1975) (Fig. 3).

In the absence of external Na, a reduction of the Na efflux was observed

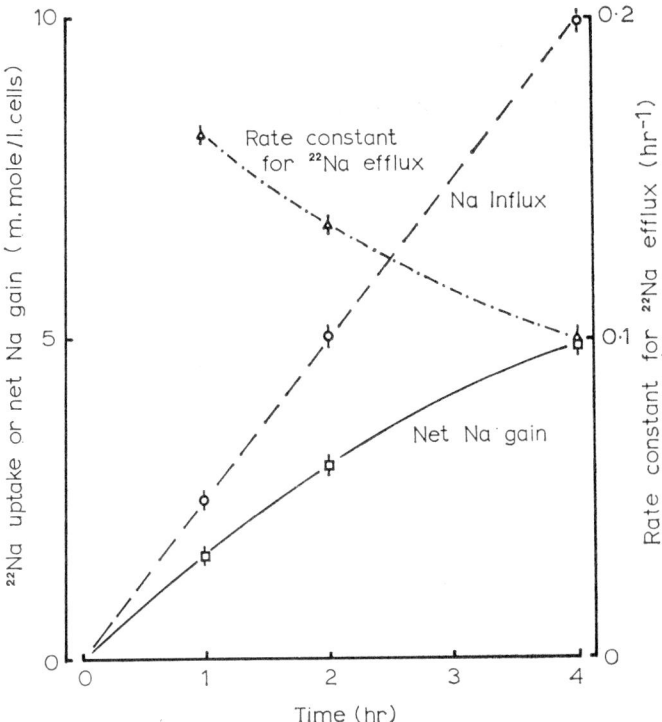

FIG. 3. The effects of internal Na concentration on Na influx, net Na gain and Na efflux in human red cells incubated in K-free Na media containing ouabain. Prior to the flux measurements the internal Na concentration was reduced by incubating the cells in Na-free 150 mM K for 12 h at 37°C. All values are the mean ± S.E.M. of four independent and simultaneous determinations. The initial internal Na was 2·45 ± 0·05 mmol (l cells)$^{-1}$. Beaugé (1975) reproduced with permission from *Biochim. Biophys. Acta*.

only when either Mg or Mg+sucrose solutions were used as substitutes (Lubowitz and Whittam, 1969; Sachs, 1970; Rettori and Lenoir, 1972; Beaugé and Ortiz, 1973; Dunn, 1973; Lew *et al.*, 1973; Motais, 1973). Other Na substitutes failed to inhibit the Na efflux (Garrahan and Glynn, 1967; Rettori and Lenoir, 1973; Lew *et al.*, 1973; Beaugé and Del Campillo, 1976) and in rat red cells, Beaugé and Ortiz (1973) found that the Na efflux was larger in choline than in Na media. Rettori and Lenoir (1972) suggested that the reduction in Na efflux results from an inhibitory effect of Mg rather than from the removal of external Na. A direct inhibitory effect of Mg on a Na efflux was also observed by Beaugé and Mullins (1976) in normal and ATP-depleted squid axons in the presence of strophanthidin.

All these results suggest that the saturable components of the unidirectional Na fluxes in the presence of ouabain are independent of each other and it cannot be said at present whether they share a common transport path or not. If they do, the carrier has to satisfy the requirements of a facilitated diffusion mechanism (Beaugé, 1975) with similar mobilities of the free and loaded form.

In rat red cells (Beaugé and Ortiz, 1973) and in human red cells (Beaugé, 1975) incubated in K-free, high–Na media, the rate of net Na gain was reduced as the internal Na concentration increased and this reduction was much larger than that predicted by simple electrodiffusion (Fig. 3). This was seen in the presence and absence of ouabain and also in ATP-depleted cells. It was not due to a variable inhibitory effect of internal K because similar results were obtained when internal Na was replaced at constant internal K.

Haas *et al.* (1975) have recently shown that in ouabain-treated human red cells external Na reduces Li influx and that a net uphill Li transport can be produced, in both directions, by suitable manipulation of the Na gradients. These results, together with the effects observed by Beaugé (1975) on the net and unidirectional Na movements, indicate the existence of a facilitated diffusion mechanism for Na translocation which is capable of operating a Na–Li countertransport.

3.2.3 *Uphill extrusion of Na in the presence of ouabain*

Hoffman and Kregenow (1966) originally suggested the existence of an active Na extrusion mechanism in the presence of ouabain, which they named Pump II. Sachs (1971), working with human red cells, and Beaugé and Ortiz (1973), using a rat red cells, provided new and more direct experimental evidence for the existence of a mechanism capable of extruding Na against an electrochemical gradient in ouabain-poisoned cells. Beaugé and Ortiz (1973) suggested that the direct source of energy for this transport was the electrochemical gradient of another ionic species and not a chemical fuel as originally proposed by Hoffman and Kregenow (1966). Choline and Mg were originally proposed as the countertransported species (Beaugé and Ortiz, 1973) but a more likely candidate is K (Sachs *et al.*, 1974), since the uphill Na efflux was abolished when the outward K gradient was reduced by increasing the external K concentration. The effect of altering the K gradient by changing the internal K concentration has not yet been investigated.

4 Can the ouabain-poisoned Na pump perform cation translocation?

The possibility that most or all of the nondiffusional components of the Na and K fluxes in human red cell discussed above are mediated by the Na pump cannot be ruled out (see Lew and Beaugé, 1977). At present, however, this is a highly speculative possibility with no direct experimental evidence in its support.

Nevertheless, the kinetic similarities between the saturable components of the ouabain-sensitive K fluxes and the Na-dependent K fluxes in the presence of ouabain are so striking that the possibility that they are all mediated by the Na pump (Glynn et al., 1970), deserves more detailed consideration. If the ouabain-poisoned Na pump is capable of translocating K, an immediate question arises: is this a flux which remains unchanged in the presence of ouabain as it is implicitly assumed when it is referred to as an *ouabain-insensitive* flux or is this an *ouabain-induced* flux? If ouabain *induces* the saturable components of the K fluxes, the actual magnitude of the K–Na exchange through the unpoisoned pump could be twice as large as that estimated from the ouabain-sensitive flux (Glynn et al., 1970). A possible mechanism by which ouabain can induce the pump to translocate K is by stabilizing a phosphorylated intermediate (Albers and Koval, 1968). This raises the question of whether the K shuttle through the unpoisoned pump requires inorganic phosphate (Glynn et al, 1970) to sustain the level of a phosphorylated intermediate or to provide a phosphoryl exchange between the pump enzyme and internal water with each translocation cycle. Some support for the view that ouabain actually induces a K–K exchange through the pump and that the magnitude of the flux might depend on the level of a phosphorylated pump intermediate comes from the analysis of certain experimental results by Beaugé and Adragna (1971) and by Simons (1975). Beaugé and Adragna found that the Rb influx in the presence of ouabain was larger in Na media than in choline media. In the absence of ouabain, the Rb influx was the same whether choline or Na where the main external cations. This means either that the maximum ouabain-sensitive Rb influx is inhibited by Na (or stimulated by choline) or that part of the Rb influx in the presence of ouabain is actually induced by the glycoside, but only in high Na media. Simons (1975) measured the ouabain-sensitive K efflux from resealed ghosts incubated in Na-free media. His experiments show that while nonhydrolyzable ATP analogues can sustain K–K exchange, hydrolyzable substrates are substantially more efficient. This could either reflect the relative efficiency of the different nucleotides acting as allosteric activators of the K flux or be due to the contribution of the hydrolyzable substrates to raise the level of a relevant phosphorylated intermediate. If the K flux in the presence of ouabain represents the behaviour of the ouabain-poisoned pump, it ought to be possible to measure only a partial inhibitory effect of inosine on the K-dependent K efflux from intact cells into Na-free media, since ATP could sustain a certain level of phosphorylated intermediate even in the absence of inorganic phosphate. The rationale behind this experiment is that inosine always acts like a partial inhibitor and the reason why it appears to inhibit the K flux completely would result from the artefactual subtraction of an ouabain-induced component. A closer look at the results of Glynn *et al.* (1970) shows that the K efflux in the presence of ouabain is consistently lower than in the presence of inosine.

That cardiac glycosides can induce flux components which do not exist in their absence was shown by Brinley and Mullins (1968) (see also Beaugé and Mullins, 1976) in ATP-depleted squid axons where strophanthidin produced a large increase in the efflux of Na without affecting the membrane permeability.

References

ALBERS, R. W. and KOVAL, G. J. (1968). *Molec. Pharmacol.* **4**, 324–326.
BEAUGÉ, L. A. (1975) *Biochim. Biophys. Acta*, **401**, 95–108.
BEAUGÉ, L. A. and ADRAGNA, N. C. (1971). *J. Gen. Physiol.* **57**, 576–592.
BEAUGÉ, L. A. and ADRAGNA, N. C. (1974). *Biochim. Biophys. Acta*, **352**, 241–247.
BEAUGÉ, L. A. and DEL CAMPILLO, M. A. (1976). *Biochim. Biophys. Acta*, **433**, 547–554.
BEAUGÉ, L. A. and MULLINS, L. J. (1976). *Proc. Roy. Soc. B*, **194**, 279–284.
BEAUGÉ, L. A. and ORTIZ, O. (1973). *J. Membrane Biol.* **13**, 165–184.
BRINLEY, J. F. and MULLINS, L. J. (1968). *J. Gen. Physiol.* **52**, 181–211.
BLUM, R. M. and HOFFMAN, J. F. (1971). *J. Membrane Biol.* **6**, 315–328.
BLUM, R. M. and HOFFMAN, J. F. (1972). *Biochem. Biophys. Res. Comm.* **46**, 1146–1152.
CAVIERES, J. D. and GLYNN, I. M. (1976). *J. Physiol.* In press.
DUNN, M. J. (1970). *J. Clin. Invest.* **49**, 1804–1814.
DUNN, M. J. (1973). *J. Clin. Invest.* **52**, 658–670.
GARAY, R. P. and GARRAHAN, P. J. (1973). *J. Physiol.* **231**, 297–325.
GARRAHAN, P. J. and GLYNN, I. M. (1967a). *J. Physiol.* **192**, 159–174.
GARRAHAN, P. J. and GLYNN, I. M. (1967b). *J. Physiol.* **192**, 189–216.
GLYNN, I. M. (1956). *J. Physiol.* **134**, 278–310.
GLYNN, I. M. (1957). *J. Physiol.* **136**, 148–173.
GLYNN, I. M., HOFFMAN, J. P. and LEW, V. L. (1971). *Phil. Trans. Roy. Soc. B*, **262**, 91–102.
GLYNN, I. M. and KARLISH, S. J. D. (1975). *Ann. Rev. Physiol.* **37**, 13–55.
GLYNN, I. M. and LEW, V. L. (1970). *J. Physiol.* **207**, 393–402.
GLYNN, I. M., LEW, V. L. and LÜTHI, U. (1970). *J. Physiol.* **207**, 371–391.
HAAS. M., JCHOOLER, J. and TOSTESON, D. C. (1975). *Nature*, **258**, 425–427.
HLADKY, S. B., GORDON, L. G. M. and HAYDON, D. A. (1974). *Ann. Rev. Physical Chem.* **25**, 11–38.
HOFFMAN, J. F. and KREGENOW, F. M. (1966). *Ann. N.Y. Acad. Sci.* **137**, 566–576.
KLEINZELLER, A. and KNOTKOVA, A. (1964). *J. Physiol.* **175**, 172–192.
KREGENOW, F. (1971). *J. Gen. Physiol.* **58**, 396–412.
LEW, V. L. (1974). *In* "Comparative Biochemistry and Physiology of Transport"

(L. Bolis, K. Bloch, S. E. Luria and F. Lynen, eds), pp. 310–316. North-Holland Amsterdam.

LEW, V. L. and BEAUGÉ, L. (1977). *In* "Transport Across Biological Membranes" (G. Giebisch, D. C. Tosteson and H. H. Ussing, eds), vol. II. Springer-Verlag, Berlin, Heidelberg, New York. In press.

LEW, V. L., GLYNN I. M. and ELLORY, J. C. (1970). *Nature*, **225**, 865–866.

LEW, V. L., HARDY, M. A. and ELLORY, J. C. (1973). *Biochim. Biophys. Acta*, **323**, 251–266.

LUBOWITZ, H. and WHITTAM, R. (1969). *J. Physiol.* **202**, 111–131.

MOTAIS, R. (1973). *J. Physiol.* **233**, 395–422.

REGA, A. F., RICHARDS D. E. and GERRAHAN, P. J. (1973). *Biochem. J.* **136**, 185–194.

RETTORI, O. and LENOIR, J. P. (1972). *Amer. J. Physiol.* **222**, 880–884.

SACHS, J. R. (1970). *J. Gen. Physiol.* **56**, 322–341.

SACHS, J. R. (1971). *J. Gen. Physiol.* **57**, 259–282.

SACHS. J. R., KNAUF P. A. and DUNHAM, P. B. (1974). *In* "The Red Blood Cell" (D. M. Surgenor, ed), vol. 2, pp. 613–703. Academic Press, New York and London.

SCHMIDT, W. F. and MCMANUS, T. J. (1974). *Fed. Proc.* **33**, 1457, Abs.

SHAW, T. I. (1955). *J. Physiol.* **129**, 464–475.

SIMONS, T. J. B. (1974). *J. Physiol.* **237**, 123–155.

SIMONS, T. J. B. (1975). *J. Physiol.* **244**, 731–739.

SOLOMON, A. K. (1952). *J. Gen. Physiol.* **36**, 57–110.

WHITTEMBURY, G. (1968). *J. Gen. Physiol.* **51**, 303s–313s.

WIETH, J. O. (1970). *Acta Physiol. Scand.* **79**, 76–87.

WILEY, S. J. and COOPER, R. A. (1974). *J. Clin. Invest.* **53**, 745–755.

Passive Ca transport and cytoplasmic Ca buffering in intact red cells

H. G. FERREIRA and V. L. LEW
Physiological Laboratory, Cambridge University, UK

1 Introduction	53
2 The human red blood cell as an experimental model for the study of Ca transport and metabolism	54
3 A few methodological points	56
4 Cytoplasmic Ca buffering	58
5 Passive Ca transport in intact red cells	63
5.1 The uptake of calcium by ATP-depleted human red blood cells	63
5.2 Ca–Ca exchange	66
5.3 Dependence of the net uptake on external calcium	68
5.4 The influence of monovalent cations on the calcium uptake	71
5.5 The efflux of calcium from calcium-loaded, ATP-depleted human red blood cells	73
5.6 Dependence of the calcium efflux on external calcium	74
5.7 Dependence of the calcium efflux on internal calcium	76
5.8 On the time-course of the calcium efflux	81
6 Calcium influx and the Ca permeability of intact red cell membranes	85
7 On the mechanism of calcium efflux from ATP-depleted red cells	86
8 The physiological importance of the regulation of the intracellular calcium concentration in red blood cells	88
Acknowledgement	90
References	90

1 Introduction

In this chapter we will present an account of work as yet largely unpublished concerning the passive Ca-permeability properties of intact human red cell membranes. For a recent account of the properties of the active Ca transport system in red cells, consult the excellent review by Schatzmann (1975a).

2 The human red blood cell as an experimental model for the study of Ca transport and metabolism

There are two main difficulties in the study of calcium transport across the plasma membranes of intact cells. First, it is in general impossible to assess the cytosolic concentration of free calcium (Ca_i^{2+}). Secondly, due to the ability of intracellular calcium-storing organelles to remove from or release into the cytosol substantial amounts of calcium at very fast rates it is impossible to control experimentally Ca_i^{2+}.

The nonnucleated mammalian red blood cell has a number of advantages for calcium transport studies:

1. It is devoid of intracellular organelles and is virtually Ca-free (see Schatzmann, 1975a).
2. By reversible lysis techniques it is possible to replace its cytoplasm with solutions of known composition.
3. The external surface of its membrane faces directly the bulk of the external suspending medium without the complication of interposed structures.
4. The human red blood cell is endowed with a powerful calcium pump which couples the hydrolysis of ATP to the uphill calcium extrusion, a mechanism which may occur in many other cells.
5. The metabolism and the biochemical and physiological role of calcium in the human erythrocyte exhibits some characteristics which are probably common to those of other cell types. For example, like other cells, the red blood cell possesses calcium-activated actin- and myosine-like proteins (Ohnishi, 1962; Rosenthal et al., 1970; Avissar et al., 1975) which may play an important role in the maintenance of its normal shape (Nakao et al., 1961; Palek et al., 1971a,b). In fact the study of the dependence of shape on calcium metabolism is now well advanced (Lionetti et al., 1968; Lionetti and McKay, 1969; Weed et al., 1969; Hoffman, 1972; LaCelle et al., 1972; Lichtmann and Marinetti, 1972).
6. The K permeability of red cells is controlled by intracellular calcium in a variety of species (Gardos, 1956; Lew, 1970; Jenkins and Lew, 1973) and similar K channels have now been identified in other cells (Meech, 1974; Krnjevic, 1974; Clusin et al., 1975; Isenberg, 1975; Ransom et al., 1975). If the calcium-dependent K channels in all these cells prove to be similar, the red blood cell offers the clear advantage of its anatomical simplicity for biochemical and pharmacological studies concerning this permeability mechanism.
7. Although no studies are available on the effect of intracellular calcium on the glycolytic metabolism of red cells, such effects probably exist, making the mammalian red cell a promising system in which the link

between calcium metabolism and some aspects of metabolic control (Bygrave, 1967) can be studied.

8. Intracellular calcium seems to control the lipid composition of the plasma membrane of red blood cells, a process which is probably related to the maintenance of normal shape (Allan and Michell, 1975; Allan et al., 1976) and to other physiological functions (Lew and Ferreira, 1976).

9. Changes in calcium permeability (Wiley and Shaller, 1974) or in the activity of the calcium pump are probably part of the mechanisms responsible for the maturation of the human erythrocyte since an increase in external calcium stimulates the mitotic activity of the bone marrow (Perris, quoted by Schatzmann, 1975b) and since in polycythaemia vera the (Ca + Mg)-ATPase activity seems to be decreased in the erythrocyte membranes (Scharff and Foder, 1975). In sickle cell disease the calcium content of the red cells is increased (Eaton and Skelton, 1973) and the calcium permeability and content are also increased in microcytic spherocytosis (Wiley and Gill, 1976). The permeability of the red cell membrane also increases after some weeks of storage (Lew, 1974; Ferreira and Lew, 1975). Thus in terms of the physiology of the erythrocyte itself the regulation of intracellular calcium content seems to be very important although we still ignore what are the tolerable limits for the intracellular free calcium concentration and which key functions are first affected.

Because of all these characteristics the human red blood cell seems to be an excellent system for the study of calcium transport. In particular, the possibility of controlling the intracellular composition by reversible haemolysis has been extremely useful (see Schatzmann, 1975a). However, a measure of caution should be introduced in this respect. Without subscribing entirely to the view that there are as many types of red blood cell membranes (ghosts) as methods of preparing them (Ponder, 1961) the experience with studies on the calcium pump has shown that it is a very labile system (Wolf, 1970, 1972a,b; Schatzmann and Rossi, 1971; Scharff, 1972; Schatzmann, 1973). Furthermore, one should not assume that all the properties of the plasma membrane of the intact cell remain untouched in the reconstituted ghost. If the (Na + K)-ATPase and the Na pump survive the procedure in good condition, the same cannot be said of the passive permeability to Na and K and the information available on the passive Ca movements across red cell membranes suggests that "resealed" ghosts and even aged bank cells are much leakier than the intact cells (Lew, 1974; Ferreira and Lew, 1975).

In view of these facts the study of the *intact* red blood cell is an important stage in the characterization of the calcium transport across the erythrocyte membrane. There are, however, certain problems. The most important is the fact that the human red blood cell is virtually calcium-free. That means that calcium accumulation or calcium release cannot be measured unless some disturbance is introduced in the calcium transport one wants to study. Unfortunately, no specific inhibitor of the calcium pump is available. Both ruthenium and lanthanum block calcium movements in general by displacing it from its binding sites. As a way of avoiding this difficulty, Lew (1970, 1971) proposed the use of metabolic inhibitors in order to deplete the cells from ATP and thus reduce the pump activity. This method is still the best available and enables us to decrease substantially the calcium pumping activity without inducing simultaneously dramatic changes in the passive permeability to calcium (Ferreira and Lew, 1975). On the other hand, a number of drugs can induce a partially reversible increase in the permeability of the cell membrane to calcium and thus be used to load the cells with calcium while the pump is still operating. Of these drugs (PCMBS, salicylates, trinitrocresol, A23187), A23187 offers the advantage of inducing a permeability change which is fairly specific to divalent cations (Ca and Mg).

A23187 can also be used in the study of intracellular calcium buffering (Ferreira and Lew, 1976) by inducing, under certain experimental conditions, almost complete equilibration between intracellular and extracellular calcium.

The present chapter is a description of the practical use of these two basic techniques, ATP-depletion and A23187-induced calcium permeability changes, in the study of the passive permeability of the human red blood cell to calcium and in the assessment of intracellular calcium buffering in intact cells.

3 A few methodological points

The composition of the solutions used in the experiments to be reported is given in Table 1. The symbols Ca_o^{2+} and Ca_i^{2+} will be used throughout the text to indicate the concentration of ionized Ca in the medium and in cell water, respectively. Ca_i will signify the total Ca concentration of cells expressed in μmole or mmole per litre original cell volume.

The Ca content of the cells was measured in two different ways, which will be referred to as method A and B. Method A is essentially identical to that reported by Lew (1971) but with the ^{45}Ca-loading or ^{45}Ca-efflux reaction terminated by the addition to the cell suspension of about 2·5 volumes of ice-cold solution A. Method B is a fast resolution technique which separates the cells contained in a largely diluted sample of the original cell suspension by centrifugation at high speed through a low-density oil (Ferreira and Lew, 1976).

This technique has the advantage of speed and simplicity but leaves within the final cell pellet a larger fraction of extracellular ^{45}Ca (about 0·1 per cent) than that remaining with method A (less than 0·001 per cent).

TABLE 1
Composition of the solutions used in the experiments reported here
(All concentrations in mM)

Code name of solution	KCl	NaCl	Tris-HCL (ph 7·5 at 37°C)	Tris-EGTA	Other major constituents
A	75	75	10	0·1	
B	80	60	10	—	Mg^{2+}, 1 (as $MgCl_2$)
Na	—	150	10	0·1	
K	150	—	10	0·1	
Li	—	—	10	0·1	LiCl, 150
Tris	—	—	160	0·1	
Ch	—	—	10	0·1	Choline Cl, 150
Sucrose	—	—	10	0·1	Sucrose, 300

When the entry of ^{45}Ca is measured in cells preloaded with tracer-free calcium as well as when the release of ^{45}Ca is determined in media containing tracer-free calcium, the specific activity of ^{45}Ca is constantly changing inside the cells while remaining practically constant outside. The determination of the ^{45}Ca activity in cells as a function of time under these conditions is, therefore, a measure of the rate at which the tracer equilibration proceeds plus the rate at which the calcium content of the cells changes. The problem arose of how to express this movement of tracer ^{45}Ca in a convenient way. It is usual to present the results in terms of the radioactivity in cells. Although such presentation can be used to calculate rate constants the comparison of the actual calcium movements is not possible unless specific activities are also given.

In order to bypass that difficulty, an apparent Ca content of the cells was calculated (ap. Ca_i) based on the original specific activity of ^{45}Ca in the external medium. It can be shown that—expressed in this way—the initial rate of change in ap. Ca_i provides a direct measure of influx or efflux. This convention, therefore, allows one to compare tracer curves at variable specific activities inside the cells with curves reporting a true Ca content of the cells.

The divalent cation ionophore A23187 (Reed and Lardy, 1972) was used in all the experiments designed to measure cytoplasmic Ca buffering. The ionophore was dissolved in absolute ethanol at a concentration of

1 mg ml^{-1} and usually about 10 μl of this or of a more diluted solution were added to about 2 ml of cell suspension.

ATP depletion was induced by preincubating the cell for about 3 h at 37°C in media containing inosine (10 mM) and iodoacetamide (6 mM) (Lew, 1971). "Fed" cells were incubated in the presence of inosine (10 mM). Depleted cells usually contained less than 2 μM ATP. The use of inosine in fed and depleted cells reduced the internal P_i concentration to the micromolar level, thus avoiding the formation of Ca precipitates.

4 Cytoplasmic Ca buffering

The measurement of the calcium content of the cells (Ca_i) does not provide in itself any information in relation to the level of intracellular free calcium ($Ca_i{}^{2+}$). This is an important shortcoming as it precludes any precise kinetic interpretation of the influence of internal calcium on the transmembrane fluxes. On the other hand it is not possible at present to measure intracellular free calcium directly in the intact human red blood cell. Although a considerable amount of data is now available on the composition of normal human red cells (Pennell, 1974) it is dangerous to extrapolate from this knowledge and from the tabulated association constants for calcium to the actual calculation of the intracellular free calcium concentration. As Berger *et al.* (1973) showed, the state of important ligands like ATP and 2,3-diphosphoglycerte is strongly dependent on factors like the state of oxygenation of the cells, and yet a detailed knowledge of the state of the different calcium ligands and thus of their apparent dissociation constants under different conditions is still lacking.

In the course of this work the results obtained on the effect of A23187 on calcium loading of ATP-depleted cells suggested an approach to this problem aiming at the measurement of the overall intracellular calcium buffering. A very suggestive experiment is shown in Fig. 1. In this figure the concentration of calcium is the external solution (open circles) and the calcium content of ATP-depleted cells (closed circles) are plotted as a function of time in an experiment in which A23187 was added three times in succession to the external medium followed by the addition of excess EGTA. After the addition of the ionophore the calcium uptake is extremely fast, reaching a plateau which is independent of the ionophore concentration. This suggests a "quasi"-equilibrium situation in relation to distribution of calcium similar to that obtained in dialysis experiments. In addition it was seen in separate experiments that the ionophore *per se* did not increase the permeability to Na and to K. The ionophore also induces an increase in the Mg permeability, and in order to avoid a massive loss of Mg from the cells all measurements performed in the

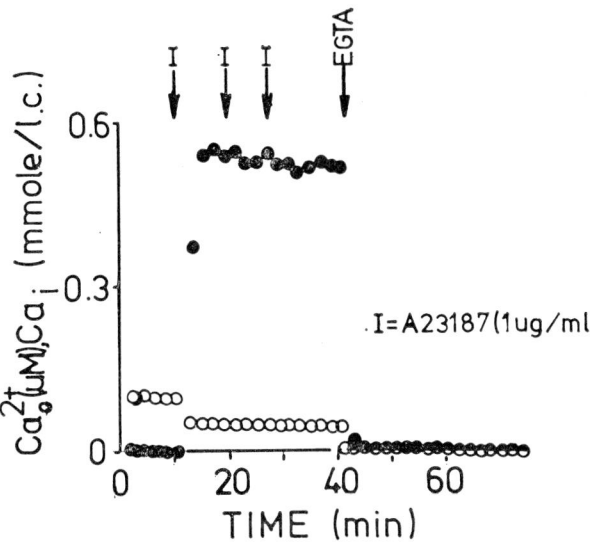

FIG. 1. Equilibration of ionized calcium across the cell membrane of ATP-depleted cells induced by A23187. Open circles = Ca_o^{2+}. Closed circles = Ca_i. Cells suspended in medium B at 37°C. Ca_i measured by method B.

presence of A23187 were done at a fixed external concentration of Mg (1 mM). On the other hand, the intracellular accumulation of calcium induces a large increase in K permeability (Gardos, 1956; Lew, 1970; Romero and Whittam, 1971) which will cause major shifts in membrane potential and in cell volume. Solution B was prepared having a mind all these factors and is aimed at clamping the membrane potential and the cell volume by keeping the external concentrations of the permeant ions (K and Cl) at electrochemical equilibrium across the membrane (corresponding to a membrane potential of −10 mV). In control experiments it was seen that neither the intracellular K or Cl concentrations nor the cell volume changed when A23187 was used to incorporate variable amounts of calcium inside the cells. The results obtained by incubating depleted cells in calcium-containing solutions (of different calcium concentrations) in the presence of A23187 are very reproducible. A typical experiment is shown in Fig. 2. The relationship between the intracellular calcium content at equilibrium and the external calcium concentration is linear over at least three decades of external concentrations (slope of the log-log plot = 0.94 between 2×10^{-6} and 10^{-3} M). The curvature downwards seen in Fig. 2 at the highest concentrations is mostly due to the haemolysis which occurs at those concentrations. In Fig. 3 the results obtained in five experiments are plotted together. In one of these experiments 0.5 mM NTA +

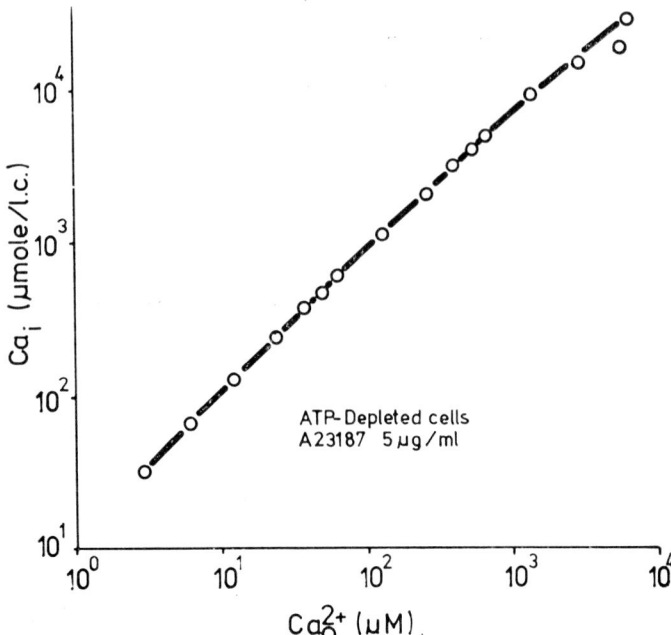

Fig. 2. Intracellular calcium buffering in ATP-depleted cells. Bank cells (4 days' storage) suspended in medium B at 37°C. Ca_i measured by method B.

1·34 mM $MgCl_2$ and 0·10 mM EDTA + 1·1 $MgCl_2$ were used together with medium B at external free calcium concentrations in the range of $0\text{--}30 \times 10^{-6}$ M. The results obtained were similar to those obtained in the absence of external buffers. The slope in Fig. 3 is again 0·94.

The calcium buffering behaviour of fed red cells is surprisingly not different from that of depleted cells. In Fig. 4 the calcium content of depleted cells (open circles) is plotted together with that of inosine-fed cells. The measurements were made at different external calcium concentrations and in the presence of A23187. As the external calcium increased, the ionophore-induced leak increased also so that above 10^{-4} M external calcium the pump fluxes became negligible and the two curves overlapped almost completely.

From a general point of view the total intracellular calcium content may be considered to be distributed between three compartments. Let us assume that one measures the calcium contained in a volume (Vc) of cells (Q_i) with a water content (Vw). Then

$$Vc\, Ca_i = Ca_i{}^{2+}\, Vw + Ca_iB\, Vc. \qquad (1)$$
$$(Q_i) \qquad (Q_i{}^2)^+ \qquad (Q_B)$$

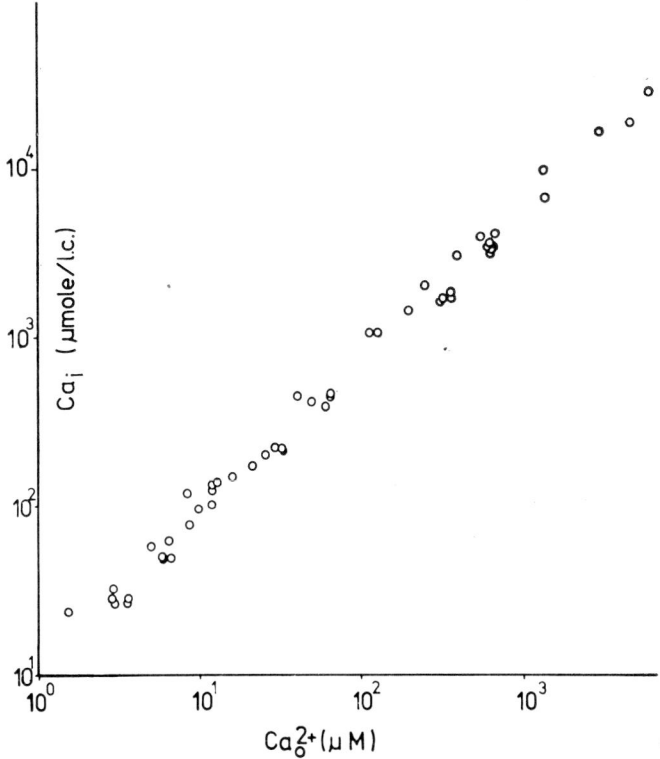

FIG. 3. Intracellular calcium buffering in ATP-depleted cells; pooled data. Five experiments similar to that of Fig. 2. Other details given in the text.

The first term on the right side (Q_i^{2+}) corresponds to the total amount of ionized calcium and the second to the total amount of calcium bound to membrane and cytosolic components (Q_B). Equation (1) can now be simplified to give:

$$\text{Ca}_i = \text{Ca}_i^{2+}\,(Vw/Vc) + \text{Ca}_iB. \tag{2}$$

In equations (1) and (2) Vw and Vc are expressed in different units (per litre cell water and per litre cells, respectively) in order to convert Ca_i and Ca_iB which are expressed in mol (l cells)$^{-1}$ into Ca_i^{2+} which is expressed in M. The fraction Vw/Vc is approximately 0·6–0·7. As a first approximation calcium may be assumed to be bound to i buffers each being characterized by its total buffering capacity (Bi (mol (l cells)$^{-1}$)) and by its apparent dissociation constant in relation to calcium (K_{iB} (M)) under the conditions prevailing inside the red blood cell cytoplasm. Then

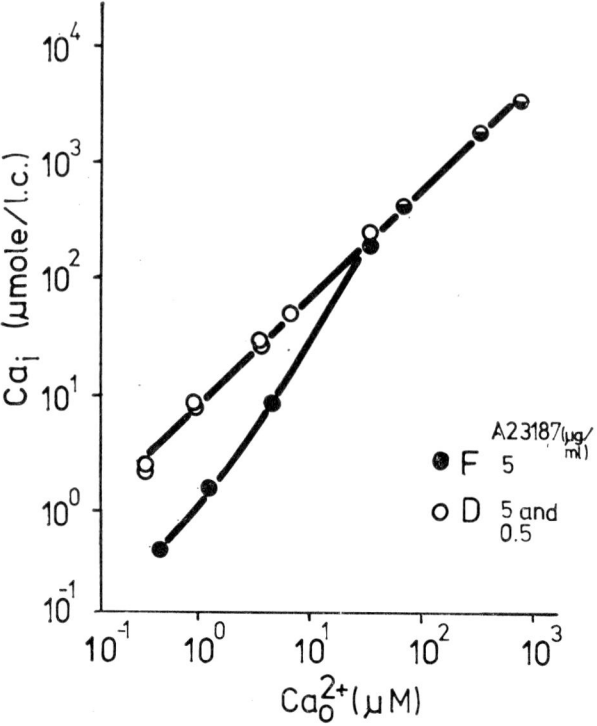

Fig. 4. Intracellular calcium buffering in inosine-fed (F) and in depleted (D) cells. Bank cells from the same donor suspended in medium B. Two concentrations of A23187 used for each Ca_o^{2+} in the case of the depleted cells.

$$Ca_iB = \sum_i Bi\, Ca_i^{2+}/(K_{iB} + Ca_i^{2+}). \tag{3}$$

If we substitute (3) into (2) and rearrange we obtain

$$Ca_i^{2+} = \alpha\, Ca_i$$

where α is given by

$$\alpha = (\sum_i Bi/K_{iB} + Ca_i^{2+}) + Vw/Vc)^{-1}.$$

In general α will depend on Ca_i but in the case of the human red blood cell experience showed that it was constant over a wide range of concentrations suggesting that

$$K_{iB} \ll Ca_i^{2+}.$$

This means that the behaviour of the intracellular buffers approached that of a single, large-capacity, low-affinity buffer. The value of α varied between 0·2 and 0·45 among cells from different donors indicating that over a very wide concentration range between 20 per cent and 45 per cent of the total Ca content of the cells is ionized.

5 Passive Ca transport in intact red cells

5.1 THE UPTAKE OF CALCIUM BY ATP-DEPLETED HUMAN RED BLOOD CELLS

When human red cells are suspended in calcium-containing solutions at 37°C no calcium uptake can be measured unless they are depleted of ATP or the calcium permeability of their plasma membrane is artificially increased. Of the published methods that can be used to lower the intracellular concentration of ATP of human erythrocytes the incubation at 37°C in a solution containing inosine plus iodoacetamide seems to be one of the most effective (Lew, 1971). The time course of the calcium uptake which is observed under these conditions depends on whether the uptake is measured during the ATP depletion period or after the ATP depletion is completed (3–4 h of incubation). If the calcium uptake is measured while the cells are being depleted of ATP the intracellular accumulation of calcium starts only after a delay of 20–30 min from the beginning of the incubation and proceeds from then onwards at a rate, depending to some extent on external calcium, but seldom exceeding 10^{-5} mol (l cells)$^{-1}$ h^{-1} (Fig. 5, curves a). When calcium is added to the external solution after the cells had been depleted of ATP (Fig. 5, curves b) one observes an initially faster rate of uptake (up to 3×10^{-5} mol (l cells)$^{-1}$ h^{-1}) which decreases gradually during the first 30–60 min and tends after this period to a constant value (up to 10^{-5} mol (l cells)$^{-1}$ h^{-1}) (see also Lew, 1974). Both initial and late uptake rates depend to some extent on external calcium but exceed only exceptionally the figures given above. When the calcium uptake is measured over long periods (more than 4 h) one observes occasionally a sudden increase in the rate of uptake. No explanation can be provided at this moment for such behaviour.

One should ask if patterns of uptake like those of Fig. 5 correspond to an intracellular accumulation of calcium or simply to the binding of this ion to the external surface of the cell membranes. Simple external binding can be discarded on the basis of the following observations:

1. Binding of calcium to red cell membranes is complete after 10–15 min (Gent et al., 1964; Forstner and Manery, 1971; Duffy and Schwarz, 1973) while the uptake of calcium measured in the same conditions as

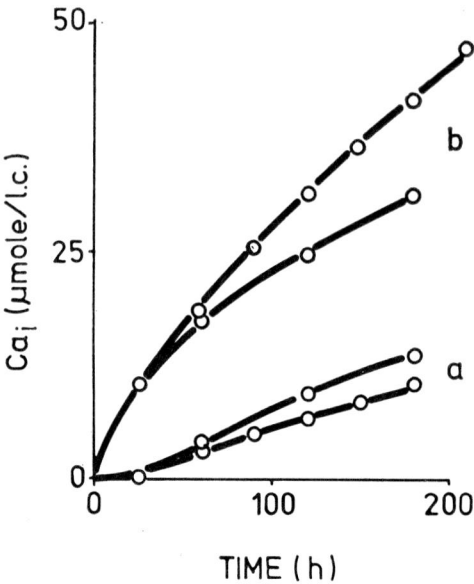

Fig. 5. Time-course of calcium uptake by human erythrocytes during ATP depletion (a) and after ATP depletion (b). Bank cells from four different donors. Cells suspended in medium A. Ca_i measured by method A. $Ca_o = 2\cdot1$ mM.

those of the experiments of Fig. 5 continues for at least 20 h, which was the longest period studied in this work.

2. The binding of calcium to the red cell membrane is not sensitive to temperature between 0°C and 37°C (Carvalho et al., 1963; Gent et al., 1964; Forstner and Manery, 1971), while the calcium uptakes reported here are very sensitive to temperature. Harrison and Long (1968) showed that more than 90 per cent of the calcium content of fresh human red cells can be removed by solutions containing calcium chelators. The calcium remaining after washing is at most $1-2 \times 10^{-6}$ mol (l cells)$^{-1}$. Since the method used in the measurements given in Fig. 5 involves four or five washes in 10–30 volumes of an isotonic solution containing 0·1 mM EGTA, most of the externally bound calcium must have been removed in the course of this procedure. Unless the preincubation with inosine plus iodoacetamide induces substantial changes in the binding affinity and in the binding capacity of the cell external membrane surface the contribution of externally located cell-associated calcium is negligible.

3. When fresh cells are treated in the same way as the ATP-depleted cells no calcium accumulation is measured.

4. Only less than 4 per cent of the radioactivity measured in the cell pellet is associated with the membrane fraction of the cell lysate (Lew, 1974).

A second possibility raised initially by Passow (quoted by Lew, 1971) and later by Schrader (1973) is that calcium is precipitated by inorganic phosphate leaking out from ATP-depleted cells. Such an explanation does not apply here since cells depleted of ATP in the presence of inosine have less than 10^{-5} mol (l cells)$^{-1}$ of intracellular P_i. Figure 6 shows clearly that practically all the calcium measured is in the cytosol. The cells were loaded with calcium during ATP depletion and were resuspended in calcium-free solution A. During the first 80 min they lost calcium at a very slow rate. The divalent cation ionophore A23187 was then added to the external solution and 30 sec afterwards the calcium content in the cell was less than 10^{-7} mol (l cells)$^{-1}$.

The results given in Fig. 5 are in good agreement with the values published by Lew (1971, see Figs 1a,b) who showed that the acceleration of the calcium uptake observed in the course of the ATP-depletion procedure coincides with the fall in the intracellular concentration of ATP. In most of the experiments reported here the calcium uptake was measured after 3–4 h of ATP depletion. The time curves obtained, although qualitatively similar, show quantitative differences depending on the experimental conditions. In every case there is an initial rapid uptake followed by a slowly decreasing rate of uptake which settles finally at a constant rate. If, as in

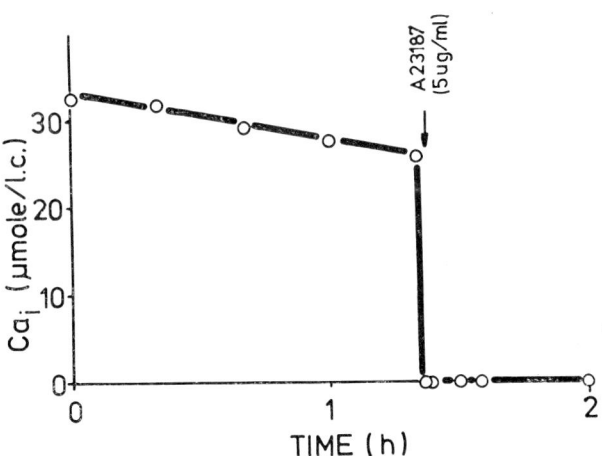

Fig. 6. Effect of A23187 on the calcium release from ATP-depleted, calcium-loaded human erythrocytes. Cells suspended in medium A (calcium-free). Ca$_i$ measured by method B.

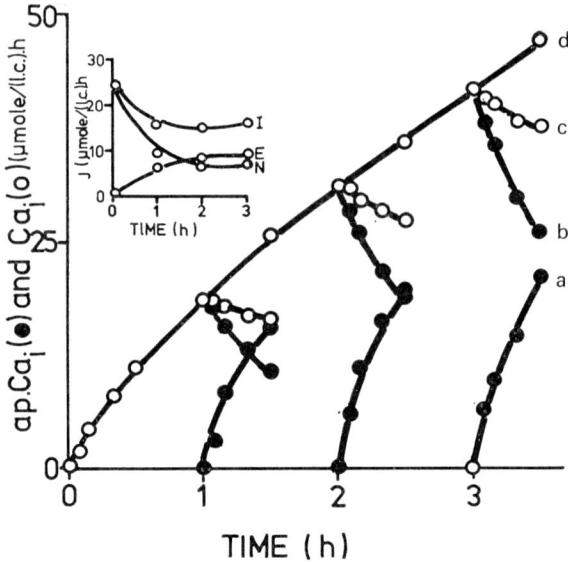

FIG. 7. Time-course of the calcium uptake and release in ATP-depleted human red blood cells. Bank blood (7 days' storage). ATP-depleted cells were resuspended in medium A and incubated at 37°C divided into two lots. Tracer-free (a) and radioactive calcium (d) were then added to the cell suspensions 1 h after the start of the incubation. 1, 2 and 3 h after the addition of calcium an aliquot of cell suspension (d) was removed, the cells washed in ice-cold medium A and resuspended in medium A (c) and in medium A containing 2·1 mM tracer-free calcium (b). At the same timings radioactive calcium was added to an aliquot of cell suspension (a). Ca_o of cell suspensions (a) and (d) was also 2·1 mM. Ca_i and ap. Ca_i was measured at the indicated times by method A. For a description of the insert see text.

the experiment of Fig. 7, the cells are first equilibrated with the incubating solution for a certain time (in this case 1 h) and calcium is added later in concentrated form, the initial rise becomes smoother. But even under these conditions the same basic pattern is obtained. A possible explanation for this pattern is that as the calcium uptake proceeds (or intracellular calcium rises) the calcium influx slows down due to a decrease in calcium permeability of the cell membrane. In the experiment of Fig. 7 the time course of the influx can be computed approximately. If one assumes that the efflux of calcium (excluding Ca–Ca exchange diffusion) is the same in the presence and in the absence of external calcium the influx can be estimated as corresponding to the sum of the net uptake with the efflux into calcium-free solution at the same internal concentration. The values obtained with this method are plotted in the insert of Fig. 7 (curve I). The figure shows simultaneously the net uptake (N) and the efflux (E) as a function of time. It is apparent that while the efflux increases (as internal calcium increases) the influx falls dramatically in the first hour. If this influx is purely diffusional it depends only on external calcium and should remain constant throughout the experiment since the external concentration of calcium is constant. On the other hand, the curve of the efflux into calcium-free solution suggests a characteristic to be analysed later, namely that this efflux saturates as a function of intracellular calcium, and this saturation explains why the uptake curve approaches a linear increase after a certain time: if the efflux saturates and if the influx after the initial transient becomes constant one should expect the net uptake to proceed at a fixed rate. This is observed most of the time.

5.2 Ca–Ca exchange

Figure 7 also shows that the efflux of ^{45}Ca is increased in the presence of external calcium (closed circles) and that the uptake of ^{45}Ca is higher in calcium-containing cells than in calcium-free cells. The first aspect will be analysed later in some detail. The second aspect can be seen in the lower curves of Fig. 7. These curves represent the apparent uptake of calcium by cells incubated in tracer-free solution identical to that used for the cells corresponding to the upper curves. At hourly intervals ^{45}Ca was added to a fraction of the tracer-free suspension and the radioactivity measured in the cells at the indicated times. For better comparison, all three curves together with the initial uptake curve (corresponding to the uptake by calcium-free cells) are plotted again in Fig. 8. The figure shows that as the initial internal calcium rises from 0 to $4 \cdot 1 \times 10^{-5}$ mol (l cells)$^{-1}$ the uptake of radioactive calcium is faster. This dependence of the influx on internal calcium probably saturates at low internal calcium since the curves obtained at 3 and $4 \cdot 1 \times 10^{-5}$ mol (l cells)$^{-1}$ of initial internal calcium are similar. That the different curves plotted in Fig. 8 result from the different initial calcium content of the cells and not from the fact that they were measured at different times is shown in Fig. 9. In this experiment three different cell suspensions were prepared simultaneously by loading ATP-depleted cells in the presence of different external calcium concentrations. After the loading period the cells were resuspended in the same solution containing radioactive calcium at the same concentration and specific activity. Again in this experiment the presence of calcium inside the cells increased the calcium influx.

5.3 Dependence of the net uptake on external calcium

Judging from these results the passive movements of calcium across the

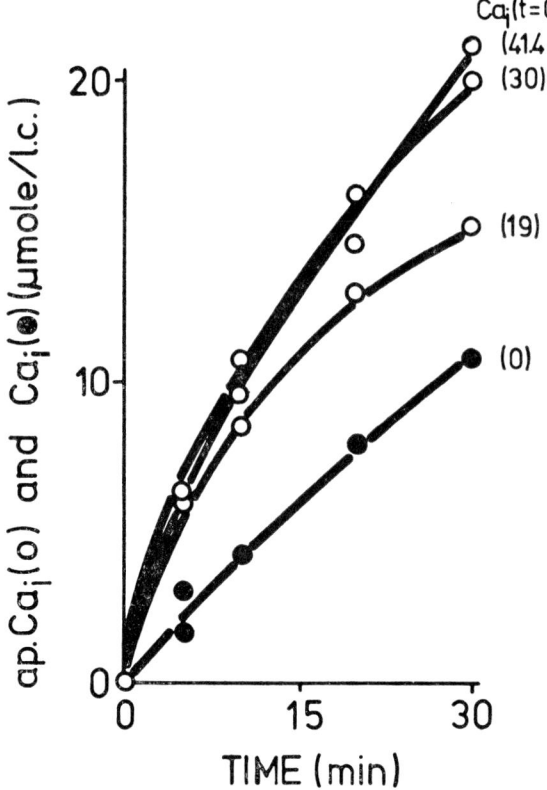

FIG. 8. The effect of internal calcium on the ^{45}Ca uptake in ATP-depleted human red blood cells. Curves (a) of Fig. 7 are replotted here. Ca_i at the time when radioactive calcium was added to the cell suspension is given in brackets.

membrane of ATP-depleted human red blood cells do not seem to be purely diffusional since at least part of the unidirectional fluxes depend on the concentration of calcium on the trans side. Romero and Whittam (1971), who measured the uptake of calcium in older bank cells depleted of ATP by a different method, reported not only much higher rates of uptake but also a linear relationship between the net influx and the external calcium concentration. Under the experimental conditions used in this work and as can be seen in Fig. 11 the calcium uptake saturated in relation to external calcium. In this figure the steady rates of uptake measured in the experiment of Fig. 10 are plotted as a function of Ca_o^{2+}. The cells were first depleted of ATP and loaded at the same time with (radioactive) calcium. The cells were then divided into nine cell suspensions containing either no calcium or 1, 2, 5 and 10 mM radioactive or nonradioactive calcium. Under

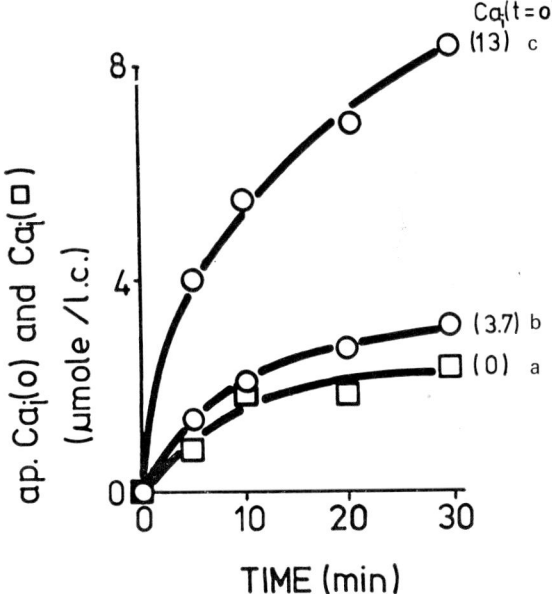

FIG. 9. The effect of internal calcium on the ^{45}Ca uptake in ATP-depleted human red blood cells. Bank blood (4 days' storage) depleted in medium A (a) and in medium A containing either 0·1 (b) or 2·0 (c) mM tracer-free calcium. The cells were then resuspended in medium A containing 3·6 mM radioactive calcium. Ca_i and ap. Ca_i measured by method A at indicated times. In brackets the calcium contents of the cells at $t = 0$.

these conditions the movements of radioactive calcium could be studied in both directions at approximately the same internal and external calcium concentrations. If one calculates the net uptake rates by fitting straight lines to the uptake curves once the initial transient is over (after the initial 60 min), and one plots these values as a function of external calcium, the curve of Fig. 11 is obtained showing clearly that the net uptake saturates above an external concentration of Ca of 5 mM. If the fast initial uptakes measured in the same experiment are plotted in a similar way, an identical curve is obtained. The same behaviour was observed in every experiment in which calcium uptakes were measured at different external calcium concentrations.

5.4 THE INFLUENCE OF MONOVALENT CATIONS ON THE CALCIUM UPTAKE

As reported earlier (Lew, 1974) the uptake of calcium depends strongly on the monovalent cationic composition of the external medium. This is

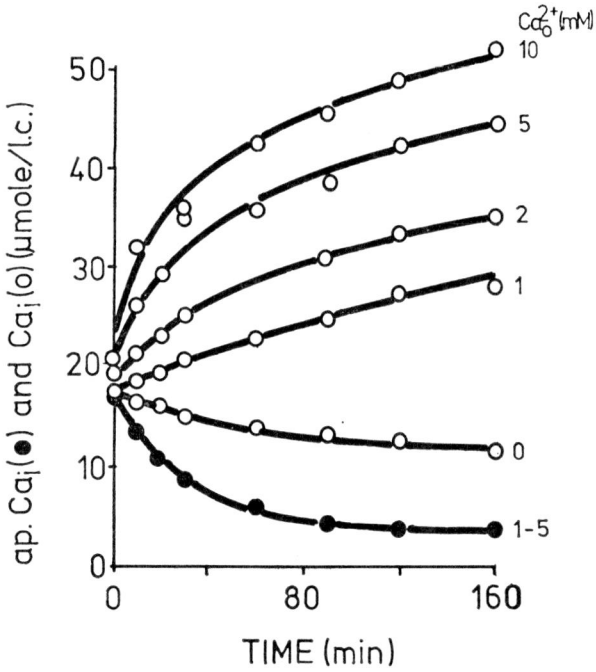

FIG. 10. The dependence on external calcium of the calcium uptake and release in ATP-depleted human red blood cells. Bank blood (4 days' storage). Cells loaded with radioactive calcium during depletion. The cells were then divided in eight lots, all suspended in medium A but containing respectively 0, 1, 2, 5, and 10 mM radioactive calcium (open circles) and 1, 2, 5 mM tracer-free calcium (closed circles). Ca_i and ap. Ca_i measured at indicated times by method A.

clearly shown in Fig. 12. The results plotted were obtained by depleting cells of ATP first and then dividing them into several cell suspensions in which the main cation (150 mM) was Li, K, Na, Tris or choline (all as chloride salts) or where chloride and cation were substituted by 300 mM sucrose.

Radioactive calcium (2 mM) was then added to the solutions and the chloride uptake measured at 37°C. These experiments are very difficult to interpret since, together with the calcium movements, there may be dramatic changes in volume and intracellular composition. The results obtained confirm the observations of other workers (Schatzmann, 1969, 1973; Porzig, 1970, 1972; Lew, 1974) that a Ca–Na exchange does not seem to play any role in the calcium movements across the red cell membrane. Figure 12 shows that the calcium uptake is actually higher in the presence of high external sodium than in the absence of external sodium.

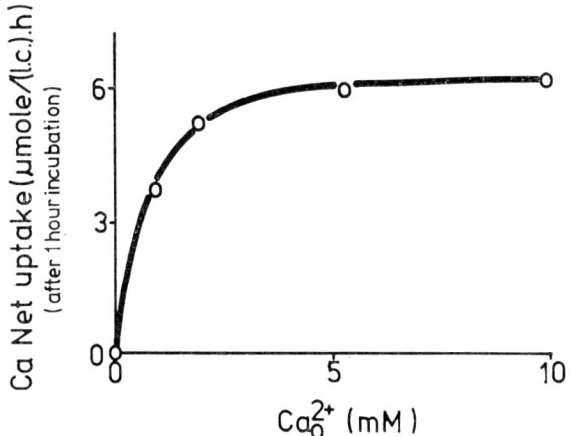

Fig. 11. Dependence on external calcium of the net calcium uptake by ATP-depleted human red blood cells. Same experiment as that of Fig. 10. The slopes of the four upper curves of that figure (between 60 and 160 min) are plotted as a function of external calcium.

This agrees with earlier reports by Lew (1971) who observed a lower uptake in media containing high potassium concentrations. Another finding that can be seen in Fig. 12 is that calcium uptake is higher in isotonic sucrose or in solutions in which the main cation is impermeable (choline or Tris). Long and Mouat (1973) and Mouat and Long (1974) reported similar observations in fresh human red blood cells incubated at 4°C. These authors showed that the uptake of calcium was correlated with the total loss of cations (Na + K) from the cells observed under those conditions. Such results cannot be interpreted as a simple K(or Na)–Ca exchange since in order to fit their data one would need to postulate a stoichiometry for the exchange of 15–160 (Na + K) ions per calcium ion. Part of the massive changes in cell volume and composition are probably due to the increase in K permeability caused by the intracellular accumulation of calcium. This increase in K permeability may produce an hyperpolarization of the membrane by shifting its potential to the K equilibrium potential and such mechanisms could explain why the *absence* of K from the external medium stimulates the calcium uptake. Yet red cells from species in which the K permeability is not sensitive to internal calcium also take up more calcium in the presence of external Na (Jenkins and Lew, 1973). Furthermore, the calcium uptake measured in the presence of external isotonic LiCi is as low as that measured in isotonic KCl.

From all these observations it seems reasonable to conclude that the inward movement of calcium across the red cell membrane takes place by a

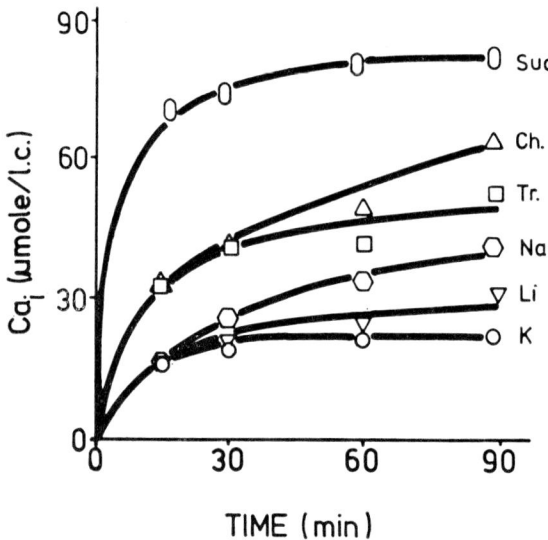

Fig. 12. The influence of external monovalent cations on the calcium uptake by ATP-depleted human red blood cells. Bank blood (6 days' storage). The cells were depleted in medium A and then resuspended in sucrose, choline, Tris, Na, Li and K media (see Table 1) containing 2·1 mM radioactive calcium. Ca_i measured by method A.

process of facilitated diffusion. At this stage it is not possible to say if there is more than one entry mechanism. For example: does the Ca–Ca exchange occur through the same mechanism as the net uptake? No Na–Ca exchange could be demonstrated and although a K–Ca exchange might be suggested this hypothesis was not tested. Should a K–Ca exchange exist one should expect a stimulation of the calcium efflux by external K. This was never observed.

5.5 THE EFFLUX OF CALCIUM FROM CALCIUM-LOADED, ATP-DEPLETED HUMAN RED BLOOD CELLS

As shown in the previous section, ATP-depleted cells can be loaded with calcium. The maximum calcium content that was obtained by such method was 10^{-4} mol (l cells)$^{-1}$, but since it is unlikely that higher concentrations can occur under physiological conditions that is not a serious limitation.

In order to obtain cells with different initial calcium contents two different procedures were used: "time loading" and "concentration loading". With the first method the cells are incubated as a single-cell suspension at a fixed external calcium concentration. At 30–60 min intervals a fraction of the cell suspension is removed, the cells are washed, resuspended and the calcium efflux is measured. In the second method the cells are divided in several cell suspensions, each containing a different external calcium concentration, incubated for 3–4 h and then processed as in the previous method. Both procedures have limitations. The "time loading" can only be used for a limited length of time since very prolonged incubations entail an increase in the rate of haemolysis which may become too high. In relation to the "concentration loading" procedure, since the uptake of calcium saturates as external calcium rises above 2–5 mM there is a limit, usually below 10^{-4} mol (l cells)$^{-1}$ as to the amount of calcium that can be loaded into the cells. As will be seen later the results obtained in terms of efflux rates were the same with both procedures.

The external solution used in most experiments was solution A, to which different amounts of calcium were added. This medium was chosen because of all the media tried it produced least haemolysis (less than 2 per cent at the end of an experiment lasting several hours). In two experiments there was a continuous increase in the efflux rate constant, in the rate of calcium uptake and in the rate of haemolysis, suggesting that there was a continuous increase in the permeability of the cell membrane.

5.6 DEPENDENCE OF THE CALCIUM EFFLUX ON EXTERNAL CALCIUM

The most striking feature of the calcium efflux from ATP-depleted cells is its dependence on external calcium. As shown in Fig. 7, the efflux of calcium into a calcium-containing solution (in the millimolar range) is more than double the efflux into calcium-free solutions. Such an effect shows that at least part of the calcium efflux is not purely diffusional. Comparison of the uptake curves in Fig. 10 (upper curves) with the efflux curves (lower curves) into calcium-containing solutions shows that the efflux increased at the same time that the internal calcium specific activity was being diluted by the entry of nonradioactive calcium. The dependence of the calcium efflux on external calcium is already saturated at 1 mM external calcium and remains constant up to 10 mM (Fig. 13), which was the highest concentration tested. Several experiments in which a range of concentrations below 1 mM was used showed that the external concentration of calcium corresponding to a half-saturation of the calcium efflux was between 1 and 2×10^{-5} M. One such experiment can be seen in Fig. 14 in which calcium-loaded cells were suspended in solution A containing calcium concentrations in the range 0–1 mM. The upper part of the figure shows the time-course of the wash-out curves and the lower part is a plot of the efflux rate constants against the external calcium concentration.

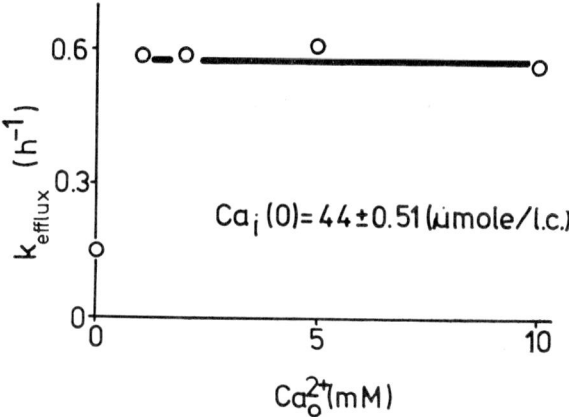

FIG. 13. Effect of external calcium on the calcium efflux from ATP-depleted human red blood cells. Bank blood (5 days' storage). Cells preloaded with radioactive calcium during ATP depletion and resuspended in solution A containing 0, 1, 2, 5 and 10 mM tracer-free calcium. The efflux rate-constants were determined by fitting single exponentials to each Ca_i or ap. Ca_i decay curve. Ca_i and ap. Ca_i measured by method A.

5.7 DEPENDENCE OF THE CALCIUM EFFLUX ON INTERNAL CALCIUM

The dependence of the calcium efflux on internal calcium was studied in a series of experiments in which the calcium efflux was measured in cells of the same donor and in the same experiment at different internal calcium contents. As referred above, two loading procedures were used. The first (time loading) is exemplified in Fig. 15. ATP-depleted cells were suspended in solution A at 37°C for 1 h, after which calcium was added to the cell suspension. At 30–60 min intervals a fraction of the cell suspension was removed, the cells were washed and divided in two lots which were resuspended in solution A and in solution A containing 2 mM of calcium. The rate constant of the calcium release was then measured in each of these cell suspensions and the initial calcium effluxes calculated. The time curves are shown in Fig. 15, and in Fig. 16 the initial calcium efflux is plotted against the initial intracellular calcium concentration. The upper curve in Fig. 16 represents the total efflux into calcium-containing solution A while the lower curve represents the efflux into calcium-free solution. The external calcium-dependent efflux (exchange efflux) was calculated as a difference between these two curves. The figure shows clearly that both the external calcium-dependent and the external calcium-independent fluxes saturate as a function of internal calcium and that in this experiment the first is six times bigger than the second. The same pattern was observed

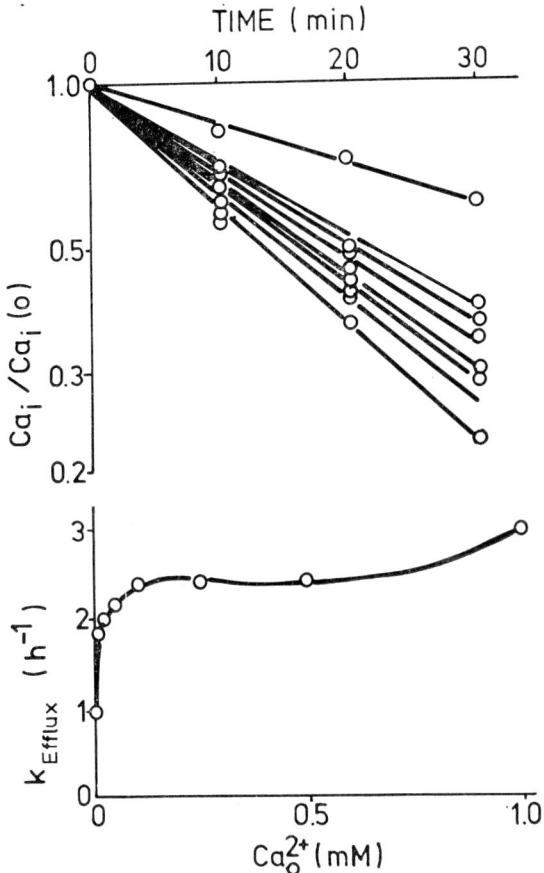

Fig. 14. Effect of external calcium on the efflux of calcium from ATP-depleted human red blood cells. Bank blood (5 days' old). Experimental design similar to that of the experiment of Fig. 13. Upper panel: semilog-plot of the fractional decay of Ca_i and ap. Ca_i as a function of time. Lower panel: similar to Fig. 13.

when the "concentration loading" procedure was used. In Fig. 17 the time curves of the release of calcium from the cells loaded by this method are shown and Fig. 18 shows, again, a dependence of the calcium efflux on internal calcium similar to that displayed by Fig. 16. In fact, patterns like those of Fig. 16 and 18 were obtained in four more experiments of similar design. The results obtained in eight such experiments together with those obtained in twenty-five other experiments in which the efflux was measured at a fixed internal concentration of calcium are pooled together in Fig. 19, where the nonexchange efflux is represented by the closed circles. The

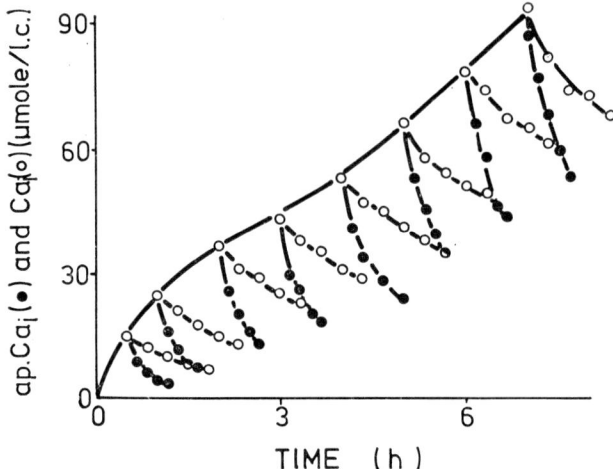

Fig. 15. "Time loading." Bank blood (8 days' storage). ATP-depleted cells suspended in 2·1 mM radioactive calcium. At $\frac{1}{2}$, 1, 2, 3, 4, 5, 6 and 7 h after the start of the incubation a fraction of the cell suspension was removed, the cells were washed and resuspended in solution A (open circles) and in solution A containing 2·1 mM tracer-free calcium. Ca_i and ap. Ca_i measured at indicated times with method A.

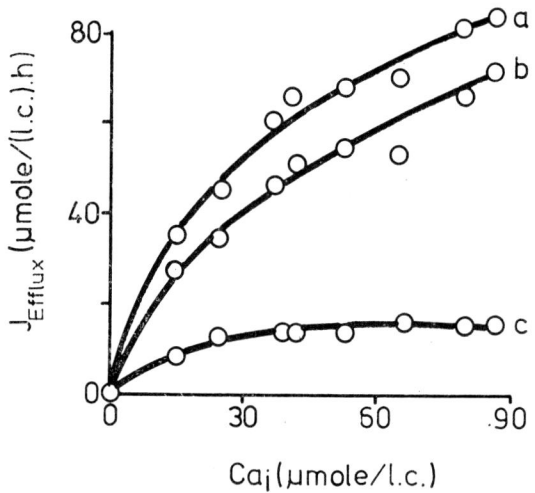

Fig. 16. Dependence on internal calcium of the calcium efflux from ATP-depleted human red blood cells. Rate constants obtained from the efflux curves of the experiment reported in Fig. 15. Curve c: efflux into medium A containing 2·1 mM calcium; curve b: difference between curves a and c.

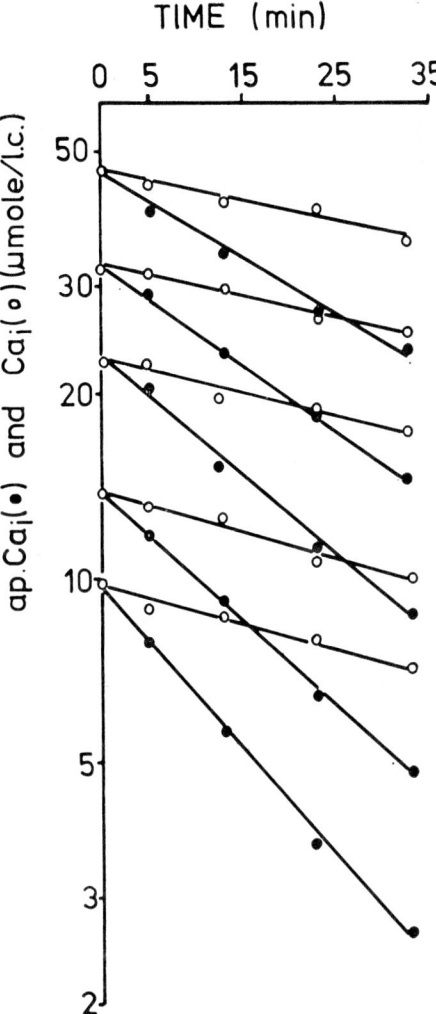

FIG. 17. "Concentration loading." Fresh cells depleted of ATP in the presence of 0·5, 1, 2, 4 and 8 mM radioactive calcium. The cells were then resuspended in medium A containing either no calcium (open circles) or 2·1 mM tracer-free calcium.

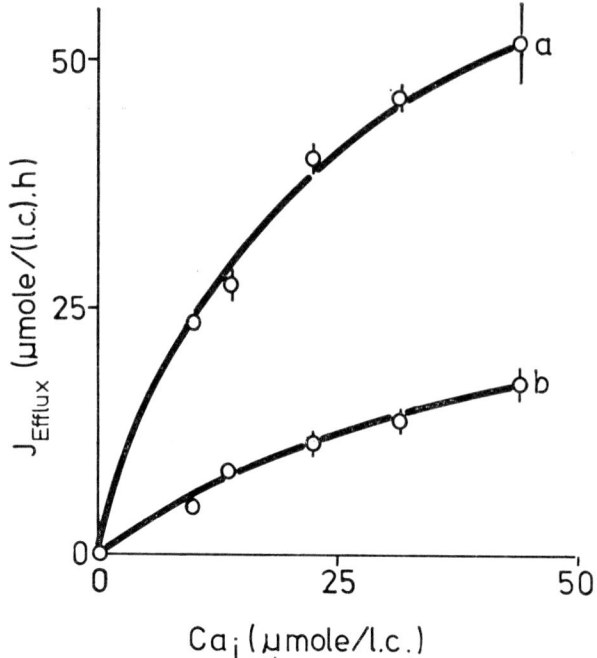

Fig. 18. Dependence on internal calcium of the calcium efflux from ATP-depleted human red blood cells. Rate-constants obtained from the efflux curves reported in Fig. 17(a). Ca efflux into Ca-containing medium; (b) Ca efflux into Ca-free medium.

corresponding curve was drawn assuming simple Michaelis kinetics with an apparent K_m of 2×10^{-5} mol (l cells)$^{-1}$ and a maximum efflux rate of 15×10^{-6} mol (l cells)$^{-1}$ h^{-1}. These figures cannot be taken as a precise parametric description of the nonexchange calcium efflux mechanism for several reasons:

a. The data obtained is insufficient to distinguish between several kinetic models, one of them being a mechanism with two or more translocating sites for calcium.

b. The internal free calcium concentration is not known for each experiment and although, as shown before, the internal free calcium is linearly related to the total calcium content, the actual fraction of free calcium may change from batch of cells to batch of cells.

Yet, despite these uncertainties, if one uses an apparent K_m of 2×10^{-5} mol (l cells)$^{-1}$ and simple (one site) Michaelis kinetics one obtains an

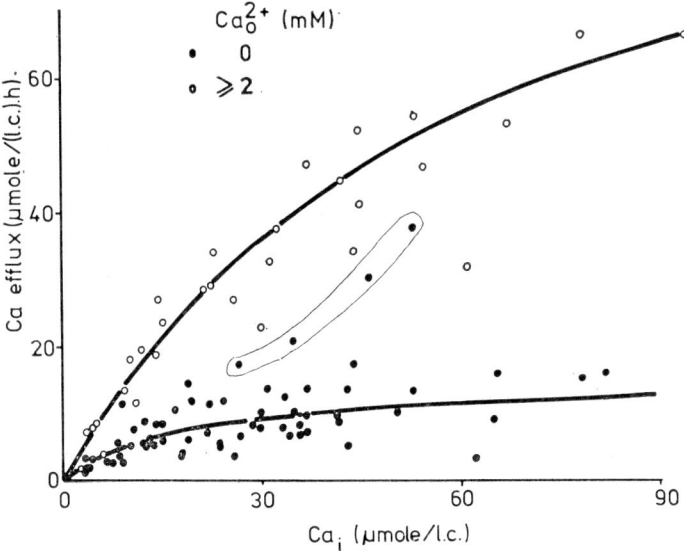

Fig. 19. Dependence on internal calcium of the calcium efflux from ATP-depleted human red blood cells. Pooled data. Open circles: efflux into solution A containing at least 2 mM calcium; closed circles: efflux into calcium-free solution A.

average value for the maximum efflux rate of $15\cdot3 \pm 1\cdot88\,(n = 6) \times 10^{-6}$ mol (1 cells)$^{-1}$ h^{-1} for six of the eight experiments in which the efflux was measured as a function of the internal calcium content. In the other two experiments the permeability of the cell membranes increased continuously in the course of the experiment. The points corresponding to one of these "odd" experiments are enclosed by a thin line in Fig. 19. Furthermore, if the same apparent K_m is used in twenty-five other experiments to calculate the maximum efflux rate from the efflux measured at only one initial internal calcium content, an average value of $14\cdot7 \pm 1\cdot54\,(n = 25) \times 10^{-6}$ mol (1 cells)$^{-1}$ h^{-1} is obtained. The dispersion of the values is thus remarkably small.

The exchange efflux is less easy to describe in parametric form for several reasons. First, because the separation between external calcium-dependent and independent efflux may not be justified. Secondly, because there is scatter in the results. Finally, because the data available is insufficient to warrant the proposal of a specific model for the Ca–Ca exchange mechanism. The exchange efflux measured in twenty-six experiments is plotted as a function of Ca$_i$ in Fig. 19. In four of these experiments the exchange efflux was measured at several different internal calcium contents (in cells from the same donor) whilst in the remaining twenty-two experiments the efflux was measured at only one initial Ca_i. The line in the figure was drawn by eye. In the four experiments in which both the apparent K_m and the maximum efflux rate could be computed, the apparent K_m was $30 \pm 11 \times 10^{-6}$ mol (1 cells)$^{-1}$ and J_m was $70 \pm 22 \times 10^{-6}$ mol (1 cells)$^{-1}$ h^{-1}.

5.8 ON THE TIME-COURSE OF THE CALCIUM EFFLUX

All the results on the efflux of calcium reported above are based on measurements of calcium efflux rates obtained by fitting single exponentials to the time curves of the radioactivity in cells. The fitting is quite good, as evidence by Fig. 17 for example. From these curves a pattern of the dependence of the calcium efflux on internal calcium emerged. Individual curves can be fitted by simple Michaelis kinetics although the lack of precise measurements at low internal calcium concentrations precludes any distinction between several kinetic alternatives. But regardless of the precise kinetic model which will ultimately fit these data the calcium efflux into calcium-free solutions seems to saturate at an internal calcium above 20–30×10^{-6} mol (1 cells)$^{-1}$. In view of this one should expect the rate constant to rise as soon as the internal calcium falls below saturation. This is shown in Fig. 20 where the computed values based on two hypothetical kinetic models are plotted. The normalized rate constant was plotted in the ordinate (k/J_m). The models considered were a simple one-site model and a model in which two calcium ions are translocated per pump cycle, both sites having the same affinity for calcium. The values of J_m, K_1 and K_2 were chosen in such way that both kinetic models will fit reasonably well the data reported in this work. The figure shows that over a wide range of Ca_i the rate constant of the efflux increases as Ca_i decreases and only at Ca_i below K_2 does the rate constant *decrease* as Ca_i decreases in the case of the two-site model. This means that in experiments in which the efflux of calcium is measured into calcium-free media the semi-log plot of the time curves of the calcium content in cells should bend *downwards* as the internal calcium falls below saturation. This was never seen and Fig. 21 shows an experiment in which the intracellular calcium content was followed during 6 h. In the same figure the thin-lined curve represents the expected behaviour (plotted assuming $J_m = 12 \times 10^{-6}$ mol (1 cells)$^{-1}$ h^{-1}; apparent K_m 2×10^{-5} mol (1 cells)$^{-1}$. The experimental curve shows a clear inflection *upwards* when Ca_i is between 2 and 3×10^{-5} mol (1 cells)$^{-1}$. Such behaviour is consistently observed if the efflux curves are followed over sufficiently long periods and is more noticeable in cells which have initially very low calcium contents.

The simplest explanation for such behaviour is to assume that calcium is

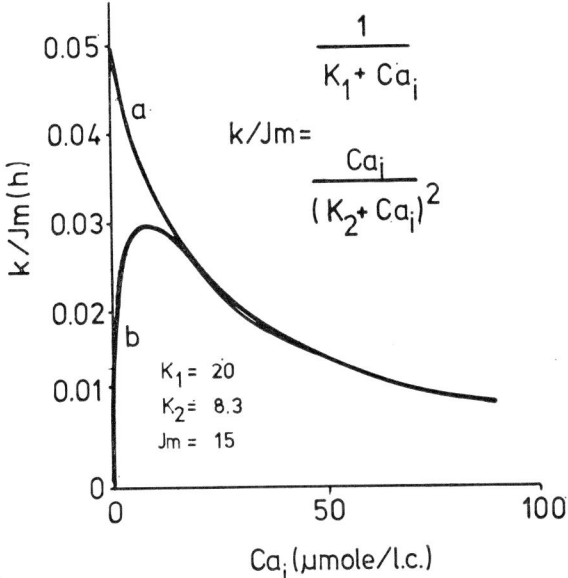

FIG. 20. The dependence of the efflux rate constant on internal calcium. It is assumed that the efflux is described by an equation of the form

$$J_e = J_m \left(\frac{Ca_i}{Ca_i + K}\right)^n.$$

The figure describes the computed curves for $n = 1$ (a) and $n = 2$ (b).

being released from two or more kinetically distinct compartments. Unless one can identify these compartments positively by an independent method this explanation is difficult to prove or disprove. It seems unlikely that if there are two compartments that release calcium at different rates they should take up calcium at the same rate. Based on this assumption two different types of experiments were designed in an attempt to identify them.

The first type of experiment is described in Fig. 22. ATP-depleted cells were first loaded with ^{45}Ca and ^{42}K. The cells were then distributed among a series of tubes containing NaCl solutions of decreasing tonicity. The incremental fraction of the cells lysed in each tube together with the incremental release (by haemolysis) of ^{45}Ca and ^{42}K were then determined and plotted in Fig. 22. The figure shows that the cells lysed in each tube have approximately the same content of ^{42}K and ^{45}Ca. That means that most cells have the same average Ca_i or alternatively that if there are cells with different Ca_i they have the same osmotic fragility.

In the second type of experiment, ATP-depleted cells were preloaded

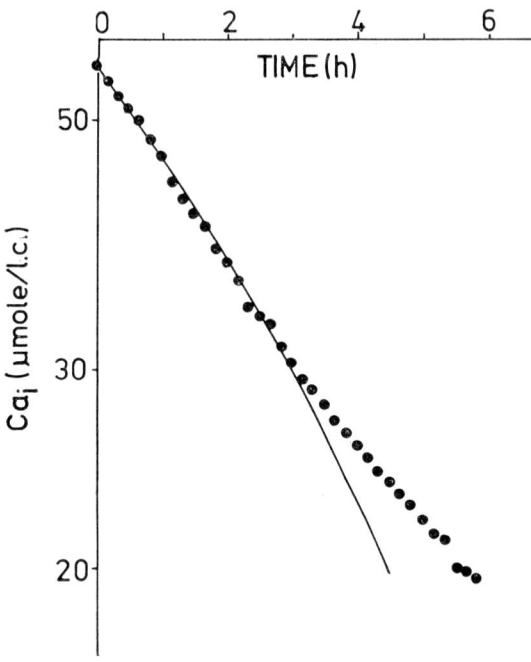

FIG. 21. Time course of the calcium efflux from ATP-depleted human red blood cells. Bank blood (5 days' storage). Cells preloaded with $5\cdot 6 \times 10^{-5}$ mol (l cells)$^{-1}$ and resuspended in calcium-free solution A. Continuous thin line: expected behaviour of Ca_i assuming that the calcium efflux is given by

$$J_e = J_m\left(\frac{Ca_i}{Ca_i + K_1}\right)$$

in which $K_1 = 2 \times 10^{-5}$ mol (l cells)$^{-1}$
$J_m = 12\cdot 6 \times 10^{-6}$ mol (l cells)$^{-1}$ h^{-1}.

with ^{45}Ca in the same way. They were then centrifuged through mixtures of ethylphthalate (s.g. 1·17) and di-*n*-butylphthalate (s.g. 1·042). A series of 1·5 ml Eppendorf tubes was prepared containing a mixture of both oils in different proportions, each tube containing 0·4 ml of the mixture. 1 ml of a 10 per cent haematocrit suspension of cells was deposited on top of the mixture and the tubes were centrifuged in an Eppendorf 3200 centrifuge (12 000 g's) during 1 min. In the tubes containing up to 7/10 of ethylphthalate all cells remained on top, while in the tubes containing only butylphthalate all the cells went to the bottom of the tube. This technique was pioneered by Danon and Marikovsky (1964) as a method of separating red blood cell populations. The results are given in Fig. 23. In this figure the incremental changes in the volume of cells that crosses the oil mixture

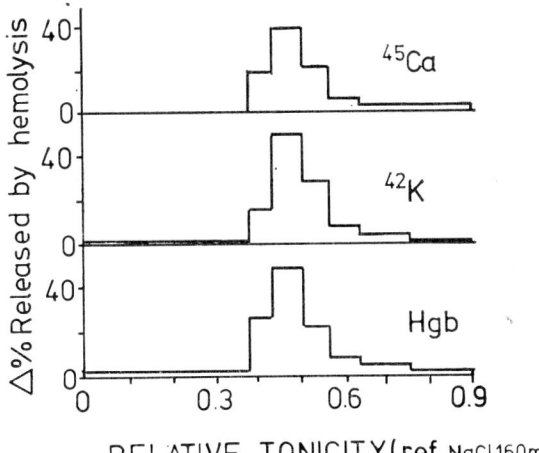

Fig. 22. Distribution of haemoglobin, ^{45}Ca and ^{42}K among different fractions of a population of ATP-depleted calcium-preloaded human red blood cells. Bank blood (8 days' storage). Cells loaded with ^{42}K and ^{45}Ca during the ATP-depletion. The cells were then delivered into tubes containing Na medium progressively diluted with distilled water. The haemoglobin, ^{45}Ca and ^{42}K were measured in the nonlysed cells and expressed as per cent of the totals. The per cent incremental release of haemoglobin, ^{45}Ca and ^{42}K was then calculated. The relative tonicity was calculated assuming that the activity coefficients of the solutes were constant at all dilutions. For more details see text.

together with its calcium contents is plotted as a function of the tube number. The tubes are numbered in such way that tube 1 contains 30 per cent and tube 8 100 per cent of di-*n*-butylphthalate and consecutive tubes contain 10 per cent increments of this compound compensated by 10 per cent decrements of ethylphthalate. The figure shows that the calcium content of cells with different densities is the same.

6 Calcium influx and the Ca permeability of intact red cell membranes

Most of the effort devoted to the study of calcium transport has gone into the study of calcium pumps, exchange mechanisms or calcium movements triggered in the course of the excitation-response coupling processes. On the other hand we know next to nothing about passive calcium movements other than those related to excitability. There seems to be a reasonable agreement between the permeability measurements done in lipid bilayers and in cell membranes of roughly similar lipid composition (de Gier, 1973; Van Deenen and de Gier, 1974). That being so, and in view of the very low permeability of lipid bilayers to calcium, it is possible that the

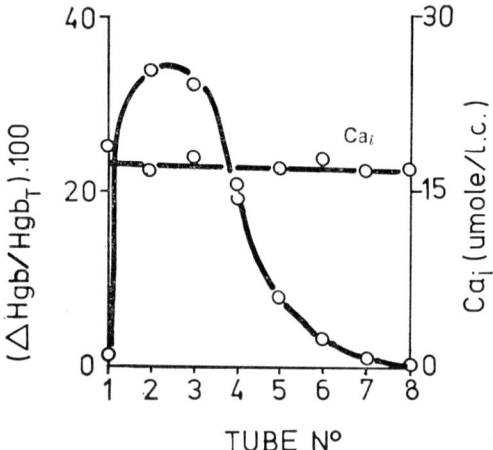

FIG. 23. Calcium content of ATP-depleted human red blood cells of different densities from a single sample. Bank blood (8 days' storage). ATP-depleted cells preloaded with radioactive calcium were suspended in medium A. 1 ml aliquots were delivered into Eppendorf tubes containing 0·4 ml of a mixture of diethylphthalate (s.q. 1·17) and di-n-butylphthalate (s.g. 1·042). The tubes were centrifuged at 12 000 g's during 1 min. Ca_i and Hb measured in cell pellet. Tube 1 contained 7/10 of diethylphthalate and consecutive tubes contained 10 per cent increments of di-n-butylphthalate and 10 per cent decrements of diethylphthalate. For more details see text.

purely diffusional movements of this ion across plasma membranes are so small that in practice they just cannot be measured.

When compared to other cells the red blood cell membrane seems to possess an extremely low permeability to calcium, probably an order of magnitude smaller than that of other cells. The results reported in this work show that the small uptake of calcium measured in the intact human red blood cells even when they are depleted from ATP is due to a low permeability to calcium and not to the fact that the cells are still pumping calcium at a substantial rate (see also Ferreira and Lew, 1975).

Several observations seem to indicate that most of the calcium uptake measured in ATP-depleted cells crosses the membrane by facilitated diffusion; it can be inhibited by strontium; it is very sensitive to temperature; it can be stimulated by internal calcium and probably by internal strontium (Ferreira and Lew, unpublished). The fact that the calcium influx saturates in relation to external calcium is also in agreement with such a hypothesis but the interpretation of these results is less simple. The external calcium concentration which produces a half-maximum rate of uptake is between 0·5 and 1 mM. A similar saturation pattern is obtained if one plots initial uptake rates, net uptake rates at steady state or influx rate, although slightly different half-maxima result from each different procedure. These observations suggest that there is genuine saturation of the entry mechanism.

There is no evidence that a Ca–Na exchange exists in the human red blood cell. It was neither seen in ghosts (Schatzmann, 1973) nor in the intact cell (this work). Although substituting K by Na (in the external medium) produces an increase in the calcium uptake, the effect is much smaller than that obtained when the main solute in the external medium is impermeant. It must be pointed out that a decrease in cell volume was not taken into account in the calculation of the results given in Fig. 12. That means that the uptake of calcium per final volume of cells was actually higher. If one can extrapolate from the observations of Plishker and Gitelmann (1976), who observed an increase in calcium uptake in fresh (fed) cells suspended in hypertonic media, this effect might be due to an increase in calcium permeability possibly due to cell shrinkage. But with such mechanism one should expect the calcium efflux into calcium-free solutions to increase, while the opposite is observed. The main difficulty in comparing the results of the efflux curves with those of the influx curves is that only exceptionally can they be measured under comparable conditions. This point is discussed below.

7 On the mechanism of calcium efflux from ATP-depleted red cells

The efflux of calcium from ATP-depleted human red blood cells displays, qualitatively, the same properties as the influx: it depends on the calcium concentration in the trans side, and both the efflux into calcium-free and calcium-containing solutions saturate as a function of internal calcium.

On the other hand, while the substitution of K by Na in the external solution stimulates the calcium uptake, no consistent pattern of the effect of such substitution was observed in relation to the calcium efflux. This was so because it is impossible to control internal calcium in intact cells without inducing pronounced changes in the calcium permeability of the membrane. These differences in experimental conditions may be one of the factors responsible for the large discrepancy between the affinity of the nonexchange efflux for internal calcium (see above) and the affinity of the influx for external calcium (5×10^{-4} M or higher). Both nonexchange efflux and influx saturate at very low flux values (below 3×10^{-5} mol (l cells)$^{-1}$ h^{-1}), the maximum influx rate being in general higher than the maximum efflux rate. The nonexchange fluxes display three puzzling characteristics:

a. The nonexchange efflux and influx are kinetically completely distinct.
b. At constant external calcium the influx slows down by at least 40 per cent during the first hour and remains constant from then onwards.
c. The calcium content of cells suspended in calcium-free solutions decreases exponentially during the first hours and yet the rate constant of the efflux decreases as the initial calcium content increases, suggesting that the efflux is already saturating.

This last aspect deserves a more detailed analysis.

In each experiment where efflux of calcium was measured the release of tracer followed, at least initially, a kinetic pattern that could reasonably be fitted by a single exponential. If anything, when more complicated patterns were observed after variable periods of time, the efflux systematically slowed down with time. There was never any evidence that as the calcium content of the cells decreased, the efflux became saturated or indeed that it was ever saturated. Moreover, in the experiments where the efflux of tracer (^{45}Ca) was measured while the cells were gaining calcium, there was never any effect due to the dilution of the internal specific activity. All these results would suggest that the calcium efflux pathway was always far below saturation. How can this be reconciled with the saturation pattern that emerges when one reports the efflux values as a function of the initial calcium content of the cells (see Fig. 19)? (In Fig. 21, Ca decreased from 56 to 20×10^{-6} mol (l cells)$^{-1}$ in about 6 h. The thin line in the same figure shows the behaviour to be expected if the influx followed saturation kinetics.) *There seems to be a conflict, therefore, between the behaviour of the efflux path as evidenced from individual time curves and as it emerges from the relation between the rate constants obtained from the same time curves and the initial calcium content* (Ca$_i$).

The most likely explanation for the upward bending of the curve would be the existence of two compartments, one of them releasing calcium at a much smaller rate. Such a situation would produce a linearization of the time curve of Ca$_i$ before the slower compartment became dominant. By manipulating numerically the size of the slow compartment and eventually its rate constant all the curves can be fitted, since they are very smooth to start with and since there are four parameters to manipulate. This approach may be numerically gratifying but unless one is able to measure separately both compartments there is a large ambiguity in the interpretation of the data. Two unsuccessful attempts were made to identify and separate such compartments.

If a fraction of the cell calcium is released at a much smaller rate the initial overall rate of release is smaller than the rate of release of the faster compartment, but it is difficult to envisage how such a system could *per se* generate saturation-like kinetics unless the slow compartment comprises a progressively larger fraction of the total calcium content as this increases. It is also difficult to envisage how a two-compartment system could explain the kinetic difference between the nonexchange influx and efflux.

Another possibility is that the intracellular calcium induces irreversible or slowly reversible alterations in the cell membrane. In that case the efflux rate becomes "imprinted" by the highest concentration of intracellular calcium that the membrane had "seen". The higher the initial calcium content of the cell, the smaller the efflux rate. Such irreversible action of calcium might not be direct but through a change in membrane composition, for example. Allan and Michell (1975) and Allan et al. (1976) have shown recently how intracellular calcium in the micromolar range can induce changes in the lipid composition of the plasma membrane. A mechanism of this sort might explain why the time course of the release curves does not show saturation while there is a clear relation between the initial cellular calcium content and the rate constant of the release, and would explain why cells which had been exposed for some hours to internal calcium (like the cells used to study calcium release) are different from the cells which were not previously exposed to internal calcium (like those used in the uptake studies). It would not explain, however, the upward bend of the release curves, which is most probably due to heterogeneity in the cell population.

8 The physiological importance of the regulation of the intracellular calcium concentration in red blood cells

No physiological process involving an acute increase of Ca_i^{2+} was yet identified in mammalian red blood cells. On the other hand, the red blood cell does not seem to possess any mechanism for rapid changes in intracellular free calcium. It lacks intracellular calcium accumulating organelles and the permeability to calcium of its cell membrane is 1 to 2 orders of magnitude lower than that of other cells in general. What, then, is the physiological importance of keeping the intracellular free calcium concentration at such low levels (probably below 10^{-7} M)? If the affinity of the calcium pump is in the micromolar range and if its J_m is as high as it seems (5–30 mmol (l cells)$^{-1}$ h^{-1}), intracellular concentrations around 10^{-6} M would produce a substantial metabolic imbalance since the supply of ATP is less than 3 mmol (l cells)$^{-1}$ h^{-1}, (McManus, 1967).

At least two types of pathological conditions have been identified in which there is a possible disturbance in the calcium metabolism. In two haemolitic conditions (Eaton and Skelton, 1973; Wiley and Gill, 1976) the human red blood cells seem to contain more calcium than normal cells, probably as a result of an abnormally increased calcium permeability.

As mentioned before, the accumulation of intracellular calcium induces changes in shape and other mechanical properties of the human erythrocyte (Weed et al., 1969) which at least in part may account for the higher fragility of these cells in those haemolytic conditions. Until now it was almost impossible to separate the effects of calcium accumulation from those of ATP depletion since it was almost impossible to obtain the former without predepleting the cells. A23187 provides a means of separating these effects. From the published work the changes in shape seem to occur when Ca_i reaches values in the range of 10^{-5} M (Weed et al., 1969) which is at least two orders of magnitude higher than the physiological Ca_i^{2+}. Other dramatic consequences of such a high intracellular calcium concentration would result from the pronounced metabolic imbalance produced by overconsumption of ATP by the calcium pump. On the other hand, the red blood cells of patients with polycythaemia vera possess less (Ca + Mg)-ATPase activity (30 per cent less) in their membranes than the erythrocytes of normal subjects (Scharff and Foder, 1975). These results were interpreted in the light of the earlier work by Perris (1971) who suggested that intracellular calcium regulates cell proliferation in mammalian tissues. Also recently Wiley and Shaller (1974) showed that the maturation of the human erythrocyte coincides with a decrease in calcium permeability. If a decrease in J_m of 30 per cent is responsible for the disturbance in cell proliferation observed in polycythaemia vera then a very precise control of the intracellular calcium concentration is required.

The K permeability of human red blood cell ghosts (Simons, 1976) and of the membrane of ATP-depleted human red cells (Lew and Ferreira, 1976) is sensitive to intracellular calcium concentrations below 10^{-6} M. In nondepleted cells the sensitivity seems to be much less, but since intracellular calcium can produce an almost thousandfold increase in K permeability even very small increases in Ca_i^{2+} may be sufficient to induce a massive K loss with a decrease in the lifespan of the cell (see chapter by Lew and Ferreira).

The inhibitory effect of intracellular calcium on the Na + K pump seems to occur in the 10^{-5} M range (Dunn, 1974) and so is again very far away from the physiological Ca_i^{2+}.

The physiological role of intracellular calcium in the red blood cell may be viewed against a more general background. Functionally, the cell membranes are anisotropic systems: they face different environments on both sides and they are responsible for vectorial processes (transport, for example). Structurally they seem also to be anisotropic. Some membrane-associated enzyme activities are located in the inner surface while other proteins can be approached only from the outside. In the red blood cell the membrane lipids facing the inside seem to be different from those facing the outside (Van Deenen and de Gier, 1974). On the other hand artificial (and thus symmetric) lipid bilayers break down when subjected to large calcium gradients (see Lee, 1975), and that results probably from the stress imposed on the film by the asymmetrical cross-linking with calcium. All these factors seem to indicate that intracellular calcium may be important because it is a component of cytosolic regulatory mechanisms (control of glycolysis, for example) and also because the maintenance of a *calcium gradient* across the plasma membrane may, in itself, be essential for the maintenance of the functional and anatomical integrity of the plasma membrane.

ACKNOWLEDGEMENT

Funds for this research were provided by a Wellcome Trust grant to V.L.L.

References

ALLAN, D., BILLAH, M. M., FINEAN, J. B. and MICHELL, R. H. (1976). *Nature*, **261**, 58–60.
ALLAN, D. and MICHELL, R. H. (1975). *Nature*, **258**, 348–349.
AVISSAR, N., DE VRIES, A., BEN-SHAUL, Y. and COHEN, I. (1975). *Biochim. Biophys. Acta*, **375**, 35–43.
BERGER, H., JANIG, G., GERBER, G., HUCKPAUL, K. and RAPOPORT, S. M. (1973). *Eur. J. Biochem.* **38**, 553–562.
BYGRAVE, F. L. (1967). *Nature*, **214**, 667–671.
CARVALHO, A. P., SANUI, H. and PACE, N. (1963). *J. Cell Comp. Physiol.* **62**, 311–317.
CLUSIN, W., SPRAY, D. C. and NENNET, M. V. L. (1975). *Nature*, **256**, 425–427.
DANON, D. and MARIKOVSKY, Y. (1964). *J. Lab. Clin. Med.* **64**, 668–674.
DUFFY, M. J. and SCHWARZ, V. (1973). *Biochim. Biophys. Acta*, **330**, 487–494.
DUNN, M. J. (1974). *Biochim. Biophys. Acta*, **352**, 97–116.
EATON, J. W. and SKELTON, T. D. (1973). *Nature*, **246**, 105–106.
FERREIRA, H. G. and LEW, V. L. (1975). *J. Physiol.* **252**, 86–97P.
FERREIRA, H. G. and LEW, V. L. (1976). *Nature*, **259**, 47–49.
FORSTNER, J. and MANERY, J. F. (1971). *Biochem. J.* **124**, 563–571.
GARDOS, G. (1956). *Acta Physiol. Hung.* **10**, 185–189.
GENT, W. L. H., TROUNCE, J. R. and WALSER, M. (1964). *Arch. Biochem. Biophys.* **105**, 582–589.
DE GIER, J. (1973). In "Erythrocytes, Trombocytes & Leucocytes" (E. Gerlach *et al.*, eds), pp. 98–100. G. Thieme, Stuttgart.
HARRISON, D. G. and LONG, C. (1968). *J. Physiol.* **199**, 367–381.
HOFFMAN, J. F. (1972). *Nouv. Rev. Franc. Hemat.* **2**, 771–774.
ISENBERG, G. (1975). *Nature*, **253**, 273–274.
JENKINS, D. M. G. and LEW, V. L. (1973). *J. Physiol.* **234**, 419–000.
KRNJEVIC, K. (1974). *Physiol. Rev.* **54**, 418–540.
LACELLE, P. L., KIRKPATRICK, F. H., UDKOW, M. P. and ARKIN, B. (1972). *Nouv. Rev. Franc. Hemat.* **12**, 789–798.

Lee, A. G. (1975). *Prog. Biophys. Mol. Biol.* **29**, 5–56.
Lew, V. L. (1970). *J. Physiol.* **206**, 35–36P.
Lew, V. L. (1971). *Biochim. Biophys. Acta*, **223**, 827–830.
Lew, V. L. (1974). In "Comparative Biochemistry and Physiology of Transport" (L. Bolis. et al., eds), pp. 310–316. North-Holland, Amsterdam.
Lew, V. L. and Ferreira, H. G. (1976). *Nature*, **263**, 336–338.
Lichtman, M. A. and Marinetti, G. V. (1972). *Nouv. Rev. Franc. Hemat.* **12**, 755–756.
Lionetti, F. J. and McKay, J. (1969). In "Modern Problems of Blood Preservation" (W. Spielman, and S. Seidl, eds), pp. 34–47. Fischer, Stuttgart.
Lionetti, F. J., McKay, J. and Gendron, H. (1968). *Microvascular Res.* **1**, 196–209.
Long, C. and Mouat, B. (1973). *Biochem. J.* **132**, 559–570.
McManus, T. J. (1967). *Fed. Proc.* **26**, 1821–1826.
Meech, R. W. (1974). *J. Physiol.* **237**, 259–277.
Mouat, B. and Long, C. C. (1974). *Biochem. J.* **142**, 629–636.
Nakao, M., Nakao, I., Yamazoe, S. and Yoshikawa, H. (1961). *J. Biochem., Tokyo*, **49**, 487–492.
Ohnishi, T. (1962). *J. Biochem., Tokyo*, **52**, 307–308.
Palek, J., Curby, W. A. and Lionetti, F. J. (1971a). *Amer. J. Physiol.* **220**, 19–26.
Palek, J., Curby, W. A. and Lionetti, F. J. (1971b). *Amer. J. Physiol.* **220**, 1028–1032.
Pennell, R. B. (1974). In "The Red Blood Cell" (D. Macn. Surgenor, ed), vol. 1, pp. 39–146. Academic Press, New York and London.
Perris, A. D. (1971). In "Cellular Mechanisms for Calcium, Transfer and Homeostasis" (G. Nichols, and R. H. Wasserman, eds), pp. 101–131. Academic Press, New York and London.
Plishker, G. and Gitelmann, H. (1976). *J. Gen. Physiol.* **68**, 29–41.
Ponder (1961). In "The Cell" (J. Brachet and A. Mirsky, eds), vol. 2, pp. 1–84. Academic Press, New York and London.
Porzig, H. (1970). *J. Membrane Biol.* **2**, 324–340.
Porzig, H. (1972). *J. Membrane Biol.* **8**, 237–258.
Ransom, B. R., Barker, J. L. and Nelson, P. G. (1975). *Nature*, **256**, 424–425.
Reed, P. W. and Lardy, H. A. (1972). *J. Biol. Chem.* **247**, 6970–6976.
Romero, P. J. and Whittam, R. (1971). *J. Physiol.* **214**, 481–507.
Rosenthal, A. S., Kregenow, F. M. and Moses, H. L. (1970). *Biochim. Biophys. Acta*, **196**, 254–262.
Scharff, O. (1972). *J. Clin. Lab. Invest.* **30**, 313–320.
Scharff, O. and Foder, B. (1975). *Scand. J. Clin. Lab. Invest.* **35**, 583–589.
Schatzmann, H. J. (1969). In "Calcium and Cellular Function" (A. W. Cuthbert, ed), pp. 85–95. MacMillan, New York.
Schatzmann, H. J. (1973). *J. Physiol.* **235**, 551–569.
Schatzmann, H. J. (1975a). In "Current Topics in Membrane Transport", vol. **5**, pp. 125–168.
Schatzmann, H. J. (1975b). Active calcium transport across the plasma membrane of erythrocytes. In Carafoli et al., (1975b), pp. 45–49.
Schatzmann, H. J. and Rossi, G. L. (1971). *Biochim. Biophys. Acta*, **241**, 379–393.
Schrader, J. (1973). In "Erythrocytes, Trombocytes & Leucocytes" (E. Gerlach et al., eds), pp. 43–45. Thieme, Stuttgart.
Simons, T. J. B. (1976). *J. Physiol.* **256**, 227–244.

VAN DEENEN, L. L. M. and DE GIER, J. (1974). *In* "The Red Blood Cell" (D. Macn. Surgenor, ed), 2nd ed., pp. 147–213. Academic Press, New York and London.
WEED, R. I., LACELLE, P. L. and MERRILL, E. W. (1969). *J. Clin. Invest.* **48**, 795–811.
WILEY, J. S. and GILL, M. (1976). *Blood*, **47**, 197–210.
WILEY, J. S. and SHALLER, C. C. (1974). *Fed. Proc.* **33**, 266.
WOLF, H. U. (1970). *Biochim. Biophys. Acta*, **219**, 521–524.
WOLF, H. U. (1972a). *Biochem. J.* **130**, 311–314.
WOLF, H. U. (1972b). *Biochim. Biophys. Acta*, **266**, 361–375.

The effect of Ca on the K permeability of red cells

V. L. LEW and H. G. FERREIRA

Physiological Laboratory, Cambridge University, UK

1 Introduction	93
2 The "Gardos effect"	94
3 ATP depletion	94
4 The gating process	95
5 Selectivity of the K pathway	97
6 The effect of inhibitors	97
7 The movement of K and the nature of the K channel	98
Acknowledgements	98
References	99

1 Introduction

It has recently become apparent that a large variety of cells possess in their membrane and K-selective channel, the gating mechanism of which is controlled by the level of ionized Ca in the cytoplasm (see Meech, 1976). This channel has a number of important physiological functions concerned with the modulation of membrane potential in excitable and nonexcitable cells (Krnjevic, 1974).

Paradoxically, the effects of Ca on the K permeability of a cell membrane were first observed in red cells (Gardos, 1956, 1957) where their function still remains unknown. The human red cell, however, has proved to be a most convenient experimental model to study the different aspects of these selective permeability mechanisms, in particular the interaction between Ca and the K gating process.

A number of different procedures have been found which produce a selective increase in the K permeability of red cells, some of them without the involvement of Ca (Passow, 1964; Riordan and Passow, 1973), but in this chapter we will concentrate on the Ca-induced effect originally observed by Gardos (1956) which, because of its important physiological potential in the control of membrane permeability, has been the most intensively investigated (Gardos, 1958; Passow, 1964; Hoffman, 1966; Riordan and Passow, 1973; Lew 1974; Lew and Beaugé, 1976).

2 The "Gardos effect"

Human red cells incubated in their own plasma in the presence of adenosine and iodoacetic acid exhibit a large selective loss of K ions within the first hour of incubation. The presence of Ca in the medium is a necessay condition for this effect to be observed since it can be prevented or reversed by the addition of a chelating agent in excess of Ca (Gardos, 1957, 1958). The mechanism by which the combination of a metabolic substrate and a metabolic inhibitor can induce this effect has now been clarified (Lew, 1974) and shown to involve a number of sequential stages. These are:

1. ATP depletion, a pre-condition for Ca entry into the cells.
2. The entry of Ca.
3. The interaction between internal ionized Ca and the K gating process.
4. The activation of the K channel.

3 ATP depletion

The addition of a metabolic substrate in the presence of iodoacetic acid or iodoacetamide largely accelerates the rate of ATP depletion (Dunham, 1957; Lew, 1971a). This is due to an increased consumption of ATP by the substrate while the synthesis of ATP is blocked by the inhibitor (Lew, 1971a). In 20–30 min at 37°C the ATP concentration is reduced to the micromolar level. ADP falls as well, although with a slightly slower time-course, and it was found that within the experimental error all the adenosine-nucleotide is stoichiometrically converted to IMP inside the cells (Lew, 1971a). With the inhibitor alone or with the use of a false substrate (2-deoxyglucose) the rate of depletion is much slower and even after 24 h the ATP content of the cells is seldom below 20 μM. By using different combinations of substrate and inhibitor one can obtain a graded control of the rate of ATP depletion.

Lew (1970, 1971a,b) observed a strict parallelism between the rate of ATP depletion, the entry of Ca and the increase in K permeability. These observations explain why Gardos was able to observe the increase in K permeability within relatively short incubation times and may also explain the findings by Hoffman (1966) that similar Ca-induced effects on the K permeability can be observed in cells simply depleted by starvation for very long periods.

The depletion of ATP is a necessary condition for Ca to enter the cells. The mechanism of Ca entry in metabolically depleted cells is discussed at length in the chapter by Ferreira and Lew in this book. The altered metabolism of the cell, however, would also seem to affect the nature of the interaction between internal Ca and the K channel.

4 The gating process

There seems now to be convincing evidence that it is the ionized Ca in the cytoplasm which interacts with the gating mechanism of the K channel (Whittam, 1968; Lew, 1970; Blum and Hoffman, 1971; Simons, 1976). Under almost all the conditions in which it was tested, the Ca site seems to exhibit a high Ca affinity, in the micromolar range (Lew, 1970; Simons, 1976). Only one exception was found in what Lew and Ferreira (1976) named the "minimally disturbed" cell. When Ca is forced into fresh intact human red blood cells (which are normally highly impermeable to Ca; see Ferreira and Lew, 1975) by the use of low concentrations of a divalent cation ionophore (A23187) the sensitivity of the K permeability process appears to be about three orders of magnitude lower than the values found previously in resealed ghosts (Simons, 1976). In the same cells, the use of higher ionophore concentrations or Mg or ATP depletion convert this response into a high sensitive one to Ca. This opens the question of what is the real affinity under physiological conditions? If Lew and Ferreira's (1976) suggestion is correct, the physiological condition is represented by a low-sentitivity gate. Since the concentration of ionized Ca in the cytoplasm of most cells seems to be about 10^{-7} M, a process with a low Ca sensitivity (in the 10^{-3} M range) may seem to be physiologically irrelevant. This need not be necessarily so. In the first place, some of the procedures which convert the gating process from a low to a high Ca sensitivity state are not particularly drastic and an attractive, though purely speculative, possibility at present is that the Ca affinity of the K channel can be subject to control by metabolism or extracellular messengers in certain cells. A second alternative suggests itself from the extremely large increase in K permeability that Ca can induce in intact red cells. The saturated effect of Ca in human red cells (Lew and Ferreira, 1976), corresponds to a K permeability of about $1.6 \; 10^{-7}$ cm sec^{-1}, a value more than three orders of magnitude higher than the ground K permeability of the red cell membrane (Lew and Beaugé, 1976). With such a large maximum effect, micromolar concentrations of Ca may induce a substantial rise in the K permeability even when the K gate is in a low-sensitivity state. The resulting effects on the membrane potential and conductance will be more pronounced the larger the contribution of K to the overall membrane conductance. Thus, in

Amphiuma red blood cells, where the K permeability is not much smaller than that of Cl (Lassen *et al.*, 1974a,b; see also chapter by Lassen, this book), a five- to tenfold increase in K permeability could easily hyperpolarize the cell, very little internal Ca being required for this effect (Lew and Ferreira, 1976; Lassen *et al.*, 1977).

When the "Gardos effect" is explored in metabolically depleted cells a striking difference is observed within samples of cells presumed to be homogeneous (Riordan and Passow, 1973). On addition of Ca to the medium, K is lost from only a fraction of the cells. This fraction may vary from 20 per cent to 80 per cent of the total K contained in any given sample of cells. Lew (1974) suggested that this may reflect heterogenicity of Ca content or intracellular Ca buffering rather than absence of K channels from part of the cells, since by increasing the external Ca concentration the proportion of K leaky cells was always increased.

The high-low Ca affinity states of the K gate provide an alternative explanation of this effect (Lew and Ferreira, 1976). Since metabolically depleted cells take up micromolar amounts of Ca (Lew, 1970, 1971a), only channels in the high Ca-affinity configuration will become activated. The transition from a low to a high Ca sensitivity may be a slow process in fresh cells undergoing depletion but would be completed in old bank cells (Romero and Whittam, 1971) and in resealed ghosts (Simons, 1976) where only a high Ca sensitivity is observed.

In red cells there is no evidence of voltage dependence or spontaneous inactivation of the K gating process. Ca seems to be the only physiological activator and a decrease in the internal Ca concentration the only inactivator. The reversible sequence of reactions from the binding of Ca to the full activation of the K channel must be very fast (probably not more than a few milliseconds). This follows from our own observations where we found that the amount of ^{42}K lost during fast, ionophore-induced Ca "peaks" (Ferreira and Lew, 1976) could only be explained by a tight time-fit of the K permeability to the varying Ca concentration inside the cell.

Lassen *et al.*, (1976) reported an interesting effect which consists in a transient hyperpolarization of *Amphiuma* red blood cells following a sudden rise in external Ca. This was accompanied by a short-lived increase in K influx but the Ca influx, if any, was unmeasurably small (less than 10 μmol (l cells)$^{-1}$ during the transient) (Lassen *et al.*, 1977). This may seem to indicate a timed inactivation of the K gate but a more likely explanation is that under certain conditions external Ca may have transient access to the gating mechanism.

Other procedures are known which induce a more or less selective increase in the K permeability of human red cell membranes (Lindemann and Passow, 1960; Passow, 1964; Lepke and Passow, 1968). Small concentrations of Pb in the medium (Henriques and Ørskov, 1936; Passow, 1964) and Mg ions acting on fluoride-poisoned cells (Lepke and Passow, 1968) will induce a large K loss only in red cells from species which have the Ca-sensitive K channel as well (Jenkins and Lew, 1973). Quinine and quinidine, which inhibit the Ca-induced effect, also inhibit the Pb-induced K loss (Armando-Hardy et al., 1975). These results suggest that all these procedures act on the same molecular apparatus to increase the K permeability. Very little is known, however, about the mechanism of these interactions and more research is needed in this field.

5 Selectivity of the K pathway

The Ca-induced permeability mechanism seems to be extremely selective to K in relation to Na. The rate constant for ^{42}K-tracer equilibration can be increased by Ca up to 10 h^{-1} without any effect on the Na permeability (Lew and Ferreira 1976). The ground Na permeability of the intact red cell membrane corresponds to a rate constant of about 0·006 h^{-1} (Lew and Beaugé, 1977) and an increase of, say, 0·001 h^{-1} would be just detectable. Even when the Na flux is slightly increased as is the case at higher Ca concentrations inside the cells, the fact that quinine only inhibits the increased K permeability (Armando-Hardy et al., 1975) suggests that the effect on the Na flux is probably mediated by a different mechanism. These considerations prompt the conclusion that the $P_K:P_{Na}$ selectivity ratio of the Ca-sensitive K channel is probably higher than 10^4.

Simons (1976) investigated the selectivity ratio of other alkali metal cations in resealed human red cell ghosts and found that the relative rates are 1(K):1·5(Rb): < 0·05 Cs. Lithium, like Na, is not transported.

6 The effect of inhibitors

Oligomycin, furosemide, ouabain, quinine and quinidine were found to inhibit the Ca- or Pb-induced K flux to different extents (Lew, 1971b, 1974; Blum and Hoffman, 1972; Riordan and Passow, 1973; Armando-Hardy et al., 1975). The mechanism of the inhibitory effect has been investigated in some detail in relation to ouabain and quinine. Blum and Hoffman (1971) found that ouabain exerts a partial inhibitory effect on the Ca-induced K flux in intact but metabolically depleted red cells. This effect is difficult to observe in other systems and, indeed, failure to observe the ouabain inhibition was reported by Simons (1976) working with resealed ghosts and by Lassen et al. (1976) in *Amphiuma* red cells. Lew (1971b) observed that the presence of ouabain during at least part of the depleting procedure can alter the levels of ATP by inhibiting the Na-pump mediated consumption or production (Lew et al., 1970) of ATP, thus varying the Ca content of the cells and consequently the K permeability. When the cells had already been fully depleted, ouabain had no effect on the K flux (Lew, 1974) but there is still no agreement as to whether ouabain acts solely through ATP or whether it has some more direct action on the K channel (Blum and Hoffman, 1971).

Quinine and quinidine seem to inhibit the K flux by blocking the K movement through the channel and not by interfering with the binding of Ca to the K gate. This follows from the fact that a tenfold change in the internal Ca content of ATP-depleted cells had no effect on the concentration of quinine which produced half-maximum inhibition of the K flux (Armando-Hardy et al., 1975).

No specific inhibitors with a high affinity for the K channel have yet been found. Such inhibitors would be extremely useful in order to explore further the similarity between the Ca-sensitivity K-permeability mechanism in different cells and the number and nature of those channels.

7 The movement of K and the nature of the K channel

Large net and exchange fluxes of K can take place through the K channel. The outward downhill gradient of ^{39}K can induce the accumulation of ^{42}K inside the cells in excess of its concentration in the medium (Joyce et al., 1954; Grigarzik and Passow, 1958; Eckman et al., 1969; Manninen, 1970; Blum and Hoffman, 1972).

This countertransport-like behaviour, together with the inhibitory action of ouabain, oligomycin and furosemide, led Blum and Hoffman (1971) to suggest the Na pump as the mechanism for the Ca-induced effect. According to them, the interaction of internal Ca with the Na pump, perhaps aided by the altered metabolism of the cells, would induce a large increase in K turnover. Glynn and Warner (1972) showed that ^{42}K accumulation could result from the coupling of diffusional fluxes and Jenkins and Lew (1973) showed that red cells from a variety of mammalian species with normal, altered (LK-type) or with no Na pump at all, all lacked the Ca-sensitive K-permeability mechanism. These results are difficult to reconcile with Blum and Hoffman's view. A cell lacking the Na pump but having the Ca-dependent K channel is, however, still to be found.

ACKNOWLEDGEMENTS

We wish to thank the Wellcome Trust Foundation and the Medical Research Council for grants to V.L.L.

References

Armando-Hardy, M., Ellory, J. C., Ferreira, H. G., Fleminger, S. and Lew, V. L. (1975). *J. Physiol.* **250**, 32–33P.
Blum, R. M. and Hoffman, J. F. (1971). *J. Membrane Biol.* **6**, 315–328.
Blum, R. M. and Hoffman, J. F. (1972). *Biochem. Biophys. Res. Commun.* **46**, 1146–1152.
Dunham, E. T. (1957). *Physiologist,* **1**, 23.
Eckman, A., Manninen, V. and Salminen, S. (1969). *Acta Physiol. Scand.* **75**, 333–344.
Ferreira, H. G. and Lew, V. L. (1975). *J. Physiol.* **252**, 86–87P.
Ferreira, H. G. and Lew, V. L. (1976). *Nature,* **259**, 47–49.
Gardos, G. (1956). *Acta Physiol. Hung.* **10**, 185–193.
Gardos, G. (1957). *Acta Physiol. Hung.* **14**, 1–5.
Gardos, G. (1958). *Acta Physiol. Hung.* **15**, 121–125.
Glynn, I. M. and Warner, A. E. (1972). *Brit. J. Pharmacol.* **44**, 271–278.
Grigarzik, H. and Passow, H. (1958). *Pflügers Archiv.* **267**, 73–92.
Henriques, V. and Ørskov, S. L. (1936). *Skand. Arch. Physiol.* **74**, 78–85.
Hoffman, J. P. (1966). *Amer. J. Med.* **41**, 666–680.
Jenkins, D. M. G. and Lew, V. L. (1973). *J. Physiol.* **234**, 41–42P.
Joyce, C. R. B., Moore, H. and Weatherhall, M. (1954). *Brit. J. Pharmacol.* **92**, 463–470.
Krnjevic, K. (1974). *Physiol. Rev.* **54**, 418–540.
Lassen, U. V., Lew, V. L., Pape, L. and Simonsen, L. O. (1977). *J. Physiol.* In press.
Lassen, U. V., Pape, L. and Vestergaard-Bogind. B. (1974a). *In* "Comparative Biochemistry and Physiology of Transport" (L. Bolis, K. Bloch, S. E. Luria and F. Lynen, eds), pp. 363–366. North-Holland, Amsterdam.
Lassen, U. V., Pape, L., Vestergaard-Bogind, B. and Bengston, O. (1974b). *J. Membrane Biol.* **18**, 125–144.
Lassen, U. V., Pape, L. and Vestergaard-Bogind, B. (1976) *J. Membrane Biol.* **26**, 51–70.
Lepke, S. and Passow, H. (1968). *J. Gen. Physiol.* **51**, 365–372s.
Lew, V. L. (1970). *J. Physiol.* **206**, 35–36P.
Lew, V. L. (1971a). *Biochim. Biophys. Acta,* **233**, 827–830.
Lew, V. L. (1971b). *Biochem. Biophys. Acta,* **249**, 236–239.
Lew, V. L. (1974). *In* "Comparative Biochemistry and Physiology of Transport" (L. Bolis, K. Bloch, S. E. Luria and F. Lynen, eds), pp. 310-316. North-Holland, Amsterdam.
Lew, V. L. and Beaugé, L. (1977). *In* "Transport Across Biological Membranes" (G. Giebisch, D. C. Tosteson and H. H. Ussing, eds), Vol. II. Springer-Verlag, Berlin, Heidelberg, New York. In press.
Lew, V. L. and Ferreira, H. G. (1976). *Nature,* **263**, 336–338.
Lew, V. L., Glynn, I. M. and Ellory, J. C. (1970). *Nature,* **225**, 865–866.
Lew, V. L., Hardy, M. A. and Ellory, J. C. (1973). *Biochim. Biophys. Acta,* **328**, 251–266.
Lindemann, B. and Passow, H. (1960). *Pflügers Archiv.* **271**, 488–496.
Manninen, V. (1970). *Acta Physiol. Scand. Suppl.* **355**, 1–74.
Meech, R. W. (1976). *In* "Calcium in Biological Systems", pp. 161–192. Cambridge University Press.

Passow, H. (1964). *In* "The Red Blood Cell" (C. Bishop and D. M. Surgenor, eds), pp. 113–120. Academic Press, New York and London.
Riordan, J. R. and Passow, H. (1973). *In* "Comparative Physiology" (L. Bolis, K. Schmidt-Nielson and S. H. P. Maddrell, eds), pp. 543–581. North-Holland, Amsterdam.
Romero, P. J. and Whittam, R. R. (1971). *J. Physiol.* **214**, 481–507.
Simons, T. J. B. (1976) *J. Physiol.* **256**, 227–244.
Whittam, R. (1968). *Nature*, **218**, 610.

Choline transport in red cells

K. MARTIN
Pharmacology Department, University of Cambridge, UK

1 The leak permeability	101
2 The "carrier-mediated" transport of choline	102
2.1 The kinetics of the carrier-mediated transport system	102
2.2 Competitive inhibitors of choline transport	106
2.3 Noncompetitive and irreversible inhibitors of choline transport; implications for the mechanism of the transport system	106
2.4 Irreversible inhibition of choline transport by low concentrations of lithium	111
2.5 Comparison between the choline transport system in erythrocytes and those in other tissues	111
References	112

1 The leak permeability

In studies of the permeabilities of cell membranes, choline and other permanently charged quaternary ammonium ions are often used when physiologically important cations such as sodium and potassium are to be replaced by a "nonpenetrating" cation. In some of these studies it is implied that choline penetrates the cell membranes much less readily than the alkali cations, yet there is little experimental evidence justifying this assumption. Askari (1966) measured the uptake of choline and tetramethylammonium by human erythrocytes and found that choline entry could be described by two mechanisms: a simple diffusion mechanism and a saturable transport system with a maximum flux that is small enough to make this route of entry negligible when choline is present at concentrations of the order of 10^{-1} M, i.e. when replacing external sodium.

According to this study the entry of choline by the simple diffusion mechanism can be described by a rate constant, $k = 0.003-0.006$ h^{-1}, i.e. it is of the same order of magnitude as that for the alkali cations. A peculiar feature of these experiments is that the uptake of choline is proportional to the time of the incubation only up to 4 h; after that, the influx of choline falls off sharply; the intracellular concentration of choline is at that time only a small fraction of the extracellular concentration. Askari (1966) observed this phenomenon with choline as well as with tetramethylammonium and found that it is independent of the external concentration of the quaternaries.

Similar leak permeabilities to choline and sodium were also found in other tissues. Kirschner (1960), using 120 mM choline, reported that the movement of choline across the short-circuited frog skin is similar to the outward diffusions of sodium. Renkin (1961) found that labelled choline enters the cell of resting frog skeletal muscle at approximately the same rate as sodium during incubation periods lasting up to 4 h.

2 The "carrier-mediated" transport of choline

It is surprising to find in human erythrocytes a transport system for which choline appears to be the physiological substrate; there is no evidence that it has a physiological role and it has been shown that labelled choline entering erythrocytes is neither incorporated into phospholipids nor converted to a metabolite (Askari, 1966; Martin, 1968). The transport system appears to be merely a vestige. This situation makes human erythrocytes as useful model for this transport system; it greatly facilitates an accurate estimate of intracellular choline concentrations which is essential for the determination of steady-state distribution ratios and for meaningful studies of choline efflux.

2.1 THE KINETICS OF THE CARRIER-MEDIATED TRANSPORT SYSTEM

At low choline concentrations—in the micromolar range—the uptake of choline by human erythrocytes is larger than that accounted for by a rate constant of about $3 \times 10^{-3} \, h^{-1}$ and it appears to follow Michaelis Menten kinetics. The choline concentration giving half-maximal influx is between 20 and 30 μM (Askari, 1966; Martin, 1968, 1972) and therefore well within the range of physiological concentrations of choline in the plasma (Bligh, 1952). The maximum capacity of the transport system is more variable and of the order of 60 μmol (l cells)$^{-1}$ h^{-1}. This means that the contribution from this facilitated transport system to the total influx of choline is very small when choline is used to replace extracellular sodium, i.e. when its concentration in the incubation medium is between 100 and 150 mM.

The parameters describing the influx of choline are not significantly altered by starving erythrocytes for 24 h, i.e it appears that the transport system is not affected by a substantial fall in the ATP level. On the other hand, at low external choline concentrations the ratio "choline concentration per volume cells: choline concentration per volume outside medium" rises above 1, suggesting that this transport system can move choline against an electrochemical gradient (assuming a transmembrane potential of 10 mV inside negative and a water content of erythrocytes of 72 per cent of the cell volume, choline should be at thermodynamic equilibrium when this ratio is about 1). This ability to concentrate choline is dependent on the composition of the extracellular medium (Fig. 1); it is considerably more pronounced when external sodium is replaced by magnesium, calcium or "Tris" but is abolished when the external sodium is replaced by another monovalent cation (potassium, lithium, rubidium or caesium). A detailed study of the effects of external cations on the movement of choline across the erythrocyte membrane (Martin, 1972) revealed that the monovalent cations inhibit the unidirectional choline influx competitively; the approximate affinity constants (M^{-1}) are: Cs 125, Rb 23, K 8, Li 4·6, Na 2–3. The unidirectional efflux of choline into a choline-free medium is, in contrast to this, smallest when no monovalent cation is present in the external medium and is *stimulated* by Cs > Rb > K > Li > Na. The implications of this are obvious when one considers that the choline transport system in erythrocytes shows a pronounced counterflux phenomenon, i.e. the unidirectional efflux of [^{14}C]-choline from loaded cells is considerably increased when unlabelled choline or other quaternary amonium compounds that can enter erythrocytes on the choline carrier are added to the external medium. On the other hand, compounds that cannot enter the cells on the choline carrier but have a high affinity for the trans-site, e.g. hemicholinium HC-3, inhibit both unidirectional influx and efflux of choline when present in the external medium. The fact that monovalent cations inhibit choline influx but stimulate the efflux indicates, therefore, that they are substrates for this transport system. Consistent with this suggestion is the fact that the stimulation of choline efflux by external monovalent cations is not observed when the external medium contains sufficient choline to saturate the carrier (Fig. 2). The choline carrier may therefore be described as a cation carrier with a high affinity for choline and affinities for Cs > Rb > K > Li > Na.

A model of this type would, in its simplest form, predict that choline should be at thermodynamic equilibrium across the cell membrane when erythrocytes are incubated in a buffer with concentrations of K and Na similar to those found in the intracellular water. Furthermore, if—after equilibrium has been reached—the extracellular K is replaced by another monovalent cation there should be a net flux of choline, i.e. a flux against an electrochemical gradient, and the direction of this net flux should depend on whether the replacing cation competes with choline for the transport site more or less effectively than K. This prediction has been tested and it has been shown that there is a net *efflux* of choline when K is replaced by Cs while the cells will accumulate choline when K is replaced by Na (Martin, 1972). This hypothesis, postulating that the K gradient is the energy source for the net influx of choline against an electrochemical gradient, will also account for the observation that choline fluxes in erythrocytes are apparently not affected by the ATP levels in the erythrocytes.

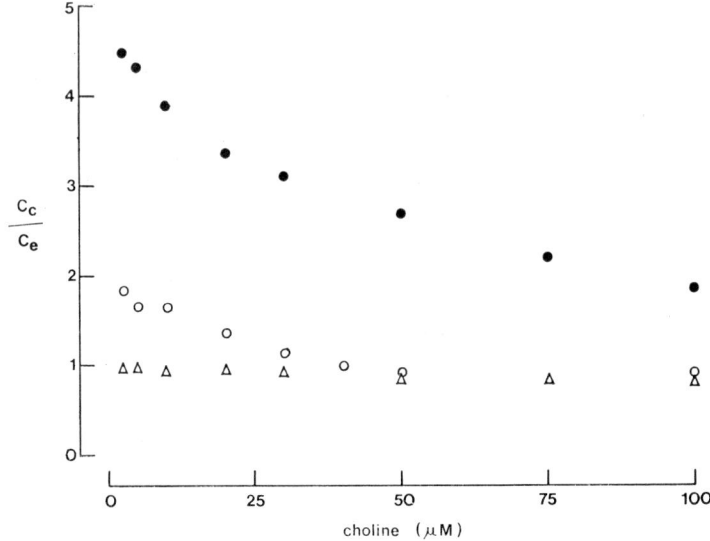

FIG. 1. The dependence of the steady-state distribution ratio on the concentration of choline in the external medium. Blood from one donor was incubated in the absence of glucose in 155 mM NaCl (○), 155 mM KCl (△) and 75 mM MgCl–75 mM sucrose (●). The cellular concentration of [^{14}C] choline is expressed as C_c/C_e, where C_c is the radioactivity per unit cell volume and C_e the radioactivity per volume external medium. The cellular radioactivity was determined after 16 h and 20 h incubation; the two values did not differ by more than 7 per cent. (From Martin, 1972.)

There is, however, an observation that cannot be reconciled with the idea that the choline transport system is a completely symmetrical cation carrier that links the downhill movement of K to the uphill movement of choline. The distribution of choline in the steady state, i.e. after prolonged incubation and when there is no more evidence of any net movement, depends very definitely on the concentration of external choline; the ratio "choline concentration per volume cells: choline concentration per volume external medium" decreases with increasing concentrations of choline in the medium (Fig. 1). Wilbrandt and Rosenberg (1961) and Stein (1967) have shown that a symmetrical carrier-mediated transport system, in which the uphill

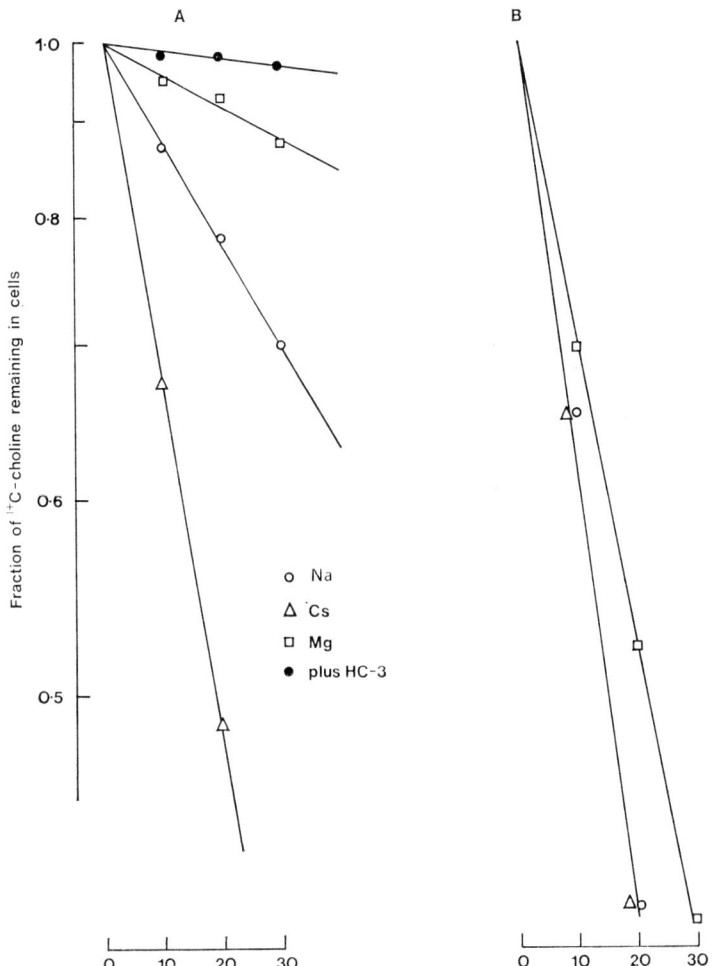

FIG. 2. The effect of external cations on the unidirectional efflux of ^{14}C-choline in the absence (A) and presence (B) of 1 mM choline in the external medium. The erythrocytes had been loaded overnight to 92 µmol choline (l cells)$^{-1}$ and, after washing, were placed in buffers containing 5 mM Tris (pH 7·4 at 37°) and 150 mM NaCl or 150 mM CsCl or 100 mM MgCl$_2$. In the presence of 1 mM hemicholinium HC-3 the efflux was as indicated and independent of the external cation.

movement of one substance is driven by the downhill movement of another, should result in a situation where the steady-state distribution of the driven molecule is independent of its concentration in the external medium.

The dependence of the steady-state distribution ratio on the concentration of external choline agrees basically with a "pump and leak" system, but if one considers as leak only the flux that cannot be blocked by a competitive inhibitor like hemicholinium HC-3, then the leak is about two orders of magnitude smaller than the one necessary to explain the situation observed.

2.2 COMPETITIVE INHIBITORS OF CHOLINE TRANSPORT

Various neuromuscular and ganglionic blocking agents inhibit choline influx competitively and reversibly; only hemicholinium HC-3 has a higher affinity for the transport site ($2 \cdot 5 \times 10^5$ M^{-1}) than choline (Askari, 1966; Martin, 1969). The affinity of the transport system for alkyltrimethylammonium compounds is considerably higher than its affinity for alkyl-bis-(trimethylammonium) compounds of similar chain length. For both series the affinity increases as the alkyl chain length is increased (Martin, 1969). Assuming that the relationship between the affinity constant (K) and the standard free energy change ($\triangle F$) on adsorption of the molecule to the carrier is given by $\triangle F = -RT\, 2 \cdot 3 \log_{10} K$, the increment in $\triangle F$ associated with the addition of a CH_2 group to the molecule has been calculated. For the monoquaternary compounds the increment in $\triangle F$ for one CH_2 group added is -360 cal mol^{-1}. For the bisquaternary compounds the increment is about -860 cal mol^{-1}. which is similar to the free energy change associated with the addition of a CH_2 group when a compound is partitioned between water and a non-polar solvent (Kauzman, 1959).

Some additional information about the transport system comes from the observation that tetramethylammonium, ethyltrimethylammonium and propyltrimethylammonium appear to enter the cells on the choline carrier while the larger monoquaternary compounds and all bisquaternary compounds bind to the carrier but are unable to cross the cell membrane. Radioactively labelled carbachol and acetylcholine do not enter the cells on the choline transport system (Martin, 1969).

2.3 NONCOMPETITIVE AND IRREVERSIBLE INHIBITORS OF CHOLINE TRANSPORT; IMPLICATIONS FOR THE MECHANISM OF THE TRANSPORT SYSTEM

A study of the effects of SH reagents on the choline transport system (Martin, 1971) revealed that not only p-chloromercuribenzene sulphonic acid (PCMBS) and N-ethylmaleimide (NEM) but also a more specific reagent like cystamine will produce an almost complete inhibition; the inhibition produced by NEM is irreversible, the one produced by cystamine can be reversed by treatment with dithioerythritol (DTE). Various SH reagents were tested for their ability to inhibit the transport system and various reducing agents for their ability to reactivate choline transport that had been completely blocked by cystamine. It emerged that the lipid solubility of the various substances is the most important factor determining the reaction with the transport system, suggesting that the reactive SH group is located in a lipophilic environment.

An interesting observation resulting from this study is that external choline increases the rate of inhibition by NEM and cystamine while intracellular choline has the opposite effect. Edwards (1973c) realized that useful information concerning the mechanism of transport might come from a detailed study of the effects of intracellular and extracellular transport substrates and inhibitors on the rate at which NEM reacts with the transport system.

The results of his study are summarized in Fig. 3. He argues that since substrate outside the cell and competitive inhibitor inside the cell both increase the rate of inactivation, they must change the conformation of the transport system. Furthermore, they probably change the conformation in

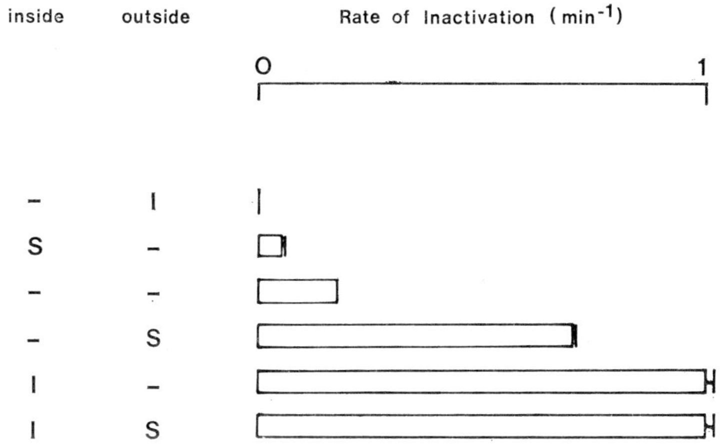

inside	outside	Rate of Inactivation (min^{-1})
		0 — 1
−	I	|
S	−	▢
−	−	▭
−	S	▭
I	−	▭ ⊢
I	S	▭ ⊢

FIG. 3. Rates of inactivation of choline transport by 1 mM N-ethylmaleimide in the presence inside or outside the cell of saturating concentrations of substrate (S) or competitive inhibitor (I). Cells were incubated with N-ethylmaleimide in the presence of substrate or competitive inhibitor, the reagent and substrate or inhibitor removed and transport assayed under standard conditions. The rate of inactivation k was obtained from $V/V' = \exp(-kt)$, where V/V' is transport in treated cells over transport in untreated cells, t is the time of incubation with N-ethylmaleimide. The rate of inactivation with a saturating concentration of the substrate or competitive inhibitor was obtained from a double-reciprocal plot of k as a function of the concentration of the substrate or inhibitor. The substrate inside was choline, outside was choline, tetramethylammonium or N-methylpyridinium. The competitive inhibitor inside was metanephrine, outside was decamethonium.

The error bars represent standard errors. (From Edwards, 1974.)

the same way because they give similar rates of inactivation, and when there is both a high concentration of competitive inhibitor inside and of substrate outside the cell, the rate of inactivation is the same as the one observed with only a saturating concentration of competitive inhibitor inside.

Competitive inhibitor outside and substrate inside have the opposite effect; they reduce the rate of inactivation by NEM, so they probably reverse the conformational change that resulted in an increased reactivity towards NEM. The simplest interpretation of the results is to assume that the transport system can exist in two conformations, of which one is at least 200 times more reactive towards NEM than the other. The rate of inactivation in any situation represents the proportion of transport sites in the more reactive conformation at any instant. Virtually all the sites are in the "non-reactive" conformation when a saturating concentration of competitive inhibitor is present on the outside while competitive inhibitor on the inside promotes the reactive conformation. Since competitive inhibitors bind to the transport site but are then not moved across the membrane, it seems reasonable to equate the reactive conformation with a conformation when the binding site faces inward and the "non-reactive" conformation with the "outside-facing" conformation of the transport system.

The effects of substrates on the rate of inactivity by NEM are entirely consistent with this interpretation. The fact that choline transport shows a pronounced counterflux phenomenon indicates that the rate at which the transport system changes from the "outside-facing" to the "inside-facing" (or "inside-facing" to "outside-facing") conformation is much faster when a substrate is bound to the transport site than when the transport site is free. As a consequence of this, substrate on one side of the membrane will make most of the transport sites face the other side (Heinz and Durbin, 1957; Martin, 1971). This explains the effects of substrate on the rate of inactivation by NEM. Also, substrate would be predicted to be less effective than competitive substrate in producing a particular conformation. A high concentration of substrate on one side will always convert only a certain proportion of the transport sites to facing the opposite side, while a saturating concentration of competitive inhibitor on one side will bind virtually all the transport sites.

The argument is considerably strengthened by the remarkable quantitative agreement between theoretical predications and experimental values. Edwards (1973a) based his theoretical treatment on a version of the carrier model that allows the carrier to be asymmetrical with respect to the outside and inside of the cell and has as the rate-limiting step for transport the change between the inward-facing and outward-facing conformations of the carrier (cf. Geck, 1971; Miller, 1971). He incorporated in this model the assumption that NEM reacts *only* with the inward-facing carrier and that the rate of this reaction is the same whether the carrier is free or complexed with substrate or competitive inhibitor. The analysis of this model shows that when the rate of inactivation by NEM is measured in the presence of various concentrations of a substrate or competitive inhibitor X, the results will give a straight line when $1/(1 - k/k_o)$ is plotted versus $1/[X]$, where k is the observed rate constant of transport inactivation by NEM and k_o is k in the absence of added substrate or competitive inhibitor. Furthermore, the theory predicts that the apparent dissociation constant for choline, calculated in this way with internal choline reducing the rate of NEM attack, should be the same as the Michaelis constant (K_m) describing the efflux of choline into a choline-free medium; the values found were 80 $\pm$ 10 μM and 72 $\pm$ 5 μM. Similarly, the external concentrations of choline giving half-maximum influx into choline-free cells and giving half-maximum accelleration of the NEM attack are predicted to be the same and were both found to be between 20 and 25 μM. An equally good agreement between the appropriate dissociation constants was obtained with another substrate, tetramethylammonium, and with the competitive inhibitors decamethonium and metanephrine.

Benzylalcohol inhibits choline transport in red cells nonspecifically and reversibly; it reduces the maximum rate of influx into choline-free cells but does not change the K_m (Clayton and Martin, 1971). Edwards (1973a) found that benzylalcohol did not effect the reaction between NEM and the transport system in any circumstances. This is consistent with the theory presented and argues against a mechanism like that postulated by Krupka (1971) to account for the accelleration by glucose of the inhibition of the glucose transport system by fluorodinitrobenzene. He suggested that a reactive conformation of the transport system was formed as a step in the transport process, so that the rate of inactivation increased with the flux of substrate.

These data provide a useful test for some models of transport. They are obviously consistent with the classical models involving a mobile carrier (Jacquez, 1961; Wilbrandt and Rosenberg, 1961). However, Vidaver (1966) has shown that identical kinetics can be obtained with models not involving a mobile carrier; he considers in this context two models. The first one is an allosteric model in which a binding site undergoes an allosteric transition between two states accessible from opposite sides of the membrane. The transition step might, for example, involve the shift in the position of a polypeptide chain, blocking access to the combining site from one direction or the other. In a "H bond" model, substrate binding involves a hydrogen bond with a combining site which can itself exist in either of two alternate hydrogen bond states. In principle similar are

Patlak's "gate" model (Patlak, 1957) and the allosteric model of Christensen (1960). All these models involve alternate states of a barrier rather than alternate locations of a carrier. The phenomenon of counterflux—very pronounced with choline transport in erythrocytes—occurs when the transition from one state to the other is facilitated by the binding of substrate to the combining site. Consequently, these models predict that substrate on the outside and competitive inhibitor on the inside should convert the transport to what might be called the "inside-facing" conformation, while substrate on the inside and competitive inhibitor on the outside will convert the carrier to the "outside-facing" conformation.

On the other hand, the models proposed by Lieb and Stein (1970, 1972) and Naftalin (1970) are not consistent with the results obtained by Edwards. Lieb and Stein suggest that a tetrameric protein binds substrate, a conformational change transfers substrate to a pool inside the tetramer, then the conformational change is reversed, releasing substrate to the other side of the membrane. The same conformational change occurs in influx and efflux, is promoted by substrate and prevented by competitive inhibitor. Unless some *ad hoc* postulates are made this model cannot account for the fact that substrate outside and competitive inhibitor inside accelerate inactivation of the choline transport system by NEM, while substrate inside and inhibitor outside have the opposite effect.

Naftalin postulates a pore through the membrane containing binding sites for substrate and postulates unstirred layers at the faces of the membrane to account for counterflux phenomena. With a saturating concentration of substrate at one face events in the unstirred layer at the other face would be the rate-limiting step, but all the binding sites in the pore would be virtually saturated with substrate. Again, the model cannot explain that the effects of substrate and competitive inhibitor should depend on whether they are present on the inside or outside of the cell membrane.

The choline transport system is particularly well suited for a study of this type; it is unusual in combining a pronounced counterflux phenomenon with a very small transport capacity. This means that choline present on one side of the membrane only will result in a large proportion of the transport system "facing the other side" and the concentration difference—and with it the particular conformation—will remain for a time that is very long compared with the rate of inactivation by NEM. Furthermore, the conformation referred to as "inside facing" is at least 200 times more reactive towards NEM than the "outside facing" one and it seems that the competitive inhibitors used—metanephrine and decamethonium—do not sterically protect the SH group attacked by NEM.

There is evidence that the reactivity of other transport systems towards irreversible inhibitors is similarly effected by substrate and competitive inhibitors. The inactivation of the glucose transport system in erythrocytes by fluorodinitrobenzene is accelerated by external glucose but retarded by internal glucose and external competitive inhibitor (Krupka, 1971; Edwards, 1973b).

Clement and Colhoun (1975) have reported that the incubation of human erythrocytes with choline mustard aziridinium results in some irreversible inhibition of the choline transport system; the rate constant for the reaction has not been determined.

2.4 IRREVERSIBLE INHIBITION OF CHOLINE TRANSPORT BY LOW CONCENTRATIONS OF LITHIUM

Following the observation that the incubation of human erythrocytes with low concentrations (below 5 mM) of lithium results in a partial but irreversible inhibition of the choline transport system, Lee *et al.* (1974) investigated the effect of lithium administration to manic-depressive patients. The results of this study show that the prolonged administration of lithium reduces choline influx into erythrocytes significantly; during the first few weeks of treatment the influx of choline is about half the normal rate, after about 2 months it has fallen to around 10 per cent. This inhibition is not dependent on the presence of lithium in the incubation medium when measuring choline influx. In a further investigation of this effect the inhibition has been shown to be also independent of the presence of lithium in the intracellular water, i.e. it is truly irreversible (Lingsch and Martin, 1976). When a patient is taken off lithium the choline transport system in the erythrocytes returns to normal over a period of 3 months, i.e. at the same rate at which erythrocytes exposed to lithium are replaced by new cells. The significance as well as the mechanism of this effect are not understood.

2.5 COMPARISON BETWEEN THE CHOLINE TRANSPORT SYSTEM IN ERYTHROCYTES AND THOSE IN OTHER TISSUES

Since the choline transport system in human erythrocytes has been studied in considerable detail and in view of its rather dramatic response to a therapeutic agent like lithium, it is clearly of interest to know how similar or dissimilar it is to other choline transport systems, in particular those in the CNS.

In contrast to the situation found with erythrocytes, tissues capable of converting choline to the transmitter acetylcholine have a so called high-affinity choline transport system ($K_m = 1-4\ \mu$M) in addition to a transport system of lower affinity ($K_m = 30$–100 μM). Investigations have concentrated on the high-affinity system since it appears to be the one associated with a marked degree of acetylcholine formation. In synaptosomes from rat brain the uptake of choline by this route is reduced to very low levels when external sodium is replaced by lithium or sucrose and is very sensitive to hemicholinium HC-3 ($K_i = 0.05$–0.1 μM) (Haga and Noda, 1973; Yamamura and Snyder, 1973). A systematic study of the inhibition of this high-affinity transport system by alkyl bisquaternary ammonium compounds confirmed that this tranport system is in many ways different from the choline transport system in erythrocytes (Holden et al., 1975).

Diamond and Kennedy (1969) found in synaptosomes from guinea-pig brain a saturating choline transport system that does not require added monovalent or divalent cations. External Na, K and Li were found to be potent inhibitors of choline influx and the system did not appear to be dependent on metabolic energy. Reagents which attack sulphhydryl groups were effective inhibitors and hemicholinium was a competitive inhibitor with a K_i of 4×10^{-5} M. The choline concentration giving half-maximum flux was 83×10^{-6} M; with synaptosomes from various parts of the rat brain the K_m values for this low-affinity, sodium-independent transport system range from 30 to 100×10^{-6} M (Haga and Noda, 1973; Yamamura and Snyder, 1973).

References

Askari, A. (1966). *J. Gen. Physiol.* **49**, 1147.
Bligh, T. (1952). *J. Physiol. (London)*, **117**, 234.
Christensen, H. N. (1960). *Adv. Prot. Chem.* **15**, 239.
Clayton, P. and Martin, K. (1971). *J. Physiol.* **218**, 50P.
Clement, J. G. and Colhoun, E. H. (1975). *Can. J. Physiol. Pharmacol.* **53**, 1089.
Diamond, I. and Kennedy, E. P. (1969). *J. Biol. Chem.* **244**, 3258.
Edwards, P. A. W. (1973a). Tests of theories of transport across cell membranes using inhibitors of the choline and glucose transport systems of the human red cell. Ph.D. thesis, Cambridge University, UK.
Edwards, P. A. W. (1973b). *Biochim. Biophys. Acta*, **307**, 415.
Edwards, P. A. W. (1973c). *Biochim. Biophys. Acta*, **311**, 123.
Edwards, P. A. W. (1974). *In* "Comparative Biochemistry and Physiology of Transport" (L. Bolis, K. Bloch, S. E. Luria and F. Lynen, eds), p. 195. North-Holland, Amsterdam.
Geck, P. (1971). *Biochim. Biophys. Acta*, **241**, 462.
Haga, T. and Noda, H. (1973). *Biochim. Biophys. Acta*, **291**, 564.
Heinz, E. and Durbin, R. P. (1957). *J. Gen. Physiol.* **41**, 101.
Holden, J. T., Rossier, J., Beaujouan, J. G., Guyenet, P. and Glowinski, J. (1975). *Molec. Pharmacol.* **11**, 19.
Jacquez, J. A. (1961). *Proc. Nat. Acad. Sci. USA*, **47**, 153.
Kauzman, W. (1959). *Adv. Prot. Chem.* **14**, 1.
Kirschner (1960). *Science*, **132**, 85.

Krupka, R. M. (1971). *Biochemistry*, **10**, 1143.
Lee, G., Lingsch, C., Lyle, P. T. and Martin, K. (1974). *Brit. J. Clin. Pharmacol.* **1**, 365.
Lieb, W. R. and Stein, W. D. (1970). *Biophys. J.* **10**, 585.
Lieb, W. R. and Stein, W. D. (1972). *Biochim. Biophys. Acta*, **265**, 187.
Lingsch, C. and Martin, K. (1976). *Brit. J. Pharmacol.* **57**, 323.
Martin, K. (1968). *J. Gen. Physiol.* **51**, 497.
Martin, K. (1969). *Brit. J. Pharmacol.* **36**, 458.
Martin, K. (1971). *J. Physiol.* **213**, 647.
Martin, K. (1972). *J. Physiol.* **224**, 207.
Miller, D. M. (1971). *Biophys. J.* **11**, 915.
Naftalin, R. J. (1970). *Biochim. Biophys. Acta*, **211**, 65.
Patlak, C. S. (1957). *Bull. Math. Biophys.* **19**, 209.
Renkin, E. M. (1961). *J. Gen. Physiol.* **44**, 1159.
Stein, W. D. (1967). "The Movement of Molecules Across Cell Membranes." Academic Press, New York and London.
Vidaver, G. A. (1966). *J. Theoret. Biol.* **19**, 301.
Wilbrandt, W. and Rosenberg, T. (1961). *Pharmacol. Rev.* **13**, 109.
Yamamura, II. I. and Snyder, S. H. (1973). *J. Neurochem.* **21**, 1355.

pH equilibrium across the red cell membrane

S. B. HLADKY and T. J. RINK

Physiological Laboratory, Cambridge University, UK

1 Introduction	115
2 The basic processes	116
3 Evidence on the nature of the anion distribution across the red cell membrane	119
4 Mechanisms of restoration of anion and pH equilibrium after perturbation	124
5 The mechanism of exchange of Cl for HCO_3	128
6 Can H or OH cross the membrane as such?	131
7 Conclusions	133
References	133

1 Introduction

The main functions of the red cell, O_2 and CO_2 transport and buffering of H, could be subserved by the contents of the cell, in particular haemoglobin (Hb) and carbonic anhydrase (CA), even if these were simply dissolved in plasma. There are, however, a number of reasons for containing these proteins within corpuscles. First, the colloid osmotic pressure of plasma with 150 g l^{-1} of dissolved Hb would be greater than 80 mmHg (10 kP) compared with the normal 25 mmHg (3 kP) due to plasma protein (Barcroft, 1922). Secondly, the viscosity of blood flowing through tubes of the dimensions of the resistance vessels of the body approaches that of plasma (Whittaker and Winton, 1933) while that of a solution of Hb in plasma would be much higher (Burton, 1969). Higher colloid osmotic pressure and higher viscosity would each have serious deleterious effects on the function of the cardiovascular system. Thirdly, the containing of Hb and CA inside corpuscles prevents loss of the proteins from the blood through filtration into tissues and into urine. Fourthly, a specialized environment can be maintained for Hb inside the corpuscles, e.g. there is a methaemoglobin reductase system which converts the continuously formed methaemoglobin (oxidized Hb) back to Hb, and the oxygenation of Hb is partly regulated by the level of 2,3-diphosphoglycerate (2, 3-DPG).

Isolating Hb and CA within an osmotic barrier has the consequence that other substances must cross the red cell membrane in order to gain access to these proteins. The passage of O_2 and CO_2 across thin lipid membranes is not importantly slower than the necessary diffusion through plasma and the cell contents, but this is not true for H or OH. It is our present purpose to examine the mechanism of H and OH transport across the membrane, and the factors affecting their distribution between the cells and surrounding medium.

2 The basic processes

From the evidence to be discussed later in this chapter it can be concluded that the physiologically important changes which occur after addition of acid, base or CO_2 to red cell suspensions can be accounted for by considering the properties of the buffers, particularly Hb, the presence of CA inside the cell and three types of passive transport across the membrane: (1) diffusion of CO_2, (2) movement of H_2O, and (3) a one-for-one electrically neutral exchange of Cl for HCO_3. The amounts of Hb, organic phosphate and cations such as K within the cells remain constant on the time scale considered here (milliseconds to minutes); or in other words, the membrane is effectively impermeable to those anions and cations. From the properties of the red cell listed above the relation between the external and internal concentrations of Cl, HCO_3 and OH can be determined. Since HCO_3 and Cl passively exchange with each other, a steady state is reached when

$$\frac{(HCO_3)_i}{(HCO_3)_o} = \frac{Cl_i}{Cl_o} \qquad (1)$$

Furthermore, the OH concentration ratio is tied to the HCO_3 ratio by the chemical reaction between CO_2 and OH. Since

$$(OH)(CO_2) = K'(HCO_3) \qquad (2)$$

and pCO_2 and K' can be taken as equal on both sides of the membrane,

$$\frac{OH_i}{OH_o} = \frac{K'(HCO_3)_i/CO_2}{K'(HCO_3)_o/CO_2} = \frac{(HCO_3)_i}{(HCO_3)_o}.$$

Furthermore, since in aqueous solutions

$$(H)(OH) = \text{constant}, \qquad (4)$$

$$\frac{\mathrm{OH}_i}{\mathrm{OH}_o} = \frac{\mathrm{H}_o}{\mathrm{H}_i}. \qquad (5)$$

Consider a cell containing B moles of univalent cation and P moles of protein and organic phosphate with mean valency z (a negative number between 3 and 4 at $\mathrm{pH}_i = 7\cdot 2$). The cell is suspended in a solution containing impermeant univalent cations at concentration b_0 and exchangeable univalent anions (Cl, HCO_3 and OH) at total concentration a_0. The total internal concentration of these anions at equilibrium is a_i. (Other species, neutral or charged, have been neglected in order to simplify the treatment.) Since in red cells some 30 per cent of the volume is occupied by Hb, internal concentrations must be expressed as moles per litre cell water. The concentrations of cell cations and of Hb plus organic phosphates are then B/V and P/V, where V is the volume of cell water at partial, i.e. anion, equilibrium.

There are two further considerations, valid regardless of the mechanisms for transport across the membrane, which allow the derivation of expres-ions for the exchangeable anion concentration ratio and the volume of water within the cells. First, the osmotic pressure must be the same on each side of the membrane since the membrane allows rapid water transfer and cannot resist appreciable hydrostatic pressure (Rand and Burton, 1964). Thus the concentration of water and hence by difference the total concentration of all the solutes (the osmolality) must be the same on both sides of the membrane, i.e. (assuming ideality)

$$B/V + P/V + a_i = b_0 + a_0 \qquad (6)$$

Under all conditions and with any membrane potential which can be achieved, in each cell and in the external solution the difference between the total number of negative charges and the total number of positive charges is negligible compared to either total. This principle of electroneutrality requires

$$a_i V = B + zP \qquad (7)$$

and

$$a_0 = b_0 \qquad (8)$$

It is important to realize that on a time scale of milliseconds to minutes any changes in the total number of exchangeable anions in the cell ($a_i V$) can and must be made using only anion exchanges (either tightly coupled or apparent as a result of the electroneutrality requirement) and diffusion of neutral molecules. For example, following exchange of one Cl from inside for one HCO_3 from outside, the new HCO_3 inside can dissociate to form CO_2, which diffuses out of the cell, and OH, which removes a H from Hb (or the phosphates), thus forming water. As a result $a_i V$ has decreased by one and zP is more negative by one and, as required, there has been no net transfer of negative charge across the membrane.

Still based on the assumption of ideality, the volume of cell water can generally be obtained from the relation

$$V = \frac{\text{sum of the number of moles of internal solutes}}{\text{sum of the concentrations of external solutes}} \qquad (9)$$

or in the present case from equations 6, 7 and 8,

$$V = \frac{B + P + a_i V}{a_0 + b_0} = \frac{2B + (z + 1)P}{2b_0}. \qquad (10)$$

The distribution ratio ($r = a_i/a_0$) for the exchangeable anions is then

$$r = \frac{2(B + zP)}{2B + (z + 1)P}. \qquad (11)$$

Thus, at anion and volume equilibrium, the anion ratio (for those anions which can exchange) is determined by the number of cations in the cell, the amount of impermeant protein and organic phosphate, and the net charge on the protein and organic phosphate, so that with z negative the anion ratio is less than 1. Thus since

$$pH_o - pH_i = \log (OH_o/OH_i) = - \log r \qquad (12)$$

$pH_i < pH_o$ and the cell interior is acid with respect to the external solution.

The net charge on the Hb and organic phosphate depends on pH_i since they have pK's in the physiological pH range. Thus as pH_i increases z becomes more negative, and as pH_i decreases z becomes less negative or even positive. From equations 10 and 11 it is clear that as z changes, the anion ratio and cell water volume will change. When pH_i increases, the negative charge on Hb and organic phosphate increases, there are fewer permeable anions inside, r decreases, cell water decreases, and thus the cell shrinks and pH_o-pH_i increases. Similarly, when pH_i decreases pH_o-pH_i becomes smaller (or reverses in sign) and the cell swells.

Practically it is pH_o and not pH_i which can be changed by adding acid or base. The change in pH_i and hence those in z, r and V can be calculated from equations 11 and 12 and the relation between z and pH_i, but the sums can become complicated. Fortunately, it is possible to see the important features of these changes by inspection of the equations given and by example. Thus when pH_o increases there will be an increase in pH_i and thus a decrease in r. From equation 12 it can be seen that the change in

pH_i will be smaller than that in pH_o because of the change in log r. For instance, in normal blood with initial pH_o 7·4, addition of sufficient base to change the final pH_o to 8·4 decreases r from 0·67 to 0·31 (Funder and Wieth, 1966a) while pH_i calculated from equation 12 increases from 7·23 to 7·9.

The partial pressure of oxygen (pO_2) is another factor which can affect the exchangeable anion distribution by changing the net charge on Hb. The binding of H by Hb is affected by its degree of oxygenation and, at physiological pH, deoxygenation increases H binding. This uptake of H on deoxygenation is known as the Haldane effect (Christiansen et al., 1914). All other things being equal, deoxygenation of blood will decrease the net negative charge on Hb, increase the anion ratio and the cell volume, and produce an alkaline shift in both the internal and external pH's. Physiologically during deoxygenation other things are not equal; CO_2 is added to the blood and the acidification thus produced roughly cancels the alkalinification due to deoxygenation.

The model presented here has been based on the characteristically clear description by Jacobs and Stewart (1947) of the application of Donnan equilibrium theory to red cells. The original paper should be consulted for consideration of more complicated examples, e.g. cells suspended in sucrose. Quantitative expressions based on the same theory can be found in Van Slyke et al. (1923) and in the detailed monograph by Siggard-Andersen (1974).

3 Evidence on the nature of the anion distribution across the red cell membrane

The fundamental description of univalent anion equilibrium in red cells was developed more than fifty years ago in classic papers by Warburg (1922) and Van Slyke et al. (1923). Much of Warburg's long paper is concerned with the physical chemistry of ionic solutions, e.g. the definition of osmolality, and is of primarily historical interest, but the final section deals explicitly with equilibria across the red cell membrane. Within this section, however, there is a serious confusion between the potential difference across the membrane and the surface potential (electrophoretic zeta potential) now known to be due to charges bound outside the membrane. The paper of Van Slyke et al., which gives a much less sophisticated theoretical treatment, is easier for the modern reader to follow.

In both the classic papers the red cell was considered to be a Donnan system with impermeant internal cations (mainly K) and anions (mainly Hb) contained within a membrane permeable to the monovalent anions and to H_2O and CO_2. It was assumed that each permeant anion separately came to equilibrium driven by its electrochemical gradient. With the conditions of equal osmolality (equation 6) and electroneutrality (equations 7 and 8), however, the final (anion) equilibrium will be the same regardless of whether it is achieved by neutral exchanges or by free, separate movement of the anions. Experimentally, these workers showed that the distribution ratios for the anions which could cross the membrane were all approximately the same, i.e.

$$\frac{Cl_i}{Cl_o} = \frac{(HCO_3)_i}{(HCO_3)_o} = \frac{OH_i}{OH_o}, \qquad (13)$$

and that these ratios varied similarly and as expected when the charge carried by the impermeant anions was varied by changing the pH. They also showed that the cell volume varied as expected with changes in Cl and HCO_3. Little has been added to our basic knowledge of the equilibrium distribution since the papers of Warburg and Van Slyke et al. The significant advances are: (1) more accurate data, (2) proper accounting for CO_2 combined directly with Hb (Roughton, 1935, 1964), (3) the finding that in many mammals including man, organic phosphate accounts for much of the impermeant anion content of the red cells (Farmer and Maizels, 1939; Rapoport and Guest, 1939), and (4) the finding of measurable leaks to cations which are, however, normally countered by active pumping which keeps the cation content of the cells constant. Normal values for the concentrations of the main substances discussed are shown in Table 1. With a plasma pH of 7·4 the internal pH of the oxygenated red cell is 7·2.

Work subsequent to that of Warburg (1922) and Van Slyke et al. (1923) has confirmed the general theory. Rapoport and Guest (1939) were able to remove certain quantitative discrepancies in the determination of HCO_3

TABLE 1

	OH	pH	HCO_3	Cl	Hb	2,3-DPG	Na	K
Red cell	$1·6 \times 10^{-7}$	7·2	16	77	7·0	6·0	16·0	134·0
Plasma	$2·5 \times 10^{-7}$	7·4	25	115	—	—	140·0	4·0

The distribution of OH and other ions between red cells and plasma in normal human arterial blood. Concentrations given in mmol (kg water)$^{-1}$. At pH 7·2 Hb bears a net charge of -3, and 2,3-DPG -4. Hb, therefore, accounts for 21 and 2,3-DPG for 24 mequiv (kg water)$^{-1}$ of impermeable anion. Data were taken from the following sources: OH, HCO_3 and Cl from Dill et al. (1937), Fitzsimons and Sendroy (1961), and Funder and Wieth (1966a); Na and K from Funder and Wieth (1966b); Hb from Gary-Bobo and Solomon (1968); and 2,3-DPG from Duhm (1971). Estimates of the charge on Hb vary from one source to the next.

ratios by allowing for CO_2 bound to Hb as carbamino groups. They also pointed out that much of the impermeant anion was in fact, 2, 3-DPG and that when cellular 2,3-DPG levels in dog blood were experimentally raised the anion ratio fell in the expected manner. 2,3-DPG is now known to alter the O_2 affinity of Hb by allosteric interaction (Benesch and Benesch, 1967). But interestingly, much of the effect of increasing 2,3-DPG levels on O_2 affinity in intact cells is due to its being an impermeant anion and thereby decreasing the anion ratio and decreasing internal pH (Battaglia et al., 1970; Duhm, 1971) as predicted by equations 11 and 12. This internal acidification then reduces the O_2 affinity of Hb (the Bohr effect). It has also been reported that changes in red cell 2,3-DPG levels in chronic acidosis and alkalosis tend to stabilize internal pH by changing the anion ratio (r) (Bellingham et al., 1971). It is worth noting that although about one-half the negative charge on the impermeant anions in normal human cells is carried by 2,3-DPG, Hb is the major internal buffer (other than HCO_3) since the charge on 2,3-DPG varies less rapidly with pH. Because of 2,3-DPG and the other organic phosphates, z will be zero at a pH somewhat to the acid side of the isoelectric point for Hb.

As noted earlier, when acid or base are added to a cell suspension, the changes in pH_o, pH_i, and r are related to each other by equation 12. It is possible to check experimentally the predictions of the Donnan theory for the relative size of the changes in pH_i and $-\log r$ for different Cl contents of the cells, $Cl_i V$. In order to change pH_i by one unit, approximately 10 mmol of HCO_3 must enter or leave the cells per mmol of Hb (Adair, 1925; Harris and Maizels, 1952; Gary-Bobo and Solomon, 1968). If $Cl_i V$ is large, the exchange of this amount of HCO_3 for Cl will result in only a small percentage change in Cl_i and thus will produce only a small change in $\log r$ (-0.34 in the example for whole blood cited earlier). If, however, the chloride content is small, the exchange of a much smaller amount of HCO_3 for Cl will cause a large percentage change in Cl_i and thus r. In effect, when the Cl content is small, the internal buffers hold pH_i constant, and changes in pH_o are reflected by changes in $-\log r$. Viewed the other way round, in order for the buffers contained in the cells to buffer the plasma, it is necessary for the cells to contain ample Cl. Lower Cl contents and hence poorer buffering of plasma by the cells can be produced (see equation 7) by increasing pH, by increasing the number of impermeant anions inside the cell, or by decreasing the number of internal impermeant cations. Results illustrating these effects are contained in reports by Dalmark (1975) and Duhm (1976). Duhm has shown that increasing the amount of internal 2,3-DPG increases the buffering capacity of the cell contents but actually decreases the buffering of the external medium by the cells at pH's greater than 7. From his Fig. 4, which shows that the ratio of the changes in internal and external pH ($\triangle pH_i/\triangle pH_o$) decreases as r decreases, from his Fig. 3 which shows that r decreases as either the 2,3-DPG level or pH_o increases, and from the universal finding that V decreases as r decreases, it is very likely that his observations can be explained by the reductions in Cl content caused by increases in 2,3-DPG and pH_o. Dalmark (1975) has altered the total internal concentration of cations using treatment with nystatin. As expected from the discussion above, he found that between pH 6·5 and 8·0 r varies from 4·4 to 0·3 at 10 mM K, but only from 1 to 0·8 at 300 mM K. The maximum value of r possible is 2 if calculated from equation 12, but much larger values are theoretically and experimentally possible whenever impermeant anions or neutral molecules such as sucrose are present outside (see Jacobs and Stewart, 1947). Dalmark's value of 4·4 at $b_0 = 10$ mM is just below the maximum theoretically possible for his conditions with $C_{sucrose} = 27$ mM.

Harris and Maizels (1952) tested directly the idea that anion distribution is passive and showed that the OH and Cl ratios were equal to each other and varied in the expected manner with pH in red cells before and after metabolic poisoning or cold storage. Fitzsimons and Sendroy (1961) in a thorough study of fresh human blood found closely similar concentration ratios for OH, Cl and HCO_3 measured with due allowance for carbamino CO_2. In another meticulous study on human blood, Funder and Wieth (1966a) demonstrated the close similarity of the OH and Cl ratios in human blood at different pH's, and also observed the expected increase in internal pH when external Cl was replaced by an impermeant substance. Qualitative changes of this kind were discussed by Jacobs and Stewart (1947).

As discussed by a number of investigators, the failure to measure exact equality between the concentration ratios for Cl, OH and HCO_3 does not invalidate the theory. The Cl ratio is determined from measured Cl concentrations while the OH ratio comes from measurements of pH. HCO_3 ratios are either taken to be equal to the OH ratio, or occasionally measured, but they are then subject to some experimental uncertainty because of combination of CO_2 with proteins. The impressive result, emphasized by almost all investigators, is that the ratios for Cl, OH and HCO_3 all vary quantitatively in the manner predicted from the effect of pH on the net charge of the impermeant anions. The finding that OH follows the Donnan equilibrium distribution in the red cell implies that it is passively distributed, i.e. that there is no active transport of OH, H or HCO_3.

It should be possible using an equation such as 10 to predict the changes in the volume of red cells which occur after changes in pH or medium osmolality. It is almost universally accepted (Williams et al., 1959;

Passow, 1964; Rand and Burton, 1964; Gary-Bobo and Solomon, 1968; Dalmark, 1976) that the osmolality and hydrostatic pressure are the same in the cell interior and the medium. Nevertheless, it has long been known (Ponder, 1948) that the changes in the volume of red cells when external osmolality is changed are not accurately predicted by relations such as equation 10 with B, P and z constant, even after allowing for all the known nonidealities. Thus at pH 7·4, if the osmolality of the medium ($2b_0$) is increased, the decrease in V is only c. 80 per cent of that expected. The variation of the osmotic coefficient of Hb in simple solution is not large enough to explain this discrepancy (Adair, 1929; Dick, 1966; Gary-Bobo and Solomon, 1968). The result would be explained if in the cell c. 20 per cent of the cell water were bound to Hb and were thus available neither to act as solvent water for the ions nor to participate in water movement across the membrane, but the arguments against the existence of so much bound water are persuasive (Gary-Bobo and Solomon, 1968), particularly since all the water in the cells is available as solvent both for nonelectrolytes and, at least in Hb solutions outside the cells, for ions.

Gary-Bobo and Solomon (1968) investigated the changes in cell water with medium osmolality at various pH's. In agreement with other workers they found at pH 7·4 that the volume changes were smaller than expected. At pH 6·1, however, they found volume changes 5 per cent larger than predicted. They argued that nonidealities or water binding would make the volume responses smaller, not larger, and thus that the behaviour at pH 6·1 and hence presumably also at pH 7·4 must reflect changes in the amount of cell Cl, i.e. that $a_i V$ depends on cell volume. To explain these Cl movements, they proposed that the magnitude of the charge on Hb decreases as Hb concentration increases and thus that Cl must move to preserve electroneutrality. In terms of the simplified model used here, at pH 7·4, as b_0 increases the cell shrinks, Hb becomes more concentrated, z which is negative becomes less so, Cl enters the cell in exchange for the OH released, the number of solute particles in the cell ($2B + (z + 1)P$), increases, and thus the decrease in V (see equation 10) is less than expected. By contrast at pH 6·1, where z is positive, as b_0 increases, z becomes less positive, Cl leaves the cell, $2B + (z + 1)P$ decreases, and the shrinkage is greater than expected.

Gary-Bobo and Solomon (1968, 1971) have presented substantial evidence that the effects just discussed are genuine. Thus (1) no other explanation is available for the larger than expected volume changes at acid pH (Fig. 5, 1968); (2) as b_0 is increased Cl enters the cells at pH 6·1 and leaves at pH 7·4 (Fig. 11, 1968); and (3) the charge on Hb in simple solutions, as measured by ion partition across a dialysis membrane, does vary with concentration (1968, 1971). Since they also found excellent agreement at pH 7·4 between measured Cl shifts and those required to explain the measured volume changes (Fig. 12, 1968), Gary-Bobo and Solomon concluded that water movements are correctly predicted when changes in cell Cl are taken into account.

Dalmark (1975) has measured the Cl and water contents of cells as functions of pH for washed cells at normal osmolality and for cells pre-equilibrated with various abnormal osmolalities in the presence of nystatin and subsequently washed to remove the nystatin. At all osmolalities the water movements in response to pH changes were 70 per cent of those predicted from the measured changes in Cl and the assumption that B and P were constant during the pH changes. At present there is no known way to reconcile these data with those of Gary-Bobo and Solomon (1968) nor has any explanation been provided for Dalmark's results (Dalmark, 1976). It is particularly difficult to imagine any type of nonideality which would predict the same ratio between the observed and expected volume changes for all osmolalities of the cell contents.

4 Mechanisms of restoration of anion and pH equilibrium after perturbation

Physiologically the most important anion and pH disequilibria result from CO_2 uptake from tissues and CO_2 loss in the lungs. In aqueous solution, CO_2 slowly hydrates to produce carbonic acid (H_2CO_3), which immediately dissociates to H and HCO_3. At equilibrium the H_2CO_3 concentration is about 1/400th that of dissolved CO_2, which in turn is about 10 μM in equilibrium with room air, and 1·3 mM in arterial blood ($pCO_2 = 40$ mmHg, 37°C). In unbuffered solution little CO_2 is converted to HCO_3 since the dissociation is stopped by the fall in pH before appreciable HCO_3 is formed. In solution buffered at pH 7·4 the reactions proceed until the HCO_3 concentration is about twenty times that of dissolved CO_2. Thus substantial uptake of CO_2 as HCO_3 requires adequate H buffering. In blood there are adequate buffers and a catalyst for CO_2 hydration, carbonic anhydrase (CA) within the cells. CO_2 uptake into blood, while more complex, is thus more rapid than in the simple solution. An outline of the mechanism is shown in Fig. 1.

On CO_2 addition, the CO_2 equilibrates rapidly across the cell membrane and some of it binds directly to Hb in the form of carbamino groups. This binding is quantitatively important in CO_2 transport from the tissues to the lungs, as described in an excellent review by Roughton in 1935 and again more recently in 1964. We shall, however, concentrate here on the mechanism which allows rapid uptake of CO_2 as HCO_3.

Within the cell in contrast to the process in plasma, the hydration of CO_2 to H_2CO_3 and dissociation to HCO_3 occurs rapidly because of the catalyst

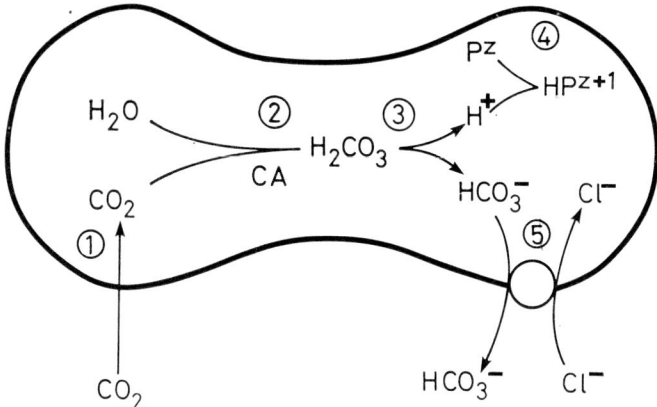

FIG. 1. Uptake of CO_2 into blood. (1) CO_2 rapidly diffuses across the red cell membrane. (2) The CO_2 is hydrated to form carbonic acid, a reaction catalysed by carbonic anhydrase. (3) The carbonic acid dissociates to H and HCO_3. (4) The H is buffered, mainly by Hb. (5) HCO_3 and Cl equilibrate across the membrane by neutral exchange. Here, and in Fig. 2, the reactions and transfers are shown, for simplicity, in the forward direction for CO_2 (or H) uptake. They are all in fact reversible as discussed in the text.

(CA) and the efficient buffering by Hb which prevents H from accumulating sufficiently to stop the dissociation. Thus as a result of CO_2 addition to the blood and the production of HCO_3 within the cell a disequilibrium for HCO_3 occurs. The equilibration of Cl and HCO_3 is achieved by Cl–HCO_3 exchange, Cl entering the cells and HCO_3 leaving, the well known Hamburger or Cl shift. In the absence of rapid Cl–HCO_3 exchange, the HCO_3 would be trapped within the cell and thus less could be formed before the increase in its concentration would stop further formation from CO_2. The exchange process allows the HCO_3 to distribute through both the cells and the plasma and in effect allows much the same uptake of CO_2 into blood as would occur were Hb and CA simply dissolved in the plasma.

Roughton (1935), however, did predict one difference in the behaviour of blood and a solution of Hb and CA. When CO_2 is added to blood, little H_2CO_3 is formed in the plasma within the time required for the steps described above to reach a pseudo-equilibrium (less than 1 sec). Thus initially pH_i decreases as H_2CO_3 is formed and dissociates inside, while pH_o does not. The subsequent adjustment of the pH's (Sirs, 1970; Forster and Crandall, 1975) and readjustment of the anion ratio takes much longer, being limited by the same factors which limit the speed of response to additions of acid or base discussed immediately below.

The processes of CO_2 diffusion and HCO_3–Cl exchange also allow equilibration of OH across the membrane and allow added acid or base to reach the intracellular buffers as shown in Fig. 2. On addition of acid to cells suspended in plasma some H_2CO_3 is formed which dehydrates at the uncatalysed rate to give CO_2. Even artificial solutions containing only the HCO_3 resulting from exposure to the CO_2 level of room air have enough HCO_3 for this effect to be important. Subsequent entry of CO_2 into the cell, catalysed conversion to H_2CO_3 and HCO_3, buffering of the H by Hb, and exchange of HCO_3 for Cl completes the equilibration process. The important catalytic role of CO_2 and HCO_3 in allowing acid or base to gain rapid access to intracellular buffers was shown by Jacobs and Stewart (1942), who found that addition of HCO_3 to HCO_3-free solutions greatly enhanced the rate of pH equilibration, which they assessed by monitoring the concomitant volume changes.

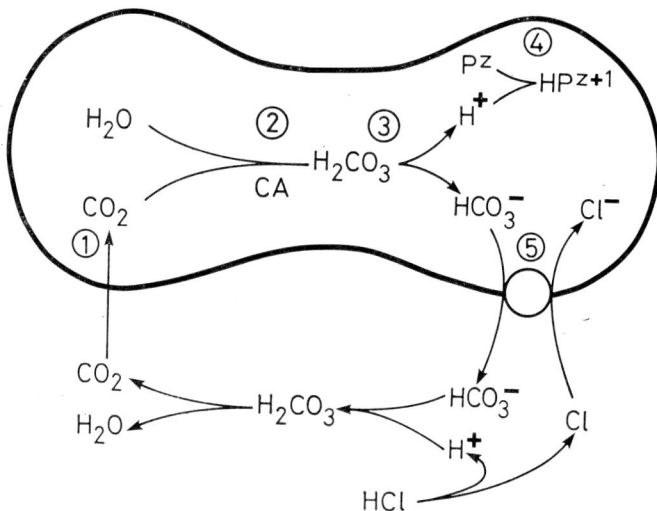

FIG. 2. Buffering of acid within the red cell. Here addition of HCl is considered. The acid not buffered externally by nonbicarbonate buffers combines with HCO_3 to form carbonic acid (6). This dehydrates, at the uncatalysed rate, to give CO_2 and H_2O (7). The next five steps are as for CO_2 uptake. The H is buffered by intracellular buffers and exchange of HCO_3 for external Cl completes the Jacobs-Stewart (1942) cycle.

The physiological event requiring rapid anion equilibration in blood is CO_2 uptake and loss. CA inside the cell allows just this. Sudden large (non-CO_2) acid and alkaline insults do not normally occur so that rapid pH equilibration is not necessary and the uncatalysed reaction between CO_2 and H_2CO_3 is sufficiently fast to deal with, for instance, the increase in acid metabolites produced during exercise. The properties of the hydration reaction and of CA are discussed in an exhaustive review by Maren (1967).

Jacobs and Stewart (1942) found that pH equilibration in a red cell suspension was more rapid after addition of acid than after addition of base. These observations can be explained by noting that the uncatalysed external reaction connecting CO_2 and H_2CO_3 is normally the slowest step in the equilibration process. At equilibrium the rate of hydration of CO_2 to H_2CO_3 and the reverse rate of dehydration are equal. After addition of acid sufficient to decrease by 1 or 2 units the pH of a cell suspension initially near pH 7, the concentration of external H_2CO_3 increases proportionally with the increase in H concentration and the rate of dehydration is likewise proportionally increased. There is sufficient HCO_3 to allow this formation of H_2CO_3, since near pH 7 the H_2CO_3 concentration is very much smaller than that of HCO_3. The decrease in external HCO_3 concentration which does occur will via steps 1–5 of Fig. 2 reduce the external CO_2 concentration and hence the uncatalysed rate of hydration. Thus, after addition of acid the net rate of dehydration is substantially faster than the initial rate of interconversion between CO_2 and H_2CO_3. Addition of sufficient base to increase the pH 1 or 2 units in the same initial cell suspension, immediately decreases proportionally the already small H_2CO_3 concentration, but since there was so little H_2CO_3, there is very little HCO_3 formed. This small amount via steps 1–5 of Fig. 2, but taken in reverse, can produce only a slight increase in external CO_2. Thus the rate of dehydration is substantially reduced and the external rate of hydration is slightly increased. Therefore, after addition of base the net rate of hydration is similar to the initial interconversion rate. The slowest step in the pH equilibration process is thus much faster after additions of acid than after additions of base.

These considerations also explain the observation of Jacobs and Stewart (1942) that adding CA to the external solution was more effective in increasing the rate of pH equilibration after additions of base than after additions of acid since the reaction catalysed was slower, before CA was added, in the former case than in the latter. After adding CA the rate-limiting step was at least partially shifted to some other stage of the cycle. Similarly explained is Jacobs and Stewart's observation that the effects of inhibiting internal CA were greater after addition of acid when the external reaction was least limiting.

To summarize this section, CA and Hb are osmotically isolated within a lipid membrane with the advantages outlined in the Introduction. For rapid access of H/OH across this membrane a special mechanism is required. The mechanism used is a rapid HCO_3–Cl exchange process, which together with rapid CO_2 transfer provides for pH equilibration.

5 The mechanism of exchange of Cl for HCO_3

Prior to the late 1960s, it was generally assumed that each species of anion separately came into equilibrium with its own electrochemical gradient (see e.g. Glynn, 1957; Roughton, 1964; Passow, 1969), though some evidence was available that anion exchange did not occur by free diffusion through aqueous pores (Tosteson, 1959; Davson, 1964; Passow, 1969). Until the late 1960s, however, no method was available to test experimentally whether the observed anion exchanges were the consequence of the requirement for electroneutrality (cations being effectively impermeant) or actually a property of the transport mechanism. The availability of substances such as valinomycin and gramicidin A (or D) which could make lipid membranes selectively permeable to cations (reviewed by Haydon and Hladky, 1972) provided the means to distinguish between these possibilities, since now a counter-ion to accompany any net anion flux was available.

If normal human red cells containing a high concentration of K and suspended in low K solution are made leaky to K then KCl loss should be exceedingly rapid if the anion transport process allows large net fluxes but very slow if only tightly coupled anion exchange is permitted. This experiment was first reported by Chappell and Crofts (1966) who added the highly selective K ionophore valinomycin to cells suspended in low K media. They found no K efflux. We now see that at that time there were two possible explanations of this result; either the anions could move only by exchange or valinomycin could not make the cells sufficiently leaky to K for measurable efflux to occur within a few minutes. The following year Harris and Pressman (1967) repeated this simple observation and demonstrated, as did Henderson and Chappell (1967), that if a H carrier was present as well as valinomycin, K efflux and H influx occurred. This demonstration of a net K flux in red cells, taken together with the demonstration of a large K conductance produced by valinomycin in black lipid membranes (Mueller and Rudin, 1967), made the second possibility most unlikely. Further confirmation came later from the finding that K tracer fluxes in red cells were enormously increased by adding valinomycin alone (Henderson et al., 1969; Hunter, 1971; Pressman and Heeb, 1971, 1972). Harris and Pressman (1967) concluded that K did not leak out of red cells exposed to valinomycin alone at an appreciable rate because the Cl present could not accompany any K loss. This demonstrated that the rapid ($t_{\frac{1}{2}}$ less than 1 sec) equilibration of labelled and unlabelled Cl across red cell membranes (Tosteson, 1959) must have resulted from a tightly coupled, electrically neutral exchange. The properties of the system which mediates this exchange are the subject of Fortes' chapter in this book.

Scarpa et al. (1968, 1970) examined the rate of swelling of cells suspended in NaCl after addition of gramicidin (D) which makes membranes permeable to Na, K and H (Henderson et al., 1969; Hladky and Haydon, 1972). They concluded that the rate of swelling was limited by electrically driven influx of Cl and that this rate was about 500 times less than that for tracer equilibration. This interpretation is incorrect. If the electrically driven Cl movements were this fast, Chappell and Crofts (1966) and Harris and Pressman (1967) would easily have measured appreciable K loss from red cells treated with valinomycin alone. The processes which occurred in the experiments of Scarpa et al. (1970) were an exchange of external Na for internal H via the gramicidin pore and an exchange of external chloride for internal OH (or HCO_3, etc.) via the anion exchange system. This dual-exchange process was proposed by Pressman and Heeb (1971, 1972) as the explanation of the cell shrinkage they observed for red cell ghosts treated with both valinomycin and FCCP.

Hunter (1971, 1973) was the first to determine the rate of the electrically driven net anion movement. He measured the rates of efflux of ^{42}K from valinomycin-treated cells into isotonic mixtures of NaCl and KCl and demonstrated that the slow ^{42}K efflux into isotonic NaCl was due to net KCl loss from the cell. Using the constant-field assumptions (Hodgkin and Katz, 1949) for the net fluxes of K and of Cl, he calculated P_{Cl}/P_{K-Val} = 0·055 and $P_{Cl} = 2·4 \times 10^{-8}$ cm sec^{-1} (37°C and pH 7·4). The anion conductance calculated from these data is c. 10^{-5} mho/cm^2. Hunter assumed that this conductance was due to Cl movements, presumably because Cl was present in much higher concentrations than HCO_3, OH or H. It should be noted, however, that a high conductance to any of these species could have given the same result since, for instance, electrically driven efflux of HCO_3, followed by HCO_3–Cl exchange, would appear as a net efflux of Cl. Hunter (1973) found that the HCO_3 constant-field permeability was insignificantly different from that of Cl. This finding leaves open as an alternative only the possibility of a surprisingly high conductance of the membrane to OH and/or H.

Tosteson et al. (1973) and Knauf and Fuhrmann (1974), using different methods for assessing KCl loss and different procedures of calculation, have confirmed Hunter's observations.

The value of the anion conductance obtained from Hunter's data is about 10^4 times less than that estimated (Tosteson, 1959) from Cl tracer equilibration. It is still, however, some 100 times larger than the upper limit of the K or Na conductance estimated from tracer fluxes (see for instance Glynn (1957) and the chapter by Beaugé and Lew). After the work of Warburg (1922) it was generally assumed, even though it had not been demonstrated, that for human red cells the membrane potential would closely follow the Cl equilibrium potential after any change in the Cl activity ratio. It follows from Hunter's results that this long-held assumption is, in fact, correct.

Measurements of the membrane potential across the human red cell membrane have established this point directly. Hoffman and Laris (1974), who first demonstrated that it is possible to use certain fluorescent dyes to assess this potential, found large changes in the expected direction when the exchangeable anion ratio was altered by replacing external Cl with inexchangeable anions such as gluconate or citrate. Hladky and Rink (1976a,b,c) have established the mechanism by which the fluorescent cation, diS-C_3-(5), reports membrane potential and have confirmed this finding of Hoffman and Laris (1974). When the Cl concentration ratio is altered the membrane potential of human red cells changes in the manner expected for a membrane whose conductance is primarily due to movements of Cl.

It is worth emphasizing that until Hunter's (1971) work it was not possible to decide whether the conductance of the human red cell membrane was due primarily to movements of cations or anions. The large anion movements could have been even more tightly coupled than they are. Interestingly in red cells of the amphibian (*Amphiuma*) the Cl conductance is of the same order as those of Na and K (see Lassen's chapter in this book) and so in this species the activities and permeability of all three ions are significant in determining the membrane potential.

Because the processes involved in pH equilibration are electrically neutral, there is no necessity for the membrane potential to affect directly the pH difference between a human red cell and the bathing medium. In fact, when the potential but not the Cl ratio is changed using valinomycin, there is initially no observable change in pH (Tosteson *et al.*, 1973; Hladky and Rink, 1976c). Thus the rapid anion exchange process maintains $Cl_i/Cl_o = OH_i/OH_o$, even in the face of substantial disequilibrium potentials. The slow change in pH which does follow occurs at the same time as the change in the chloride ratio and presumably both are due to the type of electrically driven flux of Cl, OH or H that was measured by Hunter (1973).

The low conductance of the red cell membrane in the presence of Cl, and/or HCO_3, implies that the extremely rapid Cl–HCO_3 exchange which does occur must take place via tightly coupled exchange. More generally, the low conductance of the membrane restricts the means by which any type of anion can replace Cl within the cell. Thus, even if the new type of anion could rapidly enter the cell by an independent conductance pathway, there would be no mechanism for the Cl or OH efflux required to preserve electroneutrality. This the demonstration that a normal Cl-containing cell is rapidly entered by the charged form of an anion implies that the anion has participated in a tightly coupled exchange with Cl.* Evidence, reviewed in the chapters by Motais and Fortes, is accumulating that the Cl–Cl, Cl–HCO_3 and Cl–A^- exchanges are all mediated by a single common mechanism.

It is probable that the exchange of SO_4 for Cl also occurs by an electrically neutral process even though SO_4 is divalent. Jennings (1976) has shown that the exchange of internal Cl for external SO_4 is accompanied by an equimolar shift of H into the cell. The resulting alkalinification of the medium could only be seen in rigorously CO_2- and HCO_3-free conditions ($HCO_3 < 4\,\mu M$). In the presence of traces of CO_2 and HCO_3 the Jacobs-Stewart cycle operated to maintain the partial equilibrium (Wilbrandt, 1942) between OH and Cl.

Evidence as to whether or not a particular anion can enter the cell by an electrically conducting pathway can be obtained from measurements of membrane potentials. Thus Hoffman and Laris (1974) reported that glutarate, gluconate and tartrate have constant-field permeabilities much less than that of Cl. Hladky and Rink (1976a) confirmed the earlier result for gluconate and added a rapidly exchanged anion (methylsulphate) to the list.

6 Can H or OH cross the membrane as such?

The functionally important movements of H or OH in red cells occur by the Jacobs-Stewart cycle, but it is still of some interest to enquire whether H or OH can be transported as such. An ingenious set of experiments by Jacobs and Parpart (1932) indicated that H transport was unlikely to account for pH equilibration when acid was added to cells suspended in artificial solutions. However, as Jacobs among others went on to show, even in these conditions movements of CO_2 and HCO_3 are likely to have accounted for the equilibration and their conclusion that OH was the transported species was not justified.

From the point of view presented in this chapter two questions arise. Can OH itself be transported by the anion exchange system? Is there any OH or H conductance?

Crandall *et al.* (1971) measured the time-course of the pH changes after

---

* A conceivable alternative explanation for the entry of a new species of anion is that the new species enormously enhances the Cl, HCO_3 or OH conductance of the membrane. However, the anion conductance as estimated from the rate of shrinking in the presence of valinomycin (Knauf and Fuhrmann, 1974) does not increase significantly when cells are suspended in mixtures of 125 mM NaCl with 25 mM $NaHCO_3$, Na pyruvate, Na glyoxylate, Na lactate, or Na oxalate (Hladky, unpublished). Oxalate, glyoxylate, lactate and pyruvate do enter rapidly in a charged form (Deuticke, 1972; Aubert and Motais, 1975).

large pH insults to cells suspended in HCO_3-free media. From their data, assuming that OH was the transported species, they calculated pH-dependent constant-field permeabilities for OH which were particularly large at acid pH. There are a number of difficulties which prevent acceptance of their interpretation. As was pointed out in the discussion after their symposium paper (Forster, 1972), it is unlikely that they had truly CO_2-free conditions. For the large acid insults used it is very likely that in fact pH equilibration was occurring by CO_2 entry and HCO_3–Cl exchange since, as noted earlier in this chapter, under these circumstances the Jacobs-Stewart cycle is particularly effective. For the large alkaline insults there could well have been more OH present than HCO_3 and the rate of pH change may then have been determined by Cl–OH exchange. However, even for the alkaline data which probably do relate to OH movements, the analysis must be repeated (the published data are insufficient) since a constant-field permeability is not an appropriate measure for anion exchange. Cousin *et al.* (1975), on the basis of finding very slow NH_4Cl-induced cell lysis in carefully controlled CO_2-free conditions, concluded that OH transport at pH 7·4 is very slow compared to the Jacobs-Stewart cycle in the presence of room CO_2. (In the NH_4Cl lysis a key step is Cl–HCO_3 or Cl–OH exchange, see Jacobs and Stewart, 1942). Forster and Crandall (1975), in referring to their work with Klocke, also note that OH transport is slow. It is clear that no quantitative assessment of OH movements via the exchange process is available and, indeed, except at very alkaline pH it is difficult to imagine such an assessment being achieved.

Callahan and Hoffman (1976) have suggested that the membrane anion conductance might be partly a H or OH conductance rather than a Cl conductance as normally assumed. The experimental basis for their suggestion was the observation of changes in fluorescence of a potential sensitive dye(diS-C_3-(5)) added to red cells subsequently subjected to pH disequilibria. Addition of base produced a hyperpolarization while addition of acid produced a depolarization. Hladky and Rink (unpublished) have also observed changes in dye fluorescence when such disequilibria are created and from their rapid onset and the observation that the initial changes are abolished when the membrane potential is held constant using valinomycin, it is concluded that the initial changes are indeed due to changes in the membrane potential. Thus when the OH ratio is transiently not equal to the Cl ratio, there is a shift of the membrane potential away from the Cl equilibrium potential. In the hands of the present authors these deviations were only 20–30 mV even with 2–3 pH unit gradients and therefore under these conditions the membrane potential is still dominated by the Cl ratio. Even so, the constant-field permeability for OH (or H, or both) appears to be remarkably high.

7 Conclusions

1. The distribution of the exchangeable anions in the human red blood cell, including OH, is determined by the conditions that (a) the osmolality of the cell interior must equal that of the external medium, and (b) both phases must be electrically neutral.

2. The rapid changes in cell composition which occur after addition of CO_2, acid or base to red cell suspensions are accounted for by considering the properties of the buffers, particularly haemoglobin; the presence inside the cell of carbonic anhydrase; and three types of passive transport across the membrane: (a) diffusion of CO_2, (b) movement of H_2O, and, (c) exchange of Cl for HCO_3.

3. Rapid Cl tracer equilibration and exchange of Cl for HCO_3 occur by a one for one, electrically neutral exchange process. Less than one charge is transferred for every 10^4 Cl ions which cross the membrane.

4. The rate at which OH *per se* can exchange with other anions is not known. The amount of OH transferred is in any case normally much less than that of HCO_3.

5. The conductance of the human red cell membrane is largely due to fluxes of Cl and HCO_3. The conductance due to H or OH movement appears, however, not to be negligible, which implies a surprisingly large constant-field permeability to one or the other, or both.

References

ADAIR, G. S. (1925). *J. Biol. Chem.* **63**, 517–545.
ADAIR, G. S. (1929). *Proc. Roy. Soc. (Lond.) A*, **126**, 16–24.
AUBERT, L. and MOTAIS, R. (1975). *J. Physiol.* **246**, 159–179.
BARCROFT, J. (1922). The Harvey Lectures, **17**, 146–163.
BATTAGLIA, F. C., MCGAUGHEY, H., MAKOWSKI, E. L. and MESCHIA, G. (1970). *Amer. J. Physiol.* **219**, 217–221.
BELLINGHAM, A. J., DETTER, J. C. and LENFANT, C. (1971). *J. Clin. Invest.* **50**, 70–706.
BENESCH, R. and BENESCH, R. E. (1967). *Biochem. Biophys. Res. Commun.* **26**, 162–167.
BURTON, A. C. (1969). *In* "Circulatory and Respiratory Mass Transport" (G. E. W. Wolstenholme and J. Knight, eds), pp. 67–84. Churchill, London.
CALLAHAN, T. J. and HOFFMAN, J. (1976). *Biophys. J.* **16**, 165a.
CHAPPELL, J. B. and CROFTS, A. R. (1966). In "Regulation of Metabolic Processes in Mitochondria" (J. M. Tager, S. Pape, E. Quagliariello and E. C. Slater, eds), pp. 293–316. Elsevier, Amsterdam.
CHRISTIANSEN, J., DOUGLAS, C. G. and HALDANE, J. S. (1914). *J. Physiol.* **48**, 244–271.
COUSIN, J. L., MOTAIS, R. and SOLA, F. (1975). *J. Physiol.* **253**, 385–399.
CRANDALL, E. C., KLOCKE, R. A. and FORSTER, R. E. (1971). *J. Gen. Physiol.* **57**, 664–683.

DALMARK, M. (1975). *J. Physiol.* 250, 65–84.
DALMARK, M. (1976). *Prog. Biophys. Molec. Biol.* 31, 145–164.
DAVSON, H. (1964). "A Textbook of General Physiology", 3rd edit. p. 325. Churchill, London. See also 4th edit. vol. 1, p. 466.
DEUTICKE, B. (1972). In "Oxygen Affinity of Hemoglobin and Red Cell Acid Base Status", (M. Rørth and P. Astrup, eds), Alfred Benzon Symp. IV, Munksgaard.
DICK, D. A. T. (1966). "Cell Water". Butterworth, London.
DILL, D. B., EDWARDS, H. T. and CONZOLAZIO, W. V. (1937). *J. Biol. Chem.* 118, 635–648.
DUHM, J. (1971). *Pflügers. Arch.* 326, 341–356.
DUHM, J. (1976). *Pflügers. Arch.* 363, 61–67.
FARMER, S. N. and MAIZELS, M. (1939). *Biochem. J.* 33, 280–289.
FITZSIMONS, E. J. and SENDROY, J. (1961). *J. Biol. Chem.* 236, 1565–1601.
FORSTER, R. E. (1972). In "Oxygen Affinity of Hemoglobin and Red Cell Acid-Base Status" (M. Rørth and P. Astrup, eds), Alfred Benzon Symp. IV, Munksgaard.
FORSTER, R. E. and CRANDALL, E. D. (1975). *J. Appl. Physiol.* 38, 710–718.
FUNDER, J. and WIETH, J. O. (1966a). *Acta Physiol. Scand.* 68, 234–235.
FUNDER, J. and WIETH, J. O. (1966b). *Scand. J. Clin. Lab. Invest.* 18, 167–180.
GARY-BOBO, C. M. and SOLOMON, A. K. (1968). *J. Gen. Physiol.* 52, 825–853.
GARY-BOBO, C. M. and SOLOMON, A. K. (1971). *J. Gen. Physiol.* 57, 283–289.
GLYNN, I. M. (1957). *Prog. in Biophys.* 8, 241–307.
HARRIS, E. J. and MAIZELS, M. C. (1952). *J. Physiol.* 118, 40–53.
HARRIS, E. J. and PRESSMAN, B. C. (1967). *Nature*, 216, 918–920.
HAYDON, D. A. and HLADKY, S. B. (1972). *Quart. Revs. Biophys.* 5, 187–282.
HENDERSON, P. J. F. and CHAPPELL, J. B. (1967). *Biochem. J.* 105, 16P.
HENDERSON, P. J. F., MCGIVAN, J. D. and CHAPPELL, J. B. (1969). *Biochem. J.* 111, 521–535.
HLADKY, S. B. and HAYDON, D. A. (1972). *Biochim. Biophys. Acta*, 274, 294–312.
HLADKY, S. B. and RINK, T. J. (1976a). *J. Physiol.* 258, 100P.
HLADKY, S. B. and RINK, T. J. (1976b). *J. Physiol.* 263, 287–319.
HLADKY, S. B. and RINK, T. J. (1976c). *J. Physiol.* 263, 213–214P.
HODGKIN, A. L. and KATZ, B. (1949). *J. Physiol.* 108, 37–77.
HOFFMAN, J. F. and LARIS, P. C. (1974). *J. Physiol.* 239, 519–552.
HUNTER, M. J. (1971). *J. Physiol.* 218, 49P.
HUNTER, M. J. (1973). Ph.D. Thesis, Cambridge University.
JACOBS, M. H. and PARPART, A. K. (1932). *Biol. Bull.* 62, 63.
JACOBS, M. H. and STEWART, D. R. (1942). *J. Gen. Physiol.* 25, 539–552.
JACOBS, M. H. and STEWART, D. R. (1947). *J. Cell. Comp. Physiol.* 30, 79–103.
JENNINGS, M. L. (1976). *J. Memb. Biol.* 28, 187–205.
KNAUF, P. A. and FUHRMANN, G. F. (1974). *Fed. Proc.* 33, 1591.
MAREN, T. H. (1967). *Physiol. Rev.* 47, 595–781.
MUELLER, P. and RUDIN, D. O. (1967). *Biochem. Biophys. Res. Commun.* 26, 398–404.
PASSOW, H. (1964). In "The Red Blood Cell" (E. Bishop and D. M. Surgenor, eds), pp. 71–145. Academic Press, New York and London.
PASSOW, H. (1969). *Prog. in Biophys.* 19, 423–467.
PONDER, E. (1948). "Hemolysis and Related Phenomena". Churchill, London.
PRESSMAN, B. C. and HEEB, M. J. (1971). *Biophys. J.* 11, 310a.
PRESSMAN, B. C. and HEEB, M. J. (1972). *In* "Molecular Mechanisms of Antibiotic

Action on Protein Biosynthesis and Membranes" (E. Muñoz, F. Garcia-Ferrandiz and D. Vazquez, eds), pp. 603, 614. Elsevier, Amsterdam.
RAND, R. P. and BURTON, A. C. (1964). *Biophys. J.* **4**, 115–135.
RAPOPORT, S. and GUEST, G. M. (1939). *J. Biol. Chem.* **131**, 675–689.
ROUGHTON, F. J. W. (1935). *Physiol. Rev.* **15**, 241–296.
ROUGHTON, F. J. W. (1964). *In* "Handbook of Physiology" (W. O. Fenn and H. Rahn, eds), vol. 1, pp. 767–825. Am. Physiol. Soc., Washington.
SCARPA, A. CECCHETTO, A. and AZZONE, G. F. (1968). *Nature*, **219**, 529–531.
SCARPA, A., CECCHETTO, A. and AZZONE, G. F. (1970). *Biochim. Biophys. Acta*, **219**, 179–188.
SIGGARD-ANDERSEN, O. (ed) (1974). "The Acid-Base Status of the Blood". Williams and Wilkins, Baltimore.
SIRS, J. A. (1970). *In* "Blood Oxygenation" (D. Hershey, ed). Plenum, London.
TOSTESON, D. C. (1959). *Acta Physiol. Scand.* **46**, 19–41.
TOSTESON, D. C., GUNN, R. B. and WIETH, J. O. (1973). *In* "Erythrocytes, Thrombocytes, Leucocytes" (E. Gerlach, K. Moser, E. Deutsch and E. Wilmanns, eds), pp. 62–66. Georg Thieme, Stuttgart.
VAN SLYKE, D. D., WU, H. and MCLEAN, F. C. (1923). *J. Biol. Chem.* **56**, 765–849.
WARBURG, E. J. (1922). *Biochem. J.* **XVI**, 152–340.
WHITTAKER, S. R. C. and WINTON, F. R. (1933). *J. Physiol.* **78**, 339–369.
WILBRANDT, W. (1942). *Pflüg. Archiv. Ges. Physiol.* **246**, 291–306.
WILLIAMS, T. F., FORDHAM, C. C. III, Hollander, W. Jr. and Welt, L. G. (1959). *J. Clin. Invest.* **38**, 1587–1598.

Electrical potential and conductance of the red cell membrane

U. V. LASSEN
Zoophysiological Laboratory B, August Krogh Institute, University of Copenhagen, Denmark

1 Introduction	137
2 Estimates of membrane potential of red cells	139
2.1 Microelectrode techniques	140
2.2 Equilibrium distribution of permeant ions	146
2.3 Use of fluorescent dyes to monitor membrane potential	148
3 Membrane conductance of red cells	152
3.1 Methods employing current passage	153
3.2 Indirect estimates of membrane conductance	156
4 Calcium-induced changes in membrane potential	165
5 Concluding remarks	168
Acknowledgements	169
References	170

1 Introduction

The commonly used phrase "membrane potential" in biological literature is defined as the difference in electrical potential between the cytosol and the external fluid. The membrane potential is an important driving force for passive movement of ions across the membrane. At the same time its magnitude reflects the steady-state activities of ions in cytosol and external fluid in relation to the passive conductances and possible pumps for the individual ions. The value of the membrane potential only tells the net result of the multiplicity of parameters generating it. If we can isolate one or more of these parameters, changes in membrane potential can give information about the function of the membrane not readily obtainable in other ways, the potential being a sensitive "indicator" of net charge movements.

This chapter deals with the membrane potential and to some extent with the membrane conductance of the red cell. As it will be discussed repeatedly below, the absolute magnitude of the membrane potential of red cells is different from that of almost any other cell types in being small (-10 to -15 mV). This seems to be the case regardless of whether the cell is nucleated (e.g. avian, amphibian) or nonnucleated (mammalian). What is even more astonishing is the lack of difference in calculated membrane potential between cells with high intracellular K concentration (most species) and with low intracellular K, high Na concentration (e.g. dog, cat, mutants of sheep). One then immediately asks the question if the low membrane potential is of importance for the red cell in its function. The answer may be simple: the red cell serves a function both in the transport of O_2 to the tissues and in the return of CO_2 to the lungs. During the latter process the exchange of HCO_3^- and Cl^- across the membrane plays an important role (the Hamburger shift). As has been well documented in recent years (see e.g. Gunn et al., 1973; Dalmark, 1976) this process is mediated by an ion exchange system with about equal affinities for HCO_3^- and Cl^-. In order not to have this exchange limited intracellular Cl^-, it seems desirable to have a relatively high intracellular Cl^- concentration. Quantitatively this argument may seem less important at first sight. The mean circulatory shift of Cl^- between red cells and plasma is only about 5 per cent of the intracellular pool (Siggaard-Andersen, 1974). Therefore the need for intracellular Cl^- as exchange partner for HCO_3^- could have been fulfilled at lower cytosol concentrations than actually found. However, the figure of 5 per cent is a mean for arterial blood in relation to mixed venous blood at rest. In parts of the capillary bed and during heavy exercise this figure is several times larger.

In the steady state (all concentrations constant), and in the absence of active transport of anions, the membrane potential must be created mainly by the concentration gradients for Na and K (with due allowance for possible contributions from an electrogenic Na–K pump system). If the permeabilities for these two major cations are nearly equal as in the case of red cells, the membrane potential is small in absolute magnitude This will result in an equilibrium distribution for the Cl^- (and other permeable anions) with a small concentration gradient across the membrane. Furthermore, in such a system the chloride concentration in the cells will be nearly insensitive to whether the cells are high K or low K.

If the rapid exchange transport of Cl^- was accompanied by a large membrane conductance for Cl^- in comparison to other ions, the membrane potential would also under non-steady-state situations be close to the Nernst potential for chloride. But as suggested by Tosteson in 1959, the finding of a rapid exchange does not necessarily mean a large membrane conductance for Cl^-. This very point is the background for many of the experimental findings to be discussed in the following. Important information can be deduced from the magnitude of the membrane potential in a number of conditions where the chloride ions are not in equilibrium. Of special interest is the magnitude of the chloride conductance in relation to the chloride exchange rate. The electrical measurements, performed either directly with microelectrodes, or indirectly using fluorescent dyes, confirm and extend the notion that nearly all of the transport of monovalent anions proceeds in an electrically silent fashion.

The intracellular Ca^{2+} activity has an influence on the membrane conductance to K^+ (see e.g. Riordan and Passow, 1973), thereby indirectly modifying the magnitude of the membrane potential. A number of experimental changes in potential can be related to this mechanism, which seems to be a feature of many other cell types as well (see e.g. Baker, 1975). The Ca^{2+}-induced increase in K conductance in red cells may be part of a physiological regulatory system or it may be part of a "suicide mechanism" (Lew and Beaugé, 1977) and not relevant in the normal intracellular Ca^{2+} concentration range (Lew and Ferreira, 1976). Specific ionophores for divalent cations (e.g. Reed and Lardy, 1972) have given important new data about the effect of changes in intracellular Ca^{2+}. The possibility of influencing the membrane potential in this fashion supports the concept that, at least in some red cell types, there exist latent K channels which upon full activation represent a sufficiently large conductance to cause the net loss of KCl to be limited by the Cl^- conductance.

The technical details for potential measurements in single cells such as erythrocytes are of great importance for the validity of conclusions from experimental data. The experimental possibilities and difficulties are discussed before the presentation of results and the evaluation of possible physiological implications.

A prominent feature of the present reviews is the incorporation of data that have not previously been published. It is the hope of the author hereby to update the presentation in order to make it more valuable for the specialist in the field and to draw a clearer picture for the nonspecialist.

2 Estimates of membrane potential of red cells

The rapid transport of monovalent anions across the red cell membrane (Luckner, 1939; Tosteson, 1959; Dalmark and Wieth, 1970) led for a number of years to the conclusion that the membrane potential of these cells always was equal to the equilibrium potential for Cl. As discussed in greater detail below, "this concept was supported by the lack of evidence for an active transport of Cl and by the fact that the ratio between internal and external Cl concentrations depended only on pH" (loc. cit. Cotterell and Whittam, 1971). Furthermore, this concentration ratio agrees closely with the inverse of the concentration ratio for hydrogen ions (Van Slyke *et al.*, 1923; Harris and Maizels, 1952; Funder and Wieth, 1966). These facts taken together, there seemed for a number of years to be little need for attempting measurements of the membrane potential of red cells. The determination of the chloride distribution ratio under a given experimental situation is relatively easy—certainly much more so than the potential measurements to be discussed. This may be the reason why the first published attempts to determine membrane potentials across the red cell membrane (Chang, 1966) were made primarily for the sake of comparing the electrical parameters of this cell type (*Amphiuma* erythrocytes) with those obtained in excitable cells.

The Nernst equation gives the magnitude of the equilibrium potential (E_i) for any permeable ion across the membrane:

$$E_j = \frac{RT}{z_j F} \left[\ln \frac{C_{j,\,o}}{C_{j,\,i}} + \ln \frac{\delta_{j,\,o}}{\delta_{j,\,i}} \right] \tag{1}$$

where j is the ion species, z the valency, C the concentration, δ the activity coefficient, the subscripts o and i indicating outside and inside respectively. R, T and F have their usual meanings. What is interesting in this context is that the ratio of the activity coefficients, e.g. for Cl, is not an easy figure to determine directly. On the contrary, given the magnitude of the membrane potential this ratio can be calculated. This fact led Lassen and Sten-Knudsen (1968) to investigate the membrane potential and resistance of human red cells. Shortly after Jay and Burton (1969) published similar studies. Both of these groups used microelectrodes to measure the potential difference between cytosol and suspending medium. Although the results obtained on human red cells have to be considered as questionable, this type of direct approach is the base of most of the present knowledge of membrane potential (and partially of conductance) of red cells in general.

2.1 MICROELECTRODE TECHNIQUES

The recording of a "resting" membrane potential calls for electrodes which do not themselves introduce potentials into the measurement. This requirement is met with the conventional 3 M KCl-filled glass micropipette and on Ag–AgCl rod (for a comprehensive review, see Geddes, 1972). Typically, the electrode has a tip diameter of 0·2–0·5 μm and a resistance (measured in Ringer's or plasma) of 10–30 MΩ. Even though such electrodes are the best available for the purpose, they have a number of inherent problems. First, even these small tips are large in relation to the mammalian red cell thickness of about 2 μm. Furthermore, the effect on the recorded potential of the shift in electrolyte composition and overall conductivity of the fluid around the tip before and after penetration of the membrane has to be evaluated. After using a number of simplifying assumptions and employing a Henderson regime (constant concentration gradient from microelectrode interior to surrounding fluid) Lassen and Sten-Knudsen (1968) estimated this change to be small, in the order of 1 mV. However, a strict physicochemical assessment of the absolute magnitude of the junction potentials is difficult (see e.g. Tasaki and Singer, 1968). This latter problem will not be dealt with, partly because basic questions remain to be solved and partly because several of the experimental data are related to *changes* in membrane potential. Under such circumstances the liquid junction potentials will remain essentially constant and thus have a minor influence on the recorded changes in potential.

2.1.1 Experimental procedures

The red cell membrane is readily deformable (see e.g. Braasch, 1971) and the friction between a single cell and the suspending medium is small. These two facts taken together indicate that special measures have to be taken to enable the tip of a microelectrode to penetrate the red cell membrane. In electrophysiology, the cells to be punctured are usually fixed as part of a tissue (or large, as in the case of giant axons and single muscle fibres). In the case of erythrocytes one can either mechanically fix the cells in an experimental chamber or advance the electrode rapidly so that micropuncture is performed before the cell has moved away. The latter of these two approaches was chosen by Lassen and Sten-Knudsen (1968), who devised a piezoelectric electromechanical transducer which, upon application of 50–250 V, gave an axial advancement of the microelectrode of 10–50 μm in 2 msec. The flexibility of the barium titanate piezoelectric ceramics and unintended transverse movements made the original construction less desirable in later experiments on Ehrlich ascites cells (Lassen *et al.*, 1971) and giant red cells from the salamander, *Amphiuma means* (Lassen, 1972). The movement by the piezoelectric transducer presently used in the author's laboratory is considerably more precise, at the same time sacrificing the "long" range of advancement of the version mentioned above. This transducer employs tubular piezoelectric ceramics and advances the tip of the electrode 1 μm in 50 μsec (400 V pulse, critically damped). The linear velocity of advancement is not impressive, 2 cm sec^{-1}, but the acceleration of the electrode tip, when held against the cell prior to release of the piezoelectric "gun", is sufficient for penetration of the membrane. This construction is usable when studying giant red cells, but will invariably cause mammalian red cells to burst.

Jay and Burton (1969) used the tendency of human red cells to stick to a glass surface to hold the cells fixed. By moving the microscope stage, the cells were impaled by a nonmoving microelectrode. This technique gave more stable recordings than reported by Lassen and Sten-Knudsen (1968) but with essentially the same results and the same inherent errors related to a leak in the cell membrane around the microelectrode tip. This fact will seriously influence the validity of the results as discussed below.

The larger the cell, the relatively smaller are the technical problems with micropuncture. Since the report of Gulliver (1875) on comparative morphology of red cells, it has been known that *Amphiuma* erythrocytes are probably the largest in nature. This was obviously the reason why Chang (1966) used *Amphiuma* red cells in an attempt to measure the membrane potential, resistance and capacitance of an erythrocyte. The same fact brought Hoffman and Lassen (1971) to measure the membrane potential and resistance of red cells from *Amphiuma means*, employing the above-mentioned piezoelectric device to impale the cells. Despite the large size of *Amphiuma* erythrocytes, micropuncture is difficult. Therefore, because the *Amphiuma* red cell is becoming a "cell of reference" for electrical measurements, alternative procedures for micropuncture have been attempted. Smith and Levinson (1975) fixed the cells on a La^{3+}-coated glass surface and got relatively stable recordings. Even more promising is the technique of Stoner and Kregenow (1976) who, based on the work of Burg *et al.* (1966) on kidney tubules, sucked *Amphiuma* red cells into a silicone resin-lined glass capillary. Provided the inner diameter of the glass tube was 10–15 μm, the erythrocyte was cylindrical and with hemispherical ends. Voltage across the cell membrane was measured by a microelectrode, positioned within the glass tube in such a way as to impale the entering erythrocyte. Probably due to the mechanical stability of this system, the measured potentials stayed stable for much longer periods than those reported by Hoffman and Lassen (1971), Lassen (1972) and Lassen *et al.* (1974, 1976). Furthermore, Stoner and Kregenow (1976) reported that their method allowed determination of ^{36}Cl fluxes across single cells with or without electrical current passage. This figure is of importance when evaluating the conductance of the red cell membrane in relation to anion exchange.

2.1.2 *Results and interpretations*

In the following we will first discuss the direct measurements of membrane potential in human red cells. Lassen and Sten-Knudsen (1968) reported that the potential drop upon penetration of the membrane never exceeded −14 mV. Despite the use of a piezoelectric driver as described above, it turned out to be exceedingly difficult to obtain a reasonable number of "successful" penetrations. Therefore, the published results were confined to cells in serum (pH 7·35–7·40) at 37°C. Figure 1 shows recordings from

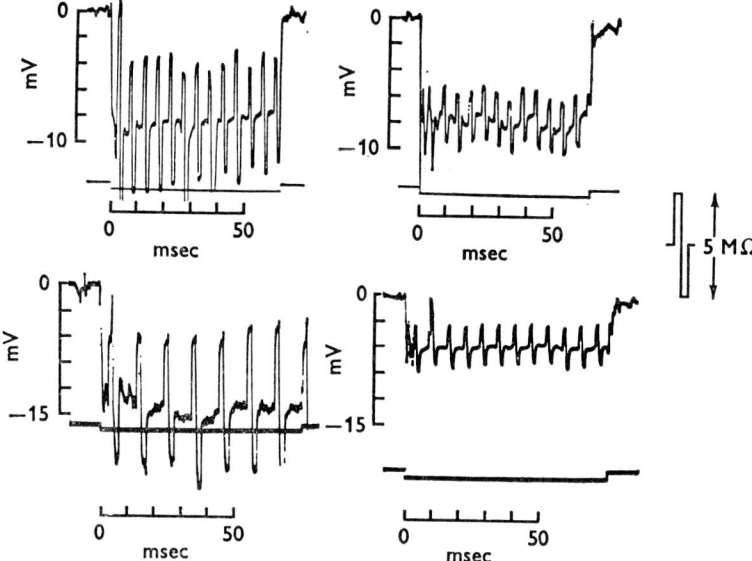

FIG. 1. Results of relatively stable potential measurements in human red cells. The lower traces in each frame indicate the voltage to the piezoelectric electromechanical transducer that advances the microelectrode. Upper traces indicate the potential changes recorded by the microelectrode. The diphasic swings indicate the increase in resistance with the electrode tip inside the cell. Abscissa: time in msec. Ordinates: upper traces mV; lower traces not calibrated. (Lassen and Sten-Knudsen, 1968, by permission.)

this work. The value of the potential drop with the electrode tip in the cell is shown. The diphasic pulses indicate the increase in resistance. Jay and Burton (1969) got more uniform potential values of -8.0 ± 0.21 mV (SEM) well in agreement with the calculated equilibrium potential for chloride at pH 7·4. Thus there was apparent conformity of the results with the values expected if the ratio of chloride activities equalled the ratio of concentrations. However, in neither of the studies was the potential studied as a function of varying equilibrium distributions for chloride. Furthermore, as mentioned by Lassen and Sten-Knudsen (1968): "Even with the very fine micropipettes used in this study, the cells are still small in size. This may in itself lead to damage of the cells during attempts at impalement. This makes it likely that the impalement often resulted in a leak between the cell and its surroundings, so that lower potentials and resistances were measured." This statement turned out to be more true than realized at the time of writing. In a microelectrode study of the membrane potential of Ehrlich ascites cells, Lassen et al. (1971) demonstrated a discharge of the membrane potential in immediate relation to the puncture. After about 0·5–2 msec the potential reached a stable value similar to that reported by other groups in studies on ascites cells. This type of recording was ascribed to a leak around the electrode tip. If the resistance of the leak pathway is much smaller than the resistance of the nonperturbed membrane, the potential across the membrane will dissipate through the low resistance. These problems may, at least in part, be related to the nature of the glass microelectrodes. The outer surface of the electrode is probably hydrated and therefore also likely to conduct current along the wall. In addition, as the cell membrane is penetrated after dimbling by the electrode tip, some of the surface coat of the cell may be drawn along the electrode surface. Both of these effects will tend to give a leak around the electrode, the magnitude of the leak being enlarged by possible vibrations of the electrode tip immediately after penetration.

In a given experimental situation, the relative damage of the cell will be smaller the larger the cell. The red cells of *Amphiuma* have a surface area of 5000 μm^2 (Chang, 1966) (or some thirty times larger than that of human red cells). Chang (1966) reported relatively small membrane potentials in the *Amphiuma* red cell ($-5·8 \pm 0·7$ mV (S.D.)), consistent with small increases in resistance with the electrode inside the cell. Both of these facts indicate that the experimental procedure caused excessive damage to the cell. Thus, the membrane potentials reported by Chang (1966) may, despite the size of the cell, have been subject to the same uncertainties as the data from human red cells.

If the leak has a certain magnitude, and provided that it can be made reasonably small, it is still of advantage to use a large cell for potential measurements. In this way the membrane capacitance to be discharged is larger, thus leading to a lower rate of discharge. Considering the data of good microelectrodes connected to an optimally neutralized "negative capacitance" input amplifier (see Lassen *et al.*, 1971), it should be possible to measure the membrane potential of *Amphiuma* red cells before the original potential was seriously influenced by the impaling electrode. This was the experimental basis for the study by Hoffman and Lassen (1971) and subsequent works by the present author and his colleagues. Figure 2 shows a typical recording from an *Amphiuma* red cell. Immediately after penetration of the cell membrane there is a sharp downward deflection of the voltage trace; after having reached a minimum the potential decays to a less negative value in about 1–2 msec. Provided that the drop in potential is fast as compared to the rate of decay, the initial drop in potential can be used as a measure of the membrane potential. The stable potential reached after a few milliseconds is presumably a diffusion potential between the cytoplasm of the damaged cell and the surrounding medium. In accordance with this view, the magnitude of the stable potential varies little with changes in the external medium (pH or ionic composition).

In the experiments on changes in membrane potential of *Amphiuma* red cells upon variation in pH of the medium, there is a very good correlation between the potentials recorded before the decay (Hoffman and Lassen, 1971; Lassen, 1972) and those recorded in the system of Stoner and Kregenow (1976) (see Fig. 4). For more comprehensive reviews of these problems see Lassen *et al.* (1971) and Lassen and Rasmussen (1977).

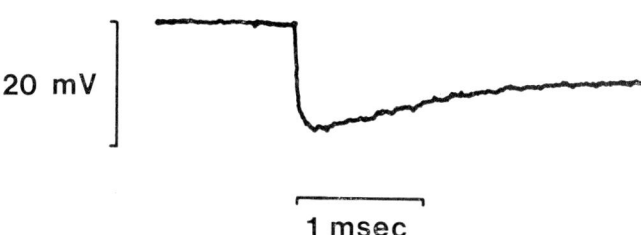

FIG. 2. After penetration of the cell membrane there is a sharp drop in potential followed by a slow decay to a less negative value. The membrane potential is taken as the magnitude of the maximal potential change immediately after impalement of the cell. Abscissa: time in msec. Ordinate: mV. 17°C, pH 7·2.

From the above arguments it may seem as if it was unconditionally desirable to obtain stable measurements. However, if a conventional microelectrode is left in a cell, the leak of KCl from the tip alters the internal concentrations of K and Cl. Nastuk and Hodgkin (1950) estimated the leak from a 0·4 µm electrode tip to be in the order of 6×10^{-14} mol sec^{-1}. If this figure is applied to an *Amphiuma* red cell (volume 13·000 µm³) and a tip diameter of the electrode of 0·2 µm, the rate of rise of intracellular KCl concentration is 1·2 mM sec^{-1}. In fast measurements of membrane potential this figure is insignificant, but in the results reported by Smith and Levinson (1975) and Stoner and Kregenow (1976) the increasing intracellular KCl concentration must be considered when evaluating membrane potentials with the microelectrode left in the cell. Apart from the leak from the electrode, the membrane potential may also be influenced by Ca leaking into the cell at the site of damage (Lassen *et al.*, 1974). This may be the reason for the unexpectedly negative potentials reported by Smith and Levinson (1975).

As evident from the above remarks, microelectrode measurements of membrane potential of mammalian red cells are not possible with the present techniques. Whether an extremely fine or even a different kind of electrode would alleviate this situation remains to be seen.

In the case of giant red cells, the measurements seem to be reliable enough to yield valuable information. However, both with these cells and any other single cells in suspension, the measurements of membrane potential and of membrane conductance with microelectrodes have to be carefully analysed in the light of possible artefacts before relying too much on the results.

In the remainder of this presentation such considerations have been taken into account. The results of experiments under a number of different conditions will be presented. As far as possible, electrical measurements will be compared to other studies of membrane properties, thereby testing the results by independent methods.

2.2 EQUILIBRIUM DISTRIBUTION OF PERMEANT IONS

It is well established that Cl is passively distributed across the red cell membrane. Allowing sufficient time for equilibrium, the ratio of the intracellular to extracellular Cl concentrations ($r_{(Cl)}$) can be used as a measure of membrane potential (with appropriate knowledge or assumptions of the ratio of activity coefficients).

In a careful study, Funder and Wieth (1966) confirmed and extended earlier works on the Cl distribution in human red cells as a function of pH of the plasma. They established an empirical, linear relation between external pH and $r_{(Cl)}$ over a range of more than two pH units

$$r_{(Cl)} = 3 \cdot 319 \pm 0 \cdot 028 \text{ (S.D.)} - (0 \cdot 359 \pm 0 \cdot 010 \text{ (S.D.)}) \times (\text{pH}_{\text{plasma}}).$$

A similar expression was found when determining extra- and intracellular *activities* of H$^+$ using glass electrodes. H$^+$ (and OH) also seems to be passively distributed across the membrane. The parallel variation with pH of $r_{(OH)}$ and $r_{(Cl)}$ is taken to indicate that the membrane potential indeed varies with the chloride distribution ratio. There was a small but significant difference between the absolute values of $r_{(Cl)}$ and $r_{(OH)}$. At identical pH values in plasma, $r_{(Cl)}$ exceeded $r_{(OH)}$ by 0·052. As justly commented by the authors: "It is not possible to determine the cause of this systematic difference. A difference in the activity coefficients of chloride in cells and plasma, protein binding of chloride, trapping of extracellular chloride between packed cells, and errors arising from liquid junction potentials in the pH measurements of lysed cells are all probable causes". However, the difference between the two types of measurements is small, at pH 7·4 the value for the membrane potential as calculated from chloride distribution is −11 mV and that calculated from glass electrode measurements −13 mV.

As no reliable direct measurements of mammalian red cells are available, it would be of interest to know the distribution of other permeable substances devoid of active transport or intracellular binding. The weak acid 5,5-dimethyl-2,4-oxazolidinedione (DMO) has been extensively employed to determine intracellular pH (see Waddell and Bates, 1969). Both with DMO and with determination of intracellular CO_2 concentration (for subsequent calculation of HCO_3^- distribution), there is a general agreement with the above calculated values for the membrane potential for human red cells. Bromberg *et al.* (1965) and Fitzsimons and Sendroy (1961) found nearly the same relation between extracellular pH and Cl–OH distribution as that reported by Funder and Wieth (1966). From all of these studies it is reasonable to conclude that the membrane potential of human red cells under physiological conditions is small, about -10 to -14 mV *provided that H^+ (OH^-) and Cl^- have reached equilibrium.* This latter statement will prove to be important when discussing experiments with sudden shifts in external Cl concentration or membrane potential. During such conditions the recently reported use of ^{31}P nuclear magnetic resonance to follow intracellular pH on intact cells (Moon and Richards, 1973) may prove applicable.

From the above considerations it is expected (see also chapters by Fortes and by Hladky and Rink, present volume) that the measured potential of red cells should follow the pH induced changes of E_{Cl}. Figure 3 shows compiled results of measurements from different sources of Cl distribution as functions of extracellular pH. On the same graph is plotted the "$r_{(Cl)}$" calculated from microelectrode measurements on *Amphiuma* red cells. It may be noted that the calculated ratios parallel the $r_{(Cl)}$ directly measured in these cells. The consistently lower values for the measured ratios in relation to the calculated (from V_m) have been ascribed by J. F. Hoffman (personal communication) to partial exclusion of Cl from the nucleus. If such an effect is taken into account, there is a close correlation between V_m and calculated E_{Cl} (from corrected values of $r_{(Cl)}$) (see Lassen, 1972). Whether or not a low nuclear concentration of Cl is a physiological fact remains to be investigated in detail. It is interesting, however, that Pietrzyk and Heinz (1974) in a study on Ehrlich ascites cells found that after fractionation of lyophilized cells in nonaqueous solvents, Na and Cl were closely associated with DNA. This was taken to indicate that Cl was present in a higher concentration in the nucleus than in the cytoplasm.

For the sake of comparison the pH dependence of $r_{(Cl)}$ in human and chicken red cells is plotted in Fig. 3. The differences is slope and absolute magnitude of $r_{(Cl)}$ at any given pH value seem to be significant but will not be discussed in the present context.

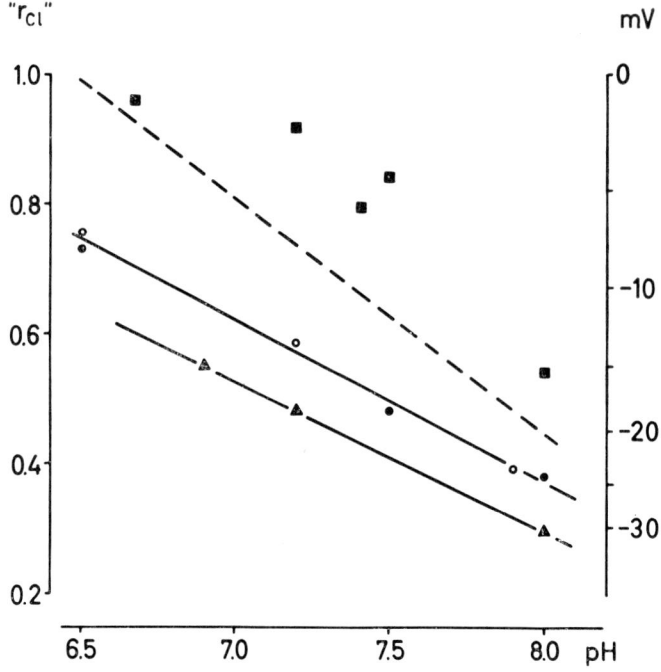

FIG. 3. Relationship between membrane potentials and chloride distribution in red cells as functions of extracellular pH (after equilibration). Measured membrane potentials in *Amphiuma* red cells: open circles, data by Hoffman and Lassen (see Lassen, 1972); filled circles, data by Stoner and Kregenow (1976). Chloride distribution ratios (r_{Cl}): triangles, *Amphiuma* red cells (Hoffman, personal communication); squares, chicken red cells (Brahm and Wieth, 1976); broken line, regression line as reported by Funder and Wieth (1966) from experiments on human red cells. Abscissa: extracellular pH. Left ordinate: ratio between intra- and extracellular chloride concentrations; right ordinate: measured membrane potentials or Nernst potentials for chloride (as calculated from "r_{Cl}" (17°C). See text for further discussion.

2.3 USE OF FLUORESCENT DYES TO MONITOR MEMBRANE POTENTIAL

Microelectrode studies are at present limited to very large red cells, and measurements of equilibrium distribution, e.g. of Cl, are confined to situations where the cells have had ample time to equilibrate with the surrounding medium. In the latter case and especially when employing inhibitors of anion transport (phloretin, phlorizin, dipyridamole) it is difficult to ascertain that equilibrium is attained.

Thus there is an obvious need for nondestructive methods for estimating membrane potential of red cells. Such a method should preferably be applicable to mammalian red cells where the magnitudes of membrane potential derived from other methods (e.g. valinomycin treatment) depend heavily on the particular model used for calculation. It was therefore a solution if the changes in birefringence, light scattering or dye-induced fluorescence as used in the study of axons (see e.g. Cohen, 1973; Davila et al., 1973; Cohen et al., 1974; Sims et al., 1974) were applicable to red cell suspensions. Birefringence and light scattering can be ruled out for a variety of reasons, and fluorescence of the commonly used 1-anilino-8-naphthalene sulphonate (ANS) has the disadvantage of being only slightly sensitive to changes in membrane potential (Conti et al., 1971). Furthermore, emitted light is strongly absorbed in a suspension of red cells. Finally, when employed in higher concentrations, ANS seems to induce a K leak in *Amphiuma* red cells (Fortes et al., unpublished) and to inhibit the anion transport in human red cells (Fortes and Hoffman, 1974). Thus it was an important observation that certain carbocyanine dyes responded to changes in membrane potential of axons with much larger changes in fluorescence than described for previously used compounds (Davila et al., 1973; Cohen et al., 1974). In the first communication, Davila et al. (1973) pointed out that this class of dyes might also prove applicable to red cells for measurement of membrane potential. Hoffman and Laris (1974) used 3,3′-dihexyl-2,2′-oxacarbocyanine (diO-C_6-(3)) and a related dye (diS-C_3-(5)) to estimate the membrane potential of human red cells and to compare the few available data from microelectrode measurements (Hoffman and Lassen, 1971) with fluorescence measurements. Figure 4 shows a typical recording from the work of Hoffman and Laris (1974) which illustrates the method of measurement. Upon addition of dye to a dilute red cell suspension, there is first an increase in fluorescence (as expected) followed by a decrease to a steady level. If the K conductance of the cell membranes is then increased by addition of valinomycin, the subsequent steady levels of fluorescence depend on the K concentration of the suspending medium. Figure 4 illustrates an important point in the method: at a certain K concentration, the fluorescence stays constant after the valinomycin addition. This "null point" is taken as the point where $E_K = E_{Cl} = V_m$ and thus represents a reference for calibrating the method. Especially with diS-C_3-(5) there was good agreement between the E_K and E_{Cl} calculated from experimentally determined concentrations at the "null point". In their study, Hoffman and Laris (1974) assumed that P_{Na} under all experimental conditions was much smaller than P_{Cl} and P_K in the presence of valinomycin. This led to a simplified version of the Goldman (constant field) equation:

$$V_m = \frac{RT}{F} \ln \frac{\alpha K_o + Cl_i}{\alpha K_i + Cl_o}$$

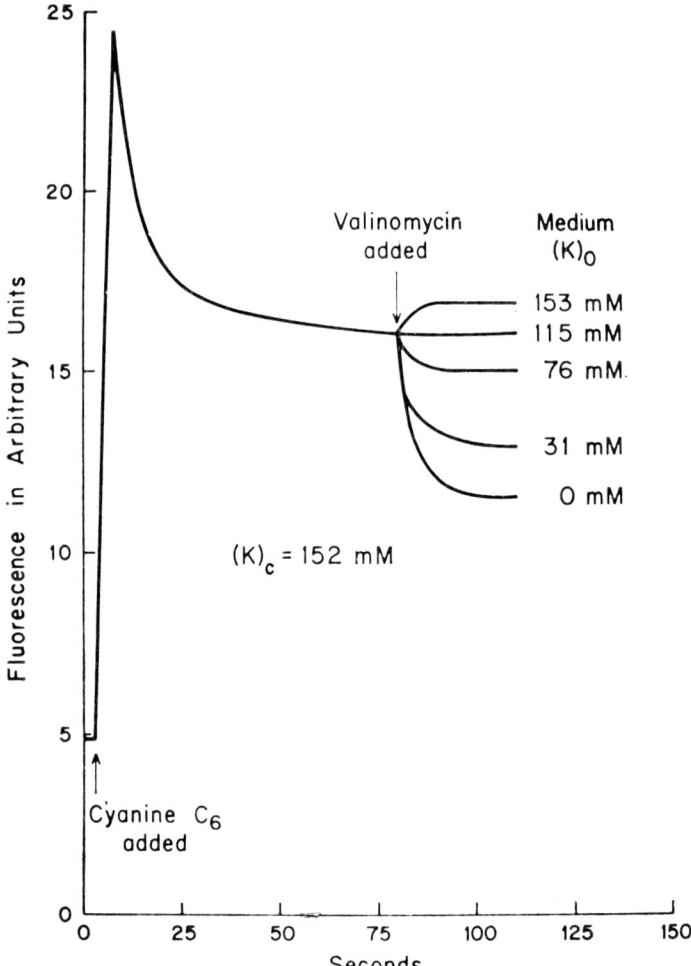

FIG. 4. Fluorescent intensity of a carbocyanine dye (DiO-C_6-(3)) in a 0·33 per cent suspension of human red cells. The figure represents tracings obtained in an experiment employing different extracellular K concentrations. After addition of valinomycin (final concentration 10^{-6} M) the shifts in fluorescence indicate changes in membrane potential, depending on K_o. Abscissa: time in sec. Ordinate: fluorescence in arbitrary units. (Hoffman and Laris, 1974, by permission.)

where α denotes $P_{K\text{-}V_{al}}/P_{Cl}$ (P being the permeabilities of the ions). Subscripts o and i indicate the extra- and intracellular phases. Furthermore, it was assumed that there was a direct proportionality between the change in fluorescence and the change in membrane potential. As the relation between fluorescence change and actual membrane potential is important, Pape and Lassen (unpublished) compared the fluorescence of diS-C_3-(5) with membrane potential in valinomycin-treated *Amphiuma* red cells. The fluorescence varied in a linear fashion with membrane potential as shown in Fig. 5. The different membrane potentials were produced by suspending the cells in media with different K concentrations. The linear relationship between fluorescence change and V_m as suggested by Hoffman and Laris (1974) is confirmed. The figure also shows another important point: there is no fixed ratio between change in membrane potential and fluorescence change. This is illustrated by the different slopes of the lines at three different cytocrits in Fig. 5. The lack of an absolute ratio is one important difficulty of the fluorescence technique. Another is that at large changes in membrane potential the relation is no longer linear (not shown).

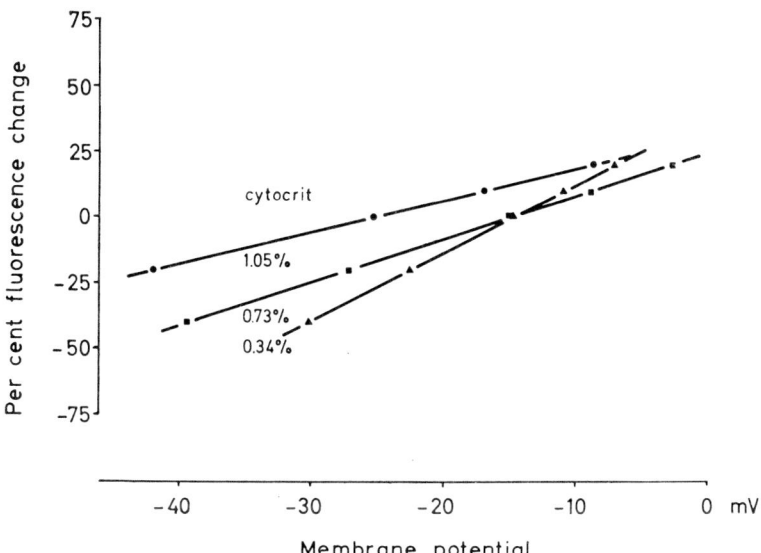

FIG. 5. Relationship between change in fluorescence intensity (ordinate, per cent change) of a fluorescent probe (DiS-C_3-(5)) (3×10^{-6} M) and membrane potential (in mV) in valinomycin-treated *Amphiuma* red cells ($1 - 3 \times 10^{-6}$ M). Three different cytocrits, as indicated in the figure, were employed. (Pape and Lassen, unpublished.)

The mechanism of fluorescence change with "potential sensitive dyes" is not clear. The equilibration of the dye between cells and medium (see Fig. 4) is slow in the case of human red cells. This process is even slower with *Amphiuma* red cells which have a surface to volume ratio that is 4·7 times smaller than in human red cells. Off-hand, the tentative explanation of Sims *et al.* (1974) for the mechanism of action seems reasonable: the membrane potential causes a distribution of the positively charged dye molecules. In the case of hyperpolarization the dye is concentrated in the cells. The larger concentration causes the formation of nonfluorescent di- and polymers of the dye molecules, thus leading to an overall quenching. the simultaneous red-shift of emitted light is ascribed to dye molecules in The hydrophobic environment of the lipid bilayer regions. These interpretations were strongly supported by the liposome experiments of Sims *et al.* (1974).

In a recent note, Hladky and Rink (1976) report that it is possible to take binding of the dye to the cell membrane, cell contents, pH, ionic strength and other variables into account when calculating the membrane potential from the fluorescence change.

3 Membrane conductance of red cells

The membrane potential of a cell in steady state reflects the stationary currents of pump ion species in relation to their conductances. If the active transport mechanisms (pumps) are electrogenic, the ensuing current has to be included in the overall picture. In human red cells, the coupling ratio of the Na–K pump is presumably different from one (see Cavieres, present volume). However, a contribution of the pump to the membrane potential has not yet been demonstrated. For this reason the pumping of Na and K is regarded only as a means of maintaining ionic gradients.

The permeable, nonpumped ion species do not directly influence the membrane potential when they are in equilibrium. But if the equilibrium is disturbed the movement of, for example, Cl will determine the magnitude of the excursion of membrane potential in response to a given perturbation. There are two obvious ways of perturbing the system: either by passage of current through the membrane or by altering the concentration gradients for a given ion species. For reasons of minimizing unwanted influences on the cell, variations of ion gradients are most often performed by altering the composition of the suspending medium. But the intracellular concentrations of ions can also be altered by, for example, addition and subsequent removal of ionophores (Cass and Dalmark, 1973) or by the PCMBS method of Garrahan and Rega (1967). The usefulness of such methods rests on the reversibility of the induced increase in permeability. Therefore it is important to check the functional integrity of the membrane after the treatment. Hoffman and Laris (1974) used the PCMBS method to obtain human red cells with a high Na and low K content. After valinomycin addition to such cells in a high K medium, there was an increase in fluorescence of the carbocyanine dye, indicating a reversal of the membrane potential (the inside now being positive with respect to the external medium). However, it is not possible at present to get unequivocal quantitative information about the membrane conductances from their experiments.

3.1 METHODS EMPLOYING CURRENT PASSAGE

The wealth of detailed information about the relation between current and voltage in excitable cells stems from the fact that current can be passed and voltage recorded with one or more electrodes inside the cell. From the considerations in previous sections, the membrane resistance of human red cells reported by Lassen and Sten-Knudsen (1968) of about 7 Ω cm² (0·14 Ω^{-1} cm^{-2}) represents an underestimate by several orders of magnitude. In giant red cells (*Amphiuma*) the relative damage upon micropuncture is smaller. Using the method of Lettvin *et al.* (1958) for passage of diphasic current pulses through the microelectrode, Hoffman and Lassen (1971) and Lassen (1972) reported specific "membrane resistances" of 1000–2000 Ω cm² (10^{-3} to 5×10^{-4} Ω^{-1} cm^{-2}). Even though this resistance value is too low, due to the leak caused by the electrode, it is interesting because it is at least three orders of magnitude larger than that expected from the exchange rate of labelled chloride. The observation is thus the first independent proof of the suggestion from valinomycin-treated red cells that net movement of chloride is much smaller than the corresponding exchange.

The requirements for sealing of the electrode *in situ* with the tip inside the cell are quite rigorous. Taking the value of the membrane resistance of *Amphiuma* red cells as discussed below (about 10^6 Ω cm²), the input resistance of one cell is 2×10^{10} Ω. Not to shunt this resistance, the sealing (and amplifier input) should have a resistance of not less than 10^{12} Ω. Resistances of this magnitude have never been reported from microelectrode studies. Whether this degree of sealing can be obtained is not clear.

When seeking information solely about the total membrane conductance, passage of current through intact cells is another possibility. Fricke (1926) and Fricke and Morse (1926) measured the electrical properties of packed dog and calf red cells by passing alternating current at frequencies ranging from 800 Hz to 4·5 MHz. Fricke was fully aware of the fact that a major part of the current at low frequencies passed through the extracellular fluid and made determination of membrane conductance difficult. At higher frequencies there was a detectable contribution by the trans-cell-current. This was rightly attributed to shunting of the membrane by its capacitance (see Cole, 1968). Even though these measurements give information about the possible state of ions in intracellular fluid, they suffer from invalidating shunting problems with respect to estimating membrane conductance of human red cells.

Johnson and Woodbury (1964) devised a method to determine the transverse resistance of a single human red cell. They sucked the cell, suspended in isotonic sucrose, into a narrow constriction at the end of a capillary. Subsequent rapid replacement of the sucrose with Ringer's at the exposed ends of the cell allowed current passage for measurement of the IV drop. The obtained values (four cells) were in the range 6–20 Ω cm^2, similar to those reported by Lassen and Sten-Knudsen (1968). However, the resistance values measured by Johnson and Woodbury (1964) would be too low if part of the current passed between the cell and the inner wall of the current passed between the cell and the inner wall of the capillary. The authors included such a possibility in their considerations and made estimates of the time needed for salt to diffuse into the "sucrose gap". It was concluded that the leakage pathway could safely be excluded from the calculations and membrane resistance. This may not be justified. LaCelle and Rothstein (1966) found a large increase in KCl permeability of human red cells suspended in low ionic strength media. The isotonic sucrose used for initial suspension of the cells in the study of Johnson and Woodbury (1964) has presumably caused the cells to leak KCl. This may influence cell volume, but more important, the "sucrose pathway" between capillary wall and cell will become conducting. In this new situation it seems likely that most of the current passes along and not through the cell as intended. Consequently the values reported may not represent the true membrane resistance.

In the author's laboratory, Rathlev (unpublished) used an approach similar to that of Johnson and Woodbury (1964). He sucked an *Amphiuma* red cell in Ringer's into a capillary with a diameter of 10–15 μm. There was a significant correlation between the observed total resistance and the length of cell sucked into the pipette. It can be shown that the resistance derived from a model in which the shunt pathway is considered as a cylindrical sheet around the cell can be expressed:

$$R_{tot} = \frac{\alpha\rho}{2\pi a \Delta} \left(\left[2 \left(\cosh \frac{L}{\alpha} - 1\right) + \frac{\alpha\rho}{R_m 2\pi a \Delta} (A_o + A_L) \sinh \frac{L}{\alpha} \right] \Big/ \left[\sinh \frac{L}{\alpha} - \frac{\alpha\rho}{R_m 2\pi a \Delta} (A_o + A_L) \cosh \frac{L}{\alpha} + \left(\frac{\alpha\rho}{R_m 2\pi a \Delta}\right)^2 A_o A_L \sinh \frac{L}{\alpha} \right] \right)$$

the symbols having the following meaning:

R_{tot} = the measured total resistance at any instance (Ω);
α = cable length constant of the cylindrical sheet of Ringer's between cell and inner wall of the pipette (cm);

ρ = specific resistivity of the Ringer's (Ω cm^{-1});
a = radius of the cylindrical part of the cell sucked into the pipette (cm);
Δ = distance from cell membrane to glass wall (cm);
L = length of sucked-in part of the cell (cm);
R_m = specific membrane resistance of the cell (Ω cm^2);
A_L = area of free end of cell inside the pipette (cm^2);
A_o = area of cell membrane outside the pipette (cm^2).

After a number of simplifying expressions and subsequent numerical solution of the resistance (R_{tot}) as a function of L, it can be shown that if the membrane of the cell is traversed by a significant part of the measuring current, the relation between R and L should depart from a straight line. This was not found, however. A rough calculation of the apparent straight line relationship compared to the measuring accuracy makes it possible to estimate a lower limit of the specific membrane resistance (L. Bass, personal communication). This lower limit value was 10^4 Ω cm^2 or nearly one order of magnitude larger than measured with passage of current through a microelectrode tip inside the cell (Lassen, 1972). Despite being a step in the right direction, the measurements did not allow a reasonably good estimate of the membrane resistance.

Therefore a slightly different method was employed (Rathlev and Lassen, unpublished). An *Amphiuma* red cell had each of its "ends" sucked into pipettes with an inner diameter of 8–14 μm. Figure 6 shows the experimental set-up in schematic form. The cell is suspended in Ringer's between the two pipettes. Subsequently the pipettes and the cell are raised into an oil droplet. In the course of few minutes the resistance from pipette to pipette is greatly increased and remains stable as the oil displaces the

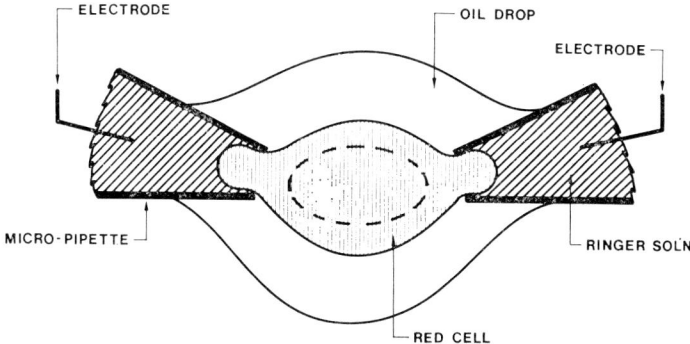

FIG. 6. Schematic diagram of set-up to measure transverse resistance of an *Amphiuma* red cell (oil gap method). See text for further details.

Ringer's at the exposed surface of the cell. The measuring situation now resembles the oil- or sucrose-gap techniques used in the study of excitable tissues. Even though simple in principle, it turned out to be extremely difficult to pass from Ringer's into the oil without pulling the cell out of the pipettes. This is the reason why only a total of four measurements were successful. In two of the experiments, analytical grade oleic acid was used as the insulating oil, in two similar experiments a silicone oil (MS 200/20) was employed. Table 1 shows the results of the measurements. Two values

TABLE 1
Oil gap measurements of membrane resistance (R_{tot}) of single *Amphiuma* red cells

Exp. no.	Type of oil	R_{tot} (Ω)	R_m (min.) (Ω cm^2)	R_m (max.) (Ω cm^2)
1	Oleic acid	5.6×10^{10}	5.9×10^4	2.4×10^5
2	Oleic acid	6.5×10^{10}	5.4×10^4	2.4×10^5
3	Silicone	5.2×10^{10}	9.1×10^4	3.2×10^5
4	Silicone	2.9×10^{10}	2.8×10^4	1.2×10^5

The length of cell sucked into each of the pipettes was measured in each case (generally about 20 μm) and the values for R_m (max.) calculated from the total area of cell in the pipettes. R_m (min.) was calculated under the assumption that the oil was creeping between the cell and capillary wall so that only the dome-shaped ends of the cells were exposed to current passage (see text for further discussion). 17°C, pH = 7.2.

for the specific membrane resistances are shown: R_m (max.) where all of membrane area sucked into the pipettes is exposed to current passage, and R_m (min.) in which it was assumed that the oil could creep along the cell inside the pipette. If the cell and pipettes were returned to the Ringer's, the total resistance immediately returned to the value before the sojourn into the oil. This indicated that Ringer's inside the pipette was not displaced by oil. R_m (max.) is thus presumably the more correct value. The mean value of R_m (max.) is *2.3 × 10^5 Ω cm^2* corresponding to a specific membrane conductance (g_m) of 4.3×10^{-6} Ω^{-1} cm^{-2}. Even this low value of specific membrane conductance of *Amphiuma* red cells may represent an upper limit as it has not been possible to correct for a narrow conducting layer along the hydrated cell wall.

3.2 INDIRECT ESTIMATES OF MEMBRANE CONDUCTANCE

From the preceding section it is obvious that determination of I/V curves for measurement of membrane resistance is not as yet possible in red cells. Even if the method of Stoner and Kregenow (1976) turns out to be promising in avoiding the most serious leak problems, there is no immediate solution in sight for direct conductance measurements on human red cells. Therefore, alternative methods have been sought in which the permeability of the membrane and/or the ionic gradients were altered. From subsequent direct or indirect measurements of membrane potential in response to these changes, estimates of membrane conductance or "single ion conductances" could be made.

3.2.1 *Data from valinomycin-treated cells*

By following the rate of KCl loss from red cells treated with ionophores for monovalent cations, it was concluded by Harris and Pressman (1967) and Scarpa *et al.* (1970) that the permeability to net loss of Cl could be limiting. This behaviour was not to be expected if the pathway for net movement of chloride was as fast as that for tracer exchange (Tosteson, 1959). Hunter (1971) reported in a short note an attempt to quantify the magnitude of Cl conductance in relation to the exchange rate. Hunter (1971) measured the rate of ^{42}K loss (from preloaded cells) after treatment with valinomycin to specifically increase the K permeability (Tosteson *et al.*, 1967). Upon variation of the external K concentration, the changes in rate constants for ^{42}K efflux were followed. It was assumed that the efflux rate was solely determined by the establishment of a diffusion potential actoss the membrane and that the magnitude of this potential could be determined by a constant field approach. From the experimental values, P_K/P_{Cl} can the, be calculated. In Hunter's words; "Although the accuracy of these values (rate constants) depends on the measurement of rather rapid K fluxes, on the validity of the constant field assumption in this system, and on the values assumed for cell K and Cl concentrations, this is the first quantitative estimate of Cl permeability in the red cell. It is about four orders of magnitude smaller than the chloride–chloride exchange permeability, which suggests that the chloride shift in the red cell is very largely mediated by a specific exchange diffusion process." This brief statement led to studies by several groups of the relation between membrane conductance on the one hand and the properties of the exchange pathway on the other. For the purpose of the present chapter it is sufficient to note that the method in principle should enable one to determine the membrane potential of red cells as perturbed by valinomycin and consequently to calculate membrane conductance for individual ion species.

A similar but still different approach was followed in a study on sheep red cells by Tosteson *et al.* (1973). These authors used the flux ratio of K before and after valinomycin addition to calculate the membrane potential according to the flux ratio equation of Ussing (1949). Knowing the concentrations inside and outside the cell, and the net fluxes of K and Cl (measured to be equal), the membrane potential and g_K and g_{Cl} could be computed. g_{Cl} was found to be about $3 \times 10^{-6} \Omega^{-1} \text{cm}^{-2}$ and g_K essentially the same depending on the valinomycin concentration employed. The most negative potentials calculated were in the range -20 to -30 mV.

Hoffman and Laris (1974) used the fluorescent dye method to monitor changes in membrane potentials under influence of valinomycin. Using a constant field approach for calculation of "P_K/P_{Cl}", Hoffman and Laris reported this ratio to be 1/100 in human red cells and 1/5 in *Amphiuma* red cells. They consider the difference between the two species to be inherent.

Very recently Hladky and Rink (1976) reported that the K conductance of human red cells dominated the membrane potential after addition of 1 μM valinomycin. Whereas the chloride concentration gradient is of importance for the membrane potential before valinomycin addition, the ionophore changes the membrane essentially into a "K electrode". The potential estimated with an improved fluorescent dye method is -60 mV as compared to E_K presumably about -80 mV. P_{Cl}/P_{K-Val} was found to be 0·055, similar to the value reported by Hunter (1971).

Figure 7 shows the variations of membrane potential in *Amphiuma* red cells as functions of the outer chloride concentration (within the experimental period the internal Cl concentration remained constant). As discussed in detail below, the potential without valinomycin in the medium is a function of the chloride gradient. However, after valinomycin addition, the potential is insensitive to changes in external Cl concentration, meaning that the K conductance must be much larger than the Cl conductance, similar to the conclusion reached by Hladky and Rink (1976) in human red cells. However, the maximal increase of K permeability induced by valinomycin in *Amphiuma* red cells in only five to ten times (Hoffman, personal communication; Hoffman and Laris, 1974). This moderate increase in relation to a Cl conductance normally twice that of K (see below) should not lead to lack of sensitivity of the membrane potential to outer Cl concentration even after valinomycin treatment. In other experiments, V_m in valinomycin-treated cells was followed as a function of the K concentration in the outer medium (Fig. 8). In this case attempts to fit the experimental observations to a constant field expression with potential and concentration independent permeabilities for K, Na and Cl did not give a good approximation to the experimental curve.

Even though the above experiments with direct or indirect measurements of membrane potential under influence of valinomycin are not entirely self-consistent, the overall message is that the chloride conductance of the membrane is four to six orders of magnitude smaller than that calculated from [35]Cl fluxes at equilibrium for Cl. This is in keeping with the direct measure-

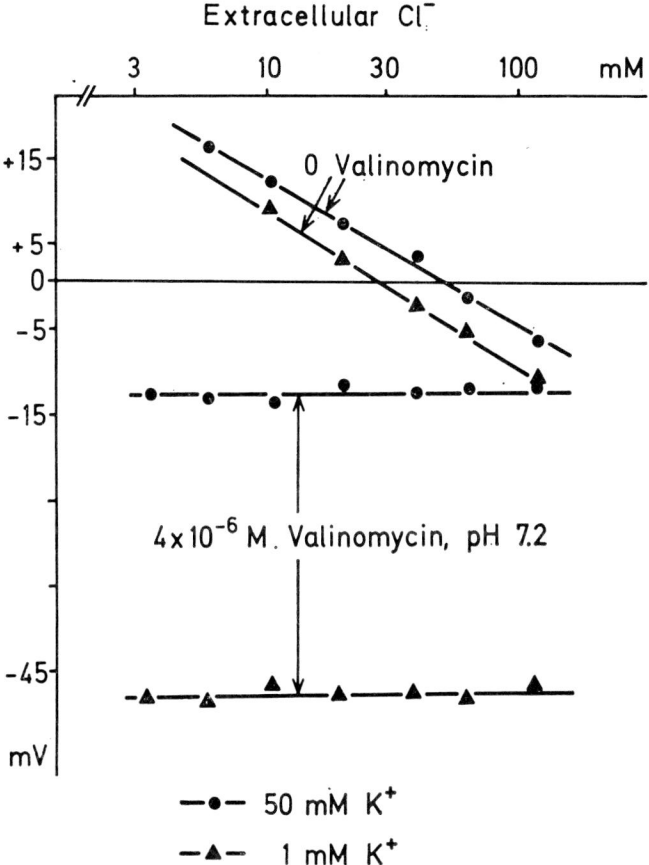

Fig. 7. Membrane potentials of *Amphiuma* red cells as function of Cl concentration of the medium (PAH used as substitute). The experiments were performed at two concentrations of K in the media, $\pm 4 \times 10^{-6}$ M valinomycin. Abscissa: external Cl concentration (log scale). Ordinate: measured potentials in mV. (Rønne, unpublished.)

ments of membrane conductance of *Amphiuma* red cells (see Lassen et al., 1975).

In sheep red cells and in human red cells there is a dramatic increase in K permeability upon addition of valinomycin. Wieth (personal communication) has estimated the increase in human red cells to be three to four orders of magnitude. This means that the situation is similar to that reported for the effect of an analogue of valinomycin on artificial liped bilayers (Ting-Beall et al., 1974). Here it was suggested that the rate of K transport was strongly influenced by the presence of a nonstirred layer of considerable thickness. The effect of stirring in a similar system has been unequivocally shown by Hladky (1973). Such an effect might well be present in the case of human red cells with the large increase in K permeability due to valinomycin and similarly in microelectrode measurements on *Amphiuma* red cells where the cells rest on a glass bottom in a nonstirred chamber. Using Laser inferometry, Lerche (1976) demonstrated that unstirred layers in an artificial system might be up to 0·5 mm in thickness (see also Ciani, *et al.*, 1975). The effect of unstirred layers can be analysed in terms of models like those presented by Haydon and Hladky (1972). Until sufficient data during massive KCl efflux from red cells are available, the effect of unstirred layers cannot be quantified. The effect might explain part of the lack of dependence of V_m on Cl_o in the case of valinomycin-treated *Amphiuma* cells. Benz and Läuger (1976) have estimated that the rate constant for movement of free valinomycin in monoolein bilayers is about ten times smaller than that of the K valinomycin complex. If present in red cells, this will lead to a diminished K sensitivity of V_m at low concentrations of K in the medium. Despite the entirely different mechanism for evoking a high K permeability, the quantitative estimates from experiments with Ca-induced K loss (see below) may suffer from similar limitations.

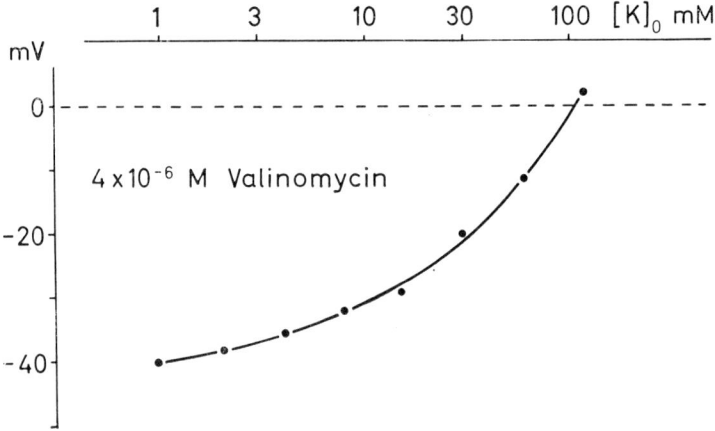

FIG. 8. Membrane potentials of *Amphiuma* red cells as function of K concentration of suspending medium (K_o) in the presence of 4×10^{-4} M valinomycin. Abscissa: K_o in mM (log scale). Ordinate: measured potentials in mV. (Rønne, unpublished.)

3.2.2 *Estimates of chloride conductance employing changes in chloride concentration gradients*

It is evident from the above considerations that the red cell has a high impedance membrane as compared to excitable cells. Until the studies with valinomycin and other ionophores, this was not believed to be the case. In the last few years, careful studies of Cl exchange and its kinetics (see e.g. Gunn *et al.*, 1973; Dalmark, 1976) have made it clear that the rapid transport of labelled Cl across the membrane is a closely coupled one-to-one exchange. Two questions then arise: (1) how much of the total membrane conductance can be accounted for by the movement of Cl and (2) is the Cl conductance part of the same system responsible for the rapid "obligatory exchange"? (as suggested by Vestergaard-Bogind and Lassen, 1974).

Before answering these questions it is necessary to know the Cl conductance (or equivalent resistance) of the red cell membrane. A number of authors changed the external Cl concentration by replacing Cl with an impermeable anion and measuring the ensuing equilibrium distribution of Cl. This type of approach (see e.g. Funder and Wieth, 1966) does not give information about chloride conductance. Hoffman and Lassen (1971) used the impermeable para-amino-hippurate (PAH) as replacement for Cl in the medium and measured a reversal of membrane potential in *Amphiuma* erythrocytes. With a fluorescent probe, Hoffman and Laris (1974) similarly showed "depolarization" both in human and *Amphiuma* red cells after a lowering of external Cl concentration. Neither of these studies was performed in a way that allowed quantitative estimates of the Cl conductance.

Lassen *et al.*, (1975), also used PAH to replace external Cl in a study of membrane potential of *Amphiuma* red cells. As shown in Fig. 9, the membrane potential varied significantly with the Cl concentration of the medium. At the lowest Cl concentrations, the curve bends markedly off. This is presumably ascribed to the fact that the reversed membrane potential caused a net movement of OH^- and HCO_3^- previously being in equilibrium. By a simultaneous lowering of external pH, these ion movements due to the change in electric driving force could be abolished. Hoffman and Lassen (1971) and Hoffman Laris (1974) lowered the pH of the medium one unit when Cl_o was lowered by a factor of 10. This size of pH change will only maintain electrochemical equilibrium for OH and HCO_3 (at constant pCO_2 and unaltered intracellular concentrations) if the membrane behaves like a Cl electrode. This is not found, however. Figure 10 shows the membrane potential of *Amphiuma* red cells as function of pH at Cl_o of 10 mM (PAH substitution). This Cl concentration is 0·08 of the normal, but at no pH value is the membrane potential 63 mV more positive than the normal of −15 mV. This would have been the case if the membrane had behaved like a Cl electrode. The change in membrane potential with pH at constant Cl_o (e.g. 10 mM) could be accounted for by varying net fluxes of OH and HCO_3. In Fig. 10, a line with a slope of −58 mV per pH unit is drawn through the point at which these ions originally (before changing Cl_o) were in equilibrium. Where this line intersects the experimental curve, there is

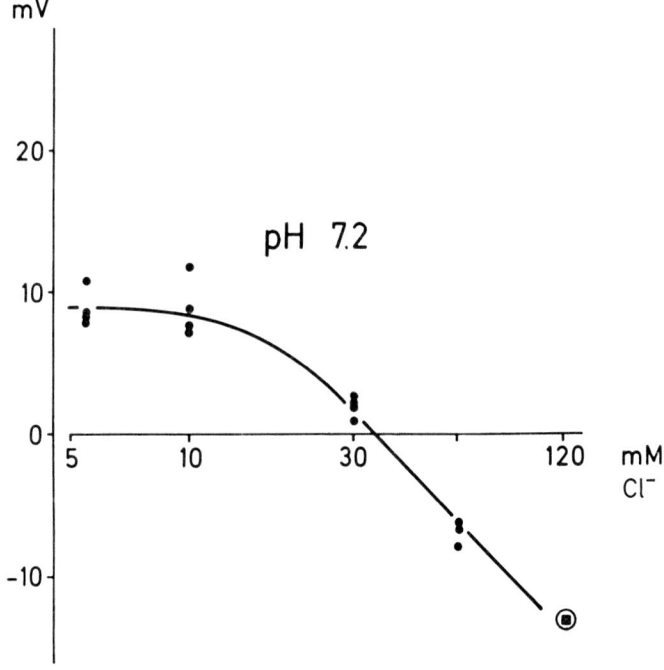

FIG. 9. Membrane potentials of *Amphiuma* red cells as function of external Cl concentration. Cells were not equilibrated at the lower Cl concentrations prior to measurements. External pH 7·2. The point at 120 mM Cl (encircled square) represents the mean value of a large number of experiments. Abscissa: Cl concentration of medium in mM (log scale). Ordinate: measured potentials in mV. Each point represents a separate experiment with some thirty to forty measurements. (Lassen et al., 1975.)

electrochemical equilibrium for OH and HCO_3 at the given Cl_o. Such experiments were performed at different values of Cl_o and the membrane potentials at the pH values for OH, HCO_3 equilibrium were plotted against log (Cl_o) in Fig. 11. The line then represents the loci of membrane potentials for which OH and HCO_3 are not contributing to the membrane current. Provided that the relationship is linear, a transport number for chloride at partial equilibrium in the system (T'_{Cl}) can be expressed (Brown et al., 1970; Christoffersen, 1973):

$$T'_{Cl} \times 0\cdot058 = \left[\frac{\delta V_m}{\delta \log(Cl)_o}\right]_{E_{Na,K}}$$

The slope of the line in Fig. 11 yields a value for T'_{Cl} of 0·48. Knowing the value of T'_{Cl}, the corresponding values of T'_{Na} and T'_K can be obtained by solving the following two equations:

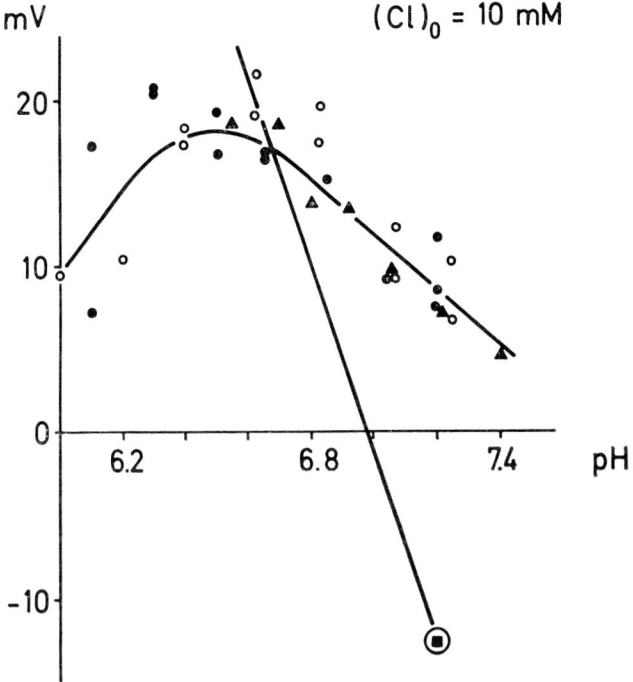

FIG. 10. Membrane potentials of *Amphiuma* red cells as function of pH medium. $Cl_o = 10$ mM. In experiments denoted by closed circles, PAH was substituting Cl; in experiments denoted by open circles, the substituent was morpholino-propane-sulphonate. Points indicated by triangles were from experiments in which 0·9 mM acetazolanide was added (PAH substitution for Cl). The straight line from the encircled point is explained in the text. Abscissa: Cl_o (log scale). Ordinate: measured potentials in mV. (Lassen *et al.*, 1975.)

$$T'_K + T'_{Na} + T'_{Cl} = 1;$$

$$V_m = E_K T'_K + E_{Na} T'_{Na} + E_{Cl} T'_{Cl}.$$

T' are the transport numbers specifically disregarding OH and HCO_3 as these ions are kept in equilibrium and consequently do not contribute to the current. It is also a prerequisite that $dV_m/dt = 0$. This condition was verified in experiments.

The transport numbers are then found to be:

$$T'_K = 0.25$$
$$T'_{Na} = 0.27$$
$$T'_{Cl} = 0.48.$$

To translate these figures into absolute values of conductance it is necessary to know one of the single ion conductances. The K conductance was obtained from the net efflux of K from ouabain-poisoned cells, using the relation:

$$(J_K^{net}) F = g_K(V_m - E_K).$$

The value of g_K determined in this way in *Amphiuma* red cells is $2 \cdot 0 \times 10^{-7} \, \Omega^{-1} \, cm^{-2}$.

Since

$$\frac{T'_{Cl}}{T'_K} = \frac{g_{Cl}}{g_K}$$

we now find:

$$g_{Cl} = 3 \cdot 9 \times 10^{-7} \, \Omega^{-1} \, cm^{-2}.$$

This conductance corresponds to a "specific Cl resistance" (R_{Cl}) of the *Amphiuma* red cell of $2 \cdot 6 \times 10^6 \, \Omega \, cm^2$. It should be noted that it is not possible to obtain the total membrane conductance of the cell by simply

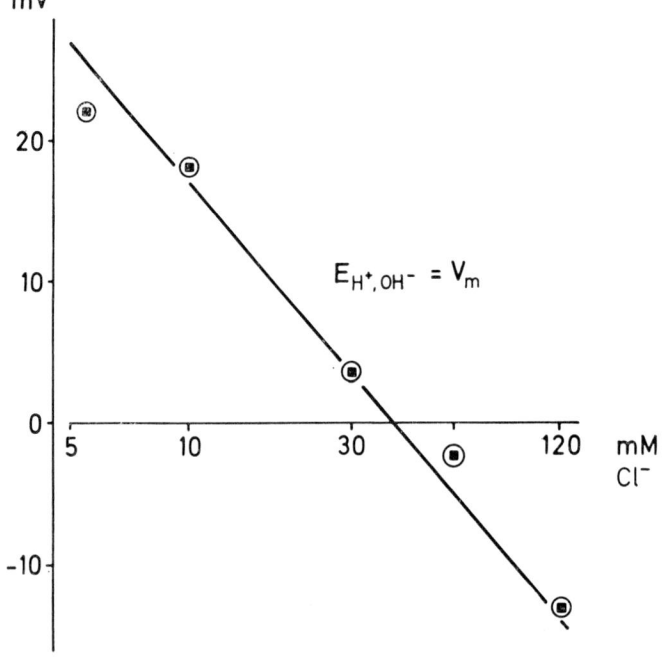

FIG. 11. Membrane potentials of *Amphiuma* red cells as function of Cl_o under conditions where E_{H^+}, E_{OH^-}, and $E_{HCO_3^-}$ equalled V_m at each value for Cl_o. See text for further discussion. Abscissa: potential in mV. Ordinate: Cl_o (log scale). (Lassen et al., 1975.)

adding g_{Cl}, g_K and g_{Na}. As stated repeatedly above, the experiments were designed to exclude currents of OH and HCO_3. Consequently, the corresponding conductances for these ions are undetermined. As g_{OH} and g_{HCO_3} contribute to the membrane conductance, these latter figures are not estimated. It is interesting, however, that $g_K + g_{Na} + g_{Cl} = 8 \cdot 1 \times 10^{-7}$ Ω^{-1} cm^{-2}, or in terms of resistance: $1 \cdot 2 \times 10^6$ Ω cm^2. There is less than one order of magnitude between this value and that determined in oil gap experiments as mentioned above. As the latter measurements probably have yielded too low resistance values, the $g_{OH} + g_{HCO_3}$ cannot be much larger than g_{Cl} (but can certainly be smaller). The value for g_{OH} in sheep red cells (about 10^{-7} Ω^{-1} cm^{-2}) reported by Tosteson et al. (1973) is not immediately applicable in the present context because of differences in experimental design, but would be compatible with the above figures from *Amphiuma* red cells.

The overall result of the measurements shown in Figs. 9–11 is that chloride does not solely *determine* the membrane potential in nonequilibrium situations (but the statement holds that it *reflects* the potential when in equilibrium).

It is still an open question whether the conductance pathway is part of the same system that mediates the rapid exchange of Cl. In this connection it is worth noting that the V_m as a function of pH shows a decline at pH values below about 6·3 (Fig. 10), Gunn et al. (1973, 1975) and Funder and Wieth (1976) have studied the rate of ^{36}Cl exchange in intact human red cells and red cell ghosts in relation to pH. The rate of exchange drops markedly at low pH values where the potential (see Fig. 10) becomes less positive at unchanged Cl_o. One might speculate that this indicates a connection between the two mechanisms.

4 Calcium-induced changes in membrane potential

An increase in intracellular (and/or membrane bound) Ca leads to increase in the K permeability of red cells. This phenomenon is discussed in detail in the chapter by Lew and Ferreira in the present volume (p. 93–99). The mechanism of the permeability increase and the influence by other cations (see e.g. Riordan and Passow, 1973) will not be discussed here.

No studies have been published concerning the membrane potential in human cells in relation to an increase in intracellular Ca activity and the consequent increase in g_K. Fluorescent probe measurements of these phenomena in human red cells are presently under investigation by the author and his colleagues.

Lassen et al. (1974, 1976) have measured the membrane potential of *Amphiuma* red cells under influence of Ca. The first of these studies reported that the membrane hyperpolarized transiently following micropuncture and withdrawal of the electrode. A second micropuncture after about 30 sec revealed a marked change of membrane potential in negative direction. This phenomenon was dependent on the presence of Ca in the external medium and it was concluded that traces of Ca had entered the cell following the first micropuncture. After resealing of the membrane, the higher intracellular Ca activity and the resulting increase in K conductance led to hyperpolarization, the magnitude of which was dependent on K_o. Probably Ca had an additional role in promoting the resealing after the first puncture. The transient nature of the hyperpolarization in this case could beyond doubt be ascribed to the activity of the Ca pump in removing the "extra" Ca from the cytosol.

In a subsequent study, Lassen et al. (1976) reported that an increase of the calcium concentration of the suspending medium of *Amphiuma* erythrocytes led to a transient hyperpolarization. In this case the hyperpolarization could be directly related to a transient net loss of K. Furthermore, the magnitude of the hyperpolarization was a function of the extracellular concentration of K. It is not clear why the hyperpolarization, which was of an all or nothing nature, vanished in time despite the maintained presence of the higher extracellular concentration of Ca.

Since the appearance of the ionophore for divalent cations (A23187) (Reed and Lardy, 1972), it has been possible to accelerate the flux of Ca across cell membranes by several orders of magnitude. This is shown in the case of human red cells by Reed and Lardy (1972), Ferreira and Lew (1975) and Sarkadi et al. (1976). Also in *Amphiuma* erythrocytes, the net influx of Ca is greatly enhanced by A23187 (Lassen et al., 1977). Dissing and Lassen (unpublished) investigated the effect of external K on the membrane potential under maximal stimulation with Ca that was introduced into the cells by means of A23187. Figure 12 shows the results of this type of experiment. There is a straight-line relationship between V_m and the logarithm of the external K concentration. As the internal K concentration stays essentially constant over the period of measurements, this would suggest that the membrane under influence of A23187 and Ca was turned into a K electrode. However, if this was the case, the slope would be 58 mV per decade and not the 30 mV found experimentally. As demonstrated in the graph, the hyperpolarizations in the ionophore experiments have the same magnitude and the same K dependence as found with a change of external Ca concentration from the normal (1·8 mM) to 15 mM. In the case of high external Ca concentration, the small slope was ascribed to the loss of hyperpolarization and consequent decrease in the mean potential (Lassen et al., 1976). This could not be the reason for the similar relation found with A23187 where the potentials were not measurably

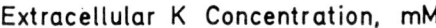
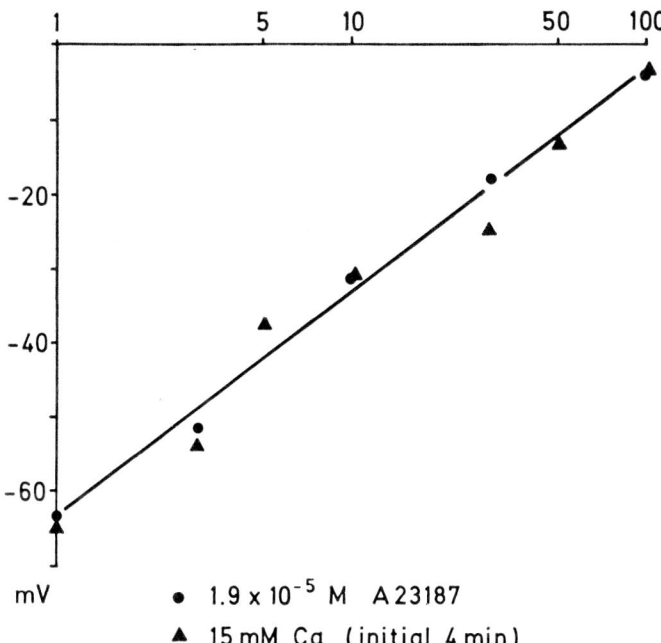

Fig. 12. Membrane potentials of *Amphiuma* red cells as funciton of external K concentration (K_o). Circles indicate experiments in which the Ca entry into the cells was promoted by the ionophore A23187 (extracellular Ca concentration 1·8 mM). Triangles show results from experiments where an increase in K permeability was induced by a rise in extracellular Ca concentration from 1·8 to 15 mM. In the latter case only, values from cells exposed less than 4 min to 15 mM Ca were included. Abscissa: K_o in mM (log scale). Ordinate: membrane potential in mV. (Dissing and Lassen, unpublished.)

changed during the period of measurement. The rapid transport of Ca-ionophore complex through the membrane may lead to a shunting effect of the Ca current on the membrane potential provided that the charged ionophore is "shuttling" back to the outer face of the membrane after delivering the Ca ion to the cytosol. Also, with the 15 mM Ca-induced hyperpolarization a Ca current might shunt part of the potential generated by K efflux. The possible effects of unstirred layers have to be considered as membrane potentials are measured under conditions of nonstirring.

Under normal conditions the Ca content of human red cells is low, probably under 1 μM (see e.g. Harrison and Long, 1968). Also, *Amphiuma* cells have a low total Ca content (10–20 μM) (Simonsen, personal communication). A maximal value for the intracellular Ca activity was obtained in *Amphiuma* cells using A23187 to accelerate Ca transport from a Ringer's containing a Ca EDTA buffering system. The cells were exposed to various extracellular Ca activities and the membrane potentials measured in the presence of A23187. The relationship between membrane potential and Ca activity is plotted in Fig. 13 (Dissing and Lassen, unpublished). It is seen that at extracellular Ca activities slightly larger than 10^{-7} M there is an onset of hyperpolarization. Disregarding the driving force by the small normal potential (-10 to -15 mV), this means that the normal intracellular Ca activity must be below 2×10^{-7} M, as this activity is sufficient to activity must be below 2×10^{-7} M, as this activity is sufficient to produce a significant hyperpolarization. A value of about 10^{-7} M is in keeping with that reported in nerve (Baker, 1975) and with a low K_m value for the Ca pump in red cells (Schatzmann, 1973, Ferreira and Lew, 1975).

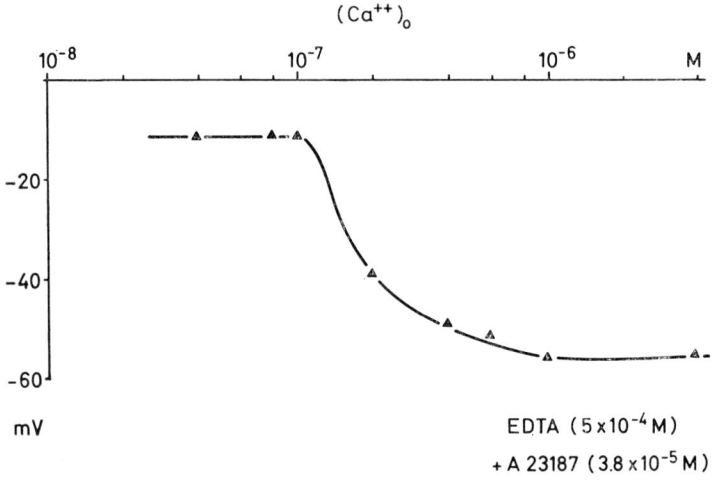

FIG. 13. Effect of extracellular Ca activity (5×10^{-4} M EDTA) in the presence of 3.8×10^{-5} M A23187 on membrane potentials of *Amphiuma* red cells. Abscissa: Ca activity of the medium. Ordinate: membrane potential in mV. (Dissing and Lassen, unpublished.)

5 Concluding remarks

The present chapter has by no means exhausted the available information on membrane potential and conductance of the red cells membrane, nor has it taken into account the future possibilities of experimental approaches to these problems.

Among the interesting facts left behind is the effect of substituted phenols on membrane properties of red cells (Gunn and Tosteson, 1971; Vestergaard-Bogind et al., 1973) and the effect of phloretin (Vestergaard-Bogind and Lassen, 1974; Wieth et al., 1974) or phlorizin (Lepke and Passow, 1973; Schnell et al., 1973). In the case of phlorizin, a "sidedness" of the effect on anion transport (see Lepke and Passow, 1973) is particularly interesting as this compound may serve to elucidate the charge separation which is the physical background for the membrane potential. Kaplan and Passow (1974) have described that whereas phlorizin inhibits Cl exchange, the combination of phlorizin and valinomycin in saturating concentrations gives a twentyfold increase in g_{Cl} in human red cells and ghosts. A similar effect on black lipid membranes using a combination of phloretin and valinomycin was observed by Andersen et al. (1976), who suggest that phloretin, by its large dipole moment and lipid solubility, changes the orientation of the polar headgroups of the phospholipids.

Other substances like local anaesthetics and tranquillizers influence the stare of "fluidity" of the lipids in natural membranes (see Seeman, 1972). It is interesting to note that some of these drugs inhibit the Ca-induced hyperpolarization of *Amphiuma* red cells (Gardos et al., 1976). Whether this effect is primarily on the state of the lipids or that compounds like chlorpromazine displace Ca from the membrane remains to be finally determined.

Active transport systems for Na–K and Ca, anion exchange, and many other "passive" transport systems are probably related to proteins imbedded in the matrix of the lipid bilayer. Following the line of thought of Lew and Beaugé (1977) the modification of the ground permeability of the bilayer by energy dissipators will be one of the main topics for research in the field. In this respect, charge separation across the membrane is one of the most sensitive indicators of transport. Consequently, new and alternative methods to measure electrical parameters of the red cell membrane have to be evolved. Not only for the sake of obtaining information about the membrane, but also about the diffuse double layer and unstirred layers outside the membrane proper.

ACKNOWLEDGEMENTS

Dr L. O. Simonsen is gratefully acknowledged for his positive criticism and valuable suggestions. Kirsten Abel has given expert technical assistance during most of the experiments performed in the author's laboratory. Elisabet Krenchel, Hanne Olesen and Villy Rasmussen have greatly facilitated the preparation of the manuscript. DiS-C_3-(5) was kindly supplied by Dr A. Waggoner, of Amherst College, USA, and ionophore A23187 by Eli Lilly Co.

References

ANDERSEN, O. S., FINKELSTEIN, A., KATZ, I. and CASS, A. (1976). *J. Gen. Physiol.* **67**, 749.
BAKER, P. F. and REUTER, H. (1975). "Calcium Movement in Excitable Cells", p. 7. Pergamon Press, Oxford.
BENZ, R. and LÄUGER, P. (1976). *J. Membrane Biol.* **27**, 171.
BRAASCH, D. (1971). *Physiol. Rev.* **51**, 679.
BRAHM, J. and WIETH, J. O. (1977). *J. Physiol.* **266**, 727.
BROMBERG, P. A., THEODORE, J., ROBIN, E. D. and JENSEN, W. N. (1965). *J. Lab. Clin. Med.* **66**, 464.
BROWN, A. M., WALKER, I. L. and SUTTON, R. B. (1970). *J. Gen. Physiol.* **56**, 559.
BURG, K., GRANTHAM, J., ABRAMOW, M. and ORLOFF, J. (1966). *Amer. J. Physiol.* **210**, 1293.
CASS, A. and DALMARK, M. (1973). *Nature New Biol.* **244**, 47.
CHANG, Y. C. (1966). *Rev. Biol.* **5**, 119.
CHRISTOFFERSEN, G. R. J. (1973). *Comp. Biochem. Physiol.* **46A**, 371.
CIANI, S., GAMBALE, F., GLIOZZI, A. and ROLANDI, R. (1975). *J. Membrane Biol.* **24**, 1.
COHEN, L. B. (1973). *Physiol. Rev.* **53**, 373.
COHEN, L. B., SALZBERG, B. M., DAVILA, H. V., ROSS, W. N., LANDOWNE, D., WAGGONER, A. S. and WANG, C. H. (1974). *J. Membrane Biol.* **19**, 1.
COLE, K. S. (1968). "Membranes, Ions and Impulses", p. 12. University of California Press, Berkeley and Los Angeles.
CONTI, F., TASAKI, I. and WANKE, E. (1971). *Biophysik*, **8**, 58.
COTTERRELL, D. and WHITTAM, R. (1971). *J. Physiol.* **214**, 509.
DALMARK, M. (1976). *J. Gen. Physiol.* **67**, 223.
DALMARK, M. and WIETH, J. O. (1970). *Biochim. Biophys. Acta*, **219**, 525.
DAVILA, H. V., SALZBERG, B. M., COHEN, L. B. and WAGGONER, A. S. (1973). *Nature New Biol.* **241**, 159.
FERREIRA, H. G. and LEW, V. L. (1976). *Nature*, **259**, 47.
FITZSIMONS, E. J. and SENDROY Jr., J. (1961). *J. Biol. Chem.* **236**, 1595.
FORTES, P. A. G. and HOFFMAN, J. F. (1974). *J. Membrane Biol.* **16**, 79.
FRICKE, H. (1926). *J. Gen. Physiol.* **9**, 137.
FRICKE, H. and MORSE, S. (1926). *J. Gen. Physiol.* **9**, 153.
FUNDER, J. and WIETH, J. O. (1966). *Acta Physiol. Scand.* **68**, 234.
FUNDER, J. and WIETH, J. O. (1976). *J. Physiol.* **262**, 679.
GARDÓS, G., LASSEN, U. V. and PAPE, L. (1976). *Biochim. Biophys. Acta.* **448**, 599.
GARRAHAN, P. J. and REGA, A. F. (1967). *J. Physiol.* **193**, 459.
GEDDES, L. A. (1972). "Electrodes and the Measurements of Bioelectric Events", p. 154. Wiley, New York.
GULLIVER, G. (1875). *Proc. Scientific Meetings Zoological Soc. London*, 474.
GUNN, R. B., DALMARK, M., TOSTESON, D. C. and WIETH, J. O. (1973). *J. Gen. Physiol.* **61**, 185.
GUNN, R. B. and TOSTESON, D. C. (1971). *J. Gen. Physiol.* **57**, 593.
GUNN, R. B., WIETH, J. O. and TOSTESON, D. C. (1975). *J. Gen. Physiol.* **65**, 731.
HARRIS, E. J. and MAIZELS, M. (1952). *J. Physiol.* **118**, 40.
HARRIS, E. J. and PRESSMAN, B. C. (1967). *Nature*, **216**, 918.
HARRISON, D. G. and LONG, C. (1968). *J. Physiol.* **199**, 367.
HAYDON, D. A. and HLADKY, S. D. (1972). *Quart. Rev. Biophys.* **5**, 188.

HLADKY, S. B. (1973). *Biochim. Biophys. Acta*, **307**, 261.
HLADKY, S. B. and RINK, T. J. (1976). *J. Physiol.* **258**, 100p.
HOFFMAN, J. F. and LARIS, P. C. (1974). *J. Physiol.* **239**, 519.
HOFFMAN, J. F. and LASSEN, U. V. (1971). XXV International Congress of Physiological Sciences, Munich. (Abstract.)
HUNTER, M. J. (1971). *J. Physiol.* **218**, 49p.
JAY, A. W. L. and BURTON, A. C. (1969). *Biophys. J.* **9**, 115.
JOHNSON, S. L. and WOODBURY, J. W. (1964). *J. Gen. Physiol.* **47**, 827.
KAPLAN, J. H. and PASSOW, H. (1974). *J. Membrane Biol.* **19**, 179.
LACELLE, P. L. and ROTHSTEIN, A. (1966). *J. Gen. Physiol.* **50**, 171.
LASSEN, U. V. (1972). *In* "Oxygen Affinity of Hemoglobin and Red Cell Acid Base Status" (M. Rørth and P. Astrup, eds), p. 291. Munksgaard, Copenhagen.
LASSEN, U. V., LEW, V. L., PAPE, L. and SIMONSEN, L. O. (1977). *J. Physiol* **266**, 72p.
LASSEN, U. V., NIELSEN, A.-M. T., PAPE, L. and SIMONSEN, L. O. (1971). *J. Membrane Biol.* **6**, 269.
LASSEN, U. V., PAPE, L. and VESTERGAARD-BOGIND, B. (1975). 5th International Biophysics Congress, Copenhagen. (Abstract.) p. 102.
LASSEN, U. V., PAPE, L. and VESTERGAARD-BOGIND, B. (1976). *J. Membrane Biol.* **26**, 51.
LASSEN, U. V., PAPE, L., VESTERGAARD-BOGIND, B., BENGTSON, O. (1974). *J. Membrane Biol.* **18**, 125.
LASSEN, U. V. and RASMUSSEN, B. E. (1977). *In* "Transport across Biological Membranes" (G. Giebisch, D. C. Tosteson and H. H. Ussing, eds), vol. 1. Springer Verlag, Berlin. In press.
LASSEN, U. V. and STEN-KNUDSEN, O. (1968). *J. Physiol.* **195**, 681.
LEPKE, S. and PASSOW, H. (1973). *Biochim. Biophys. Acta*, **298**, 529.
LERCHE, D. (1976). *J. Membrane Biol.* **27**, 193.
LETTVIN, J. Y., HOWLAND, B. and GESTELAND, R. C. (1958). *I.R.E. Trans. Medical Electronics*, **PGME-10**, 26.
LEW, V. L. and BEAUGÉ, L. (1977). *In* "Transport across Biological Membranes" G. Giebisch, D. C. Tosteson and H. H. Ussing, eds), vol. 2, Springer Verlag, Berlin. In press.
LEW, V. L. and FERREIRA, H. G. (1976). *Nature.* In press.
LUCKNER, H. (1939). *Arch. Gesam. Physiol.* **241**, 753.
MOON, R. B. and RICHARDS, J. H. (1973). *J. Biol. Chem.* **248**, 7276.
NASTUK, W. L. and HODGKIN, A. L. (1950). *J. Cell. Comp. Physiol.* **35**, 39.
PIETRZYK, C. and HEINZ, E. (1974). *Biochim. Biophys. Acta*, **352**, 397.
REED, P. W. and LARDY, H. A. (1972). *In* "The Role of Membranes in Metabolic Regulation" (M. A. Mehlman and R. W. Hanson, eds), p. 111. Academic Press, New York and London.
RIORDAN, J. R. and PASSOW, H. (1973). *In* "Comparative Physiology" (L. Bolis, K. Schmidt-Nielsen and S. H. P. Maddrell, eds), p. 543. North-Holland, Amsterdam.
SARKADI, B., SZÁSZ, I. and GARDÓS, G. (1976). *J. Membrane Biol.* **26**, 357.
SCARPA, A., CECCHETTO, A. and AZZONE, G. F. (1970). *Biochim. Biophys. Acta*, **219**, 179.
SCHATZMANN, H. J. (1973). *J. Physiol.* **235**, 551.
SCHNELL, K. F., GERHARDT, S., LEPKE, S. and PASSOW, H. (1973). *Biochim. Biophys. Acta*, **318**, 474.

SEEMAN, P. (1972). *Pharmacol. Rev.* **24**, 583.
SIGGAARD-ANDERSEN, O. (1974). *In* "The Acid-Base Status of the Blood", p. 106. Munksgaard, Copenhagen.
SIMS, P. J., WAGGONER, A. S., WANG, C.-H. and HOFFMAN, J. F. (1974). *Biochemistry*, **13**, 3315.
SMITH, T. C. and LEVINSON, C. (1975). *J. Membrane Biol.* **23**, 349.
STONER, L. C. and KREGENOW, F. M. (1967). *Biophys. J.* **16**, 170a.
TASAKI, I. and SINGER, I. (1968). *Ann. N.Y. Acad. Sci.* **148**, 36.
TING-BEALL, H. P., TOSTESON, M. T., GISIN, B. F. and TOSTESON, D. C. (1974). *J. Gen. Physiol.* **63**, 492.
TOSTESON, D. C. (1959). *Acta Physiol. Scand.* **46**, 19.
TOSTESON, D. C., COOK, P., ANDREOLI, T. and TIEFFENBERG, M. (1967). *J. Gen. Physiol.* **50**, 2513.
TOSTESON, D. C., GUNN, R. B. and WIETH, J. O. (1973). *In* "Erythrocytes, Thrombocytes, Leukocytes" (E. Gerlach, K. Moser, E. Deutsch and W. Wilmanns, eds), p. 62. Georg Thieme, Stuttgart.
USSING, H. H. (1949). *Acta Physiol. Scand.* **19**, 43.
VAN SLYKE, D. D., WU, H. and MCLEAN, F. C. (1923). *J. Biol. Chem.* **56**, 765.
VESTERGAARD-BOGIND, B. and LASSEN, U. V. (1974). *In* "Comparative Biochemistry and Physiology of Transport" (L. Bolis, K. Block, S. E. Luria and F. Lynen, eds), p. 346. North-Holland, Amsterdam.
VESTERGAARD-BOGIND, B., PAPE, L. and LASSEN, U. V. (1973). *In* "Erythrocytes, Thrombocytes, Leukocytes" (E. Gerlach, K. Moser, E. Deutsch and W. Wilmanns, eds), p. 37. Georg Thieme, Stuttgart.
WADDELL, W. J. and BATES, R. G. (1969). *Physiol. Rev.* **49**, 285.
WIETH, J. O., FUNDER, J., GUNN, R. B. and BRAHM, J. (1974). *In* "Comparative Biochemistry and Physiology of Transport" (L. Bolis, K. Block, S. E. Luria and F. Lynen, eds), p. 317. North-Holland, Amsterdam.

A comment on the semantics of the "determination" of membrane potential

S. B. HLADKY
Physiological Laboratory, Cambridge University, UK

The membrane potential of a cell ($\Delta V = V_i - V_o$) may always be calculated, at least in principle, from the condition that the total current into the cell is zero, i.e.

$$0 = -C \frac{dV}{dt} + \sum_i z_i FJ_i, \qquad (1)$$

where C is the membrane capacitance;
 dV/dt the rate of change of the membrane potential;
 $-CdV/dt$ the displacement current (positive inwards);
 F the Faraday;
 z_i the charge on the ith species of permeant ion;
 J_i the net flux of the ith species (positive inwards);
 and $\sum_i z_i FJ_i$ the total ionic current.

The net fluxes depend on the permeability of the membrane, on the ion concentrations, on the membrane potential, and, for ions which are pumped, on the metabolic state of the cell.

For all known experimental conditions with red cells, the potential changes so slowly that CdV/dt is negligible. Equation (1) can then be rewritten in a more convenient form if it is assumed that any electrogenic pump currents are negligible and that the current-carrying components of the ion movements are independent of each other (Goldman, 1943; Hodgkin and Katz, 1949; Patlak, 1960). If, for simplicity, the fluxes of ions other than Na, K and Cl are ignored, then

$$V = \frac{RT}{F} \ln \frac{P_K K_o + P_{Na} Na_o + P_{Cl} Cl_i}{P_K K_i + P_{Na} Na_i + P_{Cl} Cl_o}, \qquad (2)$$

where P_{Cl}, which in general may vary with potential, is the membrane permeability to Cl (current-carrying component), etc.

In human red cells P_{Cl} is much larger than either P_K or P_{Na} (see Chapters 6 and 7 for references) and thus as a good approximation for cells in Cl-containing media,

$$\Delta V \simeq \Delta V_{Cl} = \frac{RT}{F} \ln (Cl_i/Cl_o) \qquad (3)$$

whether or not the cells are in a steady state. In *Amphiuma* cells, P_{Cl}, P_K and P_{Na} may be similar (see Chapter 7, by Lassen) and except in the steady state, equation (2) should be used in full.

In red cells the exchangeable anions Cl, HCO_3 and OH, are not actively transported (references in Chapter 6). Thus in the steady state where all ion concentrations are constant, Cl must be at equilibrium with the membrane potential. Equation (3) is then exact and from equations (2) and (3)

$$\Delta V = \Delta V_{\text{steady state}} = \frac{RT}{F} \ln \frac{P_K K_o + P_{Na} Na_o}{P_K K_i + P_{Na} Na_i}. \qquad (4)$$

In his chapter Lassen has chosen to emphasize the interpretation of the membrane potential corresponding to equation (4). Even though it is only applicable in the steady state, equation (4) has the advantage of focusing attention on the fluxes of the activity-transported ions which are responsible for the long-term maintenance of the resting potential (cf. Adrian and Hodgkin's analysis of the resting potential of muscle given in Hodgkin (1958)).

While for human red cells recently disturbed from a steady-state the membrane potential is close to the Cl potential, the small difference between ΔV and ΔV_{Cl} is important. This difference, which exists because of the fluxes of Na and K, drives the small flux of Cl necessary to bring the cell eventually to a new steady state. Thus even though the dominant factor in determining the membrane potential at any instant is the Cl activity ratio, in the long term the Cl ratio must come into equilibrium with that potential at which the Na and K contents of the cell can remain constant This long-term steady potential is determined by the compositions of the cell and the bathing medium and by the permeabilities of the membrane to Na and K but it does not depend on the permeability to Cl.

References

GOLDMAN, D. E. (1943). *J. Gen. Physiol.* **27**, 37–60.
HODGKIN, A. L. (1958). *Proc. Roy. Soc. B*, **148**, 1–37.
HODGKIN, A. L. and KATZ B. (1949). *J. Physiol.* **108**, 37–77.
PATLAK, C. S. (1960). *Nature*, **188**, 944–945.

Anion movements in red blood cells

P. A. GEORGE FORTES

Department of Biology, University of California, San Diego, La Jolla, California 92093

1 Introduction	175
2 Brief historical background	176
3 Anion conductance and anion exchange	177
4 Kinetics of anion exchange	179
5 Effect of pH on anion exchange	181
6 Inhibitors of anion transport	182
6.1 Reversible inhibitors	182
6.2 Electrostatic factors in inhibition of anion transport	185
6.3 Chemical modification	187
7 Molecular mechanisms of anion transport	190
Acknowledgements	192
References	192

1 Introduction

The main physiological role of anion transport across the red cell membrane is to facilitate CO_2 removal from the tissues and its delivery to the alveoli. In tissue capillaries gaseous CO_2 diffuses into the red cell where it is hydrated to HCO_3^- in a reaction catalysed by carbonic anhydrase. The intracellular HCO_3^- is then exchanged for extracellular Cl^-. Thus, the bulk of the CO_2 produced by metabolism is transported to the lung in the form of plasma HCO_3^-. In the lung capillary the process is reversed: plasma HCO_3^- enters the red cell in exchange for intracellular Cl^-, carbonic acid is produced and dehydrated to CO_2 which diffuses into the alveolar space. Since the average time spent by a red cell in the lung capillary is less than 1 sec at rest and as short as $\frac{1}{4}$ sec during exercise, the above exchanges must proceed at a very fast rate. Sufficiently rapid entry and exit of HCO_3^- in red cells would be possible if the membrane were freely permeable to ions. However, this would require an energetically costly ion pumping system in order to balance the accumulation of ions and water caused by the high concentration of hemoglobin in the cell, otherwise swelling and eventual lysis of the cell would occur. Nature solved the dilemma of requiring both a low ionic permeability and fast anion movements by having a permselective membrane with low permeability to cations and a specialized system for rapid exchange of anions.

Although the actual mechanism of the anion transport system in red cells is not known, an explosive increase in information ranging from kinetic and pharmacological data to the characterization of the membrane components involved in anion transport has occurred within the last five years. Current information and ideas on the structure and organization of biological membranes and their components have provided new outlooks and methodologies. All this has led to radical changes in many traditional concepts. The purpose of this chapter is to review the salient characteristics of the anion transport system that have become available through various experimental approaches. The hope is to provide a critical, albeit biased, synthesis of current information and concepts, and pose certain questions that may be helpful to unravel the remaining mysteries of this fascinating system. Obsolescence of a review in this field is unavoidable. The information includes papers published up to the summer of 1976. An excellent recent review is available (Sachs *et al.*, 1975).

2 Brief historical background

Na and K cross the red cell membrane about 10^6 times slower than Cl^-, even if they have similar hydrated radii. To explain this selectivity for anions over cations, Mond (1927) postulated that positive charges in the membrane exclude cations and concentrate anions by a Donnan effect. Mond suggested that dissociable groups were the bearers of positive charge since the anion-cation selectivity decreased with increasing pH in solutions of low ionic strength. A quantitative development of the fixed charge hypothesis using the theory developed by Meyer and Sievers (1936) and Teorell (1952) for collodion membranes with fixed charges was introduced by Passow (1964). Assuming that the fixed charges were amino groups with a pK of 9 and located in narrow aqueous channels in the membrane at a concentration of 2·5 M, the fixed charge hypothesis could explain quantitatively the variations of sulfate fluxes with H^+, Cl^- and $SO_4^=$ concentrations in the medium over a limited pH range (Passow, 1969). However, recent information has suggested that anions do not cross the membrane by simple diffusion through aqueous channels. Anions appear to cross in association with protein components through the hydrophobic parts of the membrane, and independently from the cation channels. These findings have seriously challenged the basic postulates of the original fixed-charge hypothesis.

3 Anion conductance and anion exchange

The first type of evidence that anion transport in red cells does not occur by simple free diffusion came from experiments using ionophores. If the membrane permeability to K^+ were increased by an ionophore, net K^+ efflux should be observed if Cl^- were free to diffuse with K^+. Otherwise, K^+ loss would be prevented by build-up of negative charge in the cell. Contrary to expectations, valinomycin did not produce rapid K^+ loss from red cells unless a proton carrier was also added, which allowed K^+ for H^+ exchange (Harris and Pressman, 1967). Similarly, gramicidin induced K^+ for Na^+ exchange, but not net KCl loss (Chappell and Crofts, 1966; Scarpa et al., 1970). These observations indicate that although Cl^- can move rapidly across the red cell membrane, it cannot do so as a counter-ion for K^+ and its transport is largely through an obligatory exchange for another anion.

These conclusions were confirmed with measurements of membrane potentials in red cells of the salamander *Amphiuma means* using microelectrodes (Hoffman and Lassen, 1971; Lassen, 1972) and in human red cells using fluorescent probes (Hoffman and Laris, 1974; Sims et al., 1974).

The membrane potential is a function of the concentration of permeable ions on both sides of the membrane and their relative permeabilities. According to the Goldman (1943) equation as used by Hodgkin and Katz (1949), for normal red cells suspended in saline, and neglecting H^+ and OH^-, the membrane potential is given by:

$$V_m = \frac{RT}{F} \ln \frac{P_K[K]_o + P_{Na}[Na]_o + P_{Cl}[Cl]_i}{P_K[K]_i + P_{Na}[Na]_i + P_{Cl}[Cl]_o}, \quad (1)$$

where V_m is the membrane potential; R, T and F are the gas constant, absolute temperature and Faraday's constant, respectively; and P_i is the diffusional permeability to the ith ion. If $P_K \cong P_{Na} \ll P_{Cl}$ the membrane potential is dependent only on the Cl^- concentration gradient and is equal to the Cl^- equilibrium potential (E_{Cl}), so that equation (1) reduces to the Nernst equation:

$$V_m = E_{Cl} = \frac{RT}{F} \ln \frac{[Cl]_i}{[Cl]_o}. \quad (2)$$

In untreated red cells, the membrane potential is correctly determined from equation (2). P_{Cl}/P_K or P_{Cl}/P_{Na} as measured by tracer fluxes is about 10^6. Thus, even if P_K or P_{Na} increased up to 10 000-fold the membrane potential would change only about 1 per cent, since P_{Cl} would still be predominant. Surprisingly, addition of valinomycin to *Amphiuma* or human red cells suspended in NaCl causes drastic changes in their membrane potential, which moves from the Cl⁻ towards the K⁺ equilibrium potential, although P_K increases less than a thousandfold by the ionophore treatment (Hoffman and Lassen, 1971; Lassen, 1972; Hoffman and Laris, 1974). These observations confirmed the suggestion (Hunter, 1971) that the conductance of the membrane to Cl⁻ is very low and the bulk of Cl⁻ transport must proceed by electroneutral exchange diffusion.

Assuming that K⁺ efflux in valinomycin-treated red cells is limited by P_{Cl}, Hunter (1971) and Tosteson et al. (1973) estimated P_{Cl}, in human and sheep red cells respectively, from K fluxes and found that P_{Cl} was only about 100 times higher than P_K in the absence of valinomycin and that ionic diffusion constituted only 10^{-4} to 10^{-5} of the total Cl flux. Additional evidence was found by Lassen et al. (1973) who measured that the membrane resistance of *Amphiuma* red cells is at least $5 \times 10^4 \, \Omega \, cm^2$, about 10^4 times higher than the resistance calculated from Cl⁻ fluxes assuming that all the Cl⁻ moves by ionic diffusion.

In contrast to Cl⁻ conductance, which is negligibly small compared to the exchange Cl⁻ permeability, $SO_4^=$ conductance is a significant component of the total $SO_4^=$ flux as determined in $SO_4^=$-loaded cells by the valinomycin method (Gunn, et al, 1974; Knauf et al., 1977), since up to about 50 per cent of the sulfate flux carries current.

The observations mentioned above are incompatible with the idea that anions share the same permeability pathways with cations and that these pathways are aqueous channels. Instead, they suggest that anions must cross the membrane as neutral complexes, probably through a hydrophobic environment.

Wieth (1972) proposed that a membrane component could function as an anion carrier analogous to the liquid ion exchange membranes studied by Shean and Sollner (1966), which are able to discriminate between anions and cations almost as well as the red cell membrane. Thus, a hydrophobic membrane component with an amino group could be protonated and form a complex with an anion. The neutral ion pair could diffuse across the hydrophobic phase of the membrane, release the anion, form a new complex and return, catalysing a one-for-one exchange. Since neither the uncomplexed carrier nor the anion could diffuse at significant rates, no current can flow through the membrane, accounting for the high anion flux and the high membrane resistance that are observed.

4 Kinetics of anion exchange

The use of radioactive tracers allowed the study of anion transport at equilibrium. This greatly simplifies data analysis since the concentrations and driving forces for all ions are constant throughout the experiment and fluxes follow first order kinetics (Gardos et al., 1969). Tosteson (1959) measured tracer fluxes of halides using a flow apparatus and determined that Cl^- equilibrates with a half-time of 210 msec at room temperature. However, owing to the technical problems in measuring such fast fluxes most of the work on anion transport in the following decade was with sulfate and phosphate which equilibrate with half-times between minutes and hours at 37°C (Passow, 1969). The activation energy for phosphate and sulfate transport was found to be higher than 30 kcal mol^{-1} (Gerlach et al., 1964; Passow, 1969). If halide transport had a similar temperature dependence, the fluxes would be sufficiently slow at low temperatures to allow their measurement using more conventional techniques. That this was so was shown by Dalmark and Wieth (1970) who found that Cl^- fluxes, measured by an adaptation of the millipore filtration method of Mawe and Hempling (1965), has a half-time of 18 sec at 0°C. The activation energy for the monovalent anions Cl^-, Br^-, I^- and SCN^- (Dalmark and Wieth, 1972) and for small organic anions (Deuticke, 1973) ranges between 26 and 37 kcal mol^{-1}, similar to that for sulfate and phosphate, suggesting that their permeation mechanisms are similar.

Although considerable specificity of the anion transport system is indicated by the 10^4–10^5 difference in exchange rate between Cl^- and sulfate (Schnell et al., 1973) and the differences in rate for halide exchange (Tosteson, 1959; Dalmark and Wieth, 1972), this may only reflect the differences in mobility of the anion-carrier complexes across the membrane and not the specificity of interaction of a particular anion with the carrier.

In fact, it appears that if all anions utilize the same carrier, it has very low, if any, specificity towards the carried species since it will transport, in addition to the inorganic ions, a variety of organic anions such as salicylate (Wieth, 1970), PCMBS* (Knauf and Rothstein, 1971b), ANS (Fortes and Hoffman, 1974) and pyridoxal phosphate (Cabantchik et al., 1975a,b). This characteristic of the red cell anion transport system is in contrast with almost all other carrier-mediated transport systems, which are stereospecific with respect to the transported substrate.

*Abbreviations used: ANS, 1-anilino-8-naphthalene sulfonate; DIDS, 4,4'-diisothiocyano-2,2'-stilbene disulfonate; APMB, 2-(4'-aminophenyl)-6-methylbenzenethiazol-3',7-disulfonate; DAS, 4,4'-diacetamidostilbene-2,2'-disulfonate; DNFB, 2,4-dinitro-1-fluorobenzene; PCMBS, p-chloromercuribenzene sulfonate; SITS, 4-acetamido-4'-isothiocyanostilbene-2,2'-disulfonate; PDP, pyridoxal phosphate; MNT, 5-methoxynitrotropone; TNBS, trinitrobenzenesulfonate; NAP-taurine, N-(4-azido-2-nitrophenyl)-2-ethane sulfonate; TNC, trinitrocresolate.

The main evidence that all anions share the same transport system is that they act as competitive inhibitors. Cl^- exchange is inhibited by HCO_3^- (Dalmark, 1972; Gunn et al., 1973) and the halides in the sequence $F^- < Br^- < I^-$ (Dalmark, 1976). Cl^- inhibits phosphate uptake, with a K_I of about 10 mM (Lew et al., 1972, unpublished), and sulfate exchange (Passow, 1969). However, Cl^- and F^- accelerate I^- self-exchange (Passow and Wood, 1974). No explanation is available for the latter observation.

If anion exchange depends on a membrane component present in finite concentration, the fluxes should follow saturation kinetics. In earlier studies sulfate and phosphate exchange were found to *increase* exponentially with concentration with no indication of saturation (Passow, 1969; Deuticke, 1970). However, in these experiments the ionic strength was kept constant so that sulfate or phosphate concentrations were varied by substitution with Cl^-. If citrate, which is impermeant, is used instead of Cl^-, phosphate exchange exhibits Michaelis-Menten kinetics and saturates with an apparent K_m of 80 mM (Lew et al., 1972, unpublished). In experiments in which both the intra- and extracellular Cl^- concentrations were increased by addition of NH_4Cl (Gunn et al., 1973) or KCl in the presence of nystatin (Cass and Dalmark, 1973; Dalmark, 1975, 1976) the Cl^- exchange flux reached a maximum value around 120 mM and decreased when [Cl] was above 200 mM. Saturation kinetics have also been reported for Br^- and I^- (Wood and Passow, 1971; Wieth et al., 1973). Sulfate exchange shows evidence of both a linear and a saturable component (Gunn et al., 1974; Schnell et al., 1977).

The reason for the apparent exponential increase of the fluxes with concentration, with no evidence of saturation as observed in earlier experiments with sulfate and phosphate, is that the inhibitor (in this case Cl^-) was decreased at the same time as the substrate ($SO_4^=$ or $HPO_4^=$) was increased, giving a more than proportional increase in flux. When the concentration of substrate is increased at the expense of the inhibitor the flux will be concave, linear or convex when plotted against the substrate concentration depending on whether the affinity for the inhibitor is greater, the same, or lower, respectively, than the affinity for the substrate (Gunn et al., 1973; Dalmark, 1976; Schnell et al., 1977).

In addition to competitive inhibition between the different anions, Dalmark (1976) has recently shown that, at high concentrations, the halides also inhibit noncompetitively. This is seen by the decrease in Cl^- flux when Cl^- concentration is raised from 200 to 600 mM (chloride self-inhibition) and is also observed with F^-, Br^- and I^-. Dalmark has interpreted these observations postulating that the anion carrier has two sites: a substrate site that binds the ion and carries it across, and an inhibitor site which when occupied by an anion prevents translocation. The affinities of the inhibitory sites are lower than those of the substrate sites. Binding to both types of sites increases proportionately in the sequence: $F^- < Cl^- < Br^- < I^-$ (Dalmark, 1976). A similar noncompetitive inhibition by high concentrations of $SO_4^=$ is observed in sulfate self-exchange (Schnell et al., 1977).

5 Effect of pH on anion exchange

Sulfate and phosphate exchange fluxes show a maximum at about pH 6·4 and decrease above and below this pH (Deuticke, 1970; Schnell, 1972). Although both the mono- and divalent forms of phosphate are present in this pH range, phosphate exchange behaves as that of a divalent ion, since it shows the same maximum as sulfate, but different than the monovalent halides which show a broad maximum at pH 7·8 (Gunn et al., 1973; Dalmark, 1975). An important observation is that as the pH is raised from 6·5 to 8, divalent anion fluxes *decrease* whereas monovalent anion fluxes *increase*. This behavior is incompatible with the fixed-charge hypothesis that predicts a monotonic dependence of flux on pH in the region where the fixed charges are titrated and maximum flux, independent of pH, when all the groups are protonated.

A model to explain the dependence of anion transport on pH was recently formulated by Gunn (1972, 1973). The model postulates that the anion carrier is uncharged at high pH and cannot transport anions. As the pH is lowered to 7·8, the carrier becomes protonated and is able to complex monovalent anions and transport them so that the flux increases. If the pH is lowered from 7·8 and 6·4 a second group in the carrier becomes protonated. In this form the carrier can complex a divalent anion and transport it, or must complex two monovalent anions, which is less probable, so that divalent anion transport increases, while that of monovalents decreases. These predictions are supported by the observation that Cl^- for $SO_4^=$ exchange is accompanied by H^+ movements, with a stoichiometry of one Cl^- exchanged for one $SO_4^=$ plus one H^+ (Jennings, 1976). To explain the decrease in divalent anion flux below pH 6·4, Gunn postulates a third protonation of the carrier, which is unable to transport anions in this form. Reasonable fits to the experimental data are obtained with this model when appropriate values for the equilibrium constants between the different forms of the carrier are used (Gunn, 1973; Passow and Wood, 1974). However, recent experiments have shown that the behavior of the alkaline branch of the Cl^- flux v. pH curve depends on the

Cl⁻ concentration (Dalmark, 1975) and the presence of hemoglobin, since the decrease in flux at alkaline pH is greatly reduced in red cell ghosts (Funder and Wieth, 1975). Dalmark (1975) proposes that the decrease in flux at alkaline pH is due to the asymmetric distribution of carrier molecules on both sides of the membrane caused by the change in membrane potential due to ionization of hemoglobin which decreases the intracellular Cl⁻ concentration. In Dalmark's model, the carrier distribution across the membrane depends on pH, but its transport function is independent of pH between 7 and 9. It becomes pH-dependent below 7 when inhibitory groups with pK around 6 begin to be titrated (Dalmark, 1975). In contrast $SO_4^=$ self-exchange shows the same pH maximum in intact red cells and resealed ghosts (Schnell et al., 1977).

In addition, the behavior of the Cl⁻ flux at low pH, which shows a minimum near pH 5 at 0°C and increases below pH 5, suggests that diffusion of undissociated HCl contributes significantly to the observed flux at these extremes of pH (Gunn et al., 1975).

It should be mentioned that all the kinetic models so far presented have assumed that the rate-limiting step is the translocation of the anion-carrier complex. The association-dissociation reactions between the anion and the carrier are assumed to be fast enough so that the complex is at equilibrium with the ions at each side of the membrane. Other models in which the binding and/or dissociation reactions are rate-limiting, or more complex kinetics in which the rates of formation and translocation of the anion-carrier complex are similar, could presumably explain the observations as well as the available models.

6 Inhibitors of anion transport

6.1 REVERSIBLE INHIBITORS

An enormous number of compounds inhibit anion transport reversibly in red cells. The list includes alcohols, local anesthetics, sedatives, fluorescent probes, sulfonamides and several other compounds. The inhibitors are structurally unrelated, and can be neutral, positively or negatively charged. The only common characteristic is that all these compounds are amphipathic with affinity for polar-apolar interfaces (Deuticke, 1970; Fortes and Hoffman, 1974; Fortes and Ellory, 1975). The potency of different inhibitors is quite variable, since effective inhibitory concentrations vary from 10^{-7} to 10^{-1} M. The inhibitory potency appears to depend on the presence of aromatic groups with anionic or phenolic moieties and a large dipole moment of the molecule, as exemplified by ANS isomers (Fortes and Hoffman, 1973, 1974), dipyridamole (Deuticke, 1970) and phloretin (Wieth *et al.*, 1973), all of which inhibit Cl⁻ fluxes 50 per cent at 1–30 μM and more than 99·9 per cent at 250–500 μM. The existence of such a wide variety of inhibitors suggests that a multitude of mechanisms are involved. Nevertheless, at least some general patterns can be deduced from the many perturbations of red cell structure and function caused by these inhibitors. The general rules are:

a. All reversible inhibitors of anion exchange alter red cell shape to either echinocytes or stomatocytes (Deuticke, 1968, 1970; Fortes and Ellory, 1975).

b. None of the compounds is specific for the anion transport system; when tested they inhibit other transport systems, especially those thought to involve facilitated diffusion mechanisms: phloretin inhibits sugar transport (LeFevre, 1961), the Na–K pump (Schwartz *et al.*, 1975) and urea transport (Macey and Farmer, 1970; Owen and Solomon, 1972; Wieth *et al.*, 1974); TNC inhibits the Na–K pump (Gunn and Tosteson, 1971); ANS also inhibits the Na–K pump plus ouabain-insensitive, saturable K fluxes (Fortes and Ellory, 1975), and net KCl loss at low ionic strength (Fortes and Freter, 1975).

c. All the compounds increase cation leaks at high concentrations (Passow, 1969; Schnell and Passow, 1969; Wieth, 1970; Gunn and Tosteson, 1971; Fortes and Ellory, 1975).

d. Those compounds that have been tested in lipid bilayers, like ANS (McLaughlin *et al.*, 1971), phloretin (Andersen *et al.*, 1976) and salicylate (McLaughlin, 1973), cause a simultaneous and equivalent increase in cation and decrease in anion conductance.

It is difficult to conclude that the inhibition of anion permeability by the above types of compounds is solely due to direct interactions of the drugs with the anion transport system. On the contrary, it is possible that all the above perturbations of membrane function, including inhibition of anion transport, have a common denominator. Insight into these possibilities can be obtained from investigations of the nature and localization of the membrane sites where these inhibitors interact, the forces that determine the inhibitor-membrane interactions, and the changes, at the molecular level, that result from such interactions.

In this respect, fluorescent probes like ANS offer the special advantage of being only fluorescent when bound to the membrane. The interactions of ANS with the membrane and its concentration therein can be measured directly by fluorescence (Fortes and Hoffman, 1971). Furthermore, since the fluorescence parameters of ANS depend on the environment, the nature and properties of its binding sites can be studied spectroscopically. Since ANS is both a substrate and an inhibitor of the anion transport system (Fortes and Hoffman, 1974) its interaction with the red cell membrane was studied in detail, attempting to gain insight on the properties of the anion transport system and the mechanism of the membrane perturbations mentioned above.

From data obtained in nanosecond fluorescence spectroscopy studies it was concluded that ANS binds at the membrane-water interface and that 60–75 per cent of the ANS molecules are bound to phospholipid bilayer regions and the remainder are bound to membrane protein (Fortes, 1972, 1976; Fortes et al., 1972a,b).

The ubiquitous binding of ANS to both lipid and protein regions of the membrane indicates that, in addition to specific interactions between ANS and the anion carrier, it is possible that the perturbations of membrane function result from ANS binding to other lipid and protein sites. Both lipid and protein ANS binding sites bind other reversible inhibitors of anion transport, since the latter compete with ANS (Fortes and Hoffman, 1971) at both types of sites (Fortes, 1976). Phloretin also appears to distribute in lipid and protein binding sites, in similar proportions as ANS, as suggested by binding studies (Jennings and Solomon, 1976).

The interaction of the inhibitors with the lipid and, perhaps, protein results in expansion of the membrane, as evidenced by the increased resistance to hypotonic lysis in the presence of these drugs (Seeman, 1972; Sheetz and Singer, 1974; Fortes and Ellory, 1975). Sheetz and Singer (1974) proposed that the shape changes observed with these drugs are due to asymmetric expansion of the membrane caused by preferential binding of the drug to the inside or the outside half of the membrane. According to Sheetz and Singer (1974), the asymmetric binding to the two halves of the membrane is caused by electrostatic attraction or repulsion at the internal surface of cationic or anionic drugs, respectively, by the negatively charged phospholipids, which are asymmetrically distributed (Zwaal et al., 1973). Stomatocytes are caused by expansion of the inside membrane half by cationic drugs and echinocytes by expansion of the external half by anionic drugs, except with impermeable drugs, which can only bind to the outside and will cause echinocytes regardless of their charge.

Sheetz and Singer's (1974) hypothesis is strongly supported by the observations that ANS binding to red cell membranes depends mainly on electrostatic factors (Fortes and Hoffman, 1971; Fortes, 1972, 1976), and even though it is permeable in red cells (Fortes and Hoffman, 1974), ANS causes crenation and hemolysis protection, suggesting that it binds preferentially to the external membrane surface (Fortes and Ellory, 1975). If these observations can be generalized, phloretin behaves like an anionic drug, since it is permeable (Jennings and Solomon, 1976), is a crenator (Deuticke, 1970) and protects from hypotonic hemolysis (Seeman, 1972), suggesting preferential binding to the external membrane surface.

As mentioned above, it is possible that the perturbations which alter cell shape (i.e. asymmetric expansion) are related to inhibition of anion exchange. However, this is not supported by the observation that some compounds alter cell shape, but do not inhibit anion transport (Deuticke, 1970). Furthermore, we have found that addition of chlorpromazine to ANS-treated red cells in sufficient concentration to reverse the crenation or even to cause stomatocytosis does not reverse the inhibition of Cl exchange (Fortes and Freter, unpublished). Spheroechinocytes, produced by incubation of red cells in the absence of metabolizable substrates, show a 50 per cent slower rate of Cl^- exchange; if chlorpromazine is added, cell shape can change back to a disc or to a stomatocyte, but no change in Cl^- exchange rate is seen (Fortes and Pockros, unpublished).

Nevertheless, the observations on alteration of cell shape are included here because they indicate that inhibitors can interact asymmetrically with the red cell membrane as a consequence of nonspecific electrostatic interactions. This may be important for the interpretation of experiments in which inhibition depends on which side of the membrane is exposed to the inhibitor.

Phlorizin, the glycoside of phloretin, inhibits anion exchange in red cells or resealed ghosts when present in the medium, but does not inhibit anion exchange when present inside resealed ghosts, even though it remains inside the ghosts and inhibits D-xylose efflux (Lepke and Passow, 1973; Schnell et al., 1973). A similar sidedness was observed with the disulfonic stilbene derivative DAS, which inhibits Cl^- (Kaplan et al., 1976) and $SO_4^=$ exchange (Zaki et al., 1975) only when present in the extracellular medium. Another disulfonic inhibitor, APMB, inhibited on both surfaces (Zaki et al., 1975; Kaplan et al., 1976). These observations have been interpreted as indications of the existence of different binding sites for inhibitors on the inside and outside surfaces of the anion transport mechanism. Although this may be so, the lack of effect of an inhibitor on one side can simply be due to decreased affinity or accessibility, not to absence of sites, as suggested by the experiments on cell shape mentioned above. Nevertheless, the fact that APMB does inhibit on the inside, although it is a disulfonate like DAS, suggests that electrostatic factors are not the only ones ruling the affinity for the inhibitors.

6.2 ELECTROSTATIC FACTORS IN INHIBITION OF ANION TRANSPORT

Since the anionic ANS binds at the membrane-water interface and more than 10^7 ANS molecules per cell can be bound, it is reasonable to suppose that ANS binding creates a significant surface charge. That this is so is shown by direct measurements of ANS-dependent surface potentials in monolayers of red cell lipids and by electrophoresis of neuraminidase-treated red cells and lecithin liposomes, in which ANS increases the mobility towards the anode (Fortes, unpublished). The value of the surface potential due to bound ANS cannot be estimated from electrophoresis, because this method only measures the potential at the plane of shear, which is several ångströms away from the membrane surface. Since the surface potential decays with distance, only qualitative estimates can be obtained. Quantitative estimates of ANS-dependent surface potentials were attempted from studies of ANS binding to ghosts as a function of the ionic composition of the medium. It was found that the effect of ions on ANS binding could be explained, qualitatively and quantitatively, by double-layer theory when the effects of increased negative surface charge caused by ANS binding were taken into account. Thus, the increased ANS binding observed at high ionic strength or with divalent ions could be predicted by the charge-screening ability of the electrolyte in the medium, which reduces the surface potential and allows more ANS to bind. It was concluded that the main factor that controls ANS binding is the surface potential, which is made more negative by bound ANS. The surface potential was estimated with the Gouy-Chapman equation using the surface density of the bound ANS, obtained experimentally. It was estimated that 10–50 μM ANS produces surface potentials of -5 to -30 mV (Fortes, 1972, 1976; Fortes et al., 1972a,b). These findings are in agreement with the observation that ANS causes a surface potential of similar magnitude in phospholipid bilayers, as measured by the increase in nonactin-K conductance caused by ANS (McLaughlin et al., 1971).

The creation of a negative surface charge by ANS could explain its inhibitory effect by electrostatic repulsion of anions from the transport sites. This possibility was tested by Fortes and Hoffman (1973). They estimated hypothetical values of ANS-dependent surface potentials from changes in the rate coefficient for Cl^- exchange, assuming that the observed inhibition was only due to decreased Cl^- concentration at the membrane surface caused by the surface potential. This method gave values ranging from -31 mV at 50 μM ANS to -129 mV at 1 mM ANS, which are in remarkable agreement with those estimated from fluorescence studies in ghosts (Fortes, 1972, 1976). Thus, Fortes and Hoffman (1973, 1974) suggested that at least part of the inhibitory effect of anionic inhibitors and those with a high dipole moment is due to electrostatic factors. The inhibitor need not bear a net charge to modify the surface potential. A high dipole moment of the inhibitor and its appropriate orientation in the plane of the membrane, as well as reorientation of membrane components upon binding the inhibitor, can alter the potential arising from membrane dipoles. This can affect the interaction of ions with the membrane, its fluidity, and/or conformation or function of the transport system (Fortes and Hoffman, 1974). The recent studies of Andersen et al. (1976) support this suggestion, since they found that phloretin, even in its uncharged form, decreases anion and increases cation conductance of phospholipid bilayers through modification of the dipole potential at the membrane surface. Further support for the existence of electrostatic effects of phloretin in red cells arises from the observation that phloretin increases valinomycin-induced K^+ exchange (Wieth et al., 1973), although a different interpretation of this effect was given by these authors.

The possibility that the ANS surface potential alters the ion concentration at the membrane surface was tested by Fortes and Ellory (1975) with studies of the effect of ANS on cation fluxes. They found that below 0·5 mM, ANS does not increase the concentration of Na^+ and K^+ near their transport sites, since no increase in passive cation fluxes was seen with up to 0·5 mM ANS, which inhibits Cl^- exchange 99·9 per cent, and no decrease in the K_m for K^+ transport by the pump was seen with 2 mM ANS. Above 0·5 mM, Na and K fluxes increased exponentially with ANS concentration. It was concluded that the cation transport sites must be at a sufficient distance from the ANS binding sites to allow for decay of the electrostatic potential. A similar separation between ion transport sites and the location of sialic acid residues must exist, since elimination of the sialic acid charge by neuraminidase treatment does not affect ion transport (Knauf and Rothstein, 1971a, Fortes and Freter, 1975). Furthermore, the increase in cation permeability was observed at high ANS concentrations, which cause increased osmotic fragility and may represent prehemolytic membrane disruption (Fortes and Ellory, 1975).

In conclusion, although there is evidence that at least the most potent inhibitors, like ANS and phloretin, interact directly with the anion transport system, their mechanism of inhibition is complex. Indirect actions through electrostatic effects or perturbation of the membrane may be also involved. Therefore their usefulness in studying the mechanism of ion transport is limited. On the other hand, the variety of membrane perturbations they produce has yielded significant information on various aspects of membrane dynamics and a great deal of phenomenology, which may become useful as more insight into the actual mechanisms is obtained.

6.3 CHEMICAL MODIFICATION

The possibility of identifying certain chemical groups involved in anion transport and labeling the functional sites for identification and characterization has been studied with compounds of known reactivity and properties.

Sulfhydryl groups do not appear to be essential for anion transport, since PCMBS, which has a high reactivity with SH groups and enters the cell presumably via the same pathways as other anions, does not affect anion transport although it increases cation permeability (Knauf and Rothstein, 1971b).

On the other hand, several amino reagents inhibit anion transport, supporting Passow's (1964, 1965) suggestion that amino groups control anion permeability.

DNFB, MNT, TNBS, maleic anhydride, SITS, DIDS and pyridoxal phosphate are potent inhibitors of sulfate and chloride exchange (Passow, 1969; Passow and Schnell, 1969; Knauf and Rothstein, 1971a; Poensgen and Passow, 1971; Cabantchik and Rothstein, 1972, 1974a; Cabantchik et al., 1975a). The inhibitory effect of DNFB and MNT resembles that observed with reversible inhibitors in that, at high concentrations, both inhibitors increase cation permeability in addition to their inhibitory effect on anion transport (Passow and Schnell, 1969; Knauf and Rothstein, 1971a). In addition, DNFB treatment reduces the activation energy for sulfate exchange from 33 to 10 kcal mol^{-1} (Schwoch et al., 1974).

The disulfonic stilbene derivatives SITS and DIDS are of particular interest since they are impermeable in intact cells (Maddy, 1964), they react with a limited number of sites and inhibit Cl^- and $SO_4^=$ exchange without any appreciable effect on cation permeability (Knauf and Rothstein, 1971a; Cabantchik and Rothstein, 1972). These results provide further support to the idea that anion transport pathways are separate from cation channels and that sites located on the external membrane surface control anion permeability.

Using a series of stilbene disulfonate derivatives, some of which could react with amino groups and others which were unreactive, Cabantchik and Rothstein (1972) showed that reaction with amino groups was responsible for the irreversibility of inhibition, but was not a necessary condition for inhibition. Nonreactive disulfonic stilbenes inhibited reversibly. Cabantchik and Rothstein (1972) concluded that the site of action of the stilbene disulfonates must contain positive charges that interact electrostatically with the anionic inhibitors, and must be near hydrophobic regions, since the inhibitory potency of different derivatives varied over a 5000-fold range with those containing hydrophobic side groups, such as acetyl or aromatic rings, being most potent. The most potent inhibitor is the diisothiocyanate (DIDS), which inhibits 98 per cent of the sulfate or chloride fluxes at high concentration ($\sim 10^{-4}$ M) and 50 per cent below 1 μM.

One of the most important findings was that when radioactive derivatives of DIDS were used to label intact cells, and the pattern of labeling was analysed, more than 90 per cent of the radioactivity was found in a single polypeptide, of 95 000 molecular weight, as determined by polyacrylamide gel electrophoresis in the presence of sodium dodecyl sulfate (Cabantchik and Rothstein, 1972, 1974a). The rest of the label was in lipid ($\sim$1 per cent) and the major glycoprotein of the red cell membrane ($\sim$5 per cent). Mild digestion of the labeled cells with proteolytic enzymes released a small fraction of the bound DIDS, which corresponded to the label in the glycoprotein. Since the proteolytic digestion has no effect on anion transport in control cells, it was concluded that the functional sites that are inactivated by DIDS are in the 95 K protein (Cabantchik and Rothstein, 1974b). Pronase, which has been shown by Passow (1971) to inhibit sulfate transport, was found to hydrolyse the 95 K protein into two membrane-bound fragments. Only about 10 per cent of the bound DIDS was found in the smaller fragment (35 000 daltons) while the remainder was found in the 65 000 dalton fragment. This led Cabantchik and Rothstein (1974b) to conclude that the anion transport function resides in the 65 K portion of the 95 K protein.

A maximum of about 3×10^5 DIDS binding sites per cell were found. When DIDS binding was plotted against inhibition of anion transport a linear relationship was observed, indicating that reaction with DIDS renders the binding site nonfunctional (Cabantchik and Rothstein, 1974a).

The specificity of the DIDS labeling pattern of the membrane components depends on the accessibility of potentially reactive groups, rather than stereospecific interactions with the binding site. When "leaky" ghosts, instead of intact cells, are exposed to DIDS, extensive labeling of lipids and all the membrane proteins is observed (Cabantchik and Rothstein, 1974a). However, little additional DIDS binding to the 95 K protein is found in ghosts compared to intact cells, indicating that essentially all the functional DIDS binding sites are asymmetrically located on the outside surface of the protein.

Further evidence on the involvement of the 95 K protein is provided by the finding that other covalent inhibitors react with this polypeptide (Cabantchik *et al.*, 1975a,b; Ho and Guidotti, 1975; Zaki *et al.*, 1975) and some, like DNFB and PDP, decrease the number of DIDS-reacting sites, suggesting that they have a common site of action.

PDP inhibits anion transport reversibly when present either inside or outside the cell. Addition of borohydride makes PDP an irreversible inhibitor, suggesting that it forms a Schiff base with amino groups. In the presence of PDP, DIDS binding is inhibited by about 90 per cent (Cabantchik *et al.*, 1975a). If the PDP is removed by washing, DIDS binding returns to almost normal. However, if only external PDP is removed by washing in the presence of dipyridamole, which inhibits PDP efflux and thus traps PDP inside the cell, DIDS binding is still inhibited

40–50 per cent (Rothstein et al., 1976). These results suggest that the DIDS binding sites, which are external, can be affected by binding an inhibitor to the inside surface. Rothstein et al. (1976) have interpreted these observations as indication that the DIDS binding site can be trapped on the inside by PDP. However, an allosteric effect that does not necessarily involve translocation of the site is also possible. Also, this experiment requires the use of a third inhibitor, dipyridamole, to trap the PDP inside. It is puzzling that dipyridamole does not appear to inhibit DIDS binding, suggesting the participation of different sites not accessible or reactive with DIDS. The existence of sites that do not react with DIDS has also been suggested by Zaki et al. (1975) on the basis of inhibition of DNFB binding by DIDS and APMB.

Another labeling approach has recently been developed by Knauf et al. (1976). Since the photolysable nitrene, NAP-taurine, originally developed as a nonpenetrating photochemical label for membranes (Staros and Richards, 1974) was found to be a permeable anion at 37°C, but not at 0°C (Staros et al., 1975), the possibility of photochemical labeling of the transport site by NAP-taurine was investigated. It was found that NAP-taurine was a competitive inhibitor of Cl^- and $SO_4^=$ transport in the dark, but caused irreversible inhibition if exposed to ultraviolet light. Analysis of the labeled components using radioactive NAP-taurine showed extensive labeling of the 95 K protein although other membrane components were also labeled. However, competition between Cl^- and NAP-taurine was observed mainly at the 95 K protein, since labeling of this band was decreased at high Cl^- concentrations. DIDS also decreased labeling of the 95 K polypeptide by NAP-taurine (Rothstein et al., 1976).

An important observation is that all the irreversible inhibitors, particularly DIDS and SITS, inhibit both anion exchange and anion conductance (Sachs et al., 1975). This is strongly suggestive that both types of anion transport occur through the same pathway. However, it has been claimed that the anion conductance and exchange pathways are independent and, possibly, physically separate on the basis of differences in selectivity, pH dependence, sensitivity to inhibitors and energies of activation (Wieth et al., 1973; Sachs et al., 1975). Nevertheless, it should be kept in mind that anion conductance studies are difficult and must rely on the use of ionophores and putative specific inhibitors of anion exchange, such as phloretin (Wieth et al., 1973). Under these conditions, it is difficult to establish if the ionophore or inhibitor treatments do not perturb the properties of the system under study. In this respect, phloretin and phlorizin appear to increase Cl^- conductance (Wieth et al., 1973; Kaplan and Passow, 1974) as measured by net KCl fluxes in the presence of ionophores; however, in the absence of ionophores, phloretin decreases KCl fluxes (Fortes and Freter, 1975).

Thus it is difficult to decide, on the basis of the available information, whether or not the anion conductance pathway is related to the mechanism of anion exchange. The fact that both processes are specifically inhibited by reaction of DIDS with the 95 K protein suggests that they are related.

7 Molecular mechanisms of anion transport

The involvement of a 95 K polypeptide in anion transport has been further established by the reconstitution of sulfate exchange in liposomes treated with a triton X-100 extract from red cell membranes, containing this polypeptide as a major component (Rothstein et al., 1975). Also purified red cell membrane vesicles which were depleted of most of the other proteins, but which retained a major fraction of the 95 K polypeptides and the original membrane lipids, have been recently shown to exhibit the characteristic anion transport properties seen in the original cell, including energy of activation, pH dependence, anion selectivity, sensitivity to DIDS and differences in exchange and net rates of anion fluxes (Wolosin et al., 1976).

The 95 K polypeptide is an integral membrane protein that is asymmetrically distributed across the membrane, since different peptide fragments are labeled when different sides of the membrane are exposed to nonpenetrating labeling reagents (Bretscher, 1971; Cabantchik et al., 1975b), and different fragments are produced by exposure of the two membrane surfaces to proteolytic digestion (Jenkins and Tanner, 1975; Steck et al., 1976). These findings indicate that the protein cannot rotate or diffuse across the membrane.

Since DIDS is a bifunctional reagent, Rothstein and Cabantchik (1974) were able to use it to cross-link ferritin to the 95 K polypeptide and establish that this protein is part of the intramembrane particles seen in freeze-fracture electron microscopy. However, the size of these particles indicates that they must contain oligomers of the 95 K protein, probably in association with the glycoprotein that is also associated with these particles (Pinto Da Silva and Nicolson, 1974). This suggests the possibility that a variety of different functions, including sugar transport, are associated with the particles, constituted by clusters of different polypeptides.

Not all the 95 K polypeptides appear to be involved in anion transport. There are about 10^6 copies per cell of this polypeptide, and only about a third bind DIDS (Cabantchik and Rothstein, 1974a). This may reflect the presence of different proteins, of similar mass, that happen to migrate together in SDS gel electrophoresis. In addition, there is evidence that at least some of the 95 K polypeptides exist as noncovalent dimers (Steck, 1972; Wang and Richards, 1974). Such an oligomeric structure may exhibit half-site reactivity if reciprocal conformations of the sub-units exist.

A dimeric structure with sub-units which oscillate between two conformations, associated with the exchange of anions across the membrane, is an attractive model that is qualitatively consistent with the observations presented in this chapter and the current ideas on the structure and organization of membrane proteins (Singer, 1974; Rothstein et al., 1976).

However, any molecular model must be able to explain the impressive rate at which anions are transported, since the estimated turnover for Cl$^-$ exchange at 37°C is 5×10^5 to 8×10^5 ions site^{-1} sec^{-1} (Sachs et al., 1975), which is several orders of magnitude faster than that of carrier ionophores or other mediated transport systems like the Na–K pump. Since Cl$^-$ exchange is electroneutral, apparently requiring the movement of a part of the protein bearing a positive charge, the mobile component must be very small and must move a very short distance to exhibit such high turnover rates. The enormous difference in rates of transport of mono and divalent anions, and the possible association of the conductance and exchange pathways, are additional factors to be considered in this fascinating puzzle.

It is not unreasonable to expect that forthcoming information on the structure and organization of the proteins involved in anion transport and studies with reconstituted systems, in which the electrical behavior can be studied directly, will provide sufficient clues to understand the mechanism of anion transport in the red blood cell.

ACKNOWLEDGEMENTS

The author gratefully acknowledges support by a grant-in-aid from the American Heart Association and grant RR-08135-02 funded by the USPHS Division of Research Resources and the National Heart and Lung Institute.

References

ANDERSEN, O. S., FINKELSTEIN, A., KATZ, I. and CASS, A. (1976). *J. Gen. Physiol.* **67**, 749.
BRETSCHER, M. S. (1971). *J. Molec. Biol.* **59**, 351.
CABANTCHIK, Z. I., BALSHIN, M., BREUER, W. and ROTHSTEIN, A. (1975a). *J. Biol. Chem.* **250**, 5310.
CABANTCHIK, Z. I., BALSHIN, M., BREUER, W., MARCUS, H. and ROTHSTEIN, A. (1975b). *Biochim. Biophys. Acta*, **382**, 621.
CABANTCHIK, Z. I. and ROTHSTEIN, A. (1972). *J. Membrane Biol.* **10**, 311.
CABANTCHIK, Z. I. and ROTHSTEIN, A. (1974a). *J. Membrane Biol.* **15**, 207.

CABANTCHIK, Z. I. and ROTHSTEIN, A. (1974b). *J. Membrane Biol.* **15**, 227.
CASS, A. and DALMARK, M. (1973). *Nature New Biol.* **244**, 47.
CHAPPELL, J. B. and CROFTS, A. R. (1966). In "Regulations of Metabolic Processes in Mitochondria" (J. M. Tager, S. Papa, E. Quagliarello and E. C. Slater, eds), p. 293. Elsevier, Amsterdam.
DALMARK, M. (1972). In "Oxygen Affinity of Hemoglobin and Red Cell Acid Base Status" (P. Astrup and M. Rørth, eds), p. 320. Academic Press, New York and London.
DALMARK, M. (1975). *J. Physiol.* **250**, 39.
DALMARK, M. (1976). *J. Gen. Physiol.* **67**, 223.
DALMARK, M. and WIETH, J. O. (1970). *Biochim. Biophys. Acta*, **219**, 525.
DALMARK, M. and WIETH, J. O. (1972). *J. Physiol.* **224**, 583.
DEUTICKE, B. (1968). *Biochim. Biophys. Acta*, **163**, 494.
DEUTICKE, B. (1970). *Naturwiss.* **57**, 172.
DEUTICKE, B. (1973). In "Erythrocytes, Thrombocytes, Leukocytes" (E. Gerlach, K. Moser, E. Deutsch and W. Wilmanns, eds), p. 81. Georg Thieme, Stuttgart.
FORTES, P. A. G. (1972). Ph.D. thesis, University of Pennsylvania.
FORTES, P. A. G. (1976). In "Mitochondria, Bioenergetics, Biogenesis and Membrane Structure" (L. Packer and A. Gomez-Puyou, eds), pp. 327–348. Academic Press, New York and London.
FORTES, P. A. G. and ELLORY, J. C. (1975). *Biochim. Biophys. Acta*, **413**, 65.
FORTES, P. A. G. and FRETER, C. E. (1975). *Abstr. V Int. Biophys. Congr.*, Copenhagen, p. 101.
FORTES, P. A. G. and HOFFMAN, J. F. (1971). *J. Membrane Biol.* **5**, 154.
FORTES, P. A. G. and HOFFMAN, J. F. (1973). In "Erythrocytes, Thrombocytes, Leukocytes" (E. Gerlach, K. Moser, E. Deutsch and W. Wilmanns, eds), pp. 92–95. Georg Thieme, Stuttgart.
FORTES, P. A. G. and HOFFMAN, J. F. (1974). *J. Membrane Biol.* **16**, 79.
FORTES, P. A. G., YGUERABIDE, J. and HOFFMAN, J. F. (1972a). *Biophys. Soc. Abstr.*, Toronto, p. 255a.
FORTES, P. A. G., YGUERABIDE, J. and HOFFMAN, J. F. (1972b). *Abstr. IV Int. Biophys. Congr.* Moscow, **3**, 135.
FUNDER, J. and WIETH, J. O. (1975). *Abstr. V Int. Biophys. Congr.* Copenhagen, p. 102.
GARDOS, G., HOFFMAN, J. F. and PASSOW, H. (1969). In "Laboratory Techniques in Membrane Biophysics" (H. Passow and R. Stämpfli, eds). Springer-Verlag, Berlin.
GERLACH, E., DEUTICKE, B. and DUHM, J. (1964). *Arch. Ges. Physiol.* **280**, 243.
GOLDMAN, D. E. (1943). *J. Gen. Physiol.* **27**, 37.
GUNN, R. B. (1972). In "Oxygen Affinity of Hemoglobin and Red Cell Acid Base Status" (P. Astrup and M. Rørth, eds), p. 823. Academic Press, New York and London.
GUNN, R. B. (1973). In "Erythrocytes, Thrombocytes, Leukocytes" (E. Gerlach, K. Moser, E. Deutsch and W. Wilmanns, eds), p. 77. Georg Thieme, Stuttgart.
GUNN, R. B., DALMARK, M., TOSTESON, D. C. and WIETH, J. O. (1973). *J. Gen. Physiol.* **61**, 185.
GUNN, R. B., HARTLEY, P. N. and HORTON, J. M. (1974). *Fed. Proc.* **33**, 1592.
GUNN, R. B. and TOSTESON, D. C. (1971). *J. Gen. Physiol.* **57**, 593.
GUNN, R. B., WIETH, J. O. and TOSTESON, D. C. (1975). *J. Gen. Physiol.* **65**, 731.
HARRIS, E. J. and PRESSMAN, B. C. (1967). *Nature*, **216**, 918.

Ho, M. K. and GUIDOTTI, G. (1975). *J. Biol. Chem.* **250**, 675.
HODGKIN, A. L. and KATZ, B. (1949). *Biophys. J.* **9**, 115.
HOFFMAN, J. F. and LARIS, P. (1974). *J. Physiol.* **239**, 519.
HOFFMAN, J. F. and LASSEN, U. V. (1971). *Abstr. XXV Int. Congr. Physiol. Sci.* Munich, **9**, 253.
HUNTER, M. J. (1971). *J. Physiol.* **218**, 49P.
JENKINS, R. E. and TANNER, M. J. A. (1975). *Biochem. J.* **147**, 393.
JENNINGS, M. L. (1976). *J. Membrane Biol.* **28**, 187.
JENNINGS, M. L. and SOLOMON, A. K. (1976). *J. Gen. Physiol.* **67**, 381.
KAPLAN, J. H. and PASSOW, H. (1974). *J. Membrane Biol.* **19**, 179.
KAPLAN, J. H., SCORAH, K., FASOLD, H. and PASSOW, H. (1976). *FEBS Lett.* **62**, 182.
KNAUF, P. A., BREUER, W., DAVIDSON, L. and ROTHSTEIN, A. (1976). *Biophys. J.* **16**, 107a.
KNAUF, P. A., FUHRMANN, G. F. ROTHSTEIN S. and ROTHSTEIN, A. (1977). *J. Gen. Physiol.* **69**, 363.
KNAUF, P. A. and ROTHSTEIN, A. (1971a). *J. Gen. Physiol.* **58**, 190.
KNAUF, P. A. and ROTHSTEIN, A. (1971b). *J. Gen. Physiol.* **58**, 211.
LASSEN, U. V. (1972). *In* "Oxygen Affinity of Hemoglobin and Red Cell Acid Base Status" (P. Astrup and M. Rørth, eds), p. 291. Academic Press, New York and London.
LASSEN, U.V., Pape, L. and Vestergaard-Bogind, B. (1973). *In* "Erythrocytes, Thrombocytes, Leukocytes" (E. Gerlach, K. Moser, E. Deutsch and W. Wilmanns, eds) pp. 33–36. Georg Thieme, Stuttgart.
LEFEVRE, P. G. (1961). *Pharmacol. Rev.* **13**, 39.
LEPKE, S. and PASSOW, H. (1971). *J. Membrane Biol.* **6**, 158.
LEPKE, S. and PASSOW, H. (1973). *Biochim. Biophys. Acta*. **298**, 529.
MACEY, R. I. and FARMER, R. E. L. (1970). *Biochem. Biophys. Acta*, **211**, 104.
MADDY, A. H. (1964). *Biochim. Biophys. Acta*, **88**, 390.
MAWE, R. C. and HEMPLING, H. G. (1965). *J. Cell. Comp. Physiol.* **66**, 95.
MCLAUGHLIN, S. G. A. (1973). *Nature*, **243**, 234.
MCLAUGHLIN, S. G. A., SZABO, G. and EISENMAN, G. (1971). *J. Gen. Physiol.* **58**, 667.
MEYER, K. H. and SIEVERS, J. F. (1936). *Helv. Chim. Acta*, **19**, 649.
MOND, R. (1927). *Arch. Ges. Physiol.* **217**, 618.
OBAID, A. L., REGA, A. F. and GARRAHAN, P. J. (1972). *J. Membrane Biol.* **9**, 385.
OWEN, J. D. and SOLOMON, A. K. (1972). *Biochim. Biophys. Acta*, **290**, 414.
PASSOW, H. (1964). *In* "The Red Blood Cell" (C. Bishop and D. Surgenor, eds), p. 71. Academic Press, New York and London.
PASSOW, H. (1965). *Proc. XXIII Int. Congr. Physiol. Sci.*, p. 555.
PASSOW, H. (1969). *Prog. Biophys. Mol. Biol.* **19**, 425.
PASSOW, H. (1971). *J. Membrane Biol.* **6**, 233.
PASSOW, H. and SCHNELL, K. F. (1969). *Experientia*, **25**, 460.
PASSOW, H. and WOOD, P. G. (1974). *In* "Drugs and Transport Processes" (B. A. Callingham, ed), p. 149. MacMillan, London.
PINTO DA SILVA, P. and NICOLSON, G. L. (1974). *Biochim. Biophys. Acta*, **363**, 311.
POENSGEN, J. and PASSOW, H. (1971). *J. Membrane Biol.* **6**, 210.
ROTHSTEIN, A. and CABANTCHIK, Z. I. (1974). *In* "Comparative Biochemistry and Physiology of Transport" (L. Bolis, K. Bloch and S. E. Luna, eds), p. 354. American Elsevier, New York.

Rothstein, A., Cabantchik, Z. I., Balshin, M. and Juliano, R. (1975). *Biochem. Biophys. Res. Commun.* **64**, 144.
Rothstein, A., Cabantchik, Z. I. and Knauf, P. A. (1976). *Fed. Proc.* **35**, 3.
Sachs, J. R., Knauf, P. A. and Dunham, P. B. (1975). *In* "The Red Blood Cell" (D. M. Surgenor, ed), vol. II, p. 613. Academic Press, New York and London.
Scarpa, A., Cecchetto, A. and Azzone, G. F. (1970). *Biochim. Biophys. Acta*, **219**, 179.
Schnell, K. F. (1972). *Biochim. Biophys. Acta*, **282**, 265.
Schnell, K. F., Gerhardt, S., Lepke, S. and Passow, H. (1973). *Biochim. Biophys. Acta*, **318**, 474.
Schnell, K. F., Gerhardt, S. and Schöppe-Fredenburg, A. (1977). *J. Membrane Biol.* **30**: 319.
Schwartz, A., Lindenmayer, G. E. and Allen, J. C. (1975). *Pharmacol. Rev.* **27**, 3.
Schwoch, G., Rudloff, V., Wood-Guth, I. and Passow, H. (1974). *Biochim. Biophys. Acta*, **339**, 126.
Seeman, P. (1972). *Pharmacol. Rev.* **24**, 583.
Shean, G. and Sollner, K. (1966). *Ann. N.Y. Acad. Sci.* **137**, 759.
Sheetz, M. P. and Singer, S. J. (1974). *Proc. Nat. Acad. Sci.* **71**, 4457.
Sims, P. J., Waggoner, A. S., Wang, C. H. and Hoffman, J. F. (1974). *Biochemistry*, **13**, 3315.
Singer, S. J. (1974). *A. Rev. Biochem.* **43**, 805.
Staros, J. V. and Richards, F. M. (1974). *Biochemistry*, **13**, 2720.
Staros, J. V., Richards, F. M. and Haley, B. E. (1975). *J. Biol. Chem.* **250**, 8174.
Steck, T. L. (1972). *J. Molec. Biol.* **66**, 295.
Steck, T. L., Ramos, B. and Strapazon, E. (1976). *Biochemistry*, **15**, 1154.
Teorell, T. (1952). *J. Gen. Physiol.* **35**, 669.
Tosteson, D. C. (1959). *Acta Physiol. Scand.* **46**, 19.
Tosteson, D. C., Gunn, R. B. and Wieth, J. O. (1973). *In* "Erythrocytes, Thrombocytes, Leukocytes" (E. Gerlach, K. Moser, E. Deutsch and W. Wilmanns, eds), p. 62. Georg Thieme, Stuttgart.
Wang, K. and Richards, F. M. (1974). *J. Biol. Chem.* **249**, 8005.
Wieth, J. O. (1970). *J. Physiol.* **207**, 581.
Wieth, J. O. (1972).
Wieth, J. O., Dalmark, M., Gunn, R. B. and Tosteson, D. C. (1973). *In* "Erythrocytes, Thrombocytes, Leukocytes" (E. Gerlach, K. Moser, E. Deutsch and W. Wilmanns, eds), p. 71. Georg Thieme, Stuttgart.
Wieth, J. O., Funder, J., Gunn, R. B. and Brahm, J. (1974). *In* "Comparative Biochemistry and Physiology of Transport" (L. Bolis, K. Bloch and S. E. Luma, eds), p. 317. American Elsevier, New York.
Wolosin, J. M., Ginsburg, H. and Cabantchik, Z. I. (1977). *J. Biol. Chem.* **252**, 2419.
Wood, P. G. and Passow, H. (1971). *Abstr. XXV Int. Congr. Physiol. Sci.*, Munich, **9**, 608.
Zaki, L., Fasold, H., Schuhmann, B. and Passow, H. (1975). *J. Cell. Physiol.* **86**, 471.
Zwaal, R. F. A., Roelofsen, B. and Colley, C. M. (1973). *Biochim. Biophys. Acta*, **300**, 159.

Organic anion transport in red blood cells

R. MOTAIS

Laboratoire de Physiologie Cellulaire, Faculté des Sciences de Nice, Parc Valrose, 06034 Nice Cedex

1 Introduction	197
2 Discrimination between ionic and nonionic penetration of organic acids	198
2.1 Haemolysis criterion	199
2.2 External pH changes as a criterion	200
2.3 Net exchange as a criterion	201
3 The mode of penetration of organic anions	203
4 Relationship between organic and inorganic anion permeabilities	211
4.1 Inhibitory action of phenylpyruvate	211
4.2 Inhibition by covalently bound SITS	212
4.3 Sensitivity of organic and inorganic anion transport to amphiphilic inhibitors	213
4.4 Temperature dependency	215
4.5 Influence of inorganic anions on organic anion permeability	215
4.6 pH dependency of anion transfer	216
5 Summary	217
References	218

1 Introduction

Erythrocytes differ from other cells mainly in their highly selective permeability to anions; thus small hydrophilic anions such as Cl^- or HCO_3^- penetrate about one million times faster than hydrophilic cations of similar size such as Na^+ or K^+.

This anion selectivity was first tentatively explained by Mond (1927) on the ground of Michaelis' work (1925) on the ion permeability of the collodion membrane. He proposed that positive, dissociable fixed charges on the wall of water-filled pores facilitate penetration of hydrophilic anions and retard that of cations. The fixed charges concept of ion selectivity was later reinforced by experimental and theoretical works (Teorell, 1935; Meyer and Sievers, 1936; Wilbrandt, 1942). It was found to provide a satisfactory quantitative description of numerous data obtained on the penetration characteristics of slowly penetrating anions such as sulphate (Passow, 1969a,b), and thus was generally accepted (Deuticke, 1970; Wieth, 1970; Gunn and Tosteson, 1971).

However, not all the data concerning slowly penetrating anions fit well with this concept (see Passow and Wood, 1974). Moreover, some of the penetration characteristics of rapidly permeating anions, such as chloride and other halides, are inexplicable by the fixed-charges hypothesis (Gunn et al., 1973). Thus a new concept emerges which differs basically from the positive charges hypothesis: mainly it is assumed that the entry of anions into the cell does not proceed by the diffusion of free ions but needs a specific interaction of the penetrating anion with a component of the erythrocyte membrane (Gunn, 1972; Wieth, 1972; Gunn et al., 1973). In other words, in the first model, anionic permeability is controlled by the relation between the pore diameter and the size of the solute molecule, and in the second model it is mainly controlled by the nature of the interaction between anion and the facilitated transporting system. A direct approach to test the relative merits of the two proposed models is to evaluate the correlation between the penetration rates of various anions and their physico-chemical properties. Such an approach can easily be realized by using organic anions because, with these compounds, it is possible to use a large number of probing molecules of varying size and molecular configuration.

In the present paper, devoted to discussing the organic anion permeability of the red cell membrane, we shall first consider the penetration characteristics of these molecules, with a particular emphasis on this experimental approach. Then, by comparing the kinetics of penetration of organic and inorganic anions, we shall look at the specificity of the organic anion pathway.

2 Discrimination between ionic and nonionic penetration of organic acids

The interpretation of the results concerning organic anion permeability is complicated by the fact that because of the partial liposolubility and incomplete ionization of these anions, many of them can cross biological membranes in neutral undissociated form (Höber, 1936; Green, 1949; Giebel and Passow, 1960; Schanker et al., 1964; Deuticke, 1972a,b, 1973). When characterizing the ionic transfer system, therefore, a clear-cut distinction must be made between penetration of organic anion and penetration of undissociated acid: indeed the penetration of neutral undissociated acid does not require a receptor molecule but depends on the solubility of the compound in the lipid phase of the membrane. Such a distinction can be obtained by different techniques: the rate of haemolysis in ammonium salt (Aubert and Motais, 1975), the changes in external pH (Deuticke, 1972a; Aubert and Motais, 1975) and the net exchange measurements of extracellular organic anions with cellular chloride (Deuticke, 1972a; Motais and Cousin, 1976).

2.1 HAEMOLYSIS CRITERION

Osmotic haemolysis occurs when red cells are suspended in isotonic solutions of ammonium salts.

When organic acid enters the cell as an anion the process can be summarized as follows (Fig. 1a): the membrane is as poorly permeable to NH_4^+ as to other cations but highly permeable to uncharged NH_3 (Jacobs, 1924). NH_3 enters the cell in which a new equilibrium will then be established. The OH^- ions (or HCO_3^- due to hydration of CO_2 by the OH^- ion as in Fig. 1b) can exchange with external organic anions A^-. The net result is the penetration of the ammonium salt, a process which induces a swelling of the cell and finally osmotic haemolysis. The speed of haemolysis measures the penetration rate of the anion, penetration of NH_3 and dissociation of water not being the limiting factors. At the limit, if an anion does not enter, haemolysis does not occur (Jacobs and Stewart, 1942). Agents such as SITS,* which inhibit anion permeability across the red blood cell membrane (Knauf and Rothstein, 1971), inhibit haemolysis. Similarly, inhibition of carbonic anhydrase (Jacobs and Stewart, 1942; Maren and Wiley, 1970; Cousin et al., 1975; Motais et al., 1975), or removal of CO_2 (Cousin et al., 1975), considerably increases the time for swelling and haemolysis, i.e. inhibits the rate of A^-–OH^- exchange, suggesting that the transport of OH^- is a process predominantly mediated by HCO_3^- (Deuticke, 1972a; Cousin et al., 1975).

When organic acid enters the cell as undissociated acid the process of haemolysis is different (Fig. 1c); simultaneous penetration of the two uncharged molecules, undissociated acid AH and unionized NH_3, corresponds to the penetration of the external ammonium salt, inducing swelling and haemolysis of the cell. The limiting step of haemolysis is the solubility of the undissociated acid in the lipid phase of the membrane. As an exchange between organic anion and OH^- (or HCO_3^-) does not occur, SITS and carbonic anhydrase inhibitors have no effect on the rate of haemolysis.

In brief, the effect of SITS and carbonic anhydrase inhibitors can be used to distinguish penetration of organic anion from penetration of the undissociated acid and the rate of penetration of organic anion can be

*Abbreviations used: SITS, 4-acetamido-4'-isothiocyanostilbene-2,2'-disulphonic acid, DIDS, 4-4'-diisothiocyano-2,2'-stilbene disulphonate.

deduced from the speed of haemolysis. Haemolysis is followed by measuring the decrease in optical density (O.D.) of a suspension of red blood cells (Aubert and Motais, 1975).

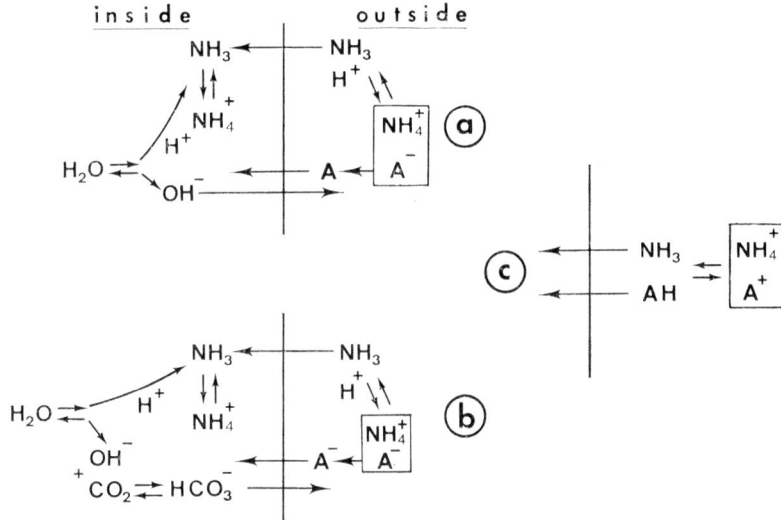

FIG. 1. Haemolysis in isotonic ammonium salt solution. The acid enters the cell as anion by exchange with intracellular OH^- (a) or HCO_3^- (b) or the acid enters the cell as undissociated acid (c).

2.2 EXTERNAL pH CHANGES AS A CRITERION

When red cells are suspended in unbuffered Cl-free Na salts of organic acids at pH 7·4, changes of pH occur and the pattern of pH shift differs according to the route of penetration of organic acid (Deuticke, 1972a). When organic acid enters the cell as anion the process can be described as follows (Fig. 2): organic anions penetrating more slowly than chloride, the external fast-moving OH^-, or more exactly HCO_3^- (Cousin et al., 1975), are exchanged for internal Cl^-, thus inducing external acidification. Then, slow re-equilibration is obtained by exchange between internal OH^- (or HCO_3^-) and external anion. Inhibition of these exchanges by SITS or carbonic anhydrase inhibitors will suppress pH changes.

When organic acid enters the cell as undissociated acid the process is as follows (Fig. 3): penetration of undissociated acid induces alkalinization of external pH. This alkalinization cannot be suppressed by SITS or carbonic anhydrase inhibitors. pH re-equilibration is obtained by exchange between internal Cl^- and external HCO_3^-. The latter process can be inhibited by SITS.

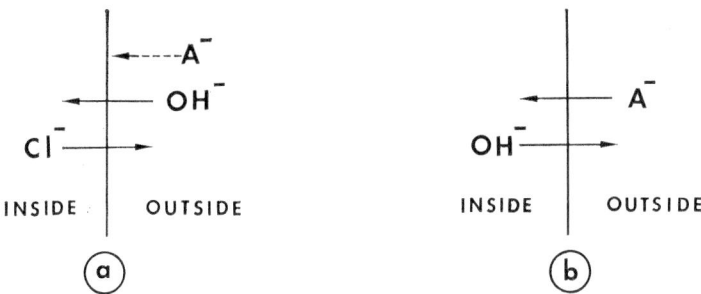

FIG. 2. Transfer processes involved in the external pH changes when organic acid penetrates as anion. (a) Ionic net movement during the decrease of pH. (b) During the re-equilibration phase.

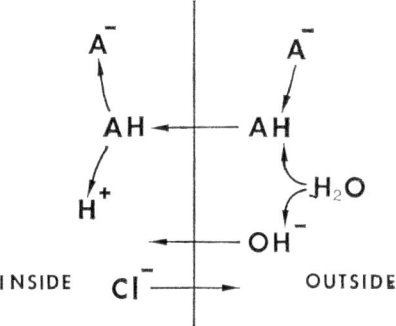

FIG. 3. Transfer processes involved in the external pH changes when organic acid penetrates as undissociated acid.

2.3 NET EXCHANGE AS A CRITERION

The discrimination between ionic and nonionic diffusion of organic acid can also be obtained, in the same experimental conditions as for measurement of external pH changes, by following the net exchange between internal chloride and external organic anion. It has been shown (Deuticke, 1972a) that the nonionic component is selectively inhibited by acetazolamide, a carbonic anhydrase inhibitor which does not influence the ionic permeability of the red cell membrane (Dalmark, 1972; Motais et al., 1975; Cousin and Motais, 1976). This inhibitory effect of acetazolamide on the penetration of undissociated acid can be explained as follows (Fig. 4): the apparent stoichiometric exchange between an external organic anion, penetrating by nonionic diffusion, and internal chloride results from two successive processes. The undissociated acid AH enters the cell, leading on increase of the external OH^- concentration. The extracellular OH^-

ions then exchange with internal chloride and inside recombine with H^+ to form water. The decrease of pH gradient thus obtained maintains a continuous transfer of AH until Donnan equilibrium for all ion species has been established. The Cl_i^-–OH_e^- exchange is mediated by HCO_3^-, which is considered to arise from OH^- and traces of CO_2 in a repetitive cycle involving carbonic anhydrase (Deuticke, 1972a). Inhibition of carbonic anhydrase by acetazolamide retards this exchange and thus also the apparent exchange Cl_i^-–A_e^- (inhibition of carbonic anhydrase cannot completely abolish the Cl^-–OH^- exchange because the uncatalysed reaction of CO_2 with OH^- provides a certain amount of HCO_3^-). It must be pointed out that in these experimental conditions, as illustrated in Fig. 7, the use of SITS cannot permit discrimination between ionic and nonionic diffusion: in ionic diffusion, of course, SITS will inhibit Cl_i–A_e^- exchange; but in nonionic diffusion, by inhibiting the exchange of Cl_i^- with OH_e^- (Fig. 4) it will impair the apparent exchange of Cl_i^- with A_e^-.

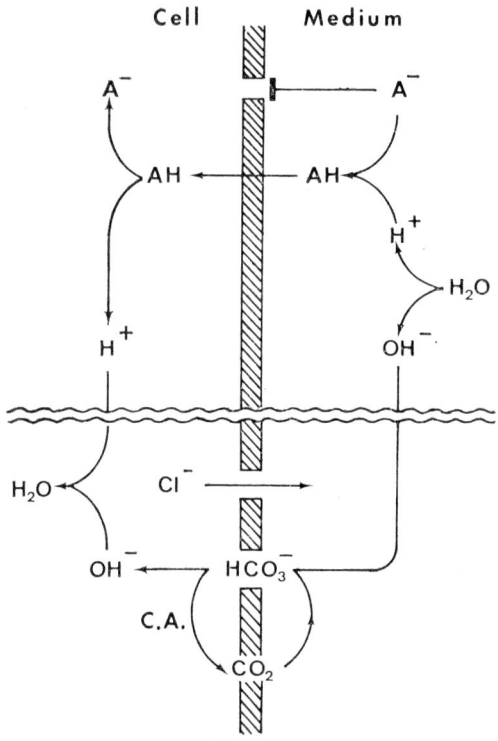

FIG. 4. Anion movements involved in the net transfer of undissociated acids across the red cell membrane (from Deuticke, 1972).

The application of these different criteria is illustrated in Figs 5–7. They allow the detection of ionic and nonionic components in mixed transfer processes (see e.g. Deuticke, 1972a, 1973; Aubert and Motais, 1975).

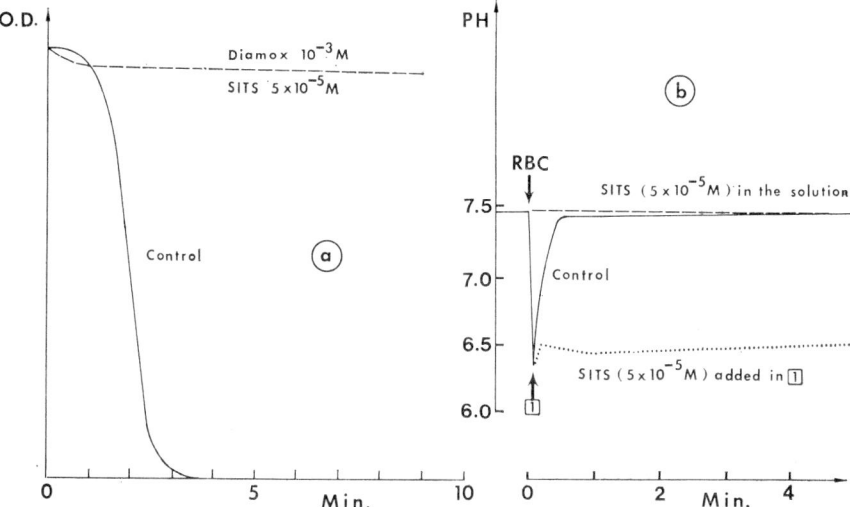

FIG. 5. Demonstration of ionic transfer of glyoxylate. (a) Haemolysis criterion—the time-course of O.D. changes of red cells suspended in isotonic ammonium glyoxylate. (b) Extracellular pH changes after addition of red cells in isotonic solution of Na glyoxylate.

3 The mode of penetration of organic anions

If penetration proceeds by simple diffusion of free anions through aqueous channels of molecular dimensions, lined with positive fixed charges, as postulated in the fixed-charges concept, two consequences must be expected: first, the penetration rate will be independent of the chemical structure of the penetrating anion species since only coulombic interactions are involved; secondly, it will depend on the respective sizes of the pore and of the penetrating anion so that a sieving effect will be observed. As long as anions can rotate freely inside the channel the difference between their penetration rates should be similar to the differences of their diffusion rates in water. When the length of the anion becomes greater than the diameter of the pore, i.e. when penetration has to occur in the direction of the longitudinal axis, a sharp decrease of the penetration rate would be observed. Moreover, for molecules of the same length but of different shape (indicated by the molar volume) large variations of penetration rates would

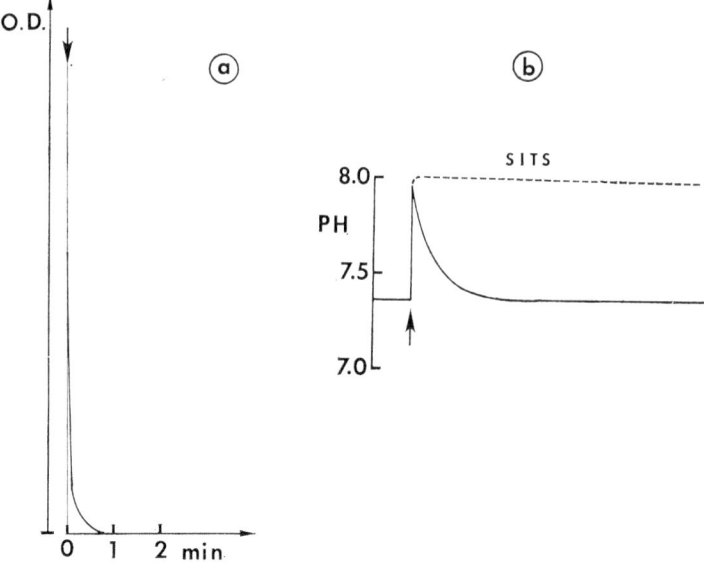

FIG. 6. Demonstration of nonionic transfer of valerate. (a) Haemolysis criterion—the time-course of O.D. changes of red cells suspended in isotonic ammonium valerate. No inhibition can be observed with SITS or Diamox. (b) Extracellular pH changes after addition of red cells in an isotonic solution of Na valerate.

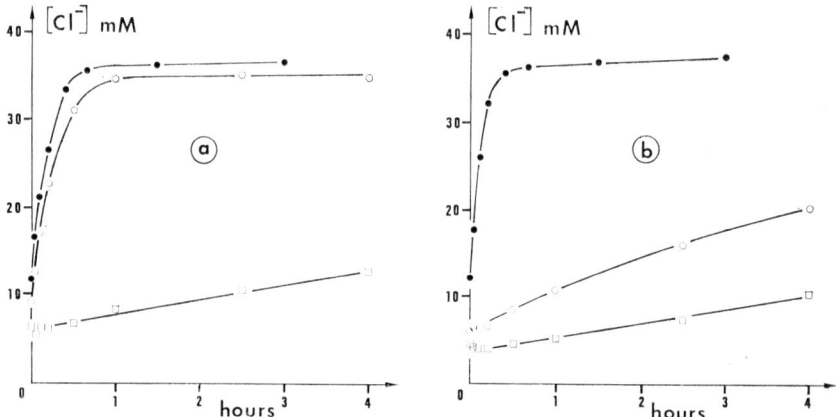

FIG. 7. Effects of SITS (5×10^{-5} M) and acetazolamide (5×10^{-3} M): (a) on exchange of extracellular pyruvate with intracellular chloride; (b) on exchange of extracellular valerate with intracellular chloride. (Haematocrit 37 per cent; 10°C.)
● Control; ○ Acetazolamide; □ SITS.

arise. Such an apparent geometrical limitation has been observed by Giebel and Passow (1960) using a series of dicarboxylic acids (Table 1). Applying the above interpretation, these data would indicate that molecules up to the length of these of malonic or hydroxymalonic acids, i.e. 7·6 Å, can rotate freely in the pore, and molecules of 9 Å length cannot (a sharp decrease in penetration rate is seen from fumaric acid, and molecules of the same length but different molar volume such as fumaric, succinic, malic and tartaric acids show large variations of diffusion rates); therefore the diameter of pores would be considered as lying in the range 7·6–9 Å.

TABLE 1
Penetration of a dicarboxylic acids in bovine red blood cells
(from Giebel and Passow, 1960)

Anion species	$t_{\frac{1}{2}}$	Molar volume cm^3	Length Å
Oxalate	1	35·8	7·6
Malonate	6	50·8	7·6
Hydroxymalonate	9	54·4	7·6
Maleate	7	59·4	6·9
Fumarate	74	59·8	8·7
Succinate	220	63·83	9·0
Malate	323	72·44	9·0
Tartrate	2200	73·90	9·0
Glutarate	1180	81·0	10·3

However, from recent data of Aubert and Motais (1975), working on about sixty organic acids, strong evidence emerges that this interpretation in terms of a geometrical limitation is not satisfactory.

1. Malate and tartrate were found to be practically impermeant, as previously demonstrated by Giebel and Passow (1960). Nevertheless, some anions which have about the same length as the "impermeant" malate or tartrate enter the cell rapidly (Fig. 8). These include aceturate, oxo-2-valerate, sulphanilate and phthalate. Moreover, hippurate and *para*-amino-hippurate, which have lengths largely exceeding that of malate and tartrate and a greater molar volume, enter the cell under ionic form.
2. The concept of a sieve effect cannot explain that benzene sulphonate enters the cell five times slower than *para*-aminobenzene-sulphonate (Fig. 9).
3. The penetration rates of chemically related anions largely depend on the relative position of a chemical group (Fig. 9). Thus, of the isomers of aminobenzene sulphonic acid it can be observed that 4-amino and 3-amino enter the cells ($t_{\frac{1}{2}}$ 20 min and 35 min, respectively), but 2-amino

cannot penetrate. Similarly, 2-carboxyl benzoic acid (phthalic acid) penetrates the cell with a half-time of 35–45 min, contrasting with 3- and 4-isomers (isophthalic and terephthalic, respectively) which cannot enter the cell.

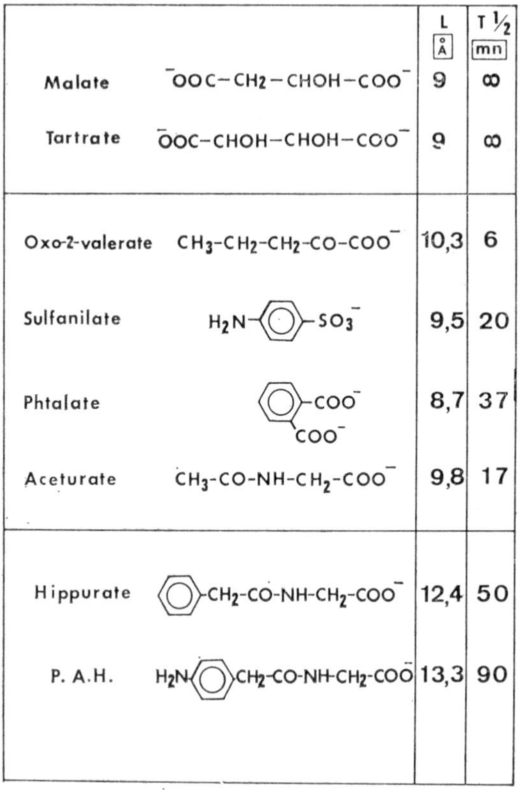

		L [Å]	T½ [mn]
Malate	⁻OOC–CH₂–CHOH–COO⁻	9	∞
Tartrate	⁻OOC–CHOH–CHOH–COO⁻	9	∞
Oxo-2-valerate	CH₃–CH₂–CH₂–CO–COO⁻	10,3	6
Sulfanilate	H₂N–⟨◯⟩–SO₃⁻	9,5	20
Phtalate	⟨◯⟩(–COO⁻)(–COO⁻)	8,7	37
Aceturate	CH₃–CO–NH–CH₂–COO⁻	9,8	17
Hippurate	⟨◯⟩–CH₂–CO–NH–CH₂–COO⁻	12,4	50
P. A. H.	H₂N–⟨◯⟩–CH₂–CO–NH–CH₂–COO⁻	13,3	90

Fig. 8. Penetration rates of some carboxylic acids.

Obviously a geometrical limitation cannot explain such a differential permeability in chemically related anions. It would seem that the erythrocyte membrane has some special property, making the anion permeability dependent on the chemical structure of the penetrating anion species. In other words, a specific interaction of the organic anion with a component of the erythrocyte membrane is involved in their transport.

What is the molecular configuration involved in the specific interaction with the anionic binding site?

The structural requirements permitting ionic transfer can be deduced from the analysis of all the data obtained by Aubert and Motais (1975).

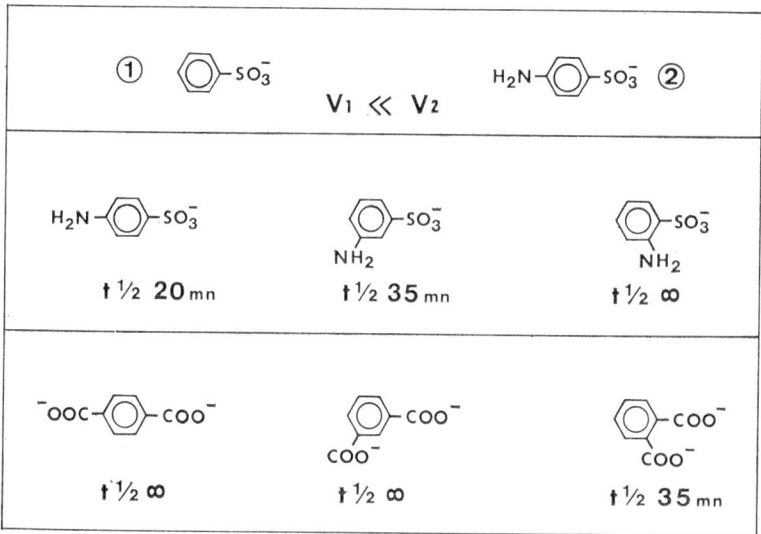

Fig. 9. Penetration rates of chemically related anions.

The example provided by the smallest carboxylic acid (formic acid) shows that carboxyl alone can account for interaction with the binding site. Some formic acid penetrates the red cell rapidly as formate anion and more slowly as undissociated acid. But analysis of the ionic transfer of all the other carboxylic acids shows that larger molecules require a more complex reactive group (however, Deuticke (1973) detects a small ionic component for acetic acid). It can be observed that for an organic acid to penetrate as an anion one of the extremities of the molecules must be strongly polar. This hydrophylic extremity can consist of (Fig. 10) either a sulphonic group or a carboxyl group, but not a carboxyl group alone. Beside the carboxyl group there has to be a complementary group: a second carboxyl group, or a keto group, or a hydroxyl group or an amide group. Among the complementary groups, OH is least efficient. Similar observa-

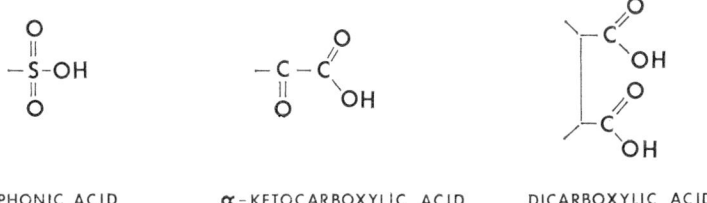

Fig. 10. Some molecular structures allowing a three-point attachment.

tions concerning the effect of α-keto and α-hydroxy substitution have been made by Deuticke (1972a, 1973).

It is important, as shown in Fig. 11, that the complementary group must be spatially close to the carboxyl group (compare 2-hydroxypropionic and 3-hydroxypropionic; 2-oxovaleric and 4-oxovaleric).

In brief, the reactive group allowing ionic transport is characteristic: it seems necessary to obtain a three-point interaction between organic anion and membrane receptor. This three-point contact involves three oxygen atoms on the anion which react by formation of ionic and hydrogen bonds with complementary loci on the membrane receptor.

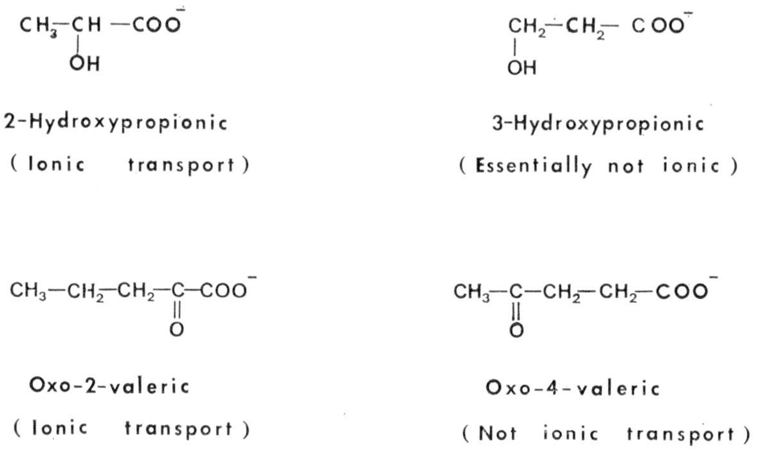

$$CH_3-CH(OH)-COO^-$$

2-Hydroxypropionic

(Ionic transport)

$$CH_2(OH)-CH_2-COO^-$$

3-Hydroxypropionic

(Essentially not ionic)

$$CH_3-CH_2-CH_2-C(=O)-COO^-$$

Oxo-2-valeric

(Ionic transport)

$$CH_3-C(=O)-CH_2-CH_2-COO^-$$

Oxo-4-valeric

(Not ionic transport)

FIG. 11. Importance of the position of the complementary group.

These requirements, however, are sufficient only when the acid is of small size; they no longer hold when the C chain length is greater than 4. It then becomes essential that the other extremity of the molecule is apolar. The necessity of such an amphiphilic structure is illustrated by the comparisons shown in Fig. 12 between 2-oxovaleric and 2-oxoglutaric acid.

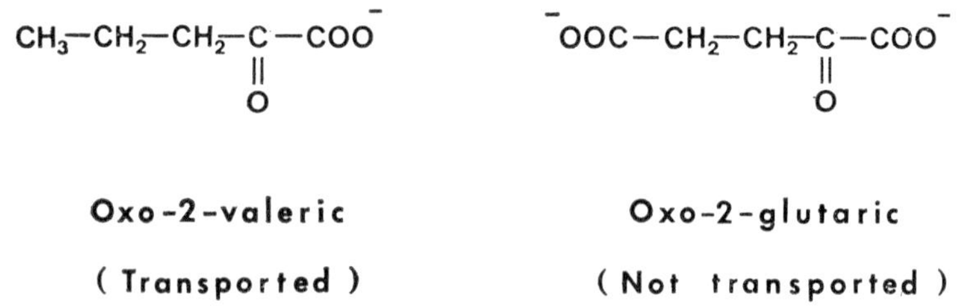

$$CH_3-CH_2-CH_2-C(=O)-COO^-$$

Oxo-2-valeric

(Transported)

$$^-OOC-CH_2-CH_2-C(=O)-COO^-$$

Oxo-2-glutaric

(Not transported)

FIG. 12. Necessity of an amphiphilic structure for the largest molecules

ORGANIC ANION TRANSPORT IN RED BLOOD CELLS 209

From the above one may consider that the structural requirement allowing for ionic transfer is a strong polar head for the smallest molecules and in addition an amphiphilic structure for acids with chain lengths greater than C4. Considering also that the transport of the substrate receptor complex occurs through lipid regions, a tentative picture of the characteristics of the transport system can be formed.

Penetration in ionic form will depend on both size and configuration of the transported molecule:

i. a small organic acid, even if highly polar, can easily enter the cell in ionic form if its molar volume fits the receptor molecule;

ii. on the other hand, a large compound would protrude its specific reacting group, which is polar, into the receptor site while its tails would lie within the lipid phase. In this situation anions would cross the membrane at rates determined mainly by the lipid solubility and volume of their tail. Thus a large compound having no polar-apolar character would not permeate the cell in ionic form. Moreover, to transport the anion across the membrane by this system the specific binding would have to be strong enough to overcome any tail resistance. Interaction between substrate and receptor, normally established by the carboxyl group (as seen with formic acid), would have to be reinforced. Experimental data suggest that reinforced interaction requires at least a three-point attachment involving three oxygen atoms in the substrate. As is to be expected, the spatial distribution of oxygen atoms is of fundamental importance.

All our data agrees with this interpretation. But we wish to lay emphasis on two particular sets of data.

First, the interesting gradation of properties displayed by the aromatic sulphonic acids can be explained by the assumed necessity of a three-point attachment for transport (Fig. 13). As shown previously, benzene sulphonic and p-aminobenzene sulphonic permeate as anions; but moving the amino group to the ortho position completely abolished permeability. These differences cannot be related to the concentration of dissociated form (pK_1 is very low for all the compounds) or to the form of the amino group (pK_2: 2·4 and 3·12 for 2- and 4-isomers). But the refractoriness to the transport of the 2-aminobenzene sulphonic acid may be explained by the capacity of this compound to form an intramolecular hydrogen bond immobilizing an oxygen of the sulphonic group essential for transport.

Second, the permeability sequence of dicarboxylic aliphatic acids, interpreted by Giebel and Passow (1960) in terms of sieving effect, readily offer an explanation on the present model. As shown in Fig. 14 there is a remarkable correlation between spatial distribution of the oxygen atoms

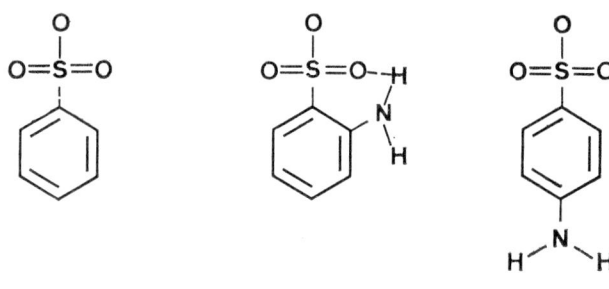

FIG. 13. Molecular structures of aromatic sulphonic acids which do or do not transfer.

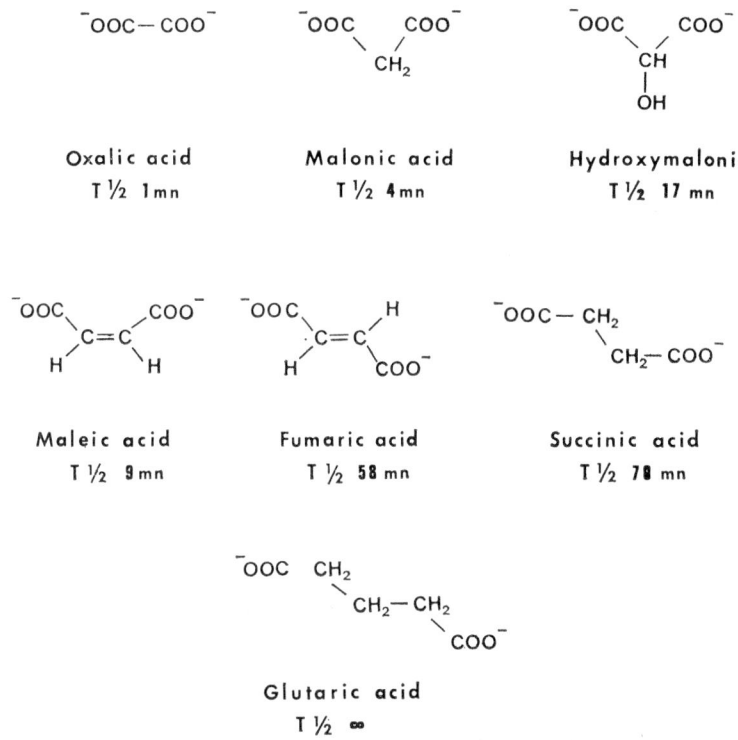

Fig. 14. Permeability sequence and molecular structures of dicarboxylic aliphatic acids.

and penetration rate: when the molecule has a polar-apolar structure and the intercharge distance is below that of maleic acid (oxalic, malonic, maleic acid) anions rapidly penetrate; if the intercharge distance exceeds that value (in correlation with this the compound has reduced amphiphilic structure) the penetration rate strongly decreases (fumaric, succinic, glutaric) even though molar volume is unchanged (maleic and fumaric).

4 Relationship between organic and inorganic anion permeabilities

The results discussed above show that the movement of organic anions does not occur by diffusion of free ions but that specific interaction of penetrating anions with a component of the erythrocyte membrane is involved in their transport. It is now well established that the transport of chloride also takes place by facilitated diffusion (Dalmark, 1972; Wieth, 1972; Gunn et al., 1973). It must be pointed out that the HCO_3^- ion, which shares the chloride transport system (Dalmark and Wieth, 1972; Dalmark, 1976), can be considered as an organic anion, and in fact fulfils the structural requirements allowing transfer across the organic transporting mechanism. Thus, the possibility that organic and inorganic anions share the same transport system must be considered. In an attempt to investigate this point a comparison of the kinetics of the penetration of organic and inorganic anions will be made in the present section. However, it is necessary to realize that, first, the available data on organic anions are rare, secondly, such a comparison between monovalent and divalent inorganic anions did not give a clear-cut answer (Passow and Wood, 1974).

4.1 INHIBITORY ACTION OF PHENYLPYRUVATE

It is expected that the movement of a molecule via a specific transport system can be inhibited by a structural analogue of the substrate. It can be demonstrated that when red cells are suspended in an isotonic pyruvate solution (140×10^{-3} M) containing phenylpyruvate (5×10^{-3} M), the exchange between external pyruvate and internal bicarbonate (Fig. 15a) or internal chloride (Fig. 15b) is markedly inhibited. The inhibiting effect of phenylpyruvate on pyruvate movements at anion equilibrium by tracer techniques (pyruvate self-exchanges) can also be observed. However, because of partial dimerization of pyruvate at physiological pH, an accurate kinetic analysis of pyruvate movement in these conditions is not realizable, so the oxalate anion, which has also been shown to permeate via the organic anion transporting system (Aubert and Motais, 1975), was chosen as a prototype substrate. The molar concentration of phenylpyruvate which inhibits the oxalate–oxalate exchange by 50 per cent (I_{50}) was found to be 9×10^{-4} M. In the same experimental conditions (0°C; pH 7·4)

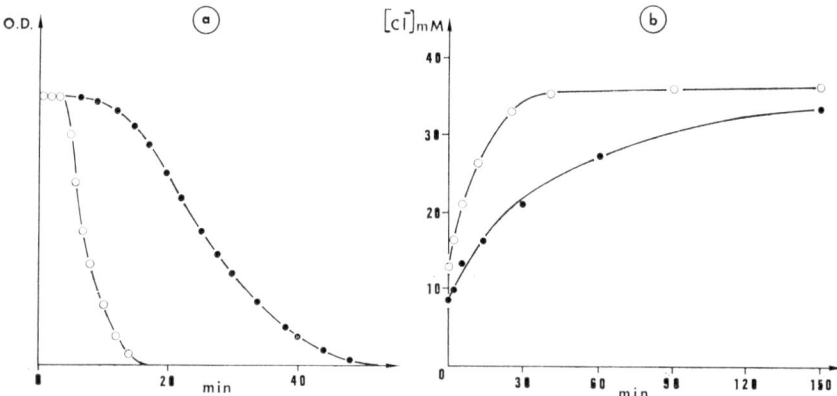

Fig. 15. Inhibition by phenylpyruvate (5×10^{-3} M) of the net exchange of external pyruvate with (a) intracellular HCO_3^- (followed by haemolysis of the cells) 34°C, (b) with intracellular chloride (followed by the change of Cl^- concentration in the medium) 10°C.

○ Control; ● With phenylpyruvate.

the chloride self-exchange is also inhibited and the I_{50} is identical (7.5×10^{-4} M).

These results could be interpreted as indicating that phenylpyruvate acts as a competitive inhibitor on a transport system shared by organic anions and chloride. However, it must be pointed out that phenylpyruvate crosses the red cell membrane essentially, if not exclusively, by nonionic diffusion (Aubert and Motais, 1975). Moreover, if phenylpyruvate acts as a competitive inhibitor, its inhibitory capacity for chloride should be very different from that for oxalate since the rate of permeation is 500 times slower for oxalate than for chloride (Cousin and Motais, 1976). Anticipating the following discussion, it seems more probable that phenylpyruvate, which is an amphiphilic compound, acts as a noncompetitive inhibitor in the same way as a great number of chemically unrelated amphiphilic substances.

4.2 INHIBITION BY COVALENTLY BOUND SITS

It is well established (Knauf and Rothstein, 1971; Cabantchik and Rothstein, 1972, 1974a,b; Rothstein et al., 1976) that some disulphonic stilbene derivatives (DIDS, SITS), which are amino-reactive agents, produce a specific and irreversible inhibition of the chloride and sulphate permeability, by interacting with sites located on the outer surface of the membrane, most of which are in the band 3 protein. This protein, which spans the membrane, contains a specific anion binding site directly involved in anion transport; recent studies indicate that the inhibitory site in band 3 is the transport site itself (Rothstein *et al.*, 1976). As illustrated in Fig. 16, after incubation in a Ringer solution containing SITS at 5×10^{-6} M (hematocrit 0·5 per cent; 0°C; pH 7·4), followed by extensive washing, the inhibition of chloride self-exchange in ox erythrocytes is total and irreversible. Below 5×10^{-6} M of SITS the per cent of inhibition decreases with SITS concentration. It can be observed that the irreversible fixation of SITS induces exactly the same inhibitory pattern on oxalate permeability, suggesting that oxalate (and more generally organic anions) share the chloride binding site allowing chloride transport. (Unpublished data from Cousin and Motais).

4.3 SENSITIVITY OF ORGANIC AND INORGANIC ANION TRANSPORT TO AMPHIPHILIC INHIBITORS

The inorganic anion permeability of erythrocytes can be reversibly and noncompetitively inhibited by a large number of chemically unrelated

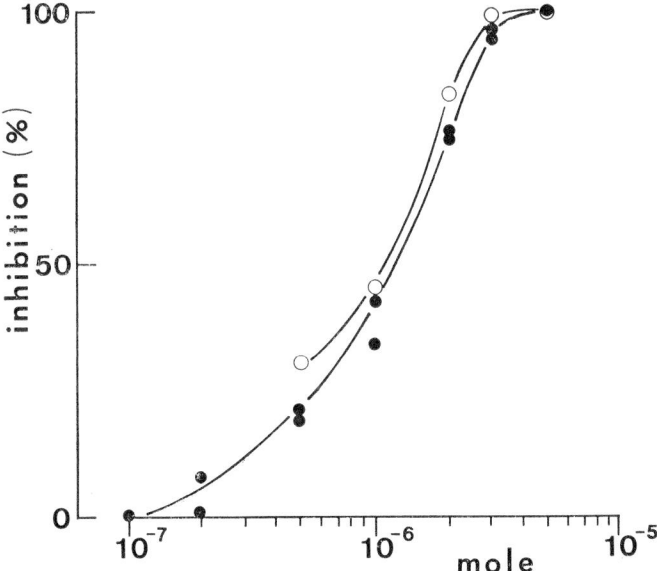

Fig. 16. Inhibition of chloride (●) and oxalate (○) equilibrium self-exchanges by covalently bound SITS at different concentrations. The cells were exposed to the various concentrations of the agent at 5°C for 2 h in darkness (haematocrit 5 per cent). Subsequently the unreacted agent was removed by washing the cells five times. (two washes with 0·5 per cent albumin in the Ringer solution). The cells were resuspended in a medium free of SITS at a haematocrit of 0·5 per cent for measuring ^{36}Cl or ^{14}C oxalate exits at 0°C.

substances, of which the only common property is the amphiphilic nature of the molecule (Passow and Schnell, 1969; Deuticke, 1970; Gunn and Tosteson, 1971; Schnell, 1972; Fortes and Hoffman, 1973; Wieth et al., 1973). For some of them (aniline, phenol, salicylate, dinitrophenol, phloridzin, dipyridamole, phenopyrazone, benzoate) the inhibitory effect on organic anion permeability has been studied and found, in all instances, positive (Schnell and Passow, 1967; Deuticke, 1972b; Schnell, 1972).

Recently it has been demonstrated that carbonic anhydrase inhibitors of the sulphonamide class (unsubstituted sulphonamides) act on the cellular membrane as specific inhibitors of anion transport in erythrocytes. (Cousin et al., 1975; Motais et al., 1975; Cousin and Motais, 1976). It is very interesting to note that when experiments are run in the same conditions of temperature (0°C) and pH (7·4), not only all sulphonamides which inhibit chloride transport inhibit that of oxalate but also that the relative potencies of the various inhibitors are strikingly identical for the two transports (Fig. 17). It was originally thought (Cousin et al., 1975; Motais et al., 1975; Cousin and Motais, 1976) that since the sulphonamide group (SO_2NH_2) of these drugs could potentially satisfy the structural requirement for organic anion transfer through the erythrocyte membrane (the electronegativities of oxygen and of nitrogen are similar), the

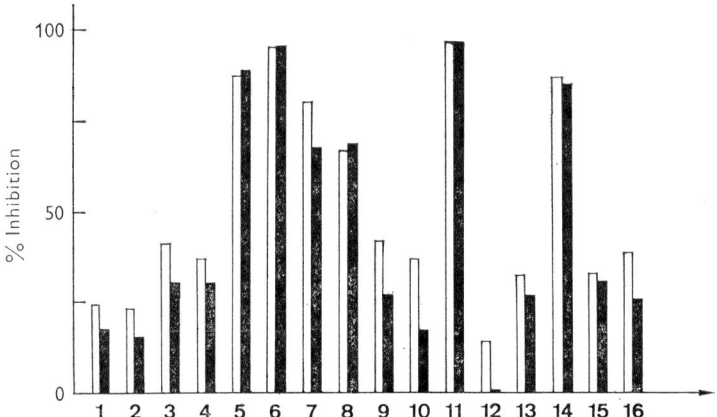

Fig. 17. Comparative inhibitory effect of sixteen sulphonamides on chloride and oxalate self-exchanges. Ordinate, per cent inhibition; abscissa: I benzene sulphonamide; II sulphanilamide; III p-nitrobenzenesulphonamide; IV p-toluene sulphonamide; V p-carboxybenzenesulphonamide; VI furosemide; VII desamide; VIII hydrochlorothiazide; IX chlorthalidone; X N-sulphanyl acetamide; XI 3-benzenesulphonamidophenol; XII acetazolamide; XIII Cl 5,343; XIV benzolamide; XV Cl 13,475; XVI Cl 13,850.
■ Chloride permeability; □ Oxalate permeability.

sulphonamides could act as competitive inhibitors. This point of view does not agree with the fact, as quoted for phenylpyruvate, that the relative potencies are identical for chloride and oxalate, of which the rates of penetration are so different. Moreover, Brazy and Gunn (1975) recently showed that one of the unsubstituted sulphonamides (furosemide) is a noncompetitive inhibitor of chloride transport.

Whatever the type of inhibition, the transport of chloride and oxalate are also influenced in a strictly identical manner by substituted sulphonamides (Motais and Cousin, 1976a) such as probenecid, which inhibits organic anion transport in kidney, or by the diuretic ethacrynic acid (Motais and Cousin, 1976b) or by 2-acetamido benzoate (unpublished data).

4.4 TEMPERATURE DEPENDENCY

In all mammalian erythrocytes the inorganic anion transport shows apparent activation enthalpies of about 29–33 kcal mol^{-1} K^{-1} (Passow, 1969a; Dalmark and Wieth, 1972; Wieth et al., 1974). Temperature dependencies of the transfer of various organic anions obtained from net exchange experiments (Deuticke, 1973; Rice and Steck, 1976) or from self-exchange measured at Donnan equilibrium (Cousin and Motais, 1976) are remarkably similar. In fact, when organic and inorganic anion self-exchanges have been measured in erythrocytes from the same mammalian species the apparent activation energies are strictly identical (compare the data from Wieth et al., 1974 and Cousin and Motais, 1976).

Of course, these similar values of temperature coefficients do not necessarily involve a similar reaction mechanism for the two types of anion; but it must be outlined that the values are unusual for a non energy dependent transfer process.

4.5 INFLUENCE OF INORGANIC ANIONS ON ORGANIC ANION PERMEABILITY

When the self-exchange fluxes of glycolate (or lactate) are determined as a function of glycolate (or lactate) concentration, they reach no saturation but increase proportionally with concentration (Deuticke, 1973). This pattern is like those of sulphate (Passow, 1969a) or phosphate (Deuticke, 1970) but in contrast to those of chloride (Cass and Dalmark, 1973; Gunn et al., 1973) and iodide (Passow and Wood, 1974). This divergence does not necessarily indicate differences between halides and other anion transport processes; it could only be due to the fact that the iso-osmotic replacement of chloride by the anion under study induces a competition between the two anion species for the same transport site, the relationship between flux and concentration depending on the relative affinities of the anions (Gunn et al., 1973). In fact, the mutual competition between organic and inorganic anions has been observed by Deuticke (1973). Moreover, typical saturation kinetics have been demonstrated for sulphate (Ho and Guidotti, 1975), pyruvate (Rice and Steck, 1976) and oxalate (Motais, unpublished data), when initial influx is measured in nonequilibrium condition without any external competitor.

4.6 pH DEPENDENCY OF ANION TRANSFER

The pH dependency of monovalent inorganic anions has been shown to be different from that of divalent anions (Dalmark, 1972; Gunn et al., 1973; Passow and Wood, 1974). This discrepancy can result from the existence of two separate pathways or from a single transport mechanism which carries monovalent or divalent anions depending on the number of its positive charges (Gunn, 1972).

A similar analysis has been made with monovalent and divalent organic anions. The permeability (expressed as the rate coefficient) of a divalent organic anion such as oxalate increases with decreasing pH from 8·5 until 6 (Fig. 18a). This agrees quite well with the pH dependency for phosphate (Deuticke, 1970) or sulphate (Passow, 1969a) permeabilities which, however, show a maximum between 6·3 and 6·5. The remarkable increase of permeability in the acidic pH range could be due to partial nonionic diffusion of oxalate. To study the possible interference of nonionic diffusion at low pH we tested the effects of SITS. As it is evident from Fig. 18a, SITS completely inhibits oxalate transfer along all the pH range, thus excluding the possibility of a nonionic transfer of oxalate.

Membrane permeability to monovalent organic anions such as glycolate, pyruvate (Deuticke, 1973) or sulphanilate (Fig. 18b) decreases when the pH is lowered from 8·5 to 6. Only ionic transfer is involved, as shown by the inhibitory action of SITS. This type of pH dependency is consistent with that of monovalent inorganic anion (Dalmark, 1972; Gunn et al., 1973; Passow and Wood, 1974). However, two results from the literature do not agree with this pattern. First, lactate permeability also diminishes when the pH is lowered from 9·0 to 7·0, but a minimum is reached and an increase occurs in the range down to 5·5 (Deuticke, 1973). It seems possible to explain this increase of permeability in the acidic pH range by a nonionic diffusion of lactic acid, the inhibitory action of SITS not being tested. Secondly, in resealed ghosts, in contrast with the results of Deuticke (1973) on whole erythrocytes, Rice and Steck (1976) showed a broad optimum for pyruvate influx between 6·0 and 7·7. It must be considered, however, that these data were obtained from net exchange experiments and not at anion equilibrium.

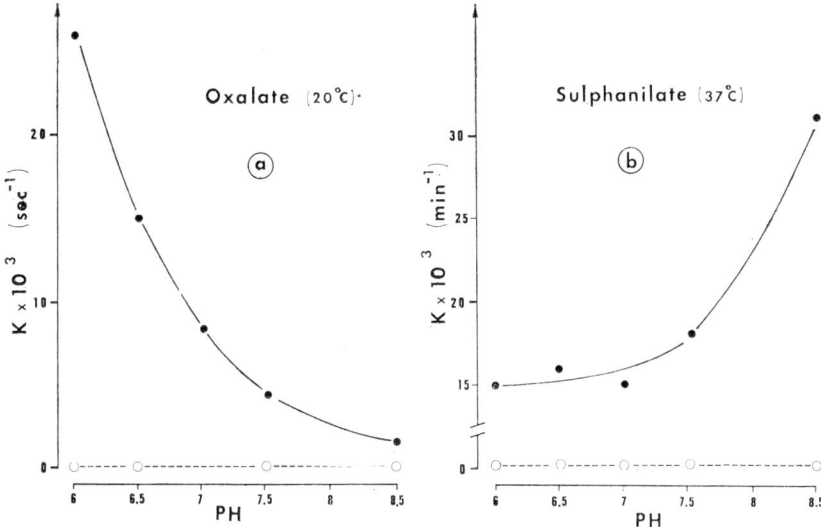

Fig. 18. The pH dependence of the equilibrium fluxes of oxalate and sulphanilate (●). Ordinate; the rate constants of the fluxes (note the difference of units between oxalate and sulphanilate). Total inhibition of oxalate and sulphanilate fluxes by SITS (○) (5×10^{-5} M) is evidence for an ionic transfer of these organic acids along all the pH range.

5 Summary

From all these results two conclusions can be made:

1. The entry of organic anions cannot be ascribed to simple diffusion of free anions across aqueous channels limited by positive charges. It needs a specific interaction of the penetrating anion with a component of the membrane as expected for a facilitated transport.
2. The facilitated transport mechanism for organic anions shows close similarities to the inorganic anion transport system(s):

   a. all of the them show saturation kinetics and organic and inorganic anions apparently compete with each other;
   b. the apparent activation energies for organic and inorganic species are very similar, although quite unusual for penetration processes;
   c. disulphonic stilbene compounds, which almost exclusively bind covalently with band 3 protein, are specific and potent inhibitors of all the anion transport systems;
   d. sensitivity of all systems to a large number of amphiphilic substances is strikingly identical;

e. an asymmetry of the transport systems can be observed. Sulphate and chloride transport are inhibited when phloretin and phloridzin are applied to the outside, but not when they are present on the inside of the ghosts (Lepke and Passow, 1973; Schnell et al., 1973). The same experiments have not been carried out with the organic anion transport system. However, this system also shows a structural asymmetry, as elegantly demonstrated by Rice and Steck (1976): pyruvate influx is stimulated by increasing ionic strength in the outer but not the inner compartment, and this stimulation is inhibited when o-phenanthroline plus $CuSO_4$ are present within the resealed ghosts, but not when added to the external medium. It is interesting to note that this reagent crosslinks band 3 selectively at the cytoplasmic surface (Steck, 1972).

Only the data on pH dependency of organic anion transport are not quite conclusive; it seems, however, reasonable to consider that monovalent organic anions and halides show the same type of pH dependency, whereas divalent organic and inorganic anions exhibit another pattern. So the question arises whether all monovalent and divalent species share a single transfer mechanism which could work differently according to the valency of the transported anion (e.g. a multi-charged site as proposed by Gunn, 1972) or whether they share parts of one pathway but not the whole pathway. It must be admitted that actually it is unknown if the fluxes of monovalent organic anion, such as the fluxes of chloride (Scarpa et al., 1970; Hunter, 1971; Lassen et al., 1974) are largely electrically silent.

References

AUBERT, L. and MOTAIS, R. (1975). *J. Physiol.* **246**, 159–179.
BRAZY, P. C. and GUNN, R. B. (1975). *Physiologist*, **18**, 151.
CABANTCHIK, Z. I. and ROTHSTEIN, A. (1972). *J. Membrane Biol.* **10**, 311–330.
CABANTCHIK, Z. I. and ROTHSTEIN, A. (1974a). *J. Membrane Biol.* **15**, 227–248.
CABANTCHIK, Z. I. and ROTHSTEIN, A. (1974b). *J. Membrane Biol.* **15**, 207–226.
CASS, A. and DALMARK, M. (1973). *Nature New Biol.* **244**, 47–49.
COUSIN, J. L. and MOTAIS, R. (1976). *J. Physiol.* **256**, 61–80.
COUSIN, J. L., MOTAIS, R. and SOLA, F. (1975). *J. Physiol.* **253**, 385–399.
DALMARK M. (1972). In "Oxygen Affinity of Hemoglobin and Red Cell Acid Base Status", pp. 320–332. Benzon Symposium IV. Munksgaard, Copenhagen.
DALMARK, M. (1976). *J. Gen. Physiol.* **67**, 223–234.
DALMARK, M. and WIETH, J. O. (1972). *J. Physiol.* **224**, 583–610.
DEUTICKE, B. (1970). *Naturwissenschaften*, **57**, 172–179.
DEUTICKE, B. (1972a). In "Oxygen Affinity of Hemoglobin and Red Cell Acid Base Status", pp. 307–316. Benzon Symposium IV. Munksgaard, Copenhagen.
DEUTICKE, B. (1972b). In "Passive Permeability of Cell Membrane" (F. Kreuzer, ed), pp. 381–391. Plenum Press, New York.
DEUTICKE, B. (1973). In "Erythrocytes, Thrombocytes, Leucocytes" (E. Gerlach,

K. Moser, E. Deutsch and W. Wilmans, eds), pp. 81–87. Thieme-Verlag, Stuttgart.
FORTES, P. and HOFFMAN, J. F. (1973). *In* "Erythrocytes, Thrombocytes, Leucocytes" (E. Gerlach, K. Moser, E. Deutsch and W. Wilmans, eds), pp. 92–96. Thieme-Berlag, Stuttgart.
GIEBEL, O. and PASSOW, H. (1960). *Pflügers Archiv.* **271**, 378–388.
GREEN, J. W. (1949). *J. Cell. Comp. Physiol.* **33**, 247–266.
GUNN, R. B. (1972). *In* "Oxygen Affinity of Hemoglobin and Red Cell Acid Base Status", pp. 823–827. Benzon Symposium IV. Munksgaard, Copenhagen.
GUNN, R. B., DALMARK, M., TOSTESON, D. C. and WIETH, J. O. (1973). *J. Gen. Physiol.* **61**, 185–206.
GUNN, R. B. and TOSTESON, D. C. (1971). *J. Gen. Physiol.* **57**, 593–609.
HO, M. K. and GUIDOTTI, G. (1975). *J. Biol. Chem.* **250**, 675–683.
HÖBER, R. (1936). *J. Cell. Comp. Physiol.* **7**, 367–391.
HUNTER, M. J. (1971). *J. Physiol.* **218**, 49P.
JACOBS, M. H. (1924). *Amer. J. Physiol.* **68**, 134.
JACOBS, M. H. and STEWART, D. R. (1942). *J. Gen. Physiol.* **25**, 539–552.
KNAUF, P. and ROTHSTEIN, A. (1971). *J. Gen. Physiol.* **58**, 190–210.
LASSEN, U. V., PAPE, L. and VESTERGAARD-BOGIND, B. (1974). *In* "Comparative Biochemistry and Physiology of Transport" (L. Bolis, K. Block, S. E. Luria, F. Lynen, eds), pp. 363–366. North-Holland, Amsterdam.
LEPKE, S. and PASSOW, H. (1973). *Biochim. Biophys. Acta*, **298**, 529–533.
MAREN, T. H. and WILEY, C. E. (1970). *Molec. Pharmacol.* **6**, 430–440.
MEYER, K. H. and SIEVERS, J. F. (1936). *Helv. Chim. Acta*, **19**, 649.
MICHAELIS, L. and FUGITA, A. (1925). *Biochem. Z.* **1961**, 47.
MOND, R. (1927). *Pflügers Archiv.* **217**, 618.
MOTAIS, R. and COUSIN, J. L. (1976a). *Biochim. Biophys. Acta*, **419**, 309–313.
MOTAIS R. and COUSIN, J. L. (1976b). *Amer. J. Physiol.* **231**, 1,485–1,489.
MOTAIS, R., COUSIN, J. L. and SOLA, F. (1975). *C. R. Séanc. Acad. Sci. Paris*, **280**, 1119–1122.
PASSOW, H. (1969a). *Prog. Biophys. Mol. Biol.* **19**, 424–467.
PASSOW, H. (1969b). *In* "The Molecular Basis of Membrane Function" (D. C. Tosteson, ed), pp. 319–351. Prentice Hall, New Jersey.
PASSOW, H. and SCHNELL, K. F. (1969). *Experientia*, **25**, 460–468.
PASSOW, H. and WOOD, P. G. (1974). *In* "Drugs and Transport Processes" (B. A. Callingham, ed), pp. 149–171. MacMillan, London.
RICE, W. R. and STECK, T. L. (1976). *Biochim. Biophys. Acta*, **433**, 39–53.
ROTHSTEIN, A., CABANTCHIK, Z. I. and KNAUF, P. (1976). *Fed. Proc.* **35**, 3–10.
SCARPA, A., CECHETTO, A. and AZZONE, G. F. (1970). *Biochim. Biophys. Acta*, **219**, 179.
SCHANKER, L. S., JOHNSON, J. M. and JEFFREY, J. J. (1964). *Amer. J. Physiol.* **207**, 503–508.
SCHNELL, K. F. (1972). *Biochim. Biophys. Acta*, **282**, 265–276.
SCHNELL, K. F., GERHARDT, S., LEPKE, S. and PASSOW, H. (1973). *Biochim. Acta*, **318**, 474–477.
SCHNELL, K. F. and PASSOW, H. (1967). *Pflügers Archiv.* **297**, R24.
STECK, T. L. (1972). *J. Molec. Biol.* **66**, 295–305.
TOERELL, T. (1935). *Proc. Soc. Exp. Biol. Med.* **33**, 282.
WIETH, J. O. (1970). *J. Physiol.* **207**, 581–609.
WIETH, J. O. (1972). *In* "Oxygen Affinity of Hemoglobin and Red Cell Acid

Base Status", pp. 265–278. Benzon Symposium IV. Munksgaard, Copenhagen.
WIETH, J. O., DALMARK, M., GUNN, R. B., TOSTESON, D. C. (1973). *In* "Erythrocytes, Thrombocytes, Leucocytes" (E. Gerlach, K. Moser, E. Deutsch, and W. Wilmans, eds), pp. 71–76. Thieme-Verlag, Stuttgart.
WIETH, J. O., FUNDER, J., GUNN, R. B. and BRAHM, J. (1974). *In* "Comparative Biochemistry and Physiology of Transport" (L. Bolis, K. Bloch, S. E. Luria and F. Lynen, eds), pp. 317–337. North-Holland, Amsterdam.
WILBRANDT, W. (1942). *Pflügers Archiv.* **246**, 274.

Note added in proof

Kinetic evidence has been presented (Halestrap, A. P. (1976). *Biochem. J.* **156**, 193–207) which suggests that the Cl^- carrier can transport pyruvate and lactate but that an additional carrier also exists.

Water and small nonelectrolyte permeation in red cells

R. I. SHA'AFI

Department of Physiology, University of Connecticut Health Center, Farmington, Connecticut 06032, USA

1 Introduction	221
2 Methods for measuring permeability coefficients of the red blood cell membrane to water and nonelectrolytes	223
2.1 Radioactive tracer movement studied with rapid-flow technique	223
2.2 Nuclear magnetic resonance technique	224
2.3 Osmotic volume changes studied with stop-flow technique	224
2.4 Hemolysis method	226
3 The permeability coefficient of red cell membrane to water	227
3.1 Relationship of water diffusion to osmotic flow	227
3.2 Reflection coefficient and its relation to the "pore" concept	230
3.3 The functional state of water in red cell membranes	232
3.4 Membrane cholesterol and water permeability	234
3.5 Effect of sulfhydryl-reactive reagents on water transport	235
3.6 Asymmetry of water flow	236
3.7 Miscellaneous factors which may influence the transport of water across red cell membrane	238
3.8 Possible structural basis for the apparent presence of hydrophilic pathway for water transport	239
4 Permeability of the red cell membrane to small nonelectrolytes	242
4.1 Is the mechanism by which small hydrophilic solutes permeate red cell membrane similar to that used by large lipophilic molecules?	243
4.2 Which inhibitors affect the movements of these small nonelectrolytes?	247
4.3 Is there a carrier-mediated mechanism for urea transport?	248
4.4 Do urea and other small molecules use the same pathways as water?	251
Acknowledgements	252
References	253

1 Introduction

One of the main functions of the plasma membrane is to permit the entry of cell food and oxygen, the exit of cell wastes and the regulation of the composition of the intracellular fluid. The intracellular fluid usually contains solutes at concentrations which are quite different from their corresponding values in the bathing medium. In fact, continued existence of the cell is critically dependent on the ability of its membrane to discriminate among various solutes so that some are allowed through, others are kept inside or outside the cell, and yet others are carried actively. The movement of water and solutes through the membrane is a dynamic process, and the living cell is never in equilibrium with the environment in terms of materials across its membrane. The cell achieves such a state of equilibrium only when it is dead.

Studies of permeability characteristics of the cell membrane have been of considerable interest to cell physiologists, since these characteristics help to define functional and structural properties of the plasma membrane and help elucidate the factors that determine the rate of movement of different substances into and out of various tissues in the body. Much of our present understanding of the cell membrane structure has been derived from the early work of Overton (1895) on the movement of water and nonelectrolytes across cell membranes. Aside from being of considerable theoretical importance, the process of water transport across biological membranes and the effect of certain hormones on this process in some tissues is of practical importance. One problem of animal life is to regulate precisely the chemical activity of water inside the organism, since this limits the dissolved ions which are critical for life (Prosser, 1973). Studies of water movement in cells allows prediction of physiological utility about the water content and can supply information about cell structure by following the water content at equilibrium and the rate of flow of water during any changes which take place (Dick, 1966). In addition, the commonly observed rectification of water flow across biological membranes is most likely due to a basic membrane structure and must be accounted for in the design of any membrane model (Sha'afi and Gary-Bobo, 1973).

Our present view of the cell membrane structure is that it is analogous to a two-dimensional oriented solution of globular lipoproteins dispersed in a discontinuous fluid bilayer of lipid solvent (Singer and Nicolson, 1972). The major fraction of the lipid is phospholipids. Both components of the membrane (proteins and lipid) are free to some degree to have lateral mobility in the plane of the membrane and in some cases are asymmetrically distributed across the two halves of the bilayer (Singer, 1974). Some proteins are peripherally attached to either of the two faces while other polypeptide chains may span the whole thickness of the membrane (Singer, 1974). These latter proteins probably correspond to the intramembranous particles seen in freeze-etch images and freeze-fracture experiments (Brayton, 1971; Branton and Daemer, 1972; Da Silva, 1973). Accordingly,

WATER AND SMALL NONELECTROLYTE PERMEATION 223

these polypeptide chains can provide a hydrophilic environment for the transport of water and certain solutes. In fact, some of them have been implicated in the transport of water (Brown *et al.*, 1975) and chloride ions (Cabantchik and Rothstein, 1974a,b; Ho and Guidotti, 1975; Rothstein *et al.*, 1976).

2 Methods for measuring permeability coefficients of the red blood cell membrane to water and nonelectrolytes

The permeability coefficients of the red blood cell membrane to water and nonelectrolytes can be measured either under steady-state conditions or under net flow of the substance under study (Sha'afi and Gary-Bobo, 1973). In the first case, cell volume remains constant during the course of the experiment, since measurements are done while net movement of neither water nor solute aside from the tracer occurs. In the second case, the permeability is obtained by measuring the rate of swelling or shrinkage of the cell under a gradient of osmotic pressure.

2.1 RADIOACTIVE TRACER MOVEMENT STUDIED WITH RAPID-FLOW TECHNIQUE

Theoretically, it is possible to use the time-course of tracer disappearance from or appearance in the medium in which red cells are suspended to measure the permeability coefficient of red cell membrane to any substance that can be labelled. Experimentally, however, the measurement becomes extremely impractical with substances whose time of equilibrium across the red cell membrane is of the order of a few seconds. In this method, red cells are mixed in a rapid-flow mixing chamber with isotonic buffered solution containing the labelled substance, and the mixture is forced down a tube with ports that permit axial sampling of the suspension medium. These ports are covered with filter paper which red cells cannot pass. Conversion of distance to time by means of velocity is the underlying principle. Since a certain minimum velocity must be exceeded in order to have efficient mixing between the red cells and the buffered solution, it becomes quite impractical to study the permeability coefficients of substances of low exchange rate ($>1 \cdot 0$ sec) (Paganelli and Solomon, 1957; Tosteson, 1959; Savitz and Solomon, 1971).

The basic equation which governs tracer diffusion between two well-stirred compartments is (Paganelli and Solomon, 1957):

$$\mathrm{d}(v_p p)/\mathrm{d}t = -k'_1 p + k'_1 q, \qquad (1)$$

Where v_p = the volume of the suspending medium (cm³);
p, q = the specific activity in the suspending medium and the cell respectively (counts per minute per ml H_2O);

k'_1 = a proportionality constant related to the permeability coefficient;
t = time

Under the usual experimental conditions when no net flow of either water or solute occurs (steady-state), the solution for equation (1) is:

$$(p/p_\infty - 1) = (p_0/p_\infty - 1)\exp(-k'_1 p_0 t / V'_0 p_\infty), \quad (2)$$

in which subscripts 0 and ∞ refer to zero and infinite time. V'_0 is the volume of cell water at time equal to zero.

2.2 NUCLEAR MAGNETIC RESONANCE TECHNIQUE

This is a simple and rapid technique for measuring the time-course for water movement across mammalian erythrocytes (Conlon and Outhred, 1972). The basis of this method is the fact that water protons can absorb energy from a radio-frequency magnetic field if the cells are placed in a static magnetic field. The decay time, which is commonly known as "spin-spin" relaxing time (T_2), of this coherent energy can be measured by standard NMR techniques. By adding a suitable concentration of a paramagnetic material such as manganese to the plasma, the spontaneous decay time (T_2) of the label for water in the plasma can be made very short (<2 msec). Since the decay time of the label for water inside is long (140 msec), the decay time within the cell will be dominated by the rate of water exit ($\simeq 8$ msec). The measurements are done under steady-state conditions and the only drawback of this technique is that only the rate of water exit can be measured. Since the cell suspension is not usually stirred in this technique, a large unstirred layer may be present. If not taken into account, this will give rise to a significantly lower value for the permeability coefficient.

2.3 OSMOTIC VOLUME CHANGES STUDIED WITH STOP-FLOW TECHNIQUE

The principle of this method is based on the use of light scattering or transmission as an index for measuring rapid changes in cell volume. Two solutions, one containing a dilute suspension of red cells and the other containing the permeating molecule, are rapidly mixed. When steady flow is achieved, the flow is stopped abruptly and the fluid is isolated in an observation tube through which light passes. The time-course of cell volume changes can be measured indirectly from the changes in the intensity of either 90° scattered light or 180° transmitted light. In the application of this principle, various approaches have been developed for rapid mixing, and for recording (Macey and Tolberg, 1966; Hempling, 1967; Sha'afi *et al.*, 1967; Blum and Forster, 1970; Sirs, 1969; Sha'afi *et al.*, 1970; Ellam and Stein, 1974).

When red cells are placed in a medium containing an iso-osmolal concentration of impermeant solute together with a suitable concentration of a permeant nonelectrolyte which enters the cell less rapidly than water, the cell initially shrinks and then returns to its initial volume after passing through a well-defined minimum. In the shrinking phase, water moves out of the cell owing to the excess of osmotically active material externally, while the nonelectrolyte moves down its concentration gradient into the cell. At the minimum point, the inward volume flow of the solute is exactly balanced by the outward volume flow of water. Subsequently, the osmotic pressure gradient reverses its direction, in part because the impermeant solute is now more concentrated in the cell than in the medium. Water enters the cell along with the permeant solute, and the volume change ends when the permeating nonelectrolyte is equally distributed between the cells and the medium. Figure 1 shows a typical time-course of cell volume changes when cells are rapidly mixed with an iso-osmolal solution containing an uncharged solute. The cell volume will respond to changes in medium osmolality (hyperosmolar) in one of four ways: (*a*) it will decrease to a new equilibrium value, (*b*) it will decrease and then increase to a new equilibrium value, (*c*) no changes in volume take place, or (*d*) the cell

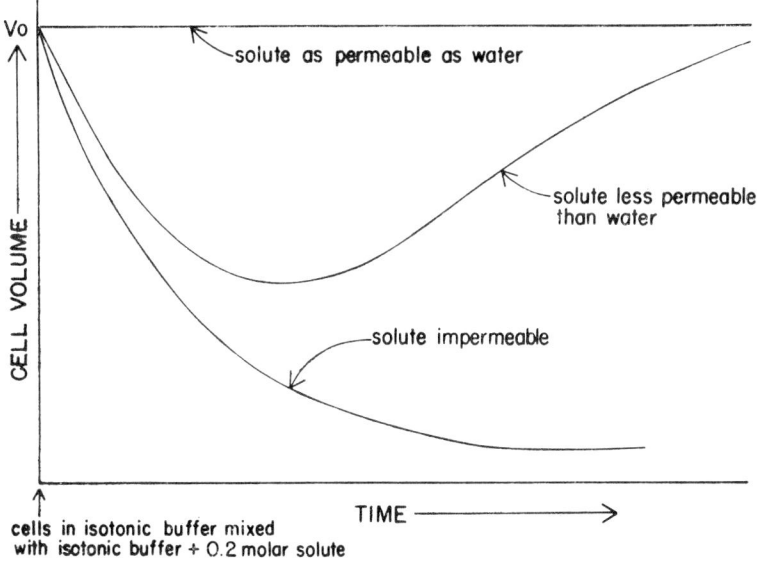

FIG. 1. Expected time-course of red cell volume.

swells and then shrinks. A mirror image is obtained when the solution is hypo-osmolar. Condition (a) is obtained when the cell membrane is completely impermeable to the solute; (b) when the solute is permeable but less so than water; (c) when both the solute and water are equally permeable; (d) when the solute is more permeable than water (usually called anomalous osmosis). We will consider only the first two conditions since the last two are less informative.

In analyses of osmotic flow and net solute movement, the two basic equations which are invariably used are those given by Kedem and Katchalsky (1958) and Katchalsky and Curran (1965). Kedem and Katchalsky give the following relations to express the relative fluxes:

$$J_v = L_p \Delta \Pi_i + L_{pd} \Delta \Pi_s, \tag{3}$$

$$J_s = (1 + L_{dp}/L_p)_s \bar{C}_s J_v + \omega_s \Delta \Pi_s, \tag{4}$$

where J_v = steady-state volume flow per unit area and time (cm^3 cm^2 sec^{-1});

L_p = the hydraulic water conductivity; it is also called water filtration coefficient (cm^3 dyn^{-1} sec^{-1});

$\Delta\Pi_i, \Delta\Pi_s$ = the osmotic pressure across the membrane due to the impermeant and permeant solutes respectively (dyn cm^{-2});

J_s = solute flow (mol cm^{-2}, sec^{-1});

ω_s = the permeability of a membrane to a particular solute (mol dyn^{-1} sec^{-1});

$\bar{C}_s$ = average concentration;

$L_{pd}=L_{dp}$ = phenomenological coefficient and have the same units as $L_p = -L_{pd}/\sigma$ where σ is the reflection coefficient.

For L_p measurements, cells are exposed to medium containing a nonpermeable solute ($\sigma = 1$). Under these conditions we have $J_v \equiv (dV'/dt) = L_p A \Delta \Pi_i$; where A is the surface area of the red cells which remains nearly constant, and V' is the volume of cell water. L_p can be easily calculated by measuring the time-course of volume change. The permeability coefficient ω_s of red cell membrane for any permeable solute can be calculated from the following relation (Sha'afi et al., 1970):

$$\omega_s = \frac{V' \min(d^2 V'/dt^2) \min}{A^2 L_p R T \Delta \Pi_c}. \tag{5}$$

2.4 HEMOLYSIS METHODS

This was first used by Hamburger (1866) (cited in Jacobs, 1931) and is based on measurement of the time required for a system of red cells to hemolyze either completely or to any specific extent when placed in a solution in which NaCl has been replaced by the permeating molecule under study. The red cells hemolyze because entry into the cell of a permeating molecule moving down its concentration gradient causes an imbalance of water activity, which drives water into the cell. The process continues until the cell hemolyzes. At this point, sufficient hemoglobin escapes from the cells so that they become invisible when viewed in their hemoglobin-containing surroundings. It is one of the simplest techniques and almost all of the early studies on permeability relied on it (Jacobs, 1931; Höber and Ørskov, 1933). In fact, its extreme simplicity contributed greatly to making erythrocytes one of the most favored cells for this type of investigation. Permeability coefficients, either for water or solutes, can be easily calculated from the time of hemolysis (Jacobs, 1952; Stein, 1967).

3 The permeability coefficient of red cell membrane to water

The transfer of water across the cell membrane has been under investigation since the days of von Limbeck, Hamburger and Henderson (cited in Jacobs, 1931). It was recognized long ago that movement of water in mammalian red cells occurs very rapidly and without a carrier-mediated mechanism. Among the many single cells and tissues studied, the rate of water movement across mammalian red cell membranes seems to be intermediate between amoeba, which is about two orders of magnitude less permeable to water, and the capillaries of the frog mesentery, which is two orders of magnitude greater (Landis, 1927; Prescott and Zeuthen, 1953; Dick, 1966; Sha'afi *et al.*, 1967). Taken together with our understanding of the lipid nature of the cell membrane, it has been difficult to explain how water which is relatively insoluble in lipid can move so rapidly across cell membranes. This is restricted not only to water but also to small hydrophilic nonelectrolytes which are more permeable than one would predict from their lipid solubility (Overton, 1895; Wright and Diamond, 1969; Naccache and Sha'afi, 1973). In the case of red blood cell membranes, the most widely proposed explanation for these results is that small water-filled "channels" exist in the membrane (Solomon, 1968). Accordingly, water and small hydrophilic solutes permeate primarily through these "pores". Since the average size of the proposed "channel" is only about twice that of a water molecule, this concept must necessarily be vague and must be considered operational.

3.1 RELATIONSHIP OF WATER DIFFUSION TO OSMOTIC FLOW

As stated earlier, the permeability of the red cell membrane to water can be measured either under steady-state conditions or as a bulk flow. The difference between these two types of measurements is not merely one of technique, for there is a fundamental molecular difference between the movement of water under these two conditions. The permeability coefficient measured under bulk flow is referred to as the hydraulic water permeability coefficient (L_p), which has the units of volume per force per time (cm³ dyn⁻¹ sec⁻¹). Other terminologies are often used, such as filtration coefficient, $P_f \equiv RTL_p/\bar{V}_w$ in cm sec⁻¹, and osmotic coefficient, $P_w \equiv RTL_p$ in cm⁴ osmol⁻¹ sec⁻¹. $\bar{V}_w$ is the partial molar volume for water. The rate of movement of water under steady-state conditions is usually referred to as the diffusional permeability coefficient ($^\omega THO$), which has the units of mol dyn⁻¹ sec⁻¹ (the symbol $P_d = {^\omega THO}\ RT$ is often used to denote the same thing). As shown in Table 1, when both coefficients are expressed in the same units, it is found that L_p is significantly higher than $^\omega THO$. This kind of comparison has since been made by numerous investigators using various kinds of cells, tissues and artificial membranes (Prescott and Zeuthen, 1953; Durbin et al., 1956; Curran and Solomon, 1957; Mauro, 1957; Pagenelli and Solomon, 1957; Villegas et al., 1958; Curran, 1960; Durbin, 1960; Robbins and Mauro, 1960; Villegas and Villegas, 1960; Hays and Leaf, 1962a; Rich et al., 1967; Solomon, 1968). The differences in the permeability to water among the various mammalian red cell membranes shown in Table 1 may be due to differences in the degree of unsaturation of membrane fatty acids. It is known that the permeability of lipid bilayer membranes increases with increasing degree of unsaturation. In addition, a positive correlation can be demonstrated in mammalian red cells between glycerol permeability and degree of unsaturation (DeGier, 1973).

TABLE 1
Permeability of mammalian red blood cell membrane to water

Species	Under osmotic flow P_f(cm sec⁻¹) × 10³	Under tracer diffusion P_d, (cm sec⁻¹) × 10³	P_f/P_d
Man	17·3[a]	5·3[d]	3·3
Beef	15·5[b]	4·7[e]	3·3
Dog	26·6[a]	5·0[f]	5·3
Cat	33·8[b]	—	—
Horse	11·5[c]	—	—
Camel	5·4[g]	—	—
Human red cell ghost	17·9[h]	—	—

Values are taken from (a) Rich et al., (1968), (b) Rich et al. (1967), (c) Blum and Forster (1970), (d) Paganelli and Solomon (1957), (e) Villegas et al. (1958), (f) Vieira et al. (1970), (g) Naccache and Sha'afi (1974), (h) Colombe et al. (1974).

In many cases, the difference between P_f and P_d can be attributed to the presence of an unstirred layer. On the other hand, in the case of human red cell membrane the difference cannot be accounted for by the presence of an unstirred layer (Sha'afi et al., 1967). Additional support for this difference between P_f and P_d comes from the work of Hays and Leaf (1962b) on toad bladder. These investigators have found that in the presence of antidiuretic hormone (ADH), the osmotic permeability coefficient of this tissue to water is 120 times greater than the diffusional coefficient.

In classical terms, any value of $P_f/P_d \equiv g$ greater than unity may be taken as evidence for bulk flow through channels, and the equality sign holds for truly nonporous membranes. Furthermore, if Poiseuille's law dealing with bulk flow down right-cylindrical pores is assumed, then the value of g is related to the average pore radius (r) (Solomon, 1968). However, classical interpretation of water movement across biological membranes cannot be truly applied due to the small size of these proposed pores. In fact, Levitt (1974) has calculated that the average number of water molecules per "pore" is about five.

The situation is quite different when water movement is treated in terms of irreversible thermodynamics. In terms of the frictional analysis of irreversible thermodynamics, g is given by the following relation (Katchalsky and Curran, 1965):

$$g = 1 + f^c{}_{ww}/f^c{}_{wm}, \qquad (6)$$

in which $f^c{}_{ww}$ and $f^c{}_{wm}$ are the coefficients of friction in the pore between water-water and water-membrane, respectively. Friction coefficients are positive and have units of dyne second per mol centimetre. A value for g greater than unity corresponds to transport in situations in which water-water friction in the membrane is more important than water-membrane friction. This means that membranes with specialized structures such as liquid membranes similar to those studied by Thau et al. (1966) can have a value of g greater than unity without an implication of porous structure. In these specialized membranes, there appear to be ways to transport water molecules in small clusters other than by bulk flow. Furthermore, Fenichel and Horowitz (1969) have pointed out recently that in these membranes g will approach unity only when both the saturation water content of the membrane and the deviations from Henry's law are small. At present, the objection raised by the latter investigators cannot be quantitatively evaluated owing to incomplete knowledge of the structural arrangement of red cell membrane.

Values of g greater than unity can be found in membranes in which the presence of porous channels is improbable. For example, in the liquid membranes which were made by coating paper with liquid or filling the apertures in polyvinyl chloride membranes with liquid, and in tributyl phosphate liquid membranes, Thau et al. (1966) found values of 2·1 and 1·8, respectively. Even in these specialized membranes, the measured value for the porosity factor is significantly lower than the corresponding value found in mammalian red cell membranes.

Even though the criticisms outlined in the preceding few paragraphs do not invalidate completely the criterion that $g > 1$ implies the existence of water-filled channels in the cell membrane, they do weaken it considerably, and its use in calculating average "pore" size becomes completely invalid. At present, the best one can say is that the intermediate values of g for red cell membranes strongly support, but do not necessarily prove, the pore model hypothesis.

3.2 REFLECTION COEFFICIENT AND ITS RELATION TO THE "PORE" CONCEPT

Since first introduced by Staverman (1951), the reflection coefficient (σ), of a membrane for a particular solute has played an important role in the field of permeability studies. It represents the discriminatory power of the membrane between water and solute. The name reflection coefficient is used to indicate that when $\sigma = 1$, all the solute is "reflected" from the membrane, while $\sigma < 1$ means that part of the solute penetrates and is not "reflected".

In red cells, this coefficient is usually measured by the zero time method of Goldstein and Solomon (1960) in which a suspension of cells in isotonic buffer is mixed rapidly with various test solutions of the probing molecule under study. The initial cell volume change $\left(\lim_{t \to 0} dV/dt\right)$ is plotted against the various concentrations of the probing molecule. The concentration of the probing molecule that gives no volume flow can be found by interpolation. The reflection coefficient (σ) can be calculated from the relation $\sigma = -\Delta \Pi_i / \Delta \Pi_s$. The results of Goldstein and Solomon have recently been criticized (Levitt, 1974) on the ground that the experimental procedure of these investigators can lead to large errors in the evaluation of σ.

The basic criticism centers around the difficulty in measuring $\left(\lim_{t \to 0} dV/dt\right)$. The work of Goldstein and Solomon does indeed suffer from this experimental difficulty, but the error is not as severe as claimed. Using continuous measurement of volume changes, Sha'afi et al. (1970) found a σ value for urea of 0·55, which is only 15 per cent less than the value reported by Goldstein and Solomon. Owen et al. (1975) have also criticized σ measurements in mammalian red cells. The main thrust of their studies is that σ values cannot be used to calculate "pore" sizes, a conclusion reached previously by others (Stein, 1967; Sha'afi and Gary-Bobo, 1973).

In 1963 Dainty and Ginzburg showed that the reflection coefficient of a given solute is related to the various frictions in the following manner:

$$1 - \sigma - \omega_s \bar{V}_s/L_p = \frac{K^c{}_s f^c{}_{sw}}{f^c{}_{sw} + f^c{}_{sm}} = \frac{A_{sf}}{A_{wf}} \quad (7)$$

in which ω_s and $\bar{V}_s$ are the diffusional permeability coefficient and partial molar volume of the solute; $f^c{}_{sw}$ and $f^c{}_{sm}$ are the coefficients of friction in the pore between solute-water and solute-membrane, respectively; $K^c{}_s$ is the partition coefficient for the solute between the water in the pore and the external solutions; A_{sf} and A_{wf} are the apparent areas for the filtration of solute and water, respectively. These authors also pointed out that if small hydrophilic solute and water molecules permeate cell membrane via commonly shared water-filled "pores", then there should be a frictional interaction between the permeating solute and the water, i.e. $f^c{}_{sw} > 0$. This gives rise to a phenomenon known as solvent drag effect. Consequently, the inequality given in equation 8 must be satisfied:

$$\sigma < 1 - \omega_s \bar{V}_s/L_p. \quad (8)$$

This relationship was found to hold true for five small hydrophilic solutes in human and dog red cells (Rich *et al.*, 1967; Sha'afi and Gary-Bobo, 1973). The presence of solvent drag has been reported in other tissues (Anderson and Ussing, 1953; Vargas, 1968; Barry and Hope, 1969; Diamond and Wright, 1969).

In general, the idea that a demonstration of solvent drag effect on solute movement implies transport across "aqueous pores" is thermodynamically sound. On the other hand, the extension of this idea to the studies on red cell or, even worse, to the studies on other tissues and the use of σ to calculate "pore" size should be re-evaluated and perhaps totally rejected for the following reasons:

a. Demonstration of the existence of solvent drag by means of a relation such as that given in equation 8 is open to question. For one thing, this is an extremely indirect method; furthermore, the relationship is necessary, but not sufficient to justify the presence of water-filled channels. It is conceivable to have a case in which $f^c{}_{sw} > 0$ and hence $\sigma < 1 - \omega_s \bar{V}_s/L_p$ without needing to postulate aqueous channels which pierce the membrane from one side to another.

b. The expression given in equation 8 holds true only when the solute under study and water permeate only through a common "pore". If the solute can partially permeate by dissolution in the membrane and/or if water molecules permeate through pores not available to the solute, then the relationship shown in equation 8 is considerably modified (Dainty and Ginzburg, 1963). It is becoming increasingly evident as will be shown later, that only a very small population of the postulated "pores" through which water permeates is available for the transport of small hydrophilic nonelectrolytes. Although this modification does not invalidate the inequality given in equation 8, it renders the use of σ for calculating "pore" size completely useless.

c. The inequality which is shown in equation 8 only proves that water molecules can use the pathway available for small hydrophilic solutes, but not the converse.

3.3 THE FUNCTIONAL STATE OF WATER IN RED CELL MEMBRANES

Relevant information concerning the physical state of membrane water and the nature of membrane water interaction can be obtained from studying the energetics of water permeation across biological membranes. In the last four decades several articles have appeared on the subject dealing with the influence of temperature on water transfer across cellular membranes and tissues (Lucke and McCutcheon, 1932; Jacobs et al., 1935; Nevis, 1958; Hempling, 1961; Hays and Leaf, 1962b; Farmer and Macey, 1970; Vieira et al., 1970). Using the data reported by Jacobs et al. (1935). one can calculate values between 3·3–7·5 kcal mol^{-1} for the apparent activation energy of water osmotic flow across various mammalian erythrocyte membranes. Probably the most systematic and complete study on the influence of temperature on water transfer in mammalian red cells is that of Vieira et al. (1970). These authors have studied the dependence on temperature of both the tracer diffusional permeability coefficient ($^{\omega}THO$) and the hydraulic conductivity (L_p) of water in human and dog red cell membranes. The apparent activation energies calculated from these results for both processes are given in Table 2. The values for the apparent activation energies for water self-diffusion and for water transport in a lipid bilayer are also included in the table. For dog red cells, the value of 4·9 kcal mol^{-1} is not significantly different from that of 4·6–4·8 kcal mol^{-1} for the apparent activation energy of the water diffusion coefficient (D_w) in free solution determined by Wang and his collaborators (Wang et al., 1953; Wang, 1965). Furthermore, it can be shown that the product $(L_p - {^{\omega}THO}\bar{V}_w)\eta_w$, where $\bar{V}_w$ is the partial molar volume of water and η_w the viscosity of water remains virtually independent of temperature for dog, but not for the human red cell membrane (Sha'afi and Gary-Bobo, 1973). The similarity of the transmembrane diffusion with bulk water diffusion and the invariance of the product $(L_p - \omega\bar{V}_w)\eta_w$ with temperature in dog red cell membranes suggests that water in these membranes behaves operationally as in bulk solution. However, in the case of the human red cell membrane, the results suggest that water-membrane interaction is relatively high. This indicates that in these cells the charged groups of membrane protein and phopholipid molecules impart unusual properties to water molecules.

TABLE 2
Comparison of apparent activation energies for water fluxes in various systems

System	Activation energies in kcal mol^{-1}	
	Under osmotic flow	Under diffusional flow
Human red cell membrane	3·3[a]	6·0[a]
Dog red cell membrane	3·7[a]	4·9[a]
Self-diffusion	—	4·8[b]
Viscous flow in water	4·2[c]	—
Lecithin/cholesterol bilayer	14·6[d]	—

Values are taken from (a) Vieira et al. (1970), (b) Wang (1965), (c) calculated from the variation of the viscosity of water over the temperature range 0–37°C, (d) Redwood and Haydon (1969).

The fact that the value of the apparent activation energy for water diffusion in lipid bilayer membranes is considerably higher than the corresponding values for red cell membranes strongly suggests that water molecules encounter a hydrophilic rather than hydrophobic environment while crossing the latter membranes. Further support for this idea is derived from the fact that if water permeates the red cell membrane by diffusion after dissolving in the lipid environment, and if one assumes that the hydrocarbon chain element in these membranes has similar properties as bulk hydrocarbons, then the calculated value for the apparent activation energy for this process will be at least twofold higher than the value given in Table 2 (Price and Thompson, 1969). In fact, as will be discussed later, when water transport through "pores" is inhibited by certain mercury compounds, the apparent activation energy for osmotic water flow increases to 11·5 kcal mol^{-1} (Macey et al., 1973). This value is in good agreement with the value of 12·4 kcal mol^{-1} calculated, assuming that water dissolves in the membrane as discrete molecules and moves across it by diffusion (Price and Thompson, 1969).

The temperature dependence of the diffusion coefficient (D_w) and the viscosity (η_w) of water are given by (Glasstone et al., 1941):

$$D_w = \lambda^2{}_4 (kT/h)\, (F^{\#}/F) \exp(-\Delta E/RT), \tag{9}$$

$$\eta_w = (\lambda_1/\lambda_2\lambda_3)(h/\lambda^2{}_4)\, (F/F^{\#}) \exp(\Delta E/RT), \tag{10}$$

in which h is Planck's constant; k, Boltzmann's constant; λ_4 is the distance between two equilibrium positions in the direction of motion; λ_1, the distance between two layers of molecules; λ_2 the distance between two adjacent molecules at right angles to direction of motion; λ_3, the distance between neighboring molecules in the same direction, F and $F^{\#}$ are partition functions of the molecule in the initial and activated states; R and T have their usual meanings and the activation energy $\Delta E = \Delta H^{\#} - T\Delta S^{\#}$ where $\Delta S^{\#}$ is the entropy and $\Delta H^{\#}$ the enthalpy of activation. In theory it is possible to analyse the data concerning the temperature effect on water transport in red cells and other membranes in terms of the apparent enthalpy and entropy of activation (Glasstone et al., 1941; Hempling, 1961) Such analysis, however, involves parameters whose values cannot be determined with certainty. Accordingly, the values reported in the literature for the apparent change in entropy of activation for water movement suffers from a great deal of inherent inaccuracy and must be taken with reservation. These parameters can be eliminated if the temperature effect on diffusion is coupled with that on viscous flow $(D_w \eta_w / T = \lambda_1 K / \lambda_2 . \lambda_3)$.

$$\frac{-\,\mathrm{d}\ln D_w}{\mathrm{d}(1/T)} + \frac{\mathrm{d}\ln \eta_w}{\mathrm{d}(1/T)} = -\frac{\mathrm{d}\ln T}{\mathrm{d}(1/T)}, \tag{11}$$

$$R\left[\frac{-\,\mathrm{d}\ln D_w}{\mathrm{d}(1/T)} + \frac{\mathrm{d}\ln 1/\eta_w}{\mathrm{d}(1/T)}\right] = RT \simeq 0\cdot 6 \text{ kcal mol}^{-1}. \tag{12}$$

In the case of the dog red cell, the difference in apparent activation energies for osmotic and diffusion flow is 1·2 kcal mol^{-1}, which is in resaonable agreement in both magnitude and direction with the value 0·6 kcal mol^{-1} given in equation 12.

3.4 MEMBRANE CHOLESTEROL AND WATER PERMEABILITY

Membrane lipids, and particularly cholesterol, are instrumental not only in the control of diffusion across biological membranes but also in the determination of the activity of membrane-bound enzymes, their modulation by hormones and other agents, and the determination of membrane fluidity (Rothfield and Finkelstein, 1968; Pohl et al., 1971; Cogan et al., 1973; Papahadjopoulos, 1973; Puchwein et al., 1974; and Rodan et al., 1974). It is generally accepted that incorporation of cholesterol in a lipid bilayer membrane tends to decrease significantly the permeability of these membranes to water (Finkelstein and Cass, 1967). Movement of water across these membranes occurs primarily by dissolution in the membrane matrix. The decrease in the rate of water transport as a result of cholesterol incorporation is due mainly to a decrease in membrane fluidity. It is found that the incorporation of cholesterol into dispersions composed of phosphatidylserine or ganglioside results in more than three-fold increase in the microviscosities of these dispersions (Feinstein et al., 1975). As a general rule, it is found that the presence of cholesterol in membranes leads to a decrease in the fluidity of the hydrocarbon chains of lipid membranes which are in the liquid-crystalline state. For example, the relative microviscosity of myelin, mitochondrial and microsomal membranes correlate well with their respective cholesterol : phospholipid ratio (Feinstein et al., 1975).

In contrast to lipid bilayer membranes, Sha'afi et al. (1969) have found that the permeability coefficient of the human red cell membrane to water did not change when the free cholesterol content in the membrane was varied from 0·84 to 1·87 mg (ml cells)$^{-1}$. Furthermore, the permeability of the human red cell membrane to sulfate and some nonelectrolytes remained constant when membrane cholesterol was partially removed (Grunze and Deuticke, 1974). These results, however, should not be taken as evidence that water transport in human red cells is independent of membrane cholesterol, since this degree of variation may be insufficient to produce alteration. In fact, extensive removal of cholesterol in these cells does increase slightly the rate of water movement, but no decrease in water movement can be achieved by increasing membrane content of cholesterol (Sha'afi, unpublished observation). These results are in agreement with the finding that extensive depletion of membrane cholesterol induces a marked increase in nonelectrolyte permeability (Grunze and Deuticke, 1974). The effect of membrane cholesterol on the transport of water is also found in other membrane systems. For example, the polyene antibiotic, Amphotericin B, which interacts specifically with serol-containing membranes, increases the permeability of the mucosal but not the serosal membrane of toad bladder to water and other solutes (Lichtenstein and Leaf, 1965; Lichtenstein and Leaf, 1966).

3.5 EFFECT OF SULFHYDRYL-REACTIVE REAGENTS ON WATER TRANSPORT

The transport of water in certain mammalian red cells as well as other cells and tissues has been shown to be inhibited by certain sulfhydryl-reactive reagents (Macey and Farmer, 1970; Naccache and Sha'afi, 1974). A summary of these studies on human red cell membranes is given in Table 3. Half-maximal inhibition is produced at a concentration of 0·25 mM. This inhibition is fully reversible by treatment with excess amount of cysteine or glutathione. As stated earlier, the finding that $P_f/P_d > 1$ is one of the most compelling pieces of evidence for the existence of "pores". This evidence disappears in the presence of PCMBS, $P_f = P_d$, suggesting that this compound acts by shutting off these "pores".

TABLE 3
Effect of p-chloromercuriphenyl sulfonate (PCMBS) on the permeability coefficients of human red cell membrane to water

Condition	Permeability coefficients (cm sec^{-1}) × 10^3		Ratio
	Under osmotic flow, P_f	Under diffusional flow, P_d	P_f/P_d
Red cells	17·30[a]	5·30[b]	3·3
+ 1 mM PCMBS	2·00[c]	1·80[c]	1·1
Ghost	17·9[d]	—	—
+ 1 mM PCMBS	≤17·9[d]	—	—

Values are taken from (a) Rich et al. (1968), (b) Paganelli and Solomon (1957), (c) Macey et al. (1972), (d) Colombe et al. (1974).

Recently the characteristics of the inhibitory site have been determined by comparing the inhibitory potency of a large number of sulfhydryl-reactive reagents (Sha'afi and Feinstein, 1976). The results are summarized in Table 4. Based on these studies, the following observations can be made:

1. Mercury-containing compounds are more effective inhibitors than disulfide reagents.
2. The inability of the compound mersalyl to act as a strong inhibitor of water movement coupled with the finding that mercury-containing compounds are very potent inhibitors of water transport suggest that the SH groups which are important for water flux are located in a hydrophobic environment. This is supported by the fact that only mercury compounds where the mercury molecule is close to the ring are potent inhibitors.
3. The presence of a nitrogen atom in the ring, in addition to an NO_2 group on the side, increases the potency of the disulfide reagent as a water transport inhibitor.
4. The effectiveness of the reagents as inhibitors of water movement parallels the electron-withdrawing capacity of the substituents.
5. Membrane sulfhydryl groups which are involved in the control of water transport are less reactive than those of a small SH-containing molecule, such as cysteine.

3.6 ASYMMETRY OF WATER FLOW

It is generally observed that the rate of red cell swelling is faster than the

TABLE 4
Effect of various sulfhydryl-reactive reagents on the transport of water across human red cell membrane

Compound	Structure	Inhibition
p-Chloromercuriphenyl sulfonate	ClHg–C$_6$H$_4$–SO$_2$–O$^-$	80
p-Chloromercuribenzoate	ClHg–C$_6$H$_4$–COO$^-$	77
Phenylmercuric chloride	C$_6$H$_5$–HgCl	61
Phenylmercuric acetate	C$_6$H$_5$–Hg–O–C(=O)–CH$_3$	57
p-Aminophenylmercuric acetate	H$_2$N–C$_6$H$_4$–Hg–O–C(=O)–CH$_3$	77
Mersalyl*	C$_6$H$_3$(OCH$_2$COOH)–C(=O)–NH–CH$_2$–CH(OCH$_3$)–CH$_2$–HgOH	30
2,2′-Dithiobis-(5-nitropyridine)	(O$_2$N–C$_5$H$_2$N)–S–S–(C$_5$H$_2$N–NO$_2$)	60
4,4′-Dithiopyridine	(C$_5$H$_4$N)–S–S–(C$_5$H$_4$N)	0
2,2′-Dipyridyldisulfide	(C$_5$H$_4$N)–S–S–(C$_5$H$_4$N)	0
6,6′-Dithiodinicotinic acid	HOOC–(C$_5$H$_2$N)–S–S–(C$_5$H$_2$N)–COOH	0
3-Nitrophenyldisulfide	(O$_2$N–C$_6$H$_4$)–S–S–(C$_6$H$_4$–NO$_2$)	30
5,5′-Dithiobis-(2-nitrobenzoic acid)	(O$_2$N,COOH–C$_6$H$_3$)–S–S–(C$_6$H$_3$–NO$_2$,COOH)	30

* Concentration is 1 mM and time of incubation is 15 min.

rate of red cell shrinkage (Rich et al., 1968; Blum and Forster, 1970; Farmer and Macey, 1970). Initially, it was suggested that these results were due to a dependence of the osmotic water permeability coefficient (L_p) on medium osmolality (Rich et al., 1968). Later, however, it was suggested that this behavior was due not to a change in medium osmolality, but rather to a rectification of water flow (inward rate being greater than outward rate) (Farmer and Macey, 1970). Asymmetry of water flow occurs also in other tissues (Loesche et al., 1970). At present, the most likely explanation of these results is to postulate that both effects, medium osmolality and rectification of water flow, are present. This rectification of water flow can be due to one or a combination of the following possibilities: (a) the behavior of the red cell membrane functionally as a double membrane (it can be shown that such an arrangement leads to rectification of water transport (Patlak et al., 1963); (b) the presence of a valve-like structure in the "aqueous channels"; (c) a change in the surface area as a result of a separation of the membrane from the adjacent layer of hemoglobin during the inward flow of water; or (d) a one-directional (from out to in) "peristaltic contraction" of the pathways used by water. Such a peristaltic behavior will give rise to a force which helps inward movement of water. Under the usual experimental conditions, this force is not taken into consideration when the permeability coefficient of red cell membrane to water is calculated. Since the hydraulic permeability coefficient (L_p) is defined as volume flow per unit driving force, such an underestimation of the driving force will give rise to an overestimation of L_p. The most likely explanation for the observed rectification of water flow is to postulate that the human red cell membrane behaves functionally as a complex system consisting of at least two barriers, one in the inner half of the membrane bilayer and another in the second half. Based on the preceding discussion, this could be due to an asymmetric distribution of cholesterol and/or the phospholipid between the two halves of the membrane bilayer. For example, if the outer half of the membrane bilayer has a higher cholesterol content than the inner half, then its permeability to water will be much lower. There is evidence suggesting that cholesterol and phospholipids are asymmetrically distributed between the two halves of the membrane bilayer in frog myelin sheath and also in human red cell membrane (Kirschner and Caspar 1972; Bretscher, 1973; Fisher, 1976).

3.7 MISCELLANEOUS FACTORS WHICH MAY INFLUENCE THE TRANSPORT OF WATER ACROSS RED CELL MEMBRANE

One of the first parameters which comes to mind among those factors which may affect membrane permeability properties in any system is pH. A study of pH effects may give some information about the role of ionizable protein groups in membrane structure on its permeability. Rich *et al.* (1968) have shown that the hydraulic water conductivity (L_p) is independent of pH in the range from 6 to 8 in human red cells. The rate of water transfer in human red cells, and probably for all other mammalian red cells, is independent of cell volume, the osmolality of the internal medium (Rich *et al.*, 1968) and membrane flexibility (Sirs, 1969). Compounds such as tetrodotoxin and valinomycin, which are known to produce selective actions on sodium and potassium transport across both biological (Rottenberg and Solomon, 1966; Tosteson *et al.*, 1967; Narahashi *et al.*, 1960) and artificial membranes (Andreoli *et al.*, 1967) have no effect on water transport across the human red cell membrane (Rich *et al.*, 1968).

Chemicals which produce an apparent effect on water movement in red cells are numerous. The word apparent is used since the results found can be attributed to changes in the membrane and not in rate of water flow. Furthermore, the nature of the changes is concentration dependent. For example, Arrhenius and Bubanovic (cited in Jacobs, 1931) have shown that substances such as chloroform, benzol, ethyl alcohol, ethyl ether and amyl alcohol have a hemolytic action at high concentration and a protective action at low concentration. They suggested that these compounds interfere with the movement of water. Jarisch (cited in Jacobs, 1931) has reported similar results and he likewise attributed them to an effect of the narcotic and other substances used upon the transfer of water. Jacobs (1931) was probably the first to recognize that this kind of study does not provide conclusive evidence that these substances change the rate of water transfer. He argued that these authors had used the hemolysis time as an index of water penetration, and thus the observed effect of these agents might be on the membrane and not on the rate of water movement. It is quite possible to treat red cells with agents so that they will be very resistive to hemolysis without changing the actual rate of water transfer (Berg *et al.*, 1965). Recently, however, it has been shown that neutral, positively and negatively charged anesthetics increase the permeability L_p of human red cell membrane to water. This increase was not related to the concentration of calcium in the membrane (Seeman *et al.*, 1970). In addition, it has been shown that tannic acid also inhibits the movement of water (Hunter, 1960).

3.8 POSSIBLE STRUCTURAL BASIS FOR THE APPARENT PRESENCE OF HYDROPHILIC PATHWAY FOR WATER TRANSPORT

There is a large body of evidence, some of which has been discussed already, which supports the view that water molecules cross the human red cell and probably other cell membranes via specialized "apparent polar regions". Figure 2 depicts schematically two possible mechanisms for water transport. Movement of water by either of these two mechanisms will have similar characteristics as movement through "aqueous pores". Although the two models shown in Fig. 2 are entirely different from the structural point of view, they both give rise to many of the observed properties of water transport in the human red cell membrane.

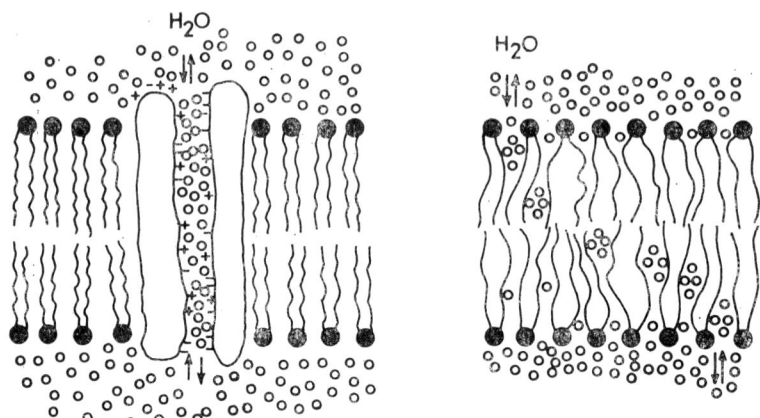

FIG. 2. Schematic representation of two possible models which may give rise for the apparent presence of hydrophilic pathways for water transport in human red cell membrane. In Fig. 2A on the left, the pores are assembled from membrane integral proteins which are aggregates of identical or nonidentical sub-units. In FIG. 2B on the right, water molecules move across the membrane by jumping into the free volume generated by the thermal fluctuations in membrane lipid.

The hydrophilic pathway shown in Fig. 2A is highly schematic and should not be taken to mean that it is a fixed right cylindrical "pore" with static structure and dimensions. It could be assembled from membrane integral proteins which are probably aggregates of identical or nonidentical sub-units. It is generally agreed that there are two known major proteins which span the human red cell membrane. In the terminology of Steck *et al.* (1971) they are band 3 (molecular weight 95 000–100 000) and PSA–1 They are also known as component *a* and glycophorin, respectively (Marchesi *et al.*, 1972; Bretscher, 1973). There are three lines of evidence which suggest that one or both of these two glycoproteins may be involved in the formation of hydrophilic pathways for water transport:

a. Marchesi *et al.* (1972) have presented evidence which indicates that glycophorin is a component of the intramembranous particles seen in freeze-fracture experiments. It has been suggested that these membrane-interrelated particles seen in human red cell membrane could provide a structural basis for the hydrophilic pathway (Da Silva, 1973).

b. Incorporation of glycophorin prepared by trypsin hydrolysis of human erythrocytes in black lipid membranes increases significantly the permeability of these membranes to water (Lea et al., 1975). This may be a nonspecific increase.

c. Using polyacrylamide gel electrophoresis, it has been shown that a band which contains band 3 and glycophorin can be selectively labelled by a water transport inhibitor (Brown et al., 1975; Sha'afi and Feinstein, 1976).

Furthermore, in a preliminary study we have found that water transport in liposomes prepared from egg lecithin and containing band 3 can be inhibited by PCMBS (Sha'afi and Feinstein, 1976). If the "aqueous pores" are made exclusively from glycophorin, then it would be difficult to understand why sulfhydryl-reactive reagents inhibit water transport. Glycophorin has been purified from human red cell membrane and sequenced (Tomita and Marchesi, 1975). It has no cysteine and, therefore, it is difficult to see how sulfhydryl-reactive reagents will interact with this protein to inhibit water transport. It must be made quite clear that band 3 is quite dispersed and that it may comprise more than one species of polypeptides. This band has been reported to contain a phosphorylated intermediate of the (Na^+-K^+)-ATPase (Avruch and Fairbanks, 1972; Knauf et al., 1974). It also binds 4,4'-diisothiocyano-2,2'-ditriostibene-disulphonates (DIDS), a specific inhibitor of anion movement (Cabantchik and Rothstein, 1974a). The heterogeneity of protein band 3 is also indicated by the observation of Cabantchik and Rothstein (1974b) that after pronase treatment the staining of this band decreased and three individual bands are revealed.

Such a mechanism for water transport with a slight modification to account for hormone-sensitive water movement is probably common to other membrane systems. In the case of the collecting duct of memmalian kidney, for example, it is conceivable to imagine that there is an interruption somewhere along the pore. This interruption can be temporarily removed through a transient conformational change brought about by ADH-induced changes in the level of cyclic AMP.

The model depicted in Fig. 2B is based on the idea that thermal fluctuations in membrane lipid can cause conformational changes in the hydrocarbon chains which lead to the generation of mobile structural defects known as "kinks" (Traüble, 1971; Traüble, 1972). These kinks can be initiated only on either side of the membrane and then migrate to the other side, giving rise to mobile packets of free volume. Water molecules on either side of the membrane can jump into this free volume and "hitch a ride" to the other side. The kink is a thermodynamically stable structure and the free volume generated by it can be of different sizes (Traüble, 1971). Although it is not intuitively obvious how such a mechanism of water movement will give rise to the finding that $P_f/P_d > 1$, it is not entirely impossible to modify the system to account for this finding. Accordingly, if water movement across the red cell membrane is to be explained in terms of the "kinks" hypothesis, then one would have to postulate that the free volume generated by the "kinks" formation should be large enough to accommodate the finding $P_f/P_d > 1$. Not only that, but one must also postulate that in a black lipid bilayer, the free volume is very small so that no water filtration can take place since $P_f = P_d$ in these membranes. The inhibitory effect of sulfhydryl-reactive reagents on water movement in red cell membrane is not entirely inconsistent with the "kink" hypothesis. It is not unreasonable to expect that interaction with membrane protein may produce a decrease either in the kink concentration and/or a decrease in the free volume formed by the "kinks". Even though the kink hypothesis is an attractive one and certainly a very good mechanism for water diffusion in a lipid bilayer, it probably accounts for only 10 per cent of water movement in the human red cell membrane. This 10 per cent is the component of water which crosses the cell membrane via the lipid region. For one thing, the permeability coefficient for water calculated on the basis of the kink hypothesis is one order of magnitude less than the experimentaly determined value in the human red cell membrane. Moreover, the kink hypothesis has to be drastically modified to account for the various properties of water transport in human red cells ($P_f/P_d = 3 \cdot 3$, inhibition of water transport by various sulfhydryl-reactive reagents, $\Delta E = \simeq 4 \text{ kcal mol}^{-1}$, possible rectification of water flow . . .).

4 Permeability of the red cell membrane to small nonelectrolytes

In this review we will restrict our discussion to small hydrophilic nonelectrolytes. However, before discussing this question in detail, it is worth noting that the value of the permeability coefficient of red cell membranes as well as of other biological membranes for a large lipophilic molecule is determined by its lipid solubility, its molecular size and shape, and the number of hydrogen bonds (N_H) it is able to form with water. The permeability coefficient increases with increasing lipid solubility and decreasing N_H, whereas it decreases with increasing molecular size and degree of branching. For example, replacement of a hydroxyl group on the molecule by a carbonyl group or an amide group tends to decrease the permeability coefficient (for a comprehensive review see Wright and Diamond, 1969; Naccache and Sha'afi, 1973). In the case of small hydrophilic molecules, we will restrict our discussion to the following points: (a) Is the mechanism by which these solutes permeate red cell membranes similar to that for large lipophilic molecules? (b) Which inhibitors affect the movements of these small nonelectrolytes? (c) Is there a carrier-mediated mechanism for urea transport? (d) Do small molecules use the same pathways as water?

4.1 IS THE MECHANISM BY WHICH SMALL HYDROPHILIC SOLUTES PERMEATE RED CELL MEMBRANE SIMILAR TO THAT USED BY LARGE LIPOPHILIC MOLECULES?

Here the problem is to decide whether these solutes permeate by dissolution in the membrane fabric or by crossing the membrane through polar pathways ("aqueous pores"). It is worth pointing out from the start that there is no conclusive evidence which enables one to decide unequivocally between these two possibilities. As will become clearer by the end of this discussion, the data at hand are merely more consistent with the postulate that these molecules permeate through polar pathways and not by dissolution in the membrane fabric. Probably the strongest evidence for this hypothesis is summarized in Table 5. The values of the diffusional perme-

TABLE 5
Values of the permeability and partition coefficients for various small hydrophilic solutes

Solute	$K_{ether}^{(a)}$	Permeability coefficient, cm sec^{-1} × 10^5	
		Human RBC[b]	Spherical bilayer[c]
Formamide	0·0014	43·7	7·8
Acetamide	0·0075	12·2	2·4
Urea	0·00047	36·5	0·49
Methylurea	0·0012	4·9	—
1,3-Dimethylurea	0·0031	2·7	—

Values are taken from (a) Collander (1949), (b) Sha'afi et al. (1971), (c) Poznansky et al. (1976).

ability coefficient for egg lecithin spherical bilayers are included in the table for comparison. Based on their lipid solubility these molecules should be quite impermeable. In fact, in the lipid bilayer, where movement of nonelectrolytes is primarily by dissolution in the membrane fabric, urea permeates these membranes very slowly. The ratio P_d:urea/P_d:H_2O is 0·0031—more than an order of magnitude smaller than the 0·11 ratio for P_d:urea/P_d:H_2O in human red cells. On the other hand, when the lipid bilayer membrane is treated with the antibiotics nystatin or Amphotericin B, the ratio P_d:urea/P_d:H_2O increases to 0·11 (Holz and Finkelstein, 1970). It has been proposed that Amphotericin B and cholesterol are complexed in lipid bilayers to form an aqueous pore of 4 Å radius (Andreoli, 1973; de Kruijff and Demel, 1974). It is very clear from Table 5 that these small solutes permeate at very high rates and that there is no apparent correlation between lipid solubility and permeability. The primary parameter which is of overwhelming importance in determining the permeability coefficient of human red cell membranes to these small hydrophilic solutes is steric hindrance. There are three parameters which are commonly used when considering steric hindrance factors. The cylindrical radius of the permeating molecule, a measure of molecular size, has been shown by Soll (1967) to be paramount in the steric interactions governing the values of the reflection coefficient (σ) in mammalian red cells. When purely geometrical factors are dominant in the members of a given homologous series, Gary-Bobo and Weber (1969) and Sha'afi et al. (1971) have found the cylindrical radius to be the parameter of choice in studies of permeation of small nonelectrolytes in both nonporous cellulose acetate and human red cell membranes. However, for small hydrophilic solutes that are members of different homologous series, a better index of geometrical factors is the molar volume, which is equal to the molecular weight divided by the density of the pure compound. The molecular weight may be construed as a measure of molecular size based on a spherical model. Division by the density modifies the strictly geometrical interpretation by introduction of the hydrogen bonding of the molecule with water because, as Pimental and McClennan (1960) have pointed out, hydrogen bonding generally increases the density and lowers the molar volume. The correlation of hydrogen bonding with density is best illustrated in series such as butanediols, propanediols, pentanediols and others. The density of the members of each series decreases as the positions of OH groups approach each other and the ability to hydrogen bond with other molecules decreases. Thus, the molar volume as a mixed parameter—a geometrical construct modified by chemical properties, primarily hydrogen bonding—is a more preferable index of geometrical factors. In fact, it provides a very good fit for the permeability coefficients of human red cell membranes to small hydrophilic solutes, as illustrated in Fig. 3. It is interesting to note that a similar relationship is found for lipid bilayer membranes treated with the antibiotics nystatin or Amphotericin B (Holz and Finkelstein, 1970; Solomon, 1972). A third index which may be used in these considerations is solute molecular weight. However, molecular weight does not differentiate between the size of two isomers. The importance of steric factors is not restricted to solutes which permeate through polar routes; it also

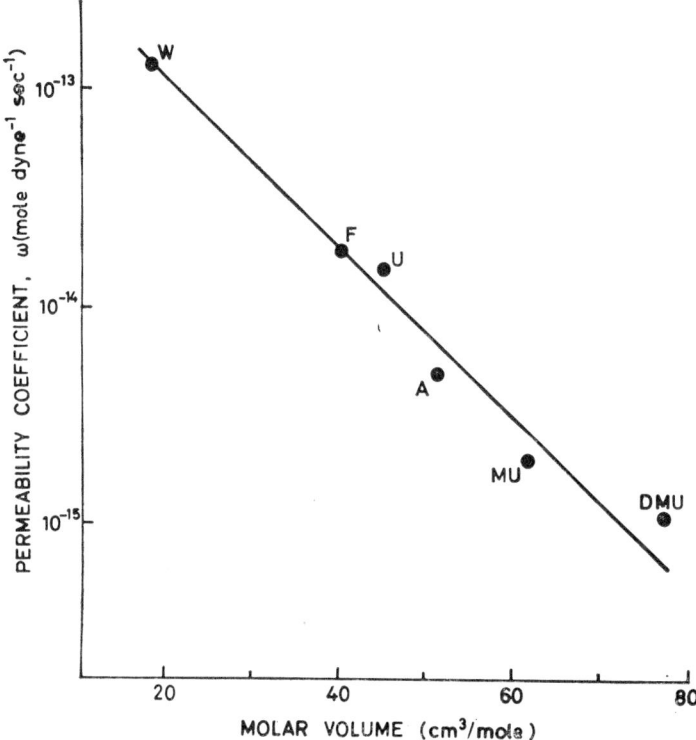

FIG. 3. Variation of the permeability coefficients of human red cell membrane to various small hydrophilic solutes with solute molar volume. The symbols are as follows: W. water; F, formamide; U, urea; A, acetamide; MU, methylurea; DMU, dimethylurea.

applies to lipophilic solutes which penetrate by dissolving in the membrane fabric.

A geometrical factor which may not be related to steric effects is the surface contact area between the permeating molecule and the membrane. This is probably more important for lipophilic solutes since lipid : lipid forces are predominantly short-range van der Waals' forces. Based on these results, one cannot escape the conclusion that these molecules will not be able to cross the membrane at such a high rate if the only mechanism is by dissolving in the membrane fabric. One is forced to conclude that they must permeate either by a specialized membrane transport system, such as a carrier-mediated mechanism, and/or through a specialized polar pathway. The temperature dependence of nonelectrolyte permeation across red cell and certain other membranes is consistent with this conclusion. It is generally found that the values of apparent activation energies for the permeation of small hydrophilic solutes are significantly lower than the corresponding values for lipophilic solutes (Galey et al., 1973; Sha'afi and Volpi, unpublished data).

A second set of experimental evidence which supports the hypothesis that small hydrophilic solutes permeate by a mechanism different than that used by lipophilic ones is given in Table 6. For a given homologous series

TABLE 6
Values of the relative permeability and partition coefficients for various small molecules

Solute	K_{ether}	N_H*	Relative permeability*
Urea	0·00047	5	1·00
Methylurea	0·0012	4	0·08
Ethylurea	0·0041	4	0·01
Thiourea	0·0063	3	0·003
Acetamide	0·0025	3	1·0
Methylacetamide	—	2	0·70
Thioacetamide	—	3	0·81
Methanol	0·14	2	1·00
Ethanol	0·26	2	0·77
n-propanol	1·90	2	0·56
n-butanol	7·70	2	0·36

* Values are taken from Naccache and Sha'afi (1973).

of small solutes, the lipid solubility of the molecule (K_{ether}) and the number of hydrogen bonds it is able to form with water (N_H) seem to exercise a very small effect on the rate of penetration. For example, the first member of the series is much more permeable than the remaining members even though it has the lowest lipid solubility and the highest value for N_H. This is also true, but to a lesser extent, for small lipophilic solutes. The most important parameters that seem to determine the rates of movement of these solutes is the molecular size. The value of the permeability coefficient decreases sharply with increasing size.

A third set of data (Sha'afi et al., 1971; Redwood et al., 1974) which are often taken as evidence that the major pathway for the permeation of small hydrophilic solutes is not by dissolution in the membrane fabric is shown in Fig. 4. The clear minimum in the curve is often taken as evidence that the two molecules which lie in the descending limb of the curve permeate through different pathways from the other solutes. Even though this explanation is possible, it is not the only one. The most likely explanation is that the presence of the minimum indicates that there are at least two controlling processes governing the movements of these solutes across human red cell membrane. Incidentally, this was the explanation put forth in the original article (Sha'afi *et al.*, 1971). The conclusion is further supported by two recent observations which show that the presence of such a minimum can be demonstrated even in systems where the presence of polar paths is extremely unlikely (Sherrill and Dietschy, 1975; Poznansky *et al.*, 1976).

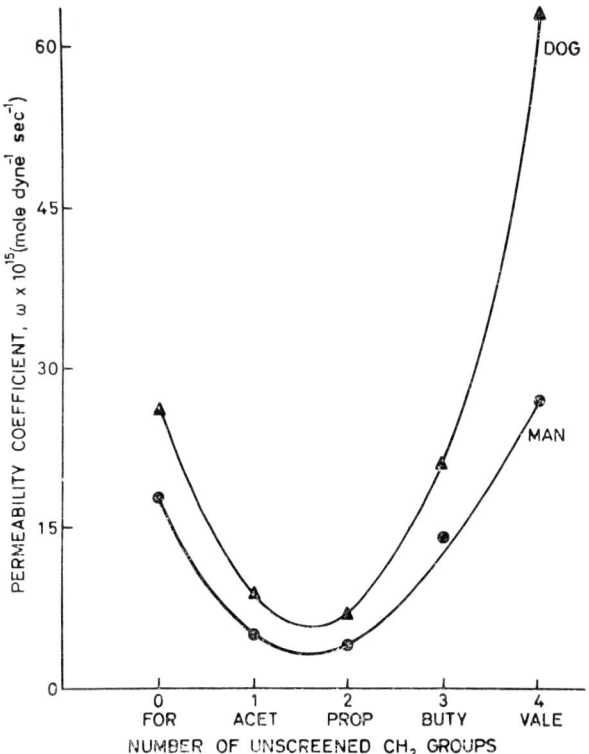

FIG. 4. The permeability coefficients of human and dog red cell membranes of a homologous series of straight chain amides as a function of the number of unscreened CH_2 groups on the compound.

4.2 WHICH INHIBITORS AFFECT THE MOVEMENTS OF THESE SMALL NON-ELECTROLYTES?

Movements of small hydrophilic solutes across human and probably other biological membranes can be affected by certain sulfhydryl-reactive reagents such as PCMBS and by phloretin. These two compounds inhibit drastically the movements of these solutes. As is evident in Table 7, the inhibitory effect of these two compounds on the permeability of these solutes decreases as the value of K_{ether} increases. Whereas the compound PCMBS has no significant effect on the permeability coefficient of the human red cell membrane to lipophilic nonelectrolytes, the compound phloretin enhances the rates of movement of these solutes. In fact, phloretin has been shown to increase significantly the permeability coefficient of pure lipid spherical bilayer (egg lecithin) to small hydrophilic solutes such as formamide (Poznansky et al., 1976). Movement across this membrane occurs only by dissolution in the membrane fabric. It is possible that this is due to an increase in the mobility of membrane lipid. The exact nature of the phloretin effect is not fully understood. It has been suggested that the effect of phloretin on nonelectrolyte permeability in red cells is actuated through an allosteric interaction with a surface extension of a membrane protein (Owen and Solomon, 1972). Other agents such as tannic acid are also known to decrease the permeability coefficients of certain mammalian red cell membranes to various small nonelectrolytes (Hunter et al., 1965).

TABLE 7
Effect of PCMBS and phloretin on the permeability coefficients of human red cell membrane to various nonelectrolytes

Molecule	K_{ether}	Relative permeability in the presence of	
		PCMBS	Phloretin
Urea	0·00047	0·10[a]	0·34[c]
Methylurea	0·0012	0·15[b]	0·30[b]
Formamide	0·0014	0·17[a]	0·55[c]
Acetamide	0·0025	0·28[a]	0·80[c]
1,3-Dimethylurea	0·003	1·00[b]	1·00[b]
Ethylurea	0·004	0·90[b]	1·00[b]
1,3-Propanediol	0·004	1·00[b]	1·30[c]
Ethylene glycol	0·005	1·00[b]	1·80[c]
Methanol	0·140	0·90[a]	—
Ethanol	0·260	0·90[a]	—
Water	0·003	0·15[a]	1·30[c]

Values are taken from (a) Naccache and Sha'afi (1974), (b) Macey and Farmer (1970), (c) Owen and Solomon (1972), (d) Gary-Bobo (private communication).

4.3 IS THERE A CARRIER-MEDIATED MECHANISM FOR UREA TRANSPORT?

The movement of urea across various mammalian red cell membranes has been studied extensively (Jacobs et al., 1935; Hunter et al)., 1965; Sha'afi et al., 1970; Macey and Wadzinski, 1974; Kaplan et al., 1975). The mechanism for urea transport in these cells has been subject to considerable debate. This controversy stems from the fact that urea is a small hydrophilic molecule which is able to form five hydrogen bonds with water and yet in spite of these properties it is extremely permeable across red cell membranes. As pointed out earlier, urea permeates lipid bilayers treated with antibiotics at a high rate. The simplest and most straightforward explanation for this is to postulate that red cell membranes behave operationally as a mosaic structure containing both lipid and polar regions. Accordingly, small hydrophilic solutes such as urea permeate through the polar route. An alternative explanation is to postulate that urea moves across these and other biological membranes from mammalian species by means of a specialized carrier-mediated mechanism. The idea that urea may be transported across human red cell membranes by means of a carrier-mediated mechanism was first advanced by Hunter et al. (1965). His conclusions were based on the finding that the movement of urea across these membranes can be inhibited by tannic acid. Recent evidence by Macey and Farmer (1970) seems to support this conclusion. They have found that the compound phloretin, a known inhibitor of facilitated transport systems, is a potent inhibitor of urea movement. Further evidence to support this view can be obtained from studies with sulfhydryl-reactive reagents. It was found that the permeability coefficient of human red cell membranes to urea and other small hydrophilic solutes was significantly reduced in the presence of PCMBS (Macey and Farmer, 1970; Naccache and Sha'afi, 1974). In addition, using the results of Sha'afi et al. (1970), Macey and Wadzinski (1974) have concluded that the movement of urea across human red cell membrane shows saturation kinetics. Incidentally, this conclusion is not entirely without equivocation. On the surface, the evidence seems to be overwhelmingly in support of a carrier-mediated mechanism for urea transport. However, these findings are also consistent with the conclusion that urea permeates membranes through specialized "aqueous pores". Even if the conclusion is correct that the movement of urea shows saturation kinetics, it implies only that the number of urea molecules is larger than the number of these pathways. If one accepts the view that the high permeability of mammalian red cell membranes to urea is due to the presence of mobile carriers for its transport, then one is forced to postulate the presence of mobile carriers for the other highly permeable small hydrophilic solutes such as formamide. In addition, the properties of these carriers must be similar to those pathways found in antibiotic-treated lipid bilayer membranes. Since there are consistent sets of arguments for the presence of "aqueous pathways" in mammalian red cell membranes, it is not possible to decide which of these two mechanisms is responsible for the high rate of urea transport.

In order to obtain a better insight into this question, we have investigated the permeability characteristics of rabbit polymorphonuclear leukocyte membranes (PMNS) to urea, methylurea and thiourea (Sha'afi and Volpi, unpublished data). These cells were chosen for two reasons. First, the value of the hydraulic permeability coefficient of the membranes to water is much lower than the corresponding value for mammalian red cell membranes (Hempling, 1973; Naccache and Sha'afi, 1974). Secondly, the value of the apparent activation energy for water transport in the former cells is much higher than the corresponding value for the latter (Hempling, 1973). These two findings suggest that rabbit polymorphonuclear leukocyte membranes do not act as a molecular sieve (absence of equivalent pores). Accordingly, it is feasible by using these membranes to decide between the two possible mechanisms for urea transport. For example, if urea is transported across biological membranes by a carrier-mediated mechanism, then the rate of urea movement across PMN membranes would be very high. On the other hand, if urea permeates through "aqueous pores", then the permeability coefficient of these membranes to urea would be very small. Furthermore, the rates of permeation of urea, methylurea and thiourea across PMN membranes would be determined mainly by the lipid solubility of each solute. The results of these studies are summarized in Table 8. The values for K_{ether}, N_H and molar volume

TABLE 8
Permeability coefficients of rabbit PMN and human red blood cell membranes to small nonelectrolytes

Solute	Molar [a] volume	K_{ether}[b]	N_H	Permeability coefficient $\times 10^5$ cm sec^{-1}	
				Rabbit PMN	Human RBC
Urea	45	0·00047	5	0·30	31·2[c]
Methylurea	61·5	0·0012	4	0·45	4·8[c]
Thiourea	54·2	0·0063	5	0·87	0·07[d]

(a) Molar volume is expressed in terms of cm^3 mol^{-1}. Values are taken from (b) Collander (1949), (c) Sha'afi et al. (1971), (d) Naccache and Sha'afi (1973).

are included in the table. The permeability coefficients of human red cell membranes to these solutes are also included in the table for comparison. It is very clear from the table that the two membranes behave quite differently with respect to the rates of permeation of these nonelectrolytes. This difference cannot be accounted for on the basis of differences in species. The pattern in the permeability coefficients of rabbit red cell membranes to urea, methylurea and thiourea is similar to that found for human erythrocyte membranes. Three conclusions can be drawn from these studies. First, there is no need to postulate a specialized mechanism (carrier-mediated) for urea transport across rabbit PMN membranes. This conclusion can probably be extended to human red cell and other biological membranes. It is very difficult to imagine why red cell membranes would have a carrier-mediated mechanism for urea transport and PMN membranes would not. Secondly, there is no need to postulate that PMN membranes contain "aqueous pores" for the transport of small hydrophilic nonelectrolytes. In these cells one can postulate that the membrane is homogeneous and permeation occurs only by dissolution in the membrane fabric. Thirdly, the idea of "aqueous pores" is not a general property of biological membranes, but is restricted only to certain ones.

These findings are not restricted to the transport of urea across leukocyte membranes. It is well known that in some red cells (fish and birds) urea is less permeable than thiourea, while in others (reptiles and mammals) the converse is true. It has been suggested that in the former cells, the membrane is homogeneous and permeation occurs only by dissolution in the membrane matrix, while in the latter cells the membrane contains both lipid and polar regions. Accordingly, thiourea (having a higher partition coefficient and lower N_H) will permeate faster than urea in the former cells, whereas in the latter cells urea is faster, owing to its smaller molecular size. The observation that phloretin enhances the movement of urea in red cells from fish and birds and inhibits the transport of urea in red cells from reptiles and mammals (Kaplan et al., 1974) is consistent with this view.

4.4 DO UREA AND OTHER SMALL MOLECULES USE THE SAME PATHWAYS AS WATER?

If one accepts the conclusion that urea and other small hydrophilic solutes permeate cell membrane through specialized "polar pathways" and not by mobile carriers, then the next question to be answered is whether or not these molecules use most of the pathways available for water movement. Considering the data available, it is hard to escape the conclusion that only a small fraction of these postulated pathways is available for the movement of urea and other small solutes. This is based on the observation that it is possible to dissociate water and solute transport in human red cell membranes. It is found (see Table 7) that while the compound phloretin significantly reduced the transport of urea and other small hydrophilic solutes, it enhances slightly the movement of water in human red cell membranes (Macey and Farmer, 1970; Owen and Solomon, 1972).

Figure 5 depicts schematically the author's current view of how water and small hydrophilic solutes permeate across red cell membranes. The model is crude, but it accounts for all the experimental data available. The basic features of this model are as follows:

1. Most of the water molecules permeate through "aqueous pores" with only a small component crossing through the membrane matrix.

2. Only a small fraction of these pores is large enough to permit the transport of small hydrophilic solutes. Some of these "pores" may be large enough to accommodate glucose molecules. This will imply that glucose transport across human red cell membrane is not by means of a mobile carrier mechanism—a not unlikely possibility.

3. A fraction of the total movement of the solute takes place through the membrane matrix. This fraction increases with increasing lipid solubility.

4. Certain sulfhydryl-reactive reagents totally abolish the movement through the "aqueous pathways" but do not affect the movement through the membrane matrix.

5. The compound phloretin is able to react allosterically only with those pathways which are large enough to permit solute penetration. This interaction can cause configurational changes in the proteins which form these pathways resulting in a significant decrease in the size of these "aqueous pores" and a change in the physical and chemical nature of the membrane matrix. The latter change can lead to an increase in the rate of solute movement through the lipid matrix.

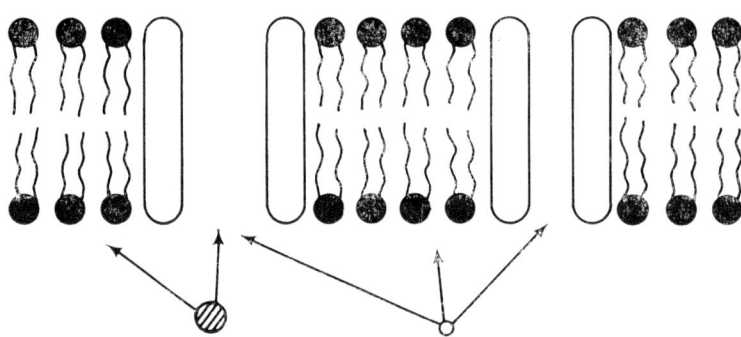

FIG. 5. Schematic representation of the various pathways available to water and small hydrophilic solutes for crossing red cell membranes. The open circle represents water molecule and the hatched circle represents the solute molecule.

Acknowledgements

Unpublished studies cited in this chapter from the author's laboratory were supported, in part, by Research Grant GM-20268-02 from the

National Institutes of General Medical Sciences. The author wishes to express his great appreciation to Ms Joan Morneault for her infinite patience in typing the manuscript.

References

ANDERSON, B. and USSING, H. H. (1953). *Acta Physiol. Scand.* **28**, 60.
ANDREOLI, T. E. (1973). *Kidney International*, **4**, 337.
ANDREOLI, T. E., TIEFFENBERG, M. and TOSTESON, D. C. (1967). *J. Gen. Physiol.* **50**, 2527.
AVRUCH, J. and FAIRBANKS, C. (1972). *Proc. Nat. Acad. Sci. USA*, **69**, 1216.
BARRY, P. H. and HOPE, H. B. (1969). *Biophys. J.* **7**, 729.
BERG, H. C., DIAMOND, J. M. and MARFEY, P. S. (1965). *Science*, **150**, 64.
BLUM, R. M. and FORSTER, P. E. (1970). *Biochim. Biophys. Acta*, **20**, 410.
BRANTON, D. (1971). *Phil. Trans. P. Soc. Lon. B*, **261**, 133.
BRANTON, D. and DAEMER, D. W. (1972). *Protoplasmatologia*, vol. II, E70.
BRETSCHER, M. S. (1973). *Science*, **181**, 622.
BROWN, A. P., FEINSTEIN, M. B. and SHA'AFI, R. I. (1975). *Nature*, **254**, 523.
CABANTCHIK, Z. I. and ROTHSTEIN, A. J. (1974a). *J. Membrane Biol.* **15**, 207.
CABANTCHIK, Z. I. and ROTHSTEIN, A. J. (1974b). *J. Membrane Biol.* **15**, 227.
COGAN, U., SHINITZKY, M., WEBER, G. and NISHIDA, T. (1973). *Biochemistry*, **12**, 521.
COLLANDER, R. (1949). *Acta Chem. Scand.* **3**, 717.
COLOMBE, B., WINOCUR and MACEY, R. I. (1974). *Biochim. Biophys. Acta*, **263**, 226.
CONLON, T. and OUTHRED, R. (1972). *Biochim. Biophys. Acta*, **288**, 354.
CURRAN, P. F. (1960). *J. Gen. Physiol.* **43**, 1137.
CURRAN, P. F. and SOLOMON, A. K. (1957). *J. Gen. Physiol.* **41**, 143.
DAINTY, J. and GINZBURG, B. Z. (1963). *J. Theoret. Biol.* **5**, 256.
DASILVA, P. P. (1973). *Proc. Nat. Acad. Sci. USA*, **70**, 1339.
DEGIER, J. (1973). *In* "Erythrocytes, Thrombocytes and Leukocytes, Recent Advances in Membrane and Metabolic" (E. Gulach, K. Moser, E. Deutsch and W. Wilmanns, eds), pp. 000. Georg Thieme, Stuttgart.
DEKRUIJFT, B. and DEMEL, R. A. (1974). *Biochim. Biophys. Acta*, **339**, 57.
DIAMOND, J. M. and WRIGHT, W. R. (1969). *A. Rev. Physiol.* **31**, 581.
DICK, D. A. T. (1966). *In* "Cell Water", chap. 6. Butterworths, London and Washington.
DURBIN, R. P. (1960). *J. Gen. Physiol.* **44**, 315.
DURBIN, R. P., FRANK, H. and SOLOMON, A. K. (1956). *J. Gen. Physiol.* **39**, 535.
ELLAM, Y. and STEIN, W. D. (1974). *In* "Methods in Membrane Biology" (E. D. Korn, ed) vol. 2, p. 283. Plenum Press, New York and London.
FARMER, R. E. L. and MACEY, R. I. (1970). *Biochim. Biophys. Acta*, **196**, 53.
FEINSTEIN, M. B., FERNANDEZ, S. M. and Sha'afi, R. I. (1975). *Biochim. Biophys. Acta*, **413**, 354.
FENICHEL, J. R. and HOROWITZ, S. B. (1969). *3rd Int. Biophys. Cong. IUPAB*, Cambridge, Mass., 240.
FINKELSTEIN, A. and CASS, A. (1967). *Nature*, **216**, 717.
FISHER, K. A. (1976). *Proc. Nat. Acad. Sci. USA*, **73**, 173.
GARY-BOBO, C. M. and WEBER, H. W. (1969). *J. Phys. Chem.* **73**, 115.

GLASSTONE, S., LAIDLER, K. J. and EYRING, H. (1941). In theory of rate processes, McGraw-Hill Book Co., New York, chapter IX.
GALEY, W. R., OWEN, J. D. and SOLOMON, A. K. (1973). *J. Gen. Physiol.* **61**, 727.
GOLDSTEIN, D. A. and SOLOMON, A. K. (1960). *J. Gen. Physiol.* **44**, 1.
GRUNZE, M. and DEUTICKE, B. (1974). *Biochim. Biophys. Acta*, **356**, 125.
HAYS, R. M. and LEAF, A. (1962a). *J. Gen. Physiol.* **45**, 905.
HAYS, R. M. and LEAF, A. (1962b). *J. Gen. Physiol.* **45**, 933.
HEMPLING, H. G. (1961). *J. Gen. Physiol.* **44**, 365.
HEMPLING, H. G. (1967). *J. Cell. Physiol.* **70**, 237.
HEMPLING H. G. (1973). *J. Cell. Physiol.* **81**, 1.
HO, M. K. and GUIDOTTI, G. (1975). *J. Biol. Chem.* **250**, 675.
HÖBER, R. and ØRSKOV, W. L. (1933). *Pflügers Archiv.* **231**, 599.
HOLZ, R. and FINKELSTEIN, A. (1970). *J. Gen. Physiol.* **56**, 125.
HUNTER, F. R. (1960). *J. Cell. Comp. Physiol.* **55**, 175.
HUNTER, F. R., GEORGE, J. and OSPINA, B. (1965). *J. Cell. Comp. Physiol.* **65**, 299.
JACOBS, M. H. (1931). *Ergebn. d. Biol.* **7**, 1.
JACOBS, M. H. (1952). In "Modern Trends in Physiology and Biochemistry" (E. S. Guzman-Barron, ed), pp. 149–172. Academic Press, New York and London.
JACOBS, M. H., GLASSMAN, H. N. and PARPART, A. K. (1935). *J. Cell. Comp.Physiol.* **7**, 197.
KAPLAN, M. A., HAYS, R. M. and BLUMENFELD, O. O. (1975). *J. Membrane Biol.* **20**, 181.
KAPLAN, M. A., HAYS, L. and HAYS, R. M. (1974). *Amer. J. Physiol.* **226**, 1327.
KATCHALSKY, A. and CURRAN, P. F. (1965). In "Nonequilibrium Thermodynamics in Biophysics", chap. 10. Harvard University Press, Cambridge, Mass.
KEDEM, O. and KATCHALSKY, A. (1958). *Biochim. Biophys. Acta*, **27**, 229.
KIRSCHNER, D. A. and CASPAR, D. L. D. (1972). *Ann. N.Y. Acad. Sci.* **195**, 309.
KNAUF, P. A., PROVERBIO, F. and HOFFMAN, J. F. (1974). *J. Gen. Physiol.* **63**, 305.
LANDIS, E. M. (1927). *Amer. J. Physiol.* **82**, 218.
LEA, E. J. A., RISH, G. T. and SEGREST, J. P. (1975). *Biochim. Biophys. Acta*, **382**, 41.
LEVITT, D. G. (1974). *Biochim. Biophys. Acta*, **373**, 115.
LICHTENSTEIN, N. S. and LEAF, A. (1965). *J. Clin. Invest.* **44**, 1328.
LICHTENSTEIN, N. S. and LEAF, A. (1966). *Ann. N.Y. Acad. Sci.* **137**, 556.
LOESCHE, K., BENTZEL, C. J. and CSAKY, T. Z. (1970). *Amer. J. Physiol.* **218**, 1723.
LUCKE, B. and MCCUTCHEON, M. (1932). *Physiol. Rev.* **12**, 68.
MACEY, R. I. and FARMER, R. E. L. (1970). *Biochim. Biophys. Acta*, **211**, 104.
MACEY, R. I., KARAN, D. M. and FARMER, R. E. L. (1973). In "Passive Permeability of Cell Membranes" (F. Kreuzer and T. F. G. Slegers, eds) vol. 3, p. 331. Plenum Press, New York, and London.
MACEY, R. I. and TALBERY, A. B. (1966). *Biochim. Biophys. Acta*, **120**, 104.
MACEY, R. I. and WADZINSKI, L. T. (1974). *Fed. Proc.* **33**, 2323.
MARCHESI, V. T. (1975). In "Cell Membranes, Hospital Practice", (G. Weissmann, ed), chap. 5. H. P. Publishing,
MARCHESI, V. T., TILLACK, T. W., JACKSON, R. L., SEGREST, J. P. and SCOTT, R. E. (1972). *Proc. Nat. Acad. Sci. USA*, **69**, 1445.
MAURO, A. (1957). *Science*, **126**, 252.
NACCACHE, P. and SHA'AFI, R. I. (1973), *J. Gen. Physiol.* **62**, 714.
NACCACHE, P. and SHA'AFI, R. I. (1974). *J. Cell. Physiol.* **83**, 449.
NARAHASHI, T., DEGUCHI, T., URAKAWA, N. and OHKUBO, Y. (1960). *Amer. J. Physiol.* **198**, 934.

NEVIS, A. H. (1958). *J. Gen. Physiol.* **41**, 927.
OVERTON, E. (1895). *Vierleljahrschr. Naturforsch. Ges. Zurich*, **40**, 159.
OWEN, JEFFRY, D. and ERYING, E. M. (1975). *J. Gen Physiol.* **66**, 251.
OWEN, J. D. and SOLOMON, A. K. (1972). *Biochim. Biophys. Acta.* **290**, 414.
PAGANELLI, C. V. and SOLOMON, A. K. (1957). *J. Gen. Physiol.* **41**, 259.
PAPAHADJOPOULOS, D., COWDEN, M. and KIMELBERG, K. (1973). *Biochim. Biophys. Acta*, **330**, 8.
PATLAK, C. S., GOLDSTEIN, D. A. and HOFFMAN, J. F. (1963). *J. Theoret. Biol.* **5**, 426.
PIMENTAL, G. C. and McCLELLAN, A. L. (1960). "The Hydrogen Bond". W. H. Freeman, San Francisco.
POHL, S. L., KRANS, H. M. J., KOZYREFF, V., BIRNBAUMER, L. and RODBELL, M. (1971). *J. Biol. Chem.* **246**, 4447.
POZNANSKY, M., TONG, S., WHITE, P. C., MILGRAM, J. M. and SOLOMON, A. K. (1976). *J. Gen. Physiol.* **67**, 45.
PRESCOTT, D. M. and ZEUTHEN, E. (1953). *Acta Physiol. Scand.* **28**, 77.
PRICE, H. D. and THOMPSON, T. E. (1969). *J. Molec. Biol.* **41**, 443.
PROSSER, C. L. (1973). In "Comparative Animal Physiology", vol. 1, 3rd edit., p. 1. W. B. Saunders Company, Philadelphia, London, Toronto.
PUCHWEIN, G., PFEUFFER, J. and HELMREICH, E. J. M. (1974). *J. Biol. Chem.* **249**, 3232.
REDWOOD, W. R. and HAYDEN, D. A. (1969). *J. Theoret. Biol.* **22**, 1.
REDWOOD, W. R., RALL, F. and PERL, W. (1974). *J. Gen. Physiol.* **64**, 706.
RICH, G. T., SHA'AFI, R. I., BARTON, T. C. and SOLOMON, A. K. (1967). *J. Gen. Physiol.* **50**, 2391.
RICH, G. T., SHA'AFI, R. I., ROMUALDEZ, A. and SOLOMON, A. K. (1968). *J. Gen. Physiol.* **52**, 941.
ROBBINS, E. and MAURO, A. (1960). *J. Gen. Physiol.* **43**, 523.
RODAN, S. B., HINTZ, R. L., SHA'AFI, R. I. and RODAN, G. A. (1974). *Nature*, **252**, 589.
ROTHFIELD, L. and FINKELSTEIN, A. (1968). *A. Rev. Biochem.* **37**, 463.
ROTHSTEIN, A., CABANTCHIK, Z. I. and KNAUF, P. (1976). *Fed. Proc.* **35**, 3.
ROTTENBERG, H. and SOLOMON, A. K. (1966). *Ann. N.Y. Acad. Sci.* **137**, 685.
SAVITZ, D. and SOLOMON, A. K. (1971). *J. Gen. Physiol.* **58**, 259.
SEEMAN, P., SHA'AFI, R. I., GALEY, W. R. and SOLOMON, A. K. (1970). *Biochim. Biophys. Acta*, **211**, 365.
SHA'AFI, R. I. and FEINSTEIN, M. (1976). *Adv. in Exp. Med. and Biol.* **80**, 67.
SHA'AFI, R. I. and GARY-BOBO, C. M. (1973). *Prog. Biophys. Mol. Biol.* **26**, 103.
SHA'AFI, R. I., GARY-BOBO, C. M. and SOLOMON, A. K. (1969). *Biochim. Biophys. Acta*, **173**, 141.
SHA'AFI, R. I., GARY-BOBO, C. M. and SOLOMON, A. K. (1971) *J. Gen. Physiol.* **58**, 238.
SHA'AFI, R. I., RICH, G. T., MIKULECKY, D. C. and SOLOMON, A. K. (1970). *J. Gen. Physiol.* **55**, 427.
SHA'AFI, R. I., RICH, G. T., SIDEL, V. W., BOSSERT, W. and SOLOMON, A. K. (1967). *J. Gen. Physiol.* **50**, 1377.
SHERRILL, B. C. and DIETSCHY, J. M. (1975). *J. Membrane. Biol.* **23**, 367.
SINGER, S. J. (1974). *A. Rev. Biochem.* **43**, 805.
SINGER, S. J. and NICOLSON, G. L. (1972). *Science*, **175**, 720.
SIRS, J. (1969). *J. Physiol. Lond.* **205**, 147.

SOLL, A. (1967). *J. Gen. Physiol.* **50**, 2565.
SOLOMON, A. K. (1968). *J. Gen. Physiol.* **51**, 335S.
SOLOMON, A. K. (1973). *In* "Passive Permeability of Cell Membranes" (F. Kreuzer and J. F. G. Sledgers, eds), vol. 3, p. 299. Plenum Press, New York and London.
STAVERMAN, A. J. (1951). *Rec. Trav. Chim.* **70**, 344.
STECK, T. L., FAIRBANKS, G. and WALLACH, D. F. H. (1971). *Biochemistry*, **10**, 2617.
STEIN, W. D. (1967). *In* "The Movement of Molecules Across Cellular Membranes", p. 113. Academic Press, New York and London.
THAU, G., BLOCH, R. and KEDEM, O. (1966). *Desalination*, **1**, 129.
TOMITA, M. and MARCHESI, V. T. (1975). *Proc. Nat. Acad. Sci. USA*, **72**, 2964.
TOSTESON, D. C. (1959). *Acta Physiol. Scand.* **46**, 19.
TOSTESON, D. C., COOK, P., ANDREOLI, T. and TIEFFENBERG, M. (1967). *J. Gen. Physiol.* **50**, 2513.
TRAÜBLE, H. (1971). *J. Membrane Biol.* **4**, 193.
TRAÜBLE, H. (1972). *In* "Passive Permeability of Cell Membranes" (F. Kreuzer, and J. F. G. Sledgers, eds), vol. 3, p. 197. Plenum Press, New York and London.
VARGAS, F. (1968). *J. Gen. Physiol.* **51**, 123S.
VIEIRA, F. L., SHA'AFI, R. I. and SOLOMON, A. K. (1970). *J. Gen. Physiol.* **55**, 451.
VILLEGAS, R., BARTON, T. C. and SOLOMON, A. K. (1958). *J. Gen. Physiol.* **42**, 355.
VILLEGAS, R. and VILLEGAS, G. M. (1960). *J. Gen. Physiol.* **43**, 73.
WANG, J. H. (1965). *J. Phys. Chem.* **69**, 4412.
WANG, J. H., ROBINSON, C. V. and EDELMAN, I. S. (1953). *J. Am. Chem. Soc.* **75**, 466.
WRIGHT, E. M. and DIAMOND, J. M. (1969). *Proc. Roy. Soc. B*, **172**, 227.

Transport of sugars in human red cells

R. J. NAFTALIN and G. D. HOLMAN

Department of Physiology, King's College, London, UK

1 Introduction	257
2 Classicial kinetics	258
2.1 Miller's investigation	259
2.2 Lattice-pore theory	265
2.3 The tetramer model	267
2.4 Geck's asymmetric carrier model	269
2.5 LeFevre's introverting hemiport model	270
2.6 Regen and Tarpley's mobile carrier with asymmetrical unstirred layers	271
2.7 Eilam's modified tetramer model	271
3 Recent specificity information	273
4 Evidence for conformational change within the red cell membrane induced by sugars	275
4.1 Effects of chemical modifiers on sugar transport kinetics	276
4.2 The effects of variation of temperature on the kinetics of sugar transport	277
4.3 Other evidence for conformational change within the transport pathway	278
4.4 Thermochemical studies	278
4.5 Absence of accelerated exchange with low-affinity sugars	279
4.6 pH dependence of net and exchange flux	279
5 The asymmetry problem	280
5.1 Studies on sugar transport in human red cell ghosts	282
5.2 The interaction of sugars with haemoglobin	282
6 Chemical studies with isolated membranes and membrane proteins	285
7 A model for facilitated diffusion and accelerated exchange of sugars relating recent physical chemical findings to transport	285
8 The sorbose problem	294
9 Summary	296
References	296

1 Introduction

Sugar transport across red cell membranes has been reviewed excellently by LeFevre (1975) and Jung (1975). Earlier reviews by Miller (1969) and

Lieb and Stein (1972) have stressed different aspects of these phenomena. Kotyk (1973) has reviewed the formal kinetics. Thus there is little need to dwell on items primarily of historical interest. In this review attention will be confined to recent developments and aspects which, in our view, require emphasis.

2 Classical kinetics

Human and also rabbit red cells—but not those of pig, ox, sheep, dog or cat (Laris, 1958) permit specific monosaccharides to move passively across their cell membranes at rates several orders of magnitude faster than would be predicted on the basis of their size relative to membrane pores (Sha'afi et al., 1971). This facilitated transport system shows a high degree of *stereospecificity* for hexose and pentose sugars in the pyranose ring form. The specificity of the sugar-membrane interactions was first systematically investigated by LeFevre and Marshall (1958) and more recently this systematic approach has been extended by Barnett et al. (1973a,b) (see section 3). Other kinetic features which establish that the sugars interact with a limited number of membrane sites are *saturation kinetics* (LeFevre, 1954; Widdas, 1954), *competitive inhibition* (LeFevre and Davies, 1951) of the rate of net transport between different sugars according to well-established rules for competitive inhibition, *and noncompetitive inhibition* of sugar transport by binding to the membrane of a relatively small number of tightly bound molecules (Bloch, 1973); $3 \cdot 3 \times 10^4$ sugar transport sites are present in each cell membrane as determined by cytochalasin B binding, which has a K_D of 2×10^{-7} M. Inhibition studies of sugar transport by $HgCl_2$, which is irreversibly bound, also indicate that there are a limited number of transport sites (Van Staveninck et al., 1965). The high Q_{10} (> 10) for net sugar entry into the red cell (Lacko et al., 1972) indicates that the reaction of sugar with the transporting elements within the membrane has a high activation energy; this is atypical of free solution diffusion (Lieb and Stein (1971b). Thus there is substantial evidence that sugars do interact in a stereospecific manner, i.e. at least three-point attachment, with some membrane constituent. *Counterflow*, first described by Rosenberg and Wilbrandt (1957), where uphill flow of labelled sugars into cells from an external solution containing sugars at low concentration is driven by the net downhill movement of unlabelled sugar present within the cells initially, at high concentrations (Table 1/Fig. 1) or vice versa, demonstrates the necessity for at least two sugar-binding sites within the transport pathway; one facing inwards on the inner surface and another facing outwards at the outer surface. Additional intermediate sites may well be present, but cannot be revealed by kinetic studies (Stein and Lieb,

1974). The counterflow phenomenon also reveals that sugars are not subject to the long-pore effect (Hodgkin and Keynes, 1955), i.e. the presence of sugar on the *trans*-side of the membrane does not retard unidirectional movement of sugar across the membrane, and suggests that the sugars can by-pass one another within the transport pathway.

This finding has led to a protracted debate as to the nature of the exchange process. Do sugars cross the membrane by being ferried to and fro complexed to a membrane carrier, as originally proposed by Wilbrandt and Rosenberg (1961), or is there sufficient freedom within the transport path for the sugar molecules to rotate and by-pass each other in constrained two- or three-dimensional diffusion process—as suggested by polar-pore theory? The finding that sugars exchange rapidly between the inside and the outside of the cell in the absence of net sugar movement (LeFevre and McGinniss, 1960) came as no surprise once counterflow had been established. However, Lacko and Burger (1962), Levine *et al.* (1965) and Mawe and Hempling (1965) showed that the exchange process was twice as fast as the rate predicted on the basis of a simple rotating carrier system. Mawe and Hempling and Levine *et al.* interpreted their data to mean that a carrier, complexed to sugar, could move across the membrane three to four times faster than the unloaded carrier.

2.1 MILLER'S INVESTIGATION

Miller (1968a,b) systematically investigated several different methods of measuring transport across red cell membranes. This study was a watershed, since it seriously challenged the validity of the mobile-carrier interpretation of the sugar transport data. Miller observed that the Michaelis-Menten parameters for sugar transport obtained by different methods were widely different. The K_m for the reduction in net efflux of D-glucose from cells containing 130 mM glucose, obtained by addition of glucose to the external bathing solution and by following the rates of cell volume change as sugars leave the cells, using the Ørskov (1935) light-scattering technique as originally applied by Sen and Widdas (1962a), was found to be 1·8 mM, the V_m 104 μmol (ml cell water)$^{-1}$. Sen and Widdas (1962a) had determined the K_m previously to be 1·86 mM and the V_m 83 μmol (ml cell water)$^{-1}$ min^{-1} at 20°C. In Lieb and Stein's (1972) terminology this experiment is called an infinite-*cis* exit experiment—for obvious reasons—and it measures the sugar affinity for the external site (Table 1). Miller (1968a) found that the K_m for equilibrium exchange of D-glucose at 20°C was 38 mM and the V_m 260 μmol (ml cell water)$^{-1}$ min^{-1}. Michaelis-Menten parameters obtained by others (see Table 1) for equilibrium exchange are not significantly different from those obtained by Miller. Miller also found

TABLE 1 and FIG. 1

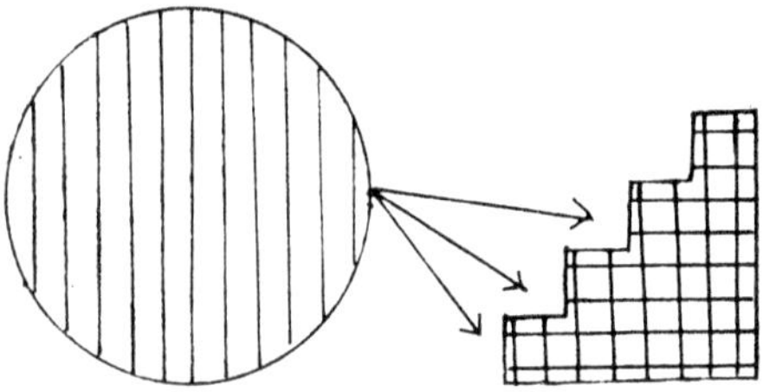

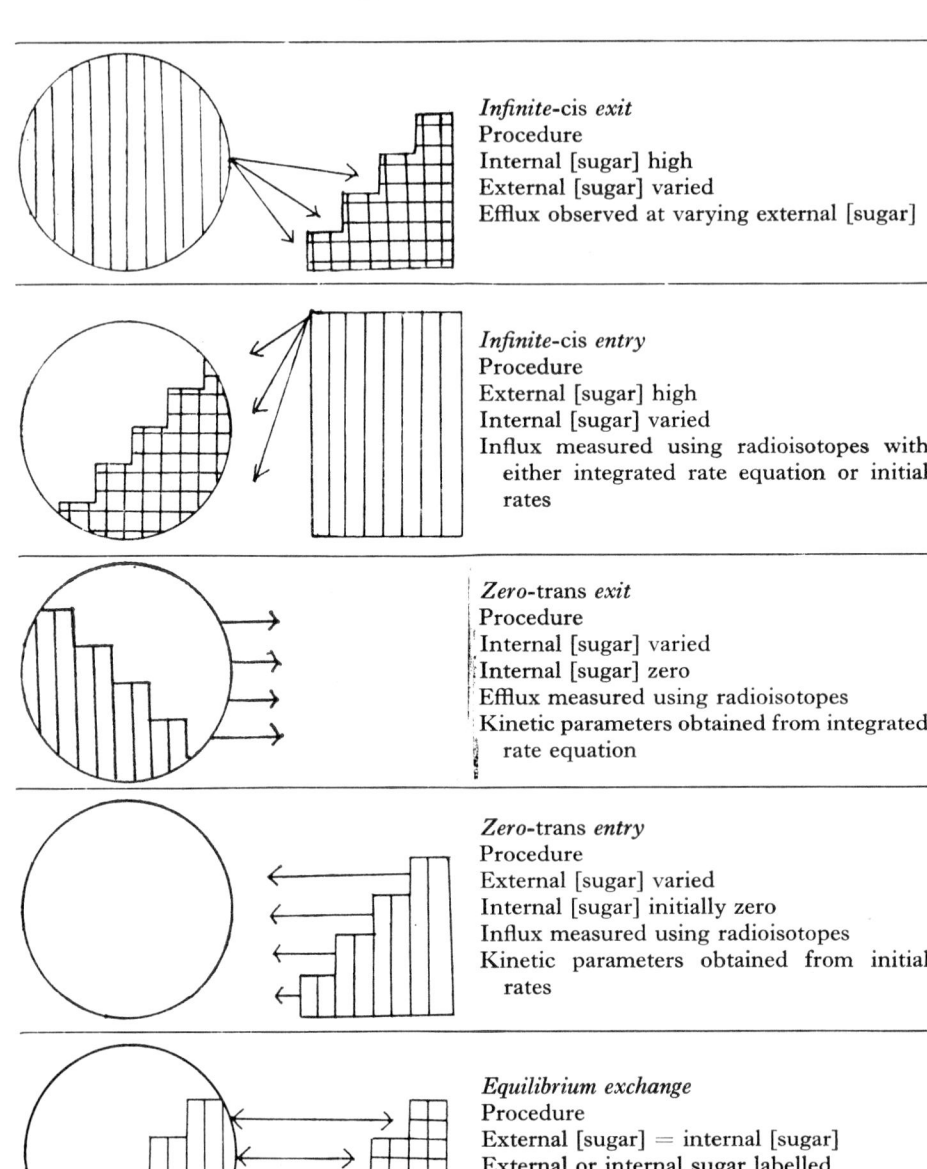

Infinite-cis *exit*
Procedure
Internal [sugar] high
External [sugar] varied
Efflux observed at varying external [sugar]

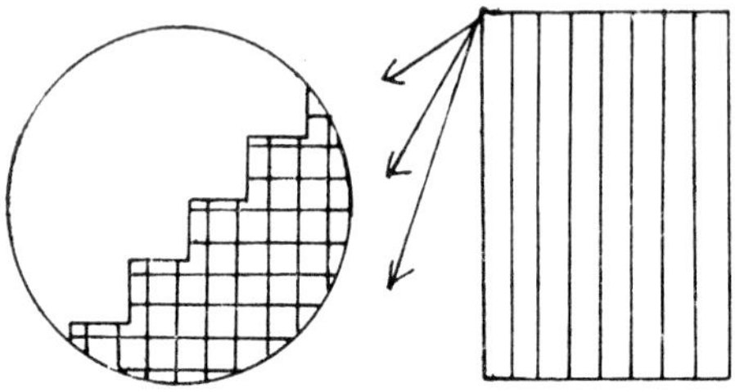

Infinite-cis *entry*
Procedure
External [sugar] high
Internal [sugar] varied
Influx measured using radioisotopes with either integrated rate equation or initial rates

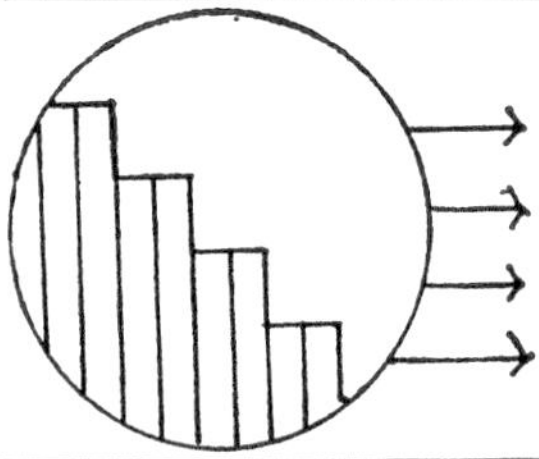

Zero-trans *exit*
Procedure
Internal [sugar] varied
Internal [sugar] zero
Efflux measured using radioisotopes
Kinetic parameters obtained from integrated rate equation

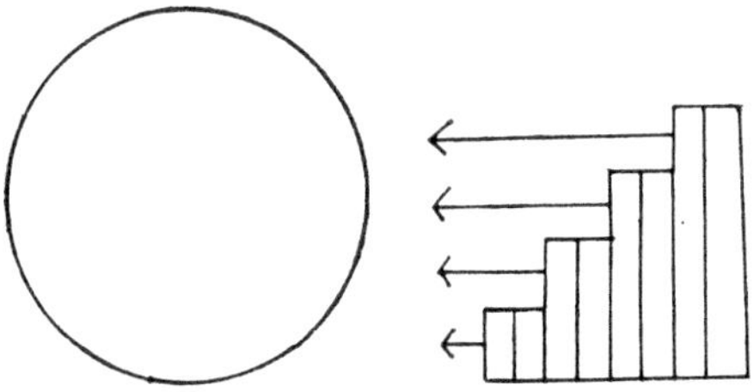

Zero-trans *entry*
Procedure
External [sugar] varied
Internal [sugar] initially zero
Influx measured using radioisotopes
Kinetic parameters obtained from initial rates

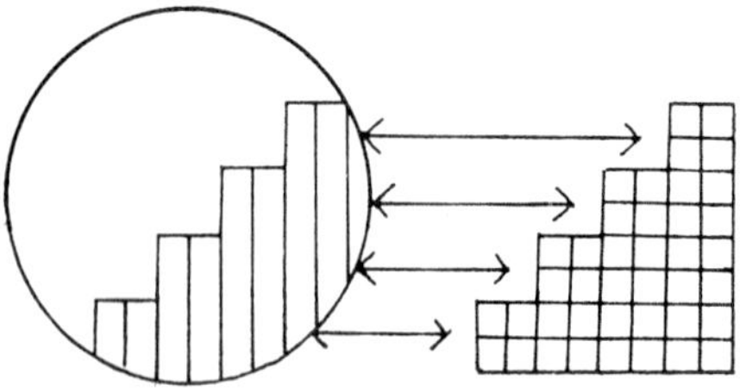

Equilibrium exchange
Procedure
External [sugar] = internal [sugar]
External or internal sugar labelled
Initial rates of exchange measured at different concentrations

	Sugar	Reference	K_m (mM)	V_m (μmol (ml cell water)$^{-1}$ min^{-1})
Measures affinity of external site and V_m for net exit	Glucose	Sen and Widdas (1962a)	1·7	83
		Harris (1964)	1·86	210
		Miller (1965)	1·8±0·3	104
	Galactose	Krupka (1971a)	12·0	—
Measures affinity of internal site and V_m for net entry	Glucose	Hankin et al. (1972)	2·8±0·6	85±2·6
	Galactose	Ginsburg and Stein (1975)	25±17	—
Measures affinity of internal site and V_m for net exit	Glucose	Karlish et al. (1972)	25±3·0	129±11
	Galactose	Ginsburg and Ram (1975)	240±5·7	255±96
Measures affinity of external site and V_m for net entry	Glucose	Lacko et al. (1972)	1·6±0·2	36±1·2
	Galactose	Ginsburg and Stein (1975) (two-parameter fit)	31·76±4·42	28·6
Measures K_m and V_m of exchange	Glucose	Miller (1968a)	38±3	260±30
		Eilam and Stein (1972)	32±1·1	357±10
		Lacko et al. (1972)	20±1·0	264±42
		Eilam (1975b)	34±0·6	360±31
	Galactose	Ginsburg and Ram (1975)	138±57	432±44
		Eilam (1976)	191±17	453±9
		Miller (1971)	75±13	180±20

TABLE 1 and FIG. 1

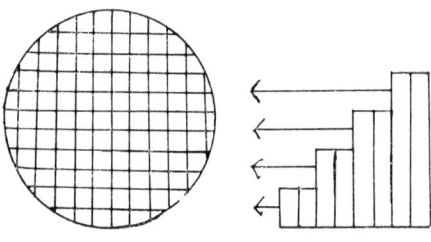

Infinite-trans *entry*
Procedure
Internal [sugar] high
External [sugar] varied
Initial influx measured using radioisotopes

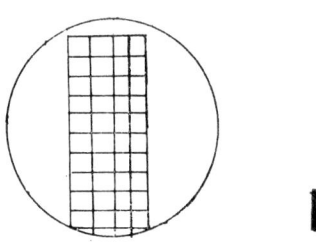

Counterflow
(A) $t = 0$
Initially high internal unlabelled (hatched) [sugar]; low external [sugar] (shaded)

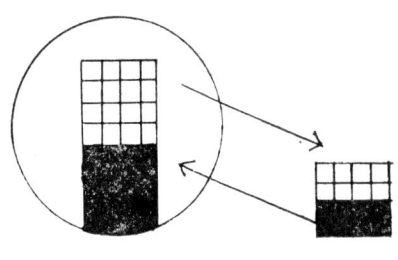

(B) $t = 1$ min
Uphill flow of isotope into cell driven by downhill flow of unlabelled sugar net loss of sugar from cell

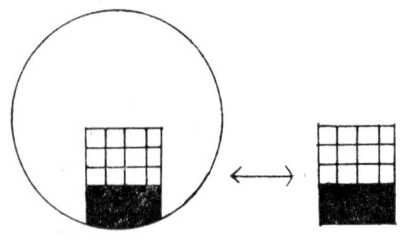

(C) $t = \infty$
Here all the sugars are equilibrated

	Sugar	Reference	K_m (mM)	V_m (μmol (ml cell water)$^{-1}$ min^{-1})
Measures affinity of external site and V_m for exchange	Glucose	Lacko et al. (1972)	1·7±0·3	174±30
	Galactose	Ginsburg and Stein (1975)	21±2·0	239±11

divergences between the observed and predicted initial rates of exchange between different sugars. The exit of glucose was accelerated more by galactose, or mannose than the exit of labelled glucose by unlabelled glucose. Galactose was accelerated less by unlabelled galactose, or mannose by unlabelled mannose, than was glucose by unlabelled glucose. Mobile-carrier kinetics predict that if the galactose-, or mannose-carrier complex moves faster than the glucose-carrier complex, as may be inferred from the fast rate of glucose–galactose heteroexchange, then the acceleration of unidirectional efflux of either galactose, or mannose by galactose and mannose, respectively, should be *more*, not less, as is observed, than the acceleration of glucose by glucose. The basis of these predictions is that there is a fixed number of carrier molecules within the membrane.

A rapid movement of the sugar-carrier complex from *cis-trans* will deplete the *cis* side of the membrane of carriers, thus limiting the *cis-trans* sugar efflux. Thus, addition of sugar to the *trans* side will increase the rate of return of carrier from *trans-cis*, increasing the number of carriers on the *cis* side, and hence will accelerate unidirectional efflux. The faster the sugar-carrier complex moves relative to the unloaded carrier, the greater will be the acceleration of exchange. Since Miller showed that this does not happen, alternative explanations to the mobile carrier theory must be considered.

Naftalin (1971) repeated the heteroexchange experiments described by Miller (1968a) in well-stirred suspensions of red cells at 20°C and found essentially the same patterns. Eilam and Stein (1972) also repeated the heteroexchange experiment of Miller and also measured efflux of radioactive galactose and mannose into solutions containing glucose. They observed, as did Naftalin (1971), that glucose substantially retards the loss of mannose, or galactose from the cells, when loss was measured over the initial 30 sec. During this interval the sugar isotopes had more than half equilibrated across the membrane. Since mannose and galactose have lower affinities for the transport system than glucose (LeFevre and Marshall, 1958), Eilam and Stein claim that the heteroexchange phenomenon results from the decreased competitive inhibition of glucose exit by galactose, or mannose entering the cells, compared with the effects of comparable intracellular concentrations of glucose. At the time interval that Eilam and Stein use (30 sec) for their reference, this is clearly valid. However, the important question—not answered by this study—is, how are the *initial* rates of heteroexchange affected? The earliest data plotted in the diagram in Eilam and Stein's paper are at 10 sec. The authors claim that at 30 sec "the difference between the predictions of the various hypotheses (the tetramer and mobile carrier) are at a maximum". This point is hard to understand, since it would be expected that the widest divergence between model predictions would occur initially. Regen and Tarpley (1974) make a similar criticism of Eilam and Stein's analysis. As no experiments have yet been described which examine rates of heteroexchange at time intervals less than 10 sec after cell suspension, the validity of Miller's findings, or of Eilam and Stein's refutation, has still to be rigorously tested. This point is no longer of crucial concern to the question of the validity of the mobile-carrier hypothesis, since other tests which are less difficult to interpret indicate that the hypothesis is invalid.

The major problem in reconciling the mobile-carrier hypothesis to the observed transport data was, and still is, the wide discrepancy between the K_m for exchange and the K_m for net flux. The mobile carrier theory predicts that the K_m for exchange should not exceed the K_m for infinite-*cis* net exit by more than the factor $K_m \text{(net)} = ((1 + r)/2r) K \text{(exchange)}$ (Levine and Stein, 1966), where r is the ratio of the rate of movement of loaded:unloaded carrier. Thus the $K_{m(ex)}$ should never exceed $K_{m(net)}$ by more than 2. Since $K_{m(ex)} = 38$ mM and $K_{m(net)} = 1 \cdot 8$ mM (see Table 1), this prediction is incorrect.

Miller's (1968a,b) papers indicating these shortcomings to the mobile-carrier hypothesis provided the stimulus for two alternative noncarrier models.

2.2 LATTICE-PORE THEORY

The lattice-pore model for sugar transport was proposed as a modification by Naftalin (1970) of Zierler's (1961) simple pore model in which saturation kinetics were simply considered to be due to a limited number of pores spanning the membrane. It was considered that sugars move across the lattice pore by "one-dimensional diffusion". The lattice pore owed much to the work of Hill and Kedem (1966), who described the kinetics of molecular movement across membranes with several different conformations of transport path. Using Monte-Carlo methods, it was shown that, provided exchange between nearest-neighbour molecules within the lattice was permitted, random walk of the sugar molecules within the pore could simulate many of the kinetic features of sugar transport system described by Miller (1968a). However, for the model to simulate accelerated exchange, it was necessary to assume that there was an "unstirred layer" effect at the external surface of the membrane. With this additional assumption the model also simulated Miller's heteroexchange phenomena. The model, like others before it, does not really explain why sugars with low affinity, e.g. ribose, fructose, erythritol or sorbose (LeFevre, 1963; La Celle and Passow, 1971), should have lower mobilities within the membrane than rapidly transported sugars such as glucose, galactose or mannose. A major assumption of the lattice-pore model is that there is a sufficiently large unstirred layer effect. There is no question that if the diffusion coefficient of sugar within the unstirred layer were the same as in free solution then its required thickness would be too large. However, it is not necessary to assume that the unstirred layer is external to the cell—it may be present in the outer part of the membrane (Naftalin, 1972; Regen and Tarpley, 1974) and hence the diffusion coefficient could conceivably be considerably lower than the free solution value. If the diffusion coefficient of glucose were 6×10^{-9} cm^2 sec^{-1}, then the unstirred layer thickness required to give the accelerated exchange observed need only be 0·1 μm.

An attempt to demonstrate this unstirred-layer effect was made by measuring maximal net efflux and exchange flux when the stirring rates of the cell suspension were varied at different temperatures. It was shown that rapid stirring increased net efflux of glucose at 0°C and at 20°C, but was less apparent at 30°C; that stirring had a negligible effect on equilibrium-exchange flux at any temperature and that stirring had a smaller effect on net efflux of galactose than of glucose. It was also shown, in a well-stirred suspension, that the ratio of exchange: net efflux fell towards unity as temperature was raised; at 30°C no acceleration of galactose exchange could be observed. Thus it was considered that the red cell transport system obeyed many of the criteria expected of a system having an external unstirred-layer effect.

The results of this paper (Naftalin, 1971) excited some adverse criticism. Hankin and Stein (1972) showed that if they dispersed cells by stirring the suspension vigorously and then at variable rates, no effect of this second period of stirring on net glucose efflux could be observed. Miller (1972) showed that his original technique of cell dispersion involves thorough mixing, hence he considered that unstirred-layer effects are not important determinants of the Michaelis-Menten parameters of sugar transport.

More recently, Edwards (1974) has suggested that a small unstirred-layer effect may have some importance at the inner surface of the red cell membrane and Regen and Tarpley (1974) have also lent support to the presence of unstirred-layer effects at both the inner and outer faces of the membrane (see below). Our present opinion is that unstirred layers do exist, but mainly inside the cell (see section 5). However, their presence does not explain acceleration of exchange flux. A critical experiment demonstrating the unimportance of the unstirred-layer effect as a determinant of accelerated exchange is the finding that chlorpromazine inhibits net efflux of glucose from red cells at 16°C without affecting exchange flux (Baker and Rogers, 1973). Since net flux is reduced, the unstirred-layer effect, which is a function of the net flux, will also be reduced. Hence, it would be predicted that the acceleration of exchange flux should be affected *more* than the net flux by any agent reducing net efflux. Since Baker and Rogers (1973) observed no effect of chlorpromazine on exchange flux, the hypothesis that the acceleration of exchange is determined by an unstirred-layer effect may be rejected. Zipper and Mawe (1972) have found that insulin increases net efflux of glucose from human red cells without affecting exchange flux. This result is also incompatible with the idea that the unstirred-layer effect determines accelerated exchange.

2.3 THE TETRAMER MODEL

The tetramer model was proposed by Licb and Stein (1970) in order to explain the differences between the operational flux parameters of net and exchange flux of D-glucose transport, i.e. the high K_m for exchange, the low K_m for net flux and the higher V_m for exchange than for net efflux. The model that Lieb and Stein proposed contains several assumptions: that the membrane component concerned in transport of glucose is a tetrameric protein embedded in the membrane; the membrane component is capable of existing in two conformations of equivalent energy; the tetramer is composed of two pairs of sub-units, one pair having a high affinity for the substrate (the H site), the other pair having a low affinity (the L site); the tetramer encloses a region within itself which is not directly accessible to either of the external bathing solutions, but substrate molecules can enter this region after first combining with the binding site; interconversion between the two forms (of the tetramer protein) occurs after, and only after, the substrate molecule interacts with the binding site; the conformational change is substrate-induced; and the substrate must leave the internal space during the conformational change that follows its entry; and finally, that the rate of interconversion between the two tetramer forms is given by 0, 1, 2, 3 or 4 times the value of a certain fundamental rate constant, respectively (Lieb and Stein, 1971a).

This model is, of course, much more complex than either the mobile carrier or the lattice-pore and hence, not surprisingly, accounts well for the primary kinetic data concerning the differences between exchange and net flux. Furthermore, the concept of a substrate-induced change in conformation, although not new (see section 4), does explain the stereo-specificity differences in the *rates* of sugar transport across the cell membrane. However, it does not simulate Miller's counterflow kinetics for labelled glucose uptake into cells containing high concentrations of unlabelled glucose, nor does it account well for the initial rates of hetero-exchange between sugars described by Miller (1968a). Stein and his co-workers have discounted the first-mentioned difference between the tetramer model predictions and observed data on technical grounds (Lieb and Stein, 1970), and the second, on the grounds that heteroexchange is due to inhibition of efflux by competing sugars entering the cells (Eilam and Stein, 1972). Like all good, and some bad, models the tetramer model is predictive—it predicts that the operational K_m for net efflux of glucose, zero-*trans* exit out of sugar-loaded cells should be determined primarily by the low-affinity site (L site), and that the K_m for net infinite-*cis* entry (net flux in the opposite direction to the Sen and Widdas experiment) should be determined by the high-affinity site (H site).

Karlish et al. (1972) determined the transport parameters for efflux by transforming data from the time-course of glucose exit into solutions containing zero sugar. The transformations were obtained using an integrated rate equation. They calculated that the K_m for zero-*trans* net glucose exit from the cells was 25 mM and the V_m 139 μmol (ml cell water)$^{-1}$ min^{-1}. Ginsburg and Ram (1975) have determined the K_m and V_m for zero-*trans* net exit of galactose at 20°C using the same method and found them to be 250 mM and 255 μmol (ml cell water)$^{-1}$ min^{-1}, respectively. Thus the first prediction of the tetramer model was verified, i.e. that the K_m for both equilibrium exchange and zero-*trans* net exit should be similar, since they are both hypothetically determined by the low-affinity L site. The K_m for infinite-*cis* net entry, which is considered to be determined by the high-affinity site at the inner surface of the membrane, has been determined by Hankin et al. (1972) using an integrated rate equation describing net entry. This was found to be 2·8 mM and the V_m was found to be 85 μmol (ml cell water)$^{-1}$ min^{-1}. Ginsburg and Stein (1975) calculated the affinity of the H site on the inner face of the membrane towards galactose to be approximately 25 mM—the V_m for galactose entry was unstated.* The infinite-*cis* exit K_m for galactose as determined by the method of Sen and Widdas (1962) is 12 mM. Thus Ginsburg and Stein (1975) have found that there are two operational affinities for sugars at the inner membrane surface, as predicted by the tetramer model, and they have also suggested that there are two operational affinities for sugars at the external surface. The evidence for this view comes from experiments in which the initial rate of galactose uptake by cells is measured at varying external galactose concentrations. Uptake was measured over a period of 5 sec, during which influx was found constant. Using a nonlinear least-square best-fit analysis they then determined the equation for net uptake using two-, three- and four-parameter Michaelis-Menten type equations. The three-parameter equation gives a significantly better fit to the data

* Foster and Jacquez (1976) consider that the K_m for infinite-*cis* entry as measured by the integrated rate equation of Hankin et al. (1972) is unreliable. This criticism may be valid for estimates of the K_m for glucose, but the absolute difference between the K_m for zero-*trans* exit and infinite-*cis* entry of D-galactose (Ginsburg and Stein, 1975) is too large to be dismissed on the basis of errors of estimation.

than the two-parameter fit; however, there is no significant improvement on fitting a four-parameter equation over the three-parameter equation. Ginsburg and Stein (1975) claim the validity of the four-parameter fit, which is the solution for two saturating transport systems in parallel, for the reason that phloretin completely inhibits uptake by both pathways, hence they say that the three-parameter fit, which corresponds to a single saturating system and a diffusion pathway in parallel, is less plausible than the four-parameter equation. They consider that phloretin in likely only to inhibit saturating sugar transport systems and phloretin inhibits influx entirely. However, it has been shown that phloretin inhibits the red cell membrane anion permeability system (Schnell, 1972) and reduces the permeability to low molecular weight nonelectrolytes (Owen *et al.*, 1972, 1974). Thus we consider that the evidence for two-carrier influx kinetics is unconvincing.

A major discrepancy between the predictions of the tetramer model and the observed results is that the tetramer model predicts that the V_m for net entry and net exit should be equal. In fact the V_m for zero-*trans* net entry of galactose is 28·6 μmol (ml cell water)$^{-1}$ min^{-1} and for zero-*trans* net exit is 255 μmol (ml cell water)$^{-1}$ min^{-1} (Ginsburg and Ram, 1975).

For glucose, the zero-*trans* V_m for net entry determined from fluxes measured during the initial 4 sec of uptake is 36 μmol (ml cell water)$^{-1}$ min^{-1} and for zero-*trans* net exit is 140 μmol (ml cell water)$^{-1}$ min^{-1} Lacko *et al.*, 1972 (Karlish *et al.*, 1972;). Thus it is clear that the maximal rate of sugar exit via the sugar transport system is five- to tenfold faster than that of net entry. As temperature is reduced below 20°C this discrepancy increases (Hankin and Stein, 1972; Lacko *et al.*, 1972).

2.4 GECK'S ASYMMETRIC CARRIER MODEL

Since sugars are not accumulated within the red cell, it follows that the Haldane relationships for net entry and exit must be the same, i.e.

$$\frac{V_i}{K_i} = \frac{V_o}{K_o}$$

where i and o refer to inside and outside, respectively. Thus the presence of asymmetric affinities implies that there also must be asymmetric V_m's.

Before the results indicating a high-affinity binding site at the inner surface were published, Geck (1971) described a model which accounted for the following data: the high K_m and V_m for net exit and the low K_m and V_m for net entry, and also the high K_m and V_m for equilibrium exchange.

Regen and Morgan (1964) had previously suggested a minimal-assumption mobile-carrier model for sugar transport in rabbit erythrocytes, where the affinities on both sides of the membrane were assumed to be equal, as this assumption fits the transport data for the rabbit sugar transport system. Geck's model is an adaptation of the Regen and Morgan model to describe the asymmetric transport in the human system. Since Geck's model assumes that there is only a single form of binding site on each side of the membrane, it cannot adequately account for the apparently low K_m found for infinite-*cis* entry of both glucose and galactose (Hankin *et al.*, 1972; Ginsburg and Stein, 1975).

2.5 LEFEVRE'S INTROVERTING HEMIPORT MODEL

LeFevre (1973) described a model for sugar transport which is hybrid between the lattice-pore and the tetramer models. This scheme proposed that the sites at both the inner and outer surfaces can face either outwards towards the adjacent pool, or inwards towards a central intramembranous compartment, which is an intermediate compartment, as in Stein's tetramer model. The probable orientation of these sites is assumed to change when sugars are bound. Following binding, the model predicts that the probability of a site facing towards the central compartment changes from 0·3 to 0·99. The features which this model has in common with the lattice-pore model are: a single species of membrane binding site; the ability of isotope species to exchange with each other between the surface sites and the adjacent pool and also between nearest-neighbour binding sites; randomness of all molecular transitions, which are all considered to be independent. The features that the model shares with the tetramer model are: the conformational transition of the binding site following interaction with the sugars—this is a positive advantage over the lattice-pore model since it provides a testable physical basis for facilitated diffusion; transmembrane interaction between monomer elements at the two interfaces; the assumption that conformational change occurs only on sugar binding; and a central intramembranous compartment which permits exchange.

It is not hard to see that this model is superior to the lattice-pore model in that it explains the high K_m for zero-*trans* exit, the low K_m for infinite-*cis* exit, the high K_m and V_m for equilibrium exchange. It can also account for the low K_m for infinite-*cis* entry, which Geck's model cannot do. However, unlike Geck's model, but like both the lattice-pore and the tetramer model, the introverting hemiport model is symmetrical and hence cannot explain why the V_m for zero-*trans* entry is less than the V_m for zero-*trans* exit.

2.6 REGEN AND TARPLEY'S MOBILE CARRIER WITH ASYMMETRIC UNSTIRRED LAYERS

There is no intrinsic reason why the unstirred-layer assumption should not be applied to the carrier as well as noncarrier models for sugar transport. Regen and Tarpley (1974) have modified the model originally proposed by Regen and Morgan (1964) (see Fig. 1) which Geck also used as the basis for his asymmetric carrier.

Regen and Tarpley assume a relatively thick unstirred layer at the inner membrane surface $1/D_i = 0.061$ min (ml cell water)$^{-1}$ and $1/D_o = 0.100$ min (ml cell water)$^{-1}$ at the external surface and also, like Geck, assign a low affinity to the internal site K_i for glucose = 12·12 mM and K_o for glucose = 0·975 mM. With this model the computed simulations fit most of the observed operational transport parameters. In particular, the model can account for the K_m and V_m for exchange, zero-*trans* net efflux, zero-*trans* net influx and infinite-*cis* net exit. This model therefore readily accounts for the observed membrane asymmetries and also for Miller's (1968a) observed maximal rates of heteroexchange. The rate-limiting step in this model is the movement of free carrier from the inside to outside. This is thirty times slower than movement of carrier in the opposite direction. Regen and Tarpley suggest that an inhibitor may be present at the inner surface which retards outward movement of the free carrier. Although this model is in many respects superior to all the others so far described (in that its predictions coincide with more data), nevertheless it is still an inadequate kinetic description of sugar movement, since it does not account for the low K_m for infinite-*cis* entry of glucose or, more obviously, of galactose: Regen and Tarpley's model requires that the affinity of the inner site should be low in all circumstances. Thus, despite the increased complexity of the mobile carrier model by two added rate constants, the internal and external unstirred-layer effects, the kinetic predictions of this model still are at variance with the experimental data.

2.7 EILAM'S MODIFIED TETRAMER MODEL

Recently, Eilam (1975a) has modified Lieb and Stein's tetramer model. She analysed the difference between simultaneous and sequential paired carriers (see Fig. 1). The sequential paired antiparallel carrier has almost identical assumptions to Regen and Morgan's (1964) minimal-assumption mobile carrier but additionally assumes a second series (β) of antiparallel elements; the ratio of $\alpha:\beta$ elements is expressed by the number n. The ratio of the K_m's in each pair of elements is expressed as the variable m. It appears that with $m = n = 10$ the following operational data

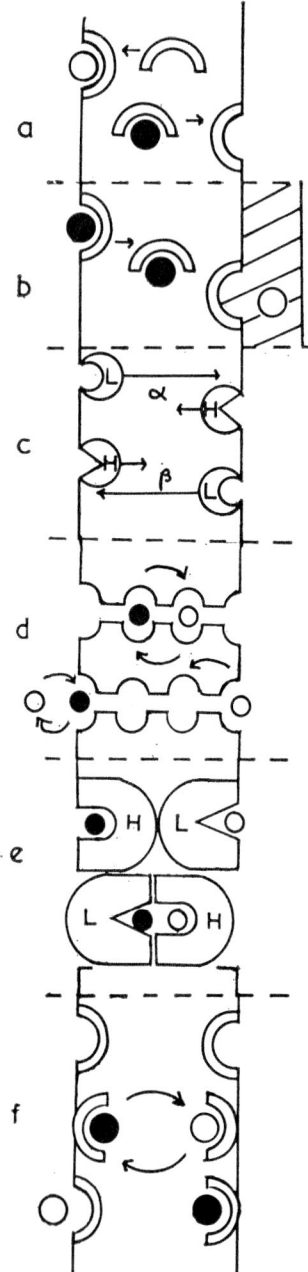

FIG. 2. (a) *The mobile carrier model* assumes (1) sugar carrier complex movement through lipid bilayer membrane is rate-limiting; (2) both sugar-carrier complex and empty carrier are mobile but movement of former is faster. (b) *The Regen-Tarpley asymmetrical carrier model* assumes (1) the carrier has asymmetric affinities for sugar $K_{m(i)} > K_{m(o)}$; (2) there is a large unstirred-layer effect inside the cell; (3) movement of empty carrier from i–o is very slow. (c) *The Eilam model* assumes (1) two sequential carriers are present [carrier α] > [carrier β]. High (H) and low (L) affinity sites are present on both sides of the membrane. (d) *The Lattice-pore model* assumed (1) sugar molecules can pass one another during transport; (2) all sites are immobile; and (3) have identical affinities for sugars. (e) *The Tetramer model* assumes (1) high (H) and low (L) affinity binding sites are present on both sides of the membrane; (2) sites are arranged in a tetramer which allows internal exchange of sugars; (3) passage from the external to the internal sites is determined by conformational changes within the protein which are induced by sugar binding to the sites. (f) *The introversion model* assumes (1) that the binding of substrate can induce the sites to change from facing outwards to inward-facing sites.

may be rationalized: the high K_m for zero-*trans* exit, the low K_m for zero-*trans* entry, the low K_m for infinite-*cis* entry, the high K_m for equilibrium exchange, the low K_m for infinite-*cis* exit, the low K_m for infinite-*trans* entry (this procedure was well described by Lacko et al. (1972)). This initial rate of uptake of labelled glucose is measured at different external concentrations into cells containing high concentrations of unlabelled sugar). Eilam's model also provides for the asymmetric V_m's for net entry and net exit and for the fast rate of equilibrium exchange. The sequential variant of the tetramer model is, unlike the Lieb and Stein (1970) model, in that each monomer element can move independently, whereas the tetramer model suggests that the sugars from either side move simultaneously. This simultaneous model predicts two site kinetics for equilibrium exchange—and hence nonlinear Lineweaver and Burk, or Hofstee, plots. Eilam (1975b) has analysed the kinetics of equilibrium exchange of both glucose and galactose over a wide concentration range and found that the Michaelis-Menten kinetic parameters are constant and give single site kinetics; hence this result is more consistent with a sequential than with a simultaneous carrier.

Kinetically, Eilam's model is consistent with all the data so far derived from studies of sugar transport. However, unlike the tetramer model, from which it derives, it provides little help towards physical interpretation of the data and is unhelpful in predicting the response of the various parameters to altered temperatures. Furthermore, it is based on the doubtful premise that there is a low-affinity external site.

3 Recent specificity information

For a transported molecule, penetration of erythrocyte by a structurally modified sugar will be related to an affinity for a recognition site, to the rate of diffusion through the membrane and to the extent of interaction with unstirred layers and intracellular protein components of the cell. In an attempt to compare sugar interaction at a single step of this process, i.e. at the membrane recognition step, Barnett et al. (1973a) measured apparent K_i values for inhibition of L-sorbose transport. The advantage of this method is that, since L-sorbose penetration is slow, the rate of entry is rate limited by the membrane. Also, the inhibiting sugar can be equilibrated to equal concentrations across the membrane, thus eliminating any compartmentalization of the inhibiting sugar at the inner cell surface. The disadvantage of this method is that L-sorbose is not a typical substrate for the sugar transport system (see section 8, below) and the K_i values are not true dissociation constants. However, by comparing a number of analogues it is possible to estimate relative selective affinities. The information obtained in this study is illustrated in Fig. 3.

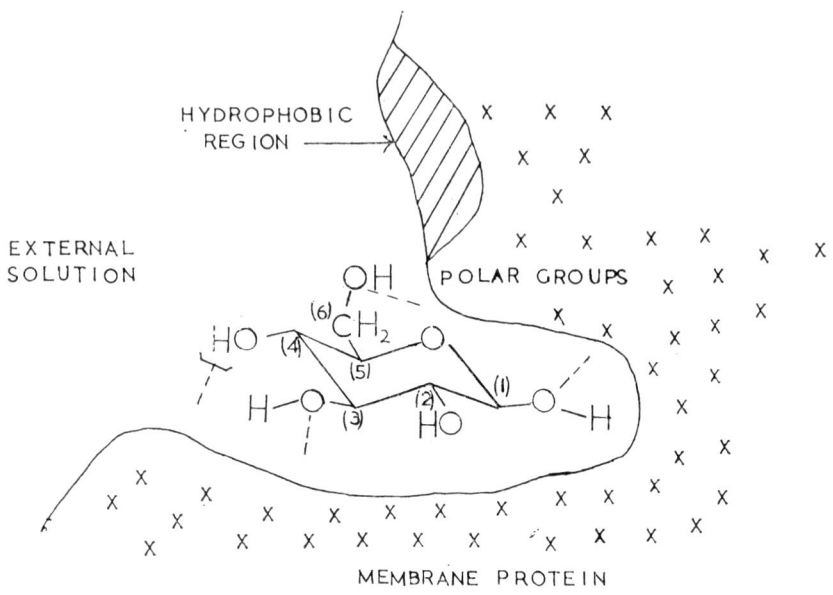

FIG. 3. After Barnett et al. (1973a). For details see text.

The important hydrogen bonding sites were determined by fluorine substitution. β-fluoro-glucose, 3-fluoro-glucose, 6-fluoro-glucose and 6-fluoro-galactose have affinities for transport higher than the corresponding deoxy sugars and sugar epimers (sugar molecules in which the hydroxyl group is axial instead of equatorial), D-galactose (the C4 epimer) has less affinity than D-glucose. The exception to these findings is that 2-deoxy-glucose and D-mannose (the C2 epimer) do not have low affinity. In fact, 2-deoxy-glucose has apparently higher affinity than D-glucose in the human red blood cell. Thus the groups postulated as being important for hydrogen bonding are at C1, C3, C6 and probably C4. Information as to the exact chemical nature of this hydrophilic bonding is still lacking as it is not clear whether direct bonds exist between membrane protons and sugar hydroxyl or fluoride groups or whether membrane proton-water-sugar complexes can totally account for the data.

Other specificity information obtained in this way is for sugar molecules that contain bulky substitutions. Steric constraint appears to be high at C1, as methyl glucosides are poor external inhibitors of transport. There is low, but measurable, affinity for the C2 O-methyl substituted sugar, while at C3 the affinity decreases in the order O-methyl-, O-ethyl-, O-propyl-glucose. At C4 and C6 steric constraint and bulky substitution do not reduce affinity but the inhibitors themselves are not transported. These results indicate the limiting structural features of the transport site and that a primary event in transport may be recognition of the unsubstituted anomeric grouping, but that any subsequent transport will depend upon the degree of substitution into other positions.

Evidence that the internal surface of the membrane has opposite limiting features which interfere with transport has been described (Barnett et al., 1973a,b, 1975) (see section 5, below) but it is clear that a distinction should be made between the specificity of nontransported molecules and of transported molecules. Transported sugars are those which are not subject to steric limitations and will interact in what is effectively a more symmetrical manner with available hydrogen bonding groups.

Another feature of Fig. 3 is the postulated presence of a hydrophobic region close to the recognition site. This might account for the high affinity of cytocholasin B, certain steroids (Taylor and Gagneja, 1976), phloretin and other inhibitors in which there is close grouping of hydrophilic and hydrophobic molecular centres (Novak and LeFevre, 1974).

4 Evidence for conformational change within the red cell membrane induced by sugars

The biochemical evidence for sugar-induced conformational change is based mainly on the changes in "dynamic accessibility" (Baldwin, 1975) of residues within the membrane which react with alkylating reagents. Bowyer and Widdas (1958) were first to show that fluoro-dinitrobenzene (FDNB) inhibits sugar transport in human red cells following alkylation of residues within the membrane. The rate of inactivation of the transport process at 20°C is relatively slow, glucose entry is inhibited by 50 per cent on incubation of cells with 1·4 mM FDNB for 132 min. However, the presence of low concentrations of glucose in the incubation medium markedly enhances the inhibitory reaction of FDNB. The K_m for the glucose-dependent increase in FDNB inactivation of glucose transport was found to be 3–5 mM. Krupka (1971a) showed that all sugars which have facilitated transport increase the rate of FDNB inactivation; the relative enhancement by each sugar is similar to their relative affinity for the sugar transport system. In a companion paper, Krupka (1971b) noted that the rate of interaction of FDNB with the sugar transport site was second order with respect to FDNB. Thus Krupka was able to suggest that the transported sugar induces a conformational change which alters the reactivity of the amino-acid residues in the vicinity of the transport site.

Jung has extended this work and shown that not only is the reactivity of the transport site to FDNB enhanced by glucose, but the activation energy for FDNB uptake is reduced by glucose from 32 kcal mol^{-1} in the absence to 17 kcal mol^{-1} in the presence of glucose. Thus at 4°C the cell membrane has hardly any reactivity to FDNB in the absence of glucose, but with glucose present there is a measurable rate of FDNB inactivation of glucose transport. Additionally, Jung showed that the pH optimum for the rate of FDNB inactivation changes from pH 9 in the absence of glucose to pH 6 in the presence of glucose.

Sugars which are bound to the transport site but not themselves transported, e.g. maltose and cellobiose, reduce the rate of inactivation. Also cytochalasin B (Bloch, 1973) and 4,6-O-benzylidene glucose (Novak and LeFevre, 1974), which are tightly bound inhibitors of the sugar transport system, markedly slow the rate of FDNB inactivation of glucose transport. These results suggest that the interaction between sugars which are rapidly transported and the membrane transport site alters the membrane conformation, thereby making sites which are normally inaccessible to alkylating reagents, or to proton exchange, accessible. It was Krupka (1971a) who first suggested that this enhanced reactivity may be related to the sugar transport process itself.

4.1 EFFECTS OF CHEMICAL MODIFIERS ON SUGAR TRANSPORT KINETICS

Bowyer and Widdas (1958) showed that FDNB had a greater effect on glucose net efflux than on net influx. Sen and Widdas (1962b) later showed that the asymmetric inhibition of entry and exit was only evident with net flux into solutions containing zero glucose. When net entry or exit rates from cells loaded with glucose into solutions with glucose present were measured no asymmetry in the inhibition of flux by FDNB was observed (Sen and Widdas, 1962b). So far no satisfactory explanation for these changes in the pattern of inhibition has been suggested. Bloch (1973), Edwards (1973) and Barnett et al. (1975) presented evidence that the inward directed face of the transport system showed more susceptibility to FDNB inactivation. This may be the case, but it does not account for greater inhibition of D-glucose exit than of entry by this agent, unless it is assumed that entry and exit are mediated by separate carrier proteins (Bloch, 1973), or as in the Eilam (1975a) model. No effect of FDNB on the operational affinity of glucose for the external membrane site was found (Sen and Widdas, 1962b).

More recently, Batt and Schachter (1973) have reported asymmetries in the inhibition of net glucose entry and exit by *para*-chlormercuribenzoic acid sulphonate (PCMBS), another alkylating agent which reacts with SH groups within the membrane, similar to those reported by Bowyer and Widdas (1958) with FDNB.

Zipper and Mawe (1974) have observed differential effects of PCMBS on exchange and net flux on glucose; exchange flux is inhibited more than is net efflux. Using a sulphydryl blocking agent, chlormedrin, which penetrates the membrane, they showed that this affected exchange and net exit to the same extent. Insulin, which until recently was thought not to affect sugar transport in red cells, has been shown to increase the maximal rate of net glucose efflux without affecting glucose exchange flux (Zipper and Mawe, 1972).

Baker and Rogers (1973) showed that chlorpromazine (a membrane stabilizer) (Roth and Seeman, 1972) inhibits net glucose efflux at 16°C without affecting exchange flux. At 36°C chlorpromazine, at a concentration of $1-2 \times 10^{-5}$ M, accelerates net efflux of glucose; above this concentration chlorpromazine inhibits glucose efflux.

A possible conclusion which may be drawn from these results is that sugar exchange and net flux can be affected to different extents by different modifiers of the membrane transport system. It is tempting to deduce from this that the membrane may adopt a different conformation in exchange from that in net flux. An alternative explanation for these results is that the exchange process is quite separate from the net flux process.

4.2 THE EFFECTS OF VARIATION OF TEMPERATURE ON THE KINETICS OF SUGAR TRANSPORT

The first systematic study of the effects of variation in temperature on the operational flux parameters of sugar transport was undertaken by Sen and Widdas (1962a). They showed that as temperature was reduced from 50°C to 5°C the V_m and K_m for net influx and efflux fell sharply between 50°C and 16°C and less steeply between 15°C and 5°C. The Q_{10} for net efflux was found to be 3·5 approximately between 20°C and 50°C, and between 5°C and 15°C approximately 1·5. The Q_{10} for the changes in K_m over the corresponding temperature ranges are 2·5 and 2·0, respectively. Levine and Stein (1966) measured the change in K_m for equilibrium exchange of glucose at 25°C, 13°C and 5°C and found these to be 11, 20 and 40 mM, respectively. Thus the effect of temperature on the K_m for exchange is opposite to its effect on the infinite-*cis* exit K_m. The V_m for exchange decreases from 400 μmol (ml cell water)$^{-1}$ min^{-1} at 25°C to 66 μmol (ml cell water)$^{-1}$ min^{-1} at 5°C. Lacko *et al.* (1972) compared the Michaelis-Menten parameters for net influx, exchange flux and infinite-*trans* influx at 0°C and 20°C; they found the Q_{20} for net influx was 170 and for exchange flux and infinite-*trans* influx 12 and 13, respectively. The Q_{20} of the K_m for exchange, net entry and infinite-*trans* net entry were 1·0, 8·0 and 2·6, respectively. These results show that the activation energy for both equilibrium exchange and infinite-*trans* exchange is considerably less than (approximately half) that of net entry. There is also a large difference between the temperature coefficient for net entry, as measured by Lacko *et al.* (1972) and that for net exit as measured by Sen and Widdas (1962a), indicating that the transport asymmetry between the V_m for net influx and efflux increases as the temperature is reduced from 37°C to 0°C.

The profound difference in the activation energy between the exchange and net flux processes, together with the opposite effects of temperature on the K_m for exchange and net flux, are additional reasons for inferring that exchange is a fundamentally different process from net flux.

4.3 OTHER EVIDENCE FOR CONFORMATIONAL CHANGE WITHIN THE TRANSPORT PATHWAY

Faust (1960), in an interesting study which has received little attention, showed that D-glucose in the β conformation entered red cells more rapidly than α-D-glucose. At pH 7 and 8, substitution of 99 per cent of the water with D_2O slows β-glucose entry, so that it enters the cells at the same rate as the α-anomer. At pH 6, in H_2O, α- and β-glucose enter the cell at the same rate. The main conclusion of this early study was that β-glucose is transported more readily than α. This finding has been confirmed by Barnett *et al.* (1973b), who showed that β-fluoro-glucose inhibits sorbose transport more than α-fluoro-glucose, and has a higher affinity for the sugar transport site. Substitutions of the C1 hydroxyl are unable to mutarotate, hence these findings allay any doubts about the validity of Faust's interpretation. It can also be inferred that uptake of glucose results in a membrane conformational change (perhaps involving a proton exchange between the membrane transport site having a pH around 7 and the water in the external solution) since removal of water, or reducing the solution pH, both reduce the permeability of the β-anomer. This result strongly suggests that sugar transport across the cell membrane may be mediated by a hydrophilic pore.

4.4 THERMOCHEMICAL STUDIES

Zala *et al.* (1974) have measured the enthalpy of interaction of D-glucose with red cell membranes free of haemoglobin. This was done by measuring the difference in enthalpy between D- and L-glucose interaction in a twin-celled batch microcalorimeter. The membrane reaction with D-glucose is endothermic (34·9 mJ g⁻¹); membrane protein is absorbed when 50 mM glucose is present. It may be inferred that other interactions besides glucose binding must be involved—namely, conformational change within the membrane involving a net increase in the number of H bonds. In the presence of FDNB the differential enthalpy of D-glucose uptake over L-glucose uptake falls to 4·0 mJ g⁻¹ protein, which indicates that the D-glucose uptake involves binding to the stereospecific sites, which may be the transport sites. (However, this view is probably an over-simplification since in the presence of 0·27 mM phloretin, the differential enthalpy of D- over L-glucose binding is 40·5 mJ g⁻¹). Interpretation of this last result is difficult, since it has been shown that phloretin binds to both high- and low-affinity sites on the membrane also (Jennings and Solomon, 1976).

4.5 ABSENCE OF ACCELERATED EXCHANGE WITH LOW-AFFINITY SUGARS

There is no rapid exchange component for transport of low-affinity sugars like D-ribose or L-sorbose (LeFevre, 1963). D-ribose has a K_m for the sugar transport system of approximately 180 mM, so it might be expected that at near saturating concentration of this sugar (approximately 2–3 M) accelerated exchange would be observed. However, no acceleration was found. Similar experiments with high concentrations of L-sorbose (Naftalin, unpublished results) have also failed to reveal any rapid exchange component. Thus, rapid exchange appears to be a characteristic confined only to sugars with high affinity for the sugar transport system. This finding suggests that rapid exchange is dependent on additional factors besides saturation of the carrier, which can be obtained as readily with high concentrations of low-affinity sugars as with low concentrations of high-affinity sugars. This again suggests that high-affinity sugars induce changes within the membrane, which make for qualitative as well as quantitative differences in the membrane transport process.

4.6 pH DEPENDENCE OF NET AND EXCHANGE FLUX

Bloch (1974a) has shown that when the pH of a cell suspension is reduced to pH 4·5, both V_m and K_m for net glucose influx rise, so that entry becomes indistinguishable from a diffusion process. Between pH 5·5 and 10 there is little effect of variation of pH on either K_m or V_m. This latter finding substantially confirms that made by Sen and Widdas (1962a). The pH-dependence of infinite-*trans* exchange differs from net influx; below pH 5 V_m decreases and K_m remains constant, while between pH 8–10, the K_m increases and V_m remains constant. These results suggest that when sugar is present at the inner surface, as well as externally, the accessibility to the external solution of the membrane protons in the vicinity of the transport site is altered.

In summary, the results described in this section suggest that sugars whose transport across the cell membrane is facilitated, induce conformational changes within the membrane which make it more readily penetrable by alkylating agents, which reduce the activation energy for alkylation and which also reduce the activation energy required for sugar passage across the membrane. It is apparent that water is an important factor in sugar recognition. It is also likely that sugar binding to the external surface is insufficient to produce the full conformational change required for acceleration of exchange flux, since sugars which are bound to the external surface but which do not themselves penetrate the membrane, e.g. maltose and cellobiose (Lacko and Burger, 1963) or 4,6-O-ethylidene glucose (Baker and Widdas, 1973a), are unable to accelerate glucose efflux. Sugars with low affinity for the membrane transport system have no capacity for rapid exchange. It therefore seems plausible that the conformational change induced by the primary recognition event may be an abbreviated form of the larger conformational change which permits facilitated transport and rapid exchange.

The evidence that net flux and exchange flux have intrinsically different mechanisms comes from a number of diverse sources. These are as follows:

1. Exchange has a higher K_m and V_m than net efflux.
2. The activation energy of exchange is approximately half that of net efflux and much less than of net influx.
3. The pH-dependent variation of exchange V_m and K_m differs from that of net flux.
4. Reduction in the temperature reduces the K_m for infinite-*cis* exit, whereas the K_m for exchange is either unaffected or raised.
5. Insulin accelerates net glucose exit without affecting exchange.
6. PCMBS inhibits exchange flux more than it affects net efflux; chloropromazine inhibits net flux more than it affects exchange flux.
7. Acceleration of exchange is not seen with high concentrations of low-affinity sugars.

5 The asymmetry problem

The primary kinetic data describing the asymmetry of the sugar transport system for glucose has already been outlined. In summary, the K_m for zero-*trans* exit exceeds the K_m for zero-*trans* entry by approximately five- to tenfold. This asymmetry increases as temperature is lowered. The V_m for zero-*trans* net exit exceeds that for zero-*trans* net entry. This asymmetry is also increased on reducing temperature. As well as low-affinity sites on the inner surface of the membrane, operationally it is apparent that there is a high-affinity site here also (Table 1). It has been suggested that there is a low-affinity site at the external membrane surface; however, the evidence for this is tenuous. Baker and Widdas (1973b) have demonstrated that 4,6,-O-ethylidene-D-glucose which is not transported by the glucose transport system inhibits D-glucose exchange six times more effectively when it is present externally than when present exclusively intracellularly. This asymmetric inhibition is shared by a large number of 6-O-alkyl substituted hexoses (Barnett et al., 1975). The K_i for external inhibition of sorbose influx decreases from 17 mM for 6-O-propyl-D-galactose to 1·5 mM and 1·2 mM for 6-O-pentyl and 6-O-benzyl-D-galactose. The K_i for internal inhibition also decreases from 200 mM for 6-O-propyl-D-galactose to 6 mM for 6-O-benzyl-D-galactose. Novak and LeFevre (1974) have examined the effect of a number of sugar acetals on net glucose exit and have shown that the K_i for 4,6-O-benzylidene-D-glucose (0·13 mM) is lower than that of 4,6-O-ethylidene-D-glucose (4 mM), supporting the suggestion from Barnett et al. (1973) that hydrophobic substitution increases the inhibitory nature of nontransported sugars. However, for a single sugar substituted at the C6/C4 position, the inhibition from the external surface is greater than from the internal surface.

Baker and Widdas (1973a) have interpreted their data in terms of a high-affinity binding site at the outer surface only. Barnett et al. (1973b, 1975) have shown that the internal site can have high affinity also, since O-alkyl glucosides inhibit net glucose and sorbose transport more when inside the cell. They suggested that the membrane has higher selectivity for the acidic portion of the sugar molecule at the external surface and accepts only unsubstituted groups at C1, C2 and C3, but can accept, but not transport, moles with a bulky group at C4 and C6. At the internal surface, they suggested that the site accepts molecules with unsubstituted C6 and C4 hydroxyl groups and can accept, but not transport, molecules with a bulky group at C1. This reciprocal behaviour may mean that the sugar is directionally polarized by the transport sites. The data of Novak and LeFevre is inconsistent with this view because molecules substituted at both ends are good inhibitors, but would be predicted to interact with neither internal nor external sites. However, O-methyl substitution of 4,6-O-benzylidene-D-glucose does reduce affinity from $K_i = 0·13$ mM to $K_i = 0·73$ mM.

It is clear from these three studies of aryl- and alkyl-substituted sugars that several factors contribute towards the extent of inhibition of sugar transport. Differences in steric constraint and hydrophobic interaction may be due to asymmetric distribution of peripheral components of the transport system. Besides the obvious differences in location of adjacent macromolecules such as haemoglobin, the band 3 protein(s) itself (which may contain the sugar transport protein, see section 6) is thought to be an irregular S shape (Jenkins and Tanner, 1975) with a 35 000 dalton sialoglycoprotein segment on the outside of the membrane and a 65 000 dalton segment buried within the membrane (Rothstein et al., 1976). Bretscher (1972) has shown differences in the lipid composition of the two sides of the membrane.

For transported molecules these antibonding factors will be less important and this leaves open the possibility that for an unsubstituted sugar there is symmetrical affinity. It has been shown by Jung and Corlson (1975) that pronase digestion of intact cells, which removes the exposed external portion of band 3 protein (Jenkins and Tanner, 1975), has no effect on glucose transport.

5.1 STUDIES ON SUGAR TRANSPORT IN HUMAN RED CELL GHOSTS

All the above results have been obtained with whole red cells; however, Benes et al. (1972) found that if phloretin was introduced into red cell ghosts there was no asymmetric inhibitor effect on sugar transport. Taverna and Langdon (1973) introduced glucose oxidase into red cell ghosts and studied the glucose movements across the membrane of the resealed ghosts by following the rate of evolution of O_2 by the preparation—glucose oxidase having been removed from the extracellular fluid. They showed that the maximum rates of entry of glucose across the ghost preparation and uptake into inside-out vesicles was the same as into normal ghosts. From this they deduced that sugar transport in ghosts is symmetrical. Jung et al. (1973) have shown that a resealed white ghost preparation, although much more permeable to slowly permeating sugars such as—glucose or mannitol than the native red cell preparation, still permits D-glucose to be transported three orders of magnitude faster than mannitol. This fast permeation of the cell membrane by glucose is inhibited by $HgCl_2$.

Thus it is evident that removal of the internal contents of the red cell has a marked effect on the symmetry of the sugar transport system. Since haemoglobin is by far the major protein constituent of the red cell interior, it may be deduced that haemoglobin may affect the sugar transport kinetics.

5.2 THE INTERACTION OF SUGARS WITH HAEMOGLOBIN

D-glucose and other rapidly transported sugars protect red cells against osmotic haemolysis (Naftalin et al., 1974) and reduce the swelling of red cells, but not red cell ghosts following immersion in hypotonic salt solutions. Direct evidence that D-glucose induces haemoglobin gel formation which stabilizes the cells comes from studies of the viscosity of haemoglobin solutions and from studies of the nuclear magnetic resonance of water bound to haemoglobin, both in solution and within the intact red cell.

Sugar-dependent increments in the viscosity of haemoglobin solutions are observed at temperatures below 25°C, increasing to a maximum near 0°C. The increments in viscosity are seen mainly with sugars which are rapidly transported across the red cell membrane. The viscosity increment of 100 mM galactose < mannose < α-D-glucose < 2-deoxy-D-glucose < β-D-glucose. No viscosity increment is observed with D-fructose and only a small increment with ribose and sorbose (Simmons and Naftalin, 1976).

At high concentrations of haemoglobin with glucose present the solution becomes visco-plastic, i.e. thixotrophy and hysteresis of the shear stress/shear strain relationship are seen. These findings indicate that glucose can induce the haemoglobin molecules to aggregate to form a loose gel. The proton magnetic resonance spectra of these solutions suggest that glucose increases the amount of water "complexed" with haemoglobin. In addition to an increase in the amount of water bound to haemoglobin, dialysis studies indicate that glucose itself is nonspecifically bound to haemoglobin (Fig 4a,b). In solutions containing 1·0 mM haemoglobin with glucose present in the concentration range 10–100 mM, approximately 50 per cent of the glucose becomes complexed. Since the concentration of haemoglobin in intact red cells is 5 mM, it is likely that at least 80 per cent of the cell glucose becomes loosely complexed to the protein. The viscosity studies indicate that the sugars bind mainly to oxyhaemoglobin, but not to deoxyhaemoglobin stabilized with 2,3-diphosphoglycerate. Thermochemical studies indicate that like the interaction of D-glucose with red cell membranes the interaction of D-glucose with haemoglobin is also endothermic. This reaction is reversible since dissociation of the glucose-water-haemoglobin complexes is a slow exothermic reaction at 20°C. The half-time is approximately 10 min in both directions (Fig. 5). Neither L-glucose, nor D-fructose interact in this way with haemoglobin. Haemoglobin is not the only polymeric material which can bind large quantities of water and sugars, gelatin (Naftalin and Symons, 1974) and agar gels (Sigler, 1974) can also bind water and sugars to form stable gels. There is a loose stereospecificity in these sugar polymer interactions which may reflect the stereospecific interactions which have been reported between glucose and water in free solution (Tait et al., 1972). The importance of these studies to transport of sugars in red cells is that they suggest a physical basis for kinetic compartmentalization of glucose within the red cell. Net sugar transport between the free and bound states involves conformational change with an alteration in the number of H bonds involved within the complex. It is clear that the rate of complexation is controlled by the rate of conformational change within the protein aggregate. Since at equilibrium the bound form is the larger portion of intracellular sugar, it seems possible that nonsaturating complexation of sugar to haemoglobin is an explanation of kinetic asymmetries of sugar transport.

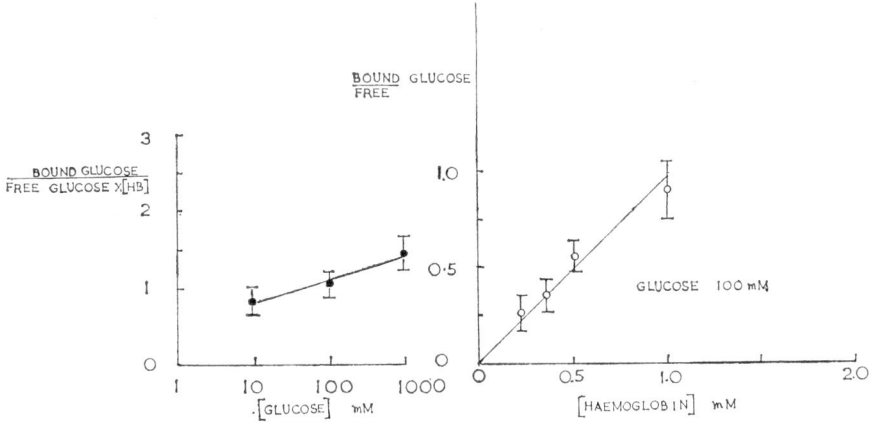

FIG. 4. (a) Shows the effects of varying concentrations of glucose on the ratio of bound : free glucose at 16°C. The concentration of free glucose was obtained by centrifuging glucose–haemoglobin solutions through Aminco-Centriflow filters which retain haemoglobin. Centrifugation was for 2 min at 600 × g. Total and free glucose were estimated from the activity of ^{14}C glucose in the filtrate and in the retained fluid following precipitation of the haemoglobin with 5 per cent trichloroacetic acid. The ratio of [bound glucose]/([free glucose] × [Hb]) as a function of glucose concentration is shown. This ratio is constant over the range of haemoglobin concentrations tested, 0·1–1 mM; however, the ratio increases from 0·8 to 1·5 as [glucose] is raised from 10 to 1000 mM. (b) The ratio of bound-free glucose increases as a linear function of [haemoglobin] in the range 0·1–1 mM. With 100 mM glucose present this ratio is 0·95 ± 0·70(5). If the [haemoglobin] is extrapolated to the intracellular level, this indicates that at equilibrium 80 per cent of the intracellular glucose is bound to haemoglobin at 16°C.

Nonspecific binding of sugars is not the only form of nonsaturating complex formed between haemoglobin and solutes. Haemoglobin and phloretin complexes (Jennings and Solomon, 1976) have also been described; however, unlike glucose, these complexes give rise to apparent accumulation of this solute within cells.

6 Chemical studies with isolated membranes and membrane proteins

Recently Kasahara and Hinkle (1976) have isolated protein from Triton X100 solubilized human red cell ghosts, which when incorporated into sonicated liposomes confers upon these structures the ability to facilitate the transport of D-glucose more than L-glucose. This transport is inhibited by both $HgCl_2$ and cytochalasin B. The protein appears to come from band 3 fraction (Steck, 1974) of the membrane proteins separated by sodium-dodecyl-sulphate polyacrylamide gels electrophoresis. Thus it is likely that the band of hydrophobic proteins which contains the Na, K, ATPase (Knauf et al., 1974), the water transport sites (Macey and Farmer, 1970), the anion binding site (Rothstein et al., 1976) and the membrane spanning protein (Jenkins and Tanner, 1975), also contains the sugar binding sites. Lin and Spudich (1974) have also shown that the cytochalasin binding protein is associated with band 3. Binding of cytochalasin B to this protein band was inhibited by high concentrations of D-glucose, but not sorbose, and also by PCMBS. Pronase digestion of the cell membrane does not prevent cytochalasin B binding nor does it inhibit sugar transport, although it destroys the external sialoproteins (band 7). Selective elution of the membrane proteins indicates that band 3, which remains undissociated from the membrane, contains the glucose binding sites (Kahlenberg, 1976).

It was indicated in section 4 that when sugars interact with the membrane transport system they induce a conformational change within the transporting complex which renders residues within this complex more reactive with alkylating reagents present in the aqueous environment.

Proton magnetic resonance studies of frozen suspensions of fragmented red cell membranes show a stereospecific sugar-dependent increase in the unfrozen water (Kuntz and Kauzmann, 1974) associated with the membrane. This sugar-dependent increase in unfrozen water can be abolished by $HgCl_2$ (Fig. 6) and reduced by cytochalasin B.

Thus it is apparent that glucose, in changing the membrane conformation, increases the amount of water associated with the membrane and presumably allows water to penetrate to regions which are normally inaccessible.

7 A model for facilitated diffusion and accelerated exchange of sugars relating recent physical chemical findings to transport

From the evidence based on dynamic accessibility studies, changes in the pH optimum for exchange compared with net flux, lack of facilitation of β-D-glucose in D_2O at pH 6 and NMR studies of glucose-dependent changes in water bound to the cell membrane, it is apparent that glucose

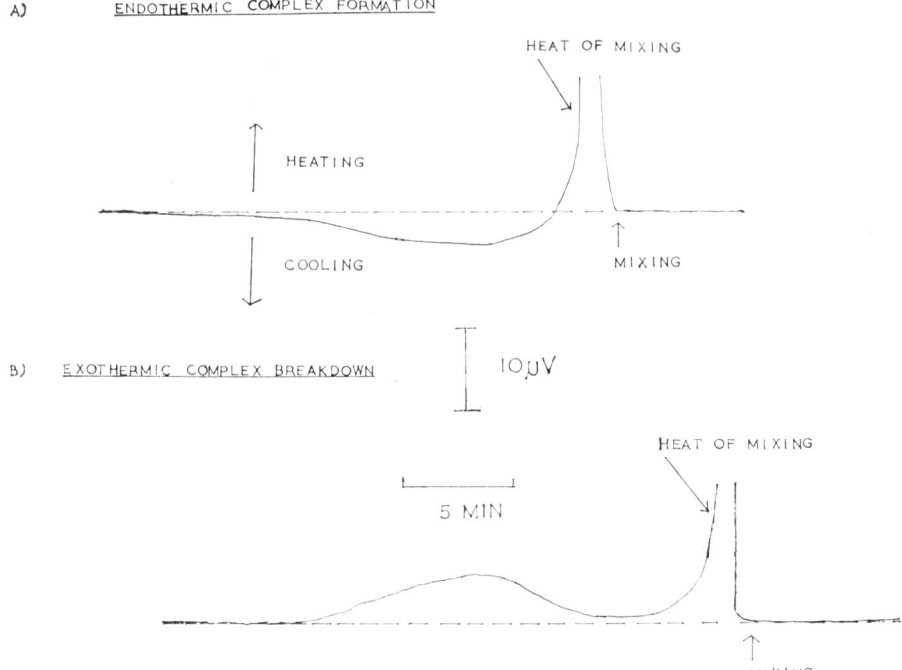

FIG. 5. (a) The time-course of the thermochemical reaction between glucose and haemoglobin at 20°C. The reaction was measured by the difference in the enthalpy of dilution of 1 ml of 2·5 mM haemoglobin into 4 ml of 500 mM D-glucose and 1 ml of 2·5 mM haemoglobin into 4 ml of water (final haemoglobin concentration 0·5 mM; final glucose concentration 400 mM). The faster reaction shows the rate of reaction between 400 mM glucose and 0·25 haemoglobin. $t_{\frac{1}{2}}$ for 0·5 mM haemoglobin 15 min, $t_{\frac{1}{2}}$ for 0·5 mM haemoglobin 9 min. (b) A trace of the time-course obtained from the chart recorder for the difference in enthalpy of dilution of 1 ml haemoglobin into 4 ml 500 mM glucose and 1 ml of 2·5 mM haemoglobin into 4 ml water. The trace was obtained using an LKB microcalorimeter with the chart set at 100 μV full scale deflection. The thermochemical response of glucose associating with haemoglobin is endothermic and slow. (c) The time-course of the exothermic dissociation between glucose and haemoglobin. This reaction was measured as the difference in heat of dilution of 1 ml of 2·5 mM haemoglobin in 500 mM glucose into 4 ml of water at 20°C and 1 mM of 2·5 mM haemoglobin into 4 ml of water at 20°C. The curve labelled 0·25 is a similar reaction in which the final haemoglobin concentration was 0·25 mM. Dissociation of the glucose-haemoglobin complex, as judged by the thermochemical response (d) is initially slow but accelerates as reaction progresses. The haemoglobin was prepared using the Drabkin method, followed by dialysis for 48 h in 10 mM *tris*-HCl pH 7·4 containing 1 mM mercaptoethanol at 4°C.

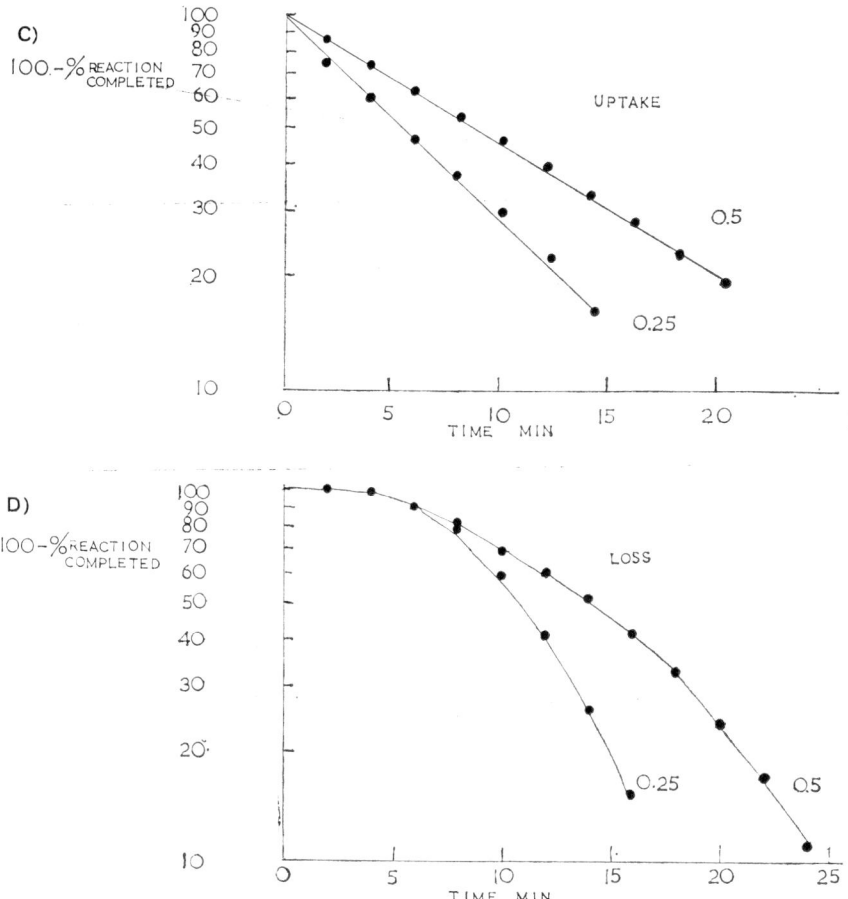

can increase the hydration at its sites of contact within the membrane; however, these sites must also include the transport sites.

An early model for sugar transport proposed by Adair (1956) suggested that sugars can induce a conformational change within the cell membrane which results in the opening of membrane pores. The new model proposed here is a small development of that proposed by Adair (1956) and also those models proposed by Stein and Danielli (1956), Burgen(1957) and Jung (1975). The transport protein consists of two sites, one at either surface. Each site can exist in one of two metastable states, closed or open, the open state consisting of the site complexed with sugar and bound water. Thus the membrane can exist in one of four possible states (see Fig. 7): closed at both ends; open at the outside; open at the inside; open at both ends. Whereas net flux across the membrane necessarily involves con-

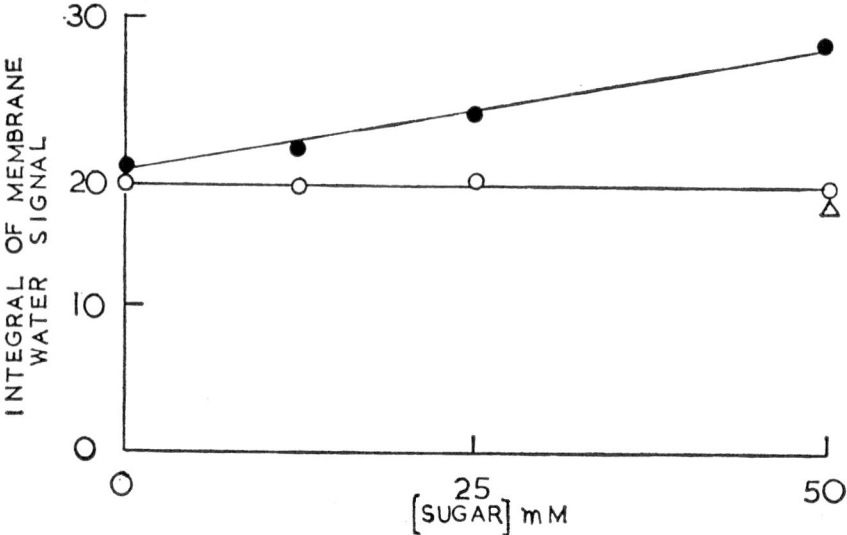

FIG. 6. Integral of unfrozen water protons at 253 °K as measured by a Bruker HFX 90/90 MHz. Fourier transform NM.R spectrometer. The amount of water is calibrated relative to the integral of the protons of an external acetone standard. Each signal was obtained from 32 scans. Human red cell membranes were obtained by the method of Dodge et al. (1963). They were freeze-dried and stored at $-20°C$ till required. The membranes were suspended in sugar solutions containing 100mM NaCl buffered to pH 7·2 with 10 mM tris-HCl to a final concentration of 15 mg ml^{-1}. They were dispersed in solution by ultrasonic disintegration.
●-● = integral of unfrozen water in membrane suspension containing D-glucose at the indicated concentrations; ○-○ = integral of the unfrozen water in membrane solutions containing D-glucose and 1 mM HgCl$_2$; △ = integral of membrane solution containing D-fructose.
(Results obtained by R. Naftalin and D. Couch at King's College based on work carried out in Leicester University by R. Naftalin, J. Harvey, G. Holman and M. C. R. Symons.)

formational change, when sugar moves from the *cis* side to open the closed *trans* site, exchange flux between open sites on opposite sides may not involve any additional conformational change within the membrane, since exchange between pairs of sugar molecules when both molecules are situated either wholly within the pore or exchange between molecules within the pore and in the adjoining solution, does not involve any net change in the number of H-bonding interactions within the system.

This model could explain the following data which have hitherto been difficult to rationalize: the lower activation energy for exchange flux than for net flux; the higher V_m for exchange flux than for net flux; the higher V_m for infinite-*trans* exchange than for net flux, also the lower activation energy for infinite-*trans* influx than for net influx; the absence of any accelerated exchange with sugars which are not rapidly facilitated by the membrane transport system; the differential effects of transport modifiers on net flux and exchange flux. This last effect could result from several mechanisms, e.g. any agent reducing the activation energy required for the sugar to induce the conformational change in the membrane protein would increase net flux more than exchange flux, since with exchange flux no new conformational change takes place; similarly, any modifier which increased the activation energy required for conformational change would reduce V_m (net flux) more than V_m (exchange flux); and finally, any agent *preventing* the total conformational change will decrease exchange flux more than net flux.

The present model has several features in common with the polar-pore model suggested by Jung (1975), who pointed out that the paucity of glucose transport sites within the cell membrane (3.5×10^5) means that their permeability to glucose must be very high. This high permeability is only consistent with the sugars whose transport is facilitated having a diffusion coefficient within the membrane approaching that in free solution. For this reason the ferry-boat protein carrier was rejected as being too slow. Jung suggests that sugars traverse a pore which is similar to the Lieb and Stein tetramer; the sugars induce a conformational change within the membrane protein which allows sugars in the external solution to pass into a central aqueous cavity, which is sufficiently large to permit two molecules to exchange between the symmetrical halves of the molecule. The kinetic behaviour of this model is similar to that of LeFevre's introversion model. Rothstein *et al.* (1976) have proposed a similar mechanism for red cell anion transport.

A difficulty with Jung's introverting-tetramer pore is that it assumes that the pore must change conformation faster during exchange than during net flux; the present modification, which assumes that the membrane remains in a metastable state, requires no further conformational changes once the membrane "gate" is fully open. This may explain the lower activation energy required for exchange than net flux.

A kinetic scheme for the gating-pore model for sugar transport which incorporates the transport asymmetry due to intracellular haemoglobin is described in Fig. 8. Kinetically the transport process involves two events:

a. *Recognition* is defined as a fast saturation process and is assumed to be symmetrical. The recognition process can be simply described in terms of the familiar Langmuir binding equations, with competitive inhibition between similar substrates for occupancy of the limited number of binding sites. Thus if there are two competing sugars (R and S), with identical affinities (K) for the sites present in the inner aqueous pool 2 and the outer infinite pool 3, then

$$\phi_{S_2} = \frac{S_2}{K + S_2 + R_2}; \quad \phi_{R_2} = \frac{R_2}{K + R_2 + S_2}$$
$$\phi_{S_3} = \frac{S_3}{K + S_3 + R_3}; \quad \phi_{R_3} = \frac{R_3}{K + R_3 + S_3}$$

where ϕ = fractional saturation of the site at 2 or 3;
ϕ max = $\sum(\phi_{S(i)} \phi_{R(i)}) = 2$.

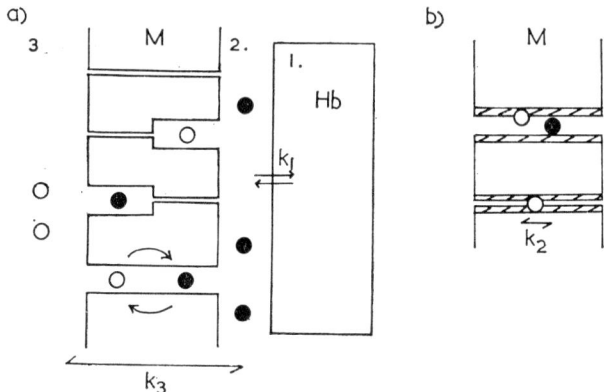

FIG. 7. (a) Gating membrane model with intracellular glucose-haemoglobin complex formation. (1) assumes that exchange is enhanced by sugar induced opening of membrane pores; (2) asymmetry of sugar transport parameters is due to a major portion of intracellular sugar slowly and reversibly complexing with haemoglobin. In (b) it is proposed that sorbose (open circles) can traverse both polar glucose-sensitive pathway and a nonpolar glucose—insensitive pathway (see text).

b. *Conformational change* which will not be subject to competition. Saturation at either side is considered to be independent of the reactions on the *trans* side since the rate of conformational change is assumed to be slow, hence the rate of sugar movement (J_s) across the membrane is defined as:

$$J_s = (k_2 + k_3(\phi_{S_2} + \phi_{R_2} + \phi_{S_3} + \phi_{R_3}))(\phi_{S_2} - \phi_{S_3}).$$

The extra constant k_2 is supplied in case the permeation process has a finite rate without any conformational change within the membrane taking place (as with sorbose transport, see section 8). As with the tetramer model, the maximal rate of exchange flux will never exceed twice the maximal rate of net flux when unimpeded by unstirred-layer effects.

The simultaneous unidirectional fluxes of two sugars, having identical affinities for the binding sites, across a three-compartment system such as postulated here, where the external compartment is infinite, can be represented by four simultaneous differential equations (Fig. 8). Since these are nonlinear they may only be solved numerically.

Solutions have been obtained which match the operational parameters of all the transport conditions described in this paper for glucose transport at 20°C. Also, exact matching of Miller's counterflow data for glucose was obtained with these parameters (Table 2 and Fig. 8).

The operational parameters for sugar transport may be rationalized in terms of the model as follows: the high operational K_m for zero-*trans* net exit results from the rapid decrease in free [glucose] in the cell water. The sugar efflux falls rapidly as the internal site desaturates; half-maximal efflux occurs when the free [sugar] present in the aqueous compartment is equal to the K_m for the membrane transport sites (symmetrical = 2 mM). At this point, the total sugar within the cell would, if it were uniformly distributed, make the concentration higher than the K_m of the inner membrane site; hence the *operational* K_m for net exit is higher than the membrane K_m. The faster the equilibration between the bound and free sugar, the nearer will the operational zero-*trans* exit K_m approach the membrane K_m. The initial rate of sugar loss from the cell is limited by the membrane transport process, since initially the free [sugar] will be high, as initially it is in equilibrium with the bound sugar; hence the operational V_m for zero-*trans* exit will be approximately the same as the V_m for infinite-*cis* net exit. The K_m for infinite-*cis* exit and for zero-*trans* net entry is determined primarily by the high-affinity membrane K_m. Similarly the K_m for infinite-*cis* net entry is determined by the membrane K_m. Since the free sugar concentration will rise more rapidly than expected on the basis of a homogeneous intracellular pool, the *operational* K_m when measured over the first milliseconds is considerably lower than the membrane K_m. However, if uptake is measured initially at 1–2 sec following entry, the K_m for infinite-*cis* entry is approximately the same as for infinite-*cis* exit. The lower *operational* V_m for entry than for exit can be explained on the basis that net entry across the membrane is reduced by the initially high concentration of "free" sugar. Influx is rate-limited by the rate of complexation of sugar with haemoglobin. The higher K_m for exchange than net influx results from the concentration-dependent conformational changes which increase the mobility of sugar within the pore as it becomes saturated. Deviations from Michaelis-Menten kinetics are too small to be detectable.

The K_m for infinite-*trans* entry is similar to the K_m for infinite-*cis* exit, because the total saturation at the internal site is identical in both procedures; the variation in the saturation in the external site on changing the sugar concentration in the external solution is also identical, the only difference being the presence of labelled sugar in the external solution with

Equations for Gating Pore with Internal Compartmentalization of D-glucose.

$$dS_1/dt = k_1 \frac{(1-V)}{V}(S_2 - S_1) \tag{1}$$

$$dR_1/dt = k_1 \frac{(1-V)}{V}(R_2 - R_1) \tag{2}$$

$$dS_2/dt = -dS_1/dt \frac{V}{1-V} + [k_2 + k_3(\phi_{S_2} + \phi_{R_2} + \phi_{S_3} + \phi_{R_3})](\phi_{S_3} - \phi_{S_2}) \tag{3}$$

$$dR_2/dt = -dR_1/dt \frac{V}{1-V} + [k_2 + k_3(\phi_{S_2} + \phi_{R_2} + \phi_{S_3} + \phi_{R_3})](\phi_{R_3} - \phi_{R_2}) \tag{4}$$

The above equations describe the model shown in Fig. 7(a). The system parameters supplied to give operational parameters shown in Table 2 are: V = haemoglobin water volume = 0·85 ml; total cell water volume = 1 ml; membrane K_m = 2 mM; k_3 = 600 μmol ml^{-1} min^{-1} for net and 1200 μmol ml^{-1} min^{-1} for exchange (referred to the 0·15 ml unbound water compartment); k_1 = 0·4 sec^{-1} (rate constant for sugar movement between bound and free compartments); k_2 = 0 for glucose experiments; $\phi_{i,j}$ = the fractional saturation of the membrane sites with solute i on the side of the membrane facing compartment j. $\phi_{i,j}$ = 2.

TABLE 2
Operational parameters for computer model of gating pore

	K_m mM	V_m μmol^{-1} ml^{-1} min^{-1}
Infinite-*cis* Exit	2·57	108
Entry	4·7	66
Zero-*trans* Exit	16·9	108
Entry	5·7	36
Infinite-*trans* Entry	3·4	142
Equilibrium exchange	37·5	192

the infinite-*trans* exchange instead of unlabelled, with the infinite-*cis* exit. Since with both these experimental procedures the internal sites remain continuously fully saturated, the total possible incremental change in conformation resulting from loading the external sites with sugars is only half that obtaining with the equilibrium exchange procedure, where *all* sites

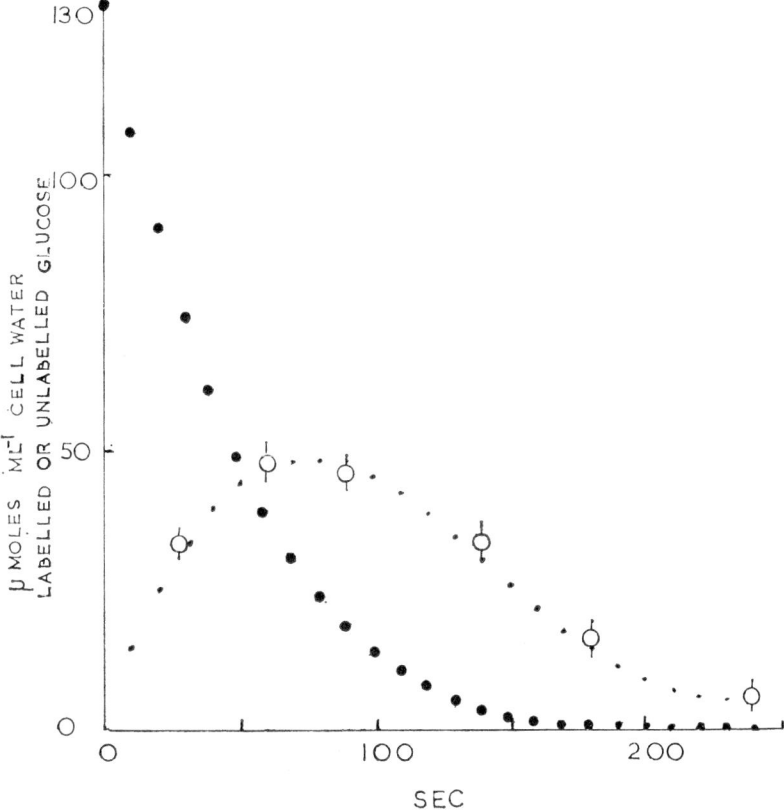

FIG. 8. Computer simulation of counterflow with system parameters as shown in table. The open circles are Miller's (1968) published data for counterflow where the cells are loaded with 130 mM glucose and the external radioactive glucose is 4·3 mM. The dotted lines are the intracellular concentrations of labelled ... and unlabelled OOO sugars.

start fully unsaturated at zero sugar and are fully saturated at high sugar concentrations. Since the high operational K_m for exchange is due to the changing mobility of the sugars within the membrane as it undergoes conformational change, it follows that with procedures involving smaller *increments* in conformational change, the operational transport K_m will approach more nearly the K_m determined by the dissociation constant of the membrane for the bound sugars. The V_m of infinite-*trans* entry is, of course, raised, since at high sugar concentration the pore is fully open; hence sugars are more mobile. Thus the present model simulates all the sugar transport parameters as well as Eilam's model does; additionally, the model explains the apparent asymmetric inhibition of sugar exit and entry by noncompetitive inhibitors.

As previously mentioned, Bowyer and Widdas (1958) showed that FDNB inhibits zero-*trans* exit of glucose more effectively than it inhibits zero-*trans* entry, yet it was found that FDNB inhibits net efflux and net influx into *trans* solutions containing substantial (30 mM) glucose concentrations to the same extent (Sen and Widdas, 1962b). These results may be explained in terms of the gating-pore model as follows: zero-*trans* exit of glucose is initially rate-limited by the V_m for the membrane transport system, hence reduction in the number of transport sites will cause a proportional decrease in efflux; glucose net uptake is rate-limited by the high concentration of "free" glucose in the aqueous intracellular phase, which occurs in the initial seconds of uptake. Reduction in the maximal rate of sugar influx across the membrane will not reduce sugar uptake rates until the rate of sugar transport across the membrane is slower than the rate of complexation of glucose by haemoglobin. When substantial concentrations of sugar are present on both sides of the membrane, net transport, in either direction, is rate-limited by the mobility of the sugar within the membrane, so here again retardation in transport by inhibitors bound irreversibly to the transport sites results in a symmetrical inhibition of net sugar flux. Of course, this solution to the problem of asymmetric transport is independent of any mechanism of membrane transport, since it depends on the slow rate of sugar complexation by haemoglobin. However, transport models which incorporate the kinetic asymmetries into the *membrane parameters* are difficult to reconcile with the inactivation data.

8 The sorbose problem

A problem stressed by Miller (1968a,b) is that the K_i for inhibition of sorbose flux by glucose is substantially larger than would be predicted on the basis of either the simple or mobile carrier model. It would be expected on the presumption that sorbose and glucose share the same simple carrier transport system that an equilibrium distribution of glucose on both sides of the membrane at a concentration sufficient to saturate half the sites on either side would reduce the flux of a low-affinity sugar like sorbose by half. However, the operational K_i at 20°C is from five to ten times (Miller, 1968a; Levine *et al.*, 1971) greater than that predicted by the mobile carrier. The tetramer model and the asymmetric carrier models all predict that the K_i for glucose inhibition of sorbose flux should be determined primarily by the low-affinity site, hence these models may be readily reconciled to this data. LeFevre's (1973) introversion model predicts that at low concentrations glucose should accelerate sorbose flux prior to it being inhibited at higher glucose concentrations. No acceleration of sorbose by low concentrations of glucose has ever been observed, hence this is a series abberation in the predictions of the introversion model.

Zimmer et al. (1972) showed with infra-red spectroscopy and gel filtration that glucose is bound mainly to membrane protein, whereas sorbose is bound mainly to other material thought to be lipoprotein. In a later paper, Zimmer et al. (1975), using viscosimetric techniques, showed that sorbose increases the fluidity of the cell membrane whereas glucose decreases the membrane fluidity. Fructose also increases the red cell membrane fluidity—this effect was found to be proportional to the concentration of fructose employed; no change in transition in membrane fluidity was found with glucose (Simmons and Naftalin, 1976). These findings all suggest that fructose and sorbose are bound to different membrane materials from those which bind glucose.

LaCelle and Passow (1971) have suggested that low-affinity sugars have two routes of permeation across the red cell membrane, one which is inhibited by glucose and another which is not.

Thus two pathways, one glucose-sensitive and one glucose-insensitive, and three events may be responsible for the mixed type of kinetics observed for sorbose transport (see Table 3). A glucose-sensitive pathway would have two characteristics: (a) inhibition by glucose of sorbose transport because the low-affinity sugar would be prevented from occupying the binding sites, and (b) some acceleration of the movement of the residual sorbose remaining in the pore, as a result of glucose-induced membrane conformational changes. Support for the view that two events occur in the

TABLE 3

	K_{is}	K_{iG}	K_{is} / K_{iG}
Glucose	7·6 [d]	2·75 [a]	2·8
3-O-methyl-glucose	13·0 [d]	5·0 [b]	2·6
Maltose	19·0 [d]	27·0 [b]	0·7
4,6-O-ethylidene-glucose	7·0 [d]	5·1 [b]	1·37
6-O-propyl-galactose	34·0 [e]	48·0 [c]	0·71
6-O-benzyl-galactose	2·4 [e]	6·0 [c]	0·4
6-O-pentyl-galactose	3·0 [e]	10·0 [c]	0·3

(a) Sen and Widdas (1962a).
(b) Inhibition of glucose net exit. G. F. Baker (personal communication)
(c) Inhibition of glucose net entry. Barnett et al. (1975).
(d) Barnett et al. (1973a).
(e) Barnett et al. (1975).

glucose-sensitive pathway is the observation that the $K_{iS} : K_{iG}$ ratio (K_{iG} is the inhibitor concentration added externally which reduces maximal exit of glucose by 50 per cent and K_{iS} is the operational K_i for inhibition of sorbose entry) for transported sugars, e.g. glucose and 3-O-methylglucose, is 2·5, whereas for nontransported, nonpenetrating sugars this ratio is nearer unity (see Table 3). Thus sugars which do not enter the membrane completely may not cause a large conformational change and the kinetics are predominated by sorbose transport via the less polar pathway and process (a). Where inhibitors have hydrophobic substitutions of their hydroxyl protons, the ratio $K_{iS} : K_{iG}$ falls below unity. The low K_{iS} values of these sugars may indicate that they can interact with hydrophobic route for sorbose transport which are inaccessible to glucose.

9 Summary

In this review we have traced the development of kinetic models of sugar transport and have also suggested a new model. This successive approximation towards definition of sugar transport illustrates the dominance of results and technique over theory. There appears to be a large measure of agreement that sugar-induced conformational changes in discrete regions of the membrane are responsible for facilitated diffusion and accelerated exchange of specific sugars via a polar pathway. The exact nature of these conformational changes remains unclear.

References

ADAIR, G. S. (1956). *Discussions Faraday Soc.* **21**, 285–286.
BAKER, G. F. and ROGERS, H. J. (1973). *J. Physiol.* **232**, 597–608.
BAKER, G. F. and WIDDAS, W. F. (1973a). *J. Physiol.* **231**, 129–142.
BAKER, G. F. and WIDDAS, W. F. (1973b). *J. Physiol.* **231**, 143–165.
BALDWIN, R. L. (1975). *A. Rev. Biochem.* **75**, 453–475.
BARNETT, J. E. G., HOLMAN, G. D., CHALKLEY, R. A. and MUNDAY, K. A. (1975). *Biochem. J.* **145**, 417–429.
BARNETT, J. E. G., HOLMAN, G. D. and MUNDAY, K. A. (1973a). *Biochem. J.* **131**, 211–221.
BARNETT, J. E. G., HOLMAN, G. D. and MUNDAY, K. A. (1973b). *Biochem. J.* **135**, 537–541.
BATT, E. R. and SCHACHTER, D. (1973). *J. Clin. Invest.* **52**, 1686–1697.
BENES, I., KOLIŃSKA, J. and KOTYK, A. (1972). *J. Membrane Biol.* **8**, 303–309.
BLOCH, R. (1973a). *Biochemistry*, **12**, 4799–4801.
BLOCH, R. (1974). *J. Biol. Chem.* **249**, 3543–3550.
BOWYER, F. and WIDDAS, W. F. (1958). *J. Physiol.* **141**, 219–232.
BRETSCHER, M. (1972). *J. Molec. Biol.* **71**, 523–528.
BURGEN, A. S. V. (1957). *Can. J. Biochem. Physiol.* **35**, 569–575.
CHEN, L. and LEFEVRE, P. G. (1965). *Fed Proc.* **24**, 465
DRABKIN, D. L. (1946). *J. Biol. Chem.* **146**, 703–711.

DODGE, J. T., MITCHELL, C. and HANAHAN, D. (1963). *Arch. Biochem. Biophys.* **100**, 119–124.
EDWARDS, P. A. W. (1973). *Biochim. Biophys. Acta*, **307**, 415–418.
EDWARDS, P. A. W. (1974). *Biochim. Biophys. Acta*, **345**, 373–386.
EILAM, Y. (1975a). *Biochim. Biophys. Acta*, **401**, 349–363.
EILAM, Y. (1975b). *Biochim. Biophys. Acta*, **401**, 364–369.
EILAM, Y. and STEIN, W. D. (1972). *Biochim. Biophys. Acta*, **266**, 161–173.
FAUST, R. G. (1960). *J. Cell. Comp. Physiol.* **56**, 103–121.
FOSTER, D. M. and JACQUEZ, J. A. (1976). *Biochim. Biophys. Acta*, **436**, 210–221.
GECK, P. (1971). *Biochim. Biophys. Acta*, **241**, 462–472.
GINSBURG, H. and RAM, D. (1975). *Biochim. Biophys. Acta*, **382**, 369–376.
GINSBURG, H. and STEIN, W. D. (1975). *Biochim. Biophys. Acta*, **382**, 353–368.
HANKIN, B. L., LIEB, W. R. and STEIN, W. D. (1972). *Biochim. Biophys. Acta*, **288**, 114–126.
HANKIN, B. L. and STEIN, W. D. (1972). *Biochim. Biophys. Acta*, **288**, 127–136.
HARRIS, E. J. (1964). *J. Physiol.* **173**, 344–353.
HILL, T. L. and KEDEM, P. (1966). *J. Theoret. Biol.* **10**, 399.
HODGKIN, A. L. and KEYNES, R. D. (1955). *J. Physiol.* **128**, 61–88.
JENKINS, R. E. and TANNER, M. J. A. (1975). *Biochem. J.* **147**, 393–399.
JENNINGS, M. L. and SOLOMON, A. K. (1976). *J. Gen. Physiol.* **67**, 381–397.
JUNG, C. Y. (1974). *J. Biol Chem.* **249**, 3568–3573.
JUNG, C. Y. (1975). In "The Red Blood Cell" (D. M. Surgenor, ed), 2nd edit., pp. 705–749. Academic Press, New York and London.
JUNG, C. Y. and CARLSON, L. M. (1975). *J. Biol. Chem.* **250**, 3217–3220.
JUNG, C. Y., CARLSON, L. M. and BALZER, C. J. (1973). *Biochim. Biophys. Acta*, **298**, 101–107.
JUNG, C. Y., CARLSON, L. M. and WHALEY, D. A. (1971). *Biochim. Biophys. Acta*, **241**, 613–627.
KAHLENBERG, A. (1976). *J. Biol. Chem.* **251**, 1582–1590.
KAHLENBERG, A., URMAN, B. and DOLANSKY, D. (1971). *Biochemistry*, **10**, 3154–3162.
KARLISH, S. J. D., LIEB, W. R., RAM, D. and STEIN, W. D. (1972). *Biochim. Biophys. Acta*, **255**, 126–132.
KASAHARA, M. and HINKLE, P. C. (1976). *Proc. Nat. Acad. Sci. USA*, **73**, 396–400.
KNAUF, P. A., PROVERBIO, F. and HOFFMAN, J. F. (1974). *J. Gen. Physiol.* **63**, 308–000.
KOTYK, A. (1973). *Biochim. Biophys. Acta*, **135**, 112–119.
KRUPKA, R. M. (1971a). *Biochemistry*, **10**, 1143–1147.
KRUPKA, R. M. (1971b). *Biochemistry*, **10**, 1148–1153.
KUNTZ, I. D. Jr. and KAUZMAN, W. (1974). "Advances in Protein Chemistry" vol. 28, pp. 239–345. Academic Press, New York and London.
LACKO, L. and BURGER, M. (1962). *Biochem. J.* **83**, 622–625.
LACKO, L. and BURGER, M. (1963). *J. Biol. Chem.* **238**, 3478–3481.
LACKO, L., WITTKE, B. and KROMPHARDT, H. (1972). *Eur. J. Biochem.* **25**, 447–454.
LACELLE, P. and PASSOW, H. (1971). *J. Membrane Biol.* **4**, 270–283.
LARIS, P. C. (1958). *J. Cell. Comp. Physiol.* **51**, 273–307.
LEFEVRE, P. G. (1948). *J. Gen. Physiol.* **31**, 505–527.
LEFEVRE, P. G. (1954). *Symp. Soc. Exp. Biol.* **8**, 118.
LEFEVRE, P. G. (1963). *J. Gen. Physiol.* **46**, 721–731.
LEFEVRE, P. G. (1973). *J. Membrane Biol.* **11**, 1–19.

LeFevre, P. G. (1975). "Current Topics in Membranes and Transport", vol. I, pp. 109–215. Academic Press, New York and London.
LeFevre, P. G. and Davis, R. I. (1951). *J. Gen. Physiol.* **34**, 515–524.
LeFevre, P. G. and Marshall, J. K. (1958). *Amer. J. Physiol.* **194**, 333–337.
LeFevre, P. G. and McGinniss, G. F. (1960). *J. Gen. Physiol.* **44**, 87–103.
Levine, M., Levine, S. and Jones, N. M. (1971). *Biochim. Biophys. Acta*, **255**, 291–300.
Levine, M., Oxender, D. L. and Stein, W. D. (1965). *Biochim. Biophys. Acta*, **109**, 151–163.
Levine, M. and Stein, W. D. (1966). *Biochim. Biophys. Acta*, **127**, 179–193.
Lieb, W. R. and Stein, W. D. (1970). *Biophys. J.* **10**, 585–609.
Lieb, W. R. and Stein, W. D. (1971a). *Nature New Biol.* **230**, 108–109.
Lieb, W. R. and Stein, W. D. (1971b). "Current Topics in Membranes and Transport", vol. 2, p. 1. Academic Press, New York and London.
Lieb, W. R. and Stein, W. D. (1972). *Biochim. Biophys. Acta*, **265**, 187–207.
Lin, S. and Spudich, J. A. (1974). *Biochem. Biophys. Res. Commun.* **61**, 1471–1476.
Macey, R. I. and Farmer, R. E. L. (1970). *Biochim. Biophys. Acta*, **211**, 104–106.
Mawe, R. C. (1956). *J. Cell. Comp. Physiol.* **47**, 177–213.
Mawe, R. C. and Hempling, H. G. (1965). *J. Cell. Comp. Physiol.* **66**, 95–104.
Miller, D. M. (1965). *Biophys. J.* **5**, 417–423.
Miller, D. M. (1968a). *Biophys. J.* **8**, 1329–1338.
Miller, D. M. (1968b). *Biophys. J.* **8**, 1339–1352.
Miller, D. M. (1969). In "Red Cell Membrane Structure and Function" (G. A. Jamieson and T. J. Greenwalt, eds). pp 240–290, Lippincott, Philadelphia.
Miller, D. M. (1971). *Biophys. J.* **11**, 915–923.
Miller, D. M. (1972). *Biochim. Biophys. Acta*, **266**, 85–90.
Naftalin, R. J. (1970). *Biochim. Biophys. Acta*, **211**, 65–78.
Naftalin, R. J. (1971). *Biochim. Biophys. Acta*, **233**, 635–643.
Naftalin, R. J. (1972). In "Biomembranes" (F. Kreutzer and J. F. G. Slegers, eds), pp. 117–126. Plenum Publishing, New York.
Naftalin, R. J., Seeman, P., Simmons, N. L. and Symons, M. C. R. (1974). *Biochim Biophys. Acta*, **352**, 146–171.
Naftalin, R. J. and Symons, M. C. R. (1974). *Biochim. Biophys. Acta*, **352**, 173–178.
Novak, R. A. and LeFevre, P. G. (1974). *J. Membrane Biol.* **17**, 383–390.
Odesser, D. and Mawe, R. C. (1967). *J. Gen. Physiol.* **50**, 2510.
Ørskov, S. L. (1935). *Biochem. Z.* **279**, 241–249.
Owen, J. D. and Solomon, A. K. (1972). *Biochim. Biophys. Acta*, **290**, 414–417.
Owen, J. D., Steggall, M. and Eyring, E. M. (1974). *J. Membrane Biol.* **19**, 79–92.
Regen, D. M. and Morgan, H. E. (1964). *Biochim. Biophys. Acta*, **79**, 151–166.
Regen, D. M. and Tarpley, H. L. (1974). *Biochim. Biophys. Acta*, **339**, 218–233.
Rosenberg, T. and Wilbrandt, W. (1957). *J. Gen. Physiol.* **41**, 289–296.
Roth, P. and Seeman, P. (1972). *Biochim. Biophys. Acta*, **255**, 190–198.
Rothstein, A., Cabantchik, Z. I., Balshin, M. and Juliano, R. (1975). *Biochem. Biophys. Res. Commun.* **64**, 144–150.
Rothstein, A., Cabantchik, Z. I. and Knauf, P. (1976). *Fed. Proc.* **35**, 3–10.
Schnell, K. F. (1972). *Biochim. Biophys. Acta*, **282**, 265–276.
Sen, A. K. and Widdas, W. F. (1962a). *J. Physiol.* **160**, 392–403.
Sen, A. K. and Widdas, W. F. (1962b). *J. Physiol.* **160**, 404–416.

SHA'AFI, R. I., GARRY-BOBO, C. M. and SOLOMON, A. K. (1971). *J. Gen. Physiol.* **58**, 238–258.
SIGLER, K. (1974). *Biopolymers*, **13**, 2553–2563.
SIMMONS, N. L. and NAFTALIN, R. J. (1976). *Biochim. Biophys. Acta*, **419**, 493–511.
STECK, T. L. (1974). *J. Cell. Biol.* **62**, 1–19.
STEIN, W. D. and DANIELLI, J. F. (1956). *Discussions Faraday Soc.* **21**, 238–251.
STEIN, W. D. and LIEB, W. R. (1974). *Israel J. Chem.* **11**, 325–339.
TAIT, M. J., SUGGETT, A., FRANKS, F., ABLETT, S. and QUICKENDEN, P. A. (1972). *J. Solution Chem.* **1**, 131–151.
TAVERNA, R. D. and LANGDON, R. G. (1973). *Biochim. Biophys. Acta*, **323**, 207–219.
TAYLOR, N. F. and GAGNEJA, G. L. (1976). *Can. J. Biochim.* **53**, 1078–1084.
VAN STAVENINCK, J., WEED, R. I. and ROTHSTEIN, A. (1965). *J. Gen. Physiol.* **48**, 617–632.
WIDDAS, W. F. (1954). *J. Physiol.* **125**, 163–180.
WILBRANDT, W. and ROSENBERG, T. (1961). *Pharmacol. Rev.* **13**, 169–183.
ZALA, C. A., JONES, M. N. and LEVINE, M. (1974). *FEBS Lett.* **48**, 196–199.
ZIERLER, K. L. (1961). *Bull. Johns Hopkins Hosp.* **109**, 35–48.
ZIMMER, G., LACKO, L. and GÜNTHER, H. (1972). *J. Membrane Biol.* **9**, 305–318.
ZIMMER, G., SCHIRMER, H. and BASTIAN, P. (1975). *Biochim. Biophys. Acta*, **410**, 244–255.
ZIPPER, H. and MAWE, R. C. (1972). *Biochim. Biophys. Acta*, **282**, 311–325.
ZIPPER, H. and MAWE, R. C. (1974). *Biochim. Biophys. Acta*, **356**, 207–218.

Note added in proof

Section 4.3. Lacko et al, (1977) have studied the thermodynamic parameters of steroid interaction with the glucose transport system. They find that the binding affinity of C-21 steroids decreases with increasing numbers of polar groups, i.e. deoxycorticosterone (tripolar) > corticosterone (tetrapolar) > cortisol (pentapolar). The authors suggest that their data implies that the disordered water surrounding the polar groups contributes to the total amount of disordered water in the region of the sugar-carrier-steroid complex. The hydrophobic moiety of the steroid decreases the amount of disordered water, thus the net inhibition by steroids is reduced by the hydrophilic groups. These results lend support to the view expressed in section 4.3 that sugars are transported via a polar channel containing randomized water molecules.

Section 6. Masiak and LeFevre (1977) report that incorporation of either trypsin, or α-chymotrypsin into erythrocyte ghosts leads to progressive inhibition of glucose transport; when present in the external solution alone, the enzymes do not affect sugar transport. Polyacrylamide-gel electrophoresis of the digested membranes shows that spectrin, which is located at the inner membrane surface, is attacked by the enzymes, but no apparent damage to band 3 proteins is observed.

On the other hand, Nickson and Jones (1977) have reconstituted a sugar transport system by incorporating red cell membrane proteins from bands 3 and 4·2 into black lipid membranes. D-glucose transport is enhanced across the membranes twenty-five-fold, is subject to competition from 2-deoxy-D-glucose, and is inhibited by the action of $HgCl_2$ PCMB, and phloretin. L-glucose transport is not facilitated. This definitive evidence for the role of membrane proteins in sugar transport is a most important landmark.

Section 7. Baker and Naftalin (1977) have obtained evidence which corroborates the view that there are multiple operational affinities for D-glucose on the inner surface of the membrane. This evidence was obtained from infinite-*trans* exit experiments of labelled D-glucose exit into solutions containing 50 mM D-galactose at 2°C. The K_m for infinite-*trans* exit is 3·8 ± 2·0 mM (S.D.) and V_m 17 mmol (1 cell water)$^{-1}$ min^{-1}. The K_m's for equilibrium-exchange and for zero-*trans* exit of D-glucose at 2°C were found to be 40 and 30 mM, respectively.

Section 8. Bowman and Levitt (1977) have proposed an asymmetric pore model which is similar to the one proposed in section 7. They show that the glucose-dependent permeabilities of a series of 4, 5 and 6 carbon polyols are inversely related to their molecular size. The authors suggest that this arises because the smaller molecules may enter the membrane pore more readily.

References

BAKER, G. F. and NAFTALIN, R. J. (1977). *J. Physiol.* (in press).
BOWMAN, R. J. and LEVITT, D. G. (1977). *Biochim. Biophys. Acta*, **466**, 68–83.
LACKO, L., WITTKE, B. and LACKO, I. (1977). *J. Cell. Physiol.* **90**, 161–168.
MASIAK, S. J. and LeFEVRE, P. G. (1977). *Biochim. Biophys. Acta*, **465**, 371–377.
NICKSON, J. K. and JONES, M. N. (1977). *Biochem. Soc. Trans.* **5**, 147–149.

Red cell amino acid transport

J. D. YOUNG and J. C. ELLORY

ARC Institute of Animal Physiology, Babraham, Cambridge, UK, and Department of Physiology, Cambridge University, UK

1 Introduction	301
2 The permeability of red cells and liposomes to amino acids	303
3 Na dependence of red cell amino acid transport	307
4 Kinetic analysis of amino acid transport in red cells	308
5 Amino acid transport in reticulocytes	316
6 The role of thiol groups in red cell amino acid transport	319
7 The physiological and biochemical significance of red cell amino acid transport systems	320
8 Conclusions	322
References	323

1 Introduction

Although the mammalian red cell has received extensive attention in membrane transport studies, information on the permeability of red cells to amino acids is surprisingly limited and fragmentary. Hence the present attempt at reviewing the field has revealed several gaps and inconsistencies, which can be contrasted with the situation for ion or glucose transport (Cavieres; Beaugé and Lew; Ferreira and Lew; Lew and Ferreira; Martin; Naftalin and Holman, this volume) or for amino acid transport in nucleated cells including avian red cells (Kregenow, this volume). This reticence to study red cell amino acid transport is puzzling since the role of amino acids in glutathione (GSH) biosynthesis may be considered as vital as the availability of glucose for preserving ATP levels. Indeed our interest in this field was originally stimulated by the possibility that amino acid availability may directly influence red cell GSH concentrations. However, it must be said that the mature red cell is biochemically limited, and does not carry out many of the functions for which there is an obvious amino acid requirement. Most amino acids are present in plasma at concentrations in the 20–500 μM range, with similar intracellular concentrations. In fact, it could be thought that the passive permeability of the red cell membrane *per se* might be enough to cater for the cell's amino acid requirement. If this were the case, amino acid uptake would show no stereospecificity, and although factors such as ionization and lipid solubility would influence the permeation of different amino acids, predictable permeability patterns should emerge, and one might expect a correlation between amino acid fluxes in red cells and liposomes. We have therefore included in this review such data on liposome amino acid permeability as we can find.

When Christensen and co-workers began to determine the permeability of red cells to amino acids in the 1950s using tracer techniques, it soon became apparent that considerable differences existed between D and L isomers, and amongst various amino acids, which could not be explained on the basis of simple diffusion. No striking concentrative accumulation of amino acids has been reported for mammalian red cells, however, and no significant evidence for energy utilization or Na dependence of amino acid transport exists. Amino acid fluxes in these cells can therefore be considered as carrier-mediated facilitated transport (for a discussion of the terminology and its implications see LeFevre, 1975), and the dissection of the nature of the systems involved has depended entirely on operational criteria. Three approaches have been adopted towards characterizing red cell amino acid transport. Initially, measurements of uptake or loss of different, radioactively labelled naturally occurring amino acids were carried out. Further manipulations involved comparing exchange and inhibition interactions between different amino acids. Unhappily the data indicated low apparent affinities and broad substrate specificities, making it difficult to define the number of systems present. A second approach, which has only been applied peripherally to mature red cells, was that adopted by Christensen and his colleagues principally for nucleated cells, where substrate analogues were designed with the idea of increasing the affinities and thus sharpening the discrimination between various transport systems. An alternative idea which we have attempted to develop uses genetic variants with different transport characteristics, a technique greatly favoured with bacterial systems. In this case, certain Finnish Landrace sheep showing a genetically controlled and selective low permeability to a number of amino acids were proposed as lacking one amino acid transport system. Thus, by comparing amino acid fluxes in these cells with normal individuals it was possible to define in detail the specificity of the transport system. Interestingly, the defect manifests its effect in several other ways in the cell, including lowering the red cell GSH concentration, raising the intracellular concentrations of certain amino acids, particularly ornithine and lysine, altering Na and K levels and markedly diminishing the potential life-span of the cell.

Red cell amino acid transport systems have been regarded as non-functional relics from the reticulocyte stage. However, the study of GSH-deficient sheep red cells has emphasized the role of amino acid transport in providing GSH precursors. A role has also been proposed for red cell amino acid transport systems in inter-organ amino acid transport, and it has been suggested that the γ-glutamyl cycle may be involved in red cell amino acid transport. Our present intention is to summarize the state of knowledge on the number, specificity, mechanism and physiological importance of amino acid transport systems in mammalian red cells, although inevitably we shall raise more questions than we shall answer.

2 The permeability of red cells and liposomes to amino acids

This section collects data for the uptake of amino acids by mammalian red cells and compares the results with amino acid flux measurements in liposomes. Although early investigators considered the red cell to be impermeable to amino acids (Gryns, 1896; Hedin, 1897), subsequent studies (Constantino, 1913; Abderhalden and Kürten, 1921; Danielson, 1933; Sbarsky, 1941; Ussing, 1943; Christensen et al., 1947, 1952) demonstrated that the red cell membrane was permeable to a number of amino acids. More recent investigations have been surprisingly limited in number, and only for human, rabbit and sheep red cells have the studies been detailed enough to permit the influence of amino acid structure on permeability to be assessed, or to allow a comparison of the permeability characteristics of cells from different species (see Table 1).

The first detailed study of amino acid uptake by red cells was that of Winter and Christensen (1964), who investigated the permeability of human red cells to a series of neutral amino acids. The initial rate of amino acid uptake was found to be a function of the size of the apolar side chain, and the presence of polar groupings markedly reduced the transport rate. Partial stereoselectivity was observed for a number of amino acids, and the cells were found to be impermeable to L-asparate and L-glutamate. Dibasic amino acid uptake by human red cells was investigated by Gardner and Levy (1972). Influx rates for L-ornithine, L-lysine and L-arginine were considerably less than those observed for neutral amino acids of comparable size, and a significant uptake of L-cystine was observed. A similar permeability pattern was found in rabbit red cells, but they exhibited faster uptake rates (Winter and Christensen, 1965; Rohrs and Archdeacon, 1967; Antonioli and Christensen, 1969; Young et al., 1975b). The uptake of L-alanine, α-aminoisobutyrate and N-methyl-α-aminoisobutyrate by rat red cells has been investigated by Wise (1976).

The amino acid permeability of sheep red cells was examined by Young

TABLE 1
Effect of amino acid structure on red cell permeability
(Initial rate of amino acid uptake: μmol min^{-1} (l cells)$^{-1}$)

	Human	Sheep (high GSH)	Sheep (low GSH)
Glycine	0·9	0·10	0·05*
L-Proline	15	0·12	0·08*
L-Alanine	5	2·57	0·04*
D-Alanine	1·4	0·08	0·03*
Sarcosine	0·2		
L-α-Amino-*n*-butyrate		11·6	0·92*
α-Aminoisobutyrate	1·2		
L-Valine	240	0·56	0·16*
D-Valine	39		
L-Norvaline	3·3		
D-Norvaline	0·9		
L-Leucine	440	0·24	0·27
L-Isoleucine		0·21	0·26
D,L-Norleucine	250		
1-Aminocyclohexane carboxylic acid	220		
3-Methyl-1-aminocyclohexane carboxylic acid	190		
1-Aminocyclopentane carboxylic acid	91		
L-Cysteine		3·82	0·58*
L-Serine	52	0·39	0·05*
L-Threonine		0·16	0·06*
L-Methionine	240	0·15	0·18
L-Phenylalanine	360	0·46	0·48
L-Tyrosine	100	0·48	0·74
L-Histidine	46	0·15	0·19
D,L-Tryptophan	39		
L-Lysine	5·0	0·25	0·08*
L-Ornithine	13	0·27	0·07*
L-Arginine	6·8	0·08	0·07
L-Cystine	3·9	0·14	0·16
L-Aspartate	†	†	†
L-Glutamate	†	†	†
L-Asparagine		0·11	0·04*
L-Glutamine		0·03	0·04

† No significant uptake.
Amino acids were present at an extracellular concentration of 1 mM, except in the sheep experiments where the concentration was 0·2 mM. Incubations were at 37°C. The human neutral amino acid data were calculated from the distribution ratios of Winter and Christensen (1964) and the dibasic amino acid uptake rates were obtained from Gardner and Levy (1972). Sheep data are reproduced from Young *et al.* (1976), but for convenience the S.E.M.'s have been omitted. Significant differences in uptake rates between high- and low-GSH cells are indicated by *. For comparison with these values, glycine, L-alanine and L-leucine uptake rates in rabbit red cells have been estimated to be 42, 65 and >600 μmol min^{-1} (l cells)$^{-1}$, respectively (Winter and Christensen, 1965) and Wise (1976) reported L-alanine, α-aminoisobutyrate and *N*-methyl-α-aminoisobutyrate uptake rates of 83, 20 and 1·4 μmol min^{-1} (l cells)$^{-1}$, respectively for rat red cells.

et al. (1975a, 1976). Alanine uptake showed a high degree of stereoselectivity, with the rate of L-alanine transport similar to that reported for human cells. However, in marked contrast to human and rabbit cells, sheep red cells were relatively impermeable to large neutral amino acids, and L-cysteine and L-α-amino-*n*-butyrate gave the highest uptake rates. Tucker and Kilgour (1970) described an inherited red cell GSH deficiency in certain animals of the Finnish Landrace breed. This GSH deficiency, which is inherited in a simple autosomal recessive manner, was subsequently shown to be associated with high intracellular concentrations of certain amino acids, particularly ornithine and lysine (Ellory *et al.*, 1972), and amino acid uptake measurements revealed that the permeability characteristics of these cells were markedly different from normal (high GSH) sheep red cells (Young *et al.*, 1975a, 1976) (see also Table 1). It was particularly interesting that the permeability difference was limited to certain amino acids. The diminished amino acid uptake by these GSH-deficient (low GSH) cells was not a secondary consequence of either the low intracellular GSH concentration or the high amino acid content of these cells, but rather represents a membrane transport defect. This amino acid transport lesion is considered in detail in subsequent sections.

The data presented in Table 1 suggest a considerable species variation in red cell amino acid permeability. These differences have been confirmed in our laboratory, and the comparison extended to include a number of additional species (Table 2). The results suggest that a low permeability

TABLE 2

Amino acid permeability of red cells from various mammalian species
(Initial rate of amino acid uptake μmol min^{-1} (l cells)$^{-1}$)

	Human	Rabbit	Rat	Sheep (high GSH)	Cattle	Goat
Glycine	1·05	7·03	5·77	0·18	0·24	0·20
L-Alanine	3·55	8·07	8·47	2·20	3·32	2·88
D-Alanine	0·58	6·10	5·77	0·20	0·21	0·20
L-Valine	40·8	147	>250	0·93	1·03	1·09
L-Leucine	80·0	>250	>250	0·37	0·49	0·45
L-Phenylalanine	91·5	>250	>250	0·69	1·05	0·89
L-Lysine	6·90	10·1	2·17	0·23	0·51	0·38
L-Glutamate	0·07	0·06	0·26	0·04	0·07	0·05

Initial amino acid uptake rates (extracellular concentration 0·2 mM, 37°C) were determined as previously described (Young *et al.*, 1976) except that extracellular isotope was removed by centrifuging the cells through a layer of dibutyl phthalate. Values are means of three animals of each species. S.E.M.'s were typically less than 10 per cent of mean values.

to large neutral amino acids may be a general characteristic of ruminant red cells.

An estimate of the amino acid permeability of artificial phospholipid bilayers may prove useful for comparison with red cell data. At least three groups have measured the permeability of liposomes to amino acids by either light-scattering or isotope techniques, and Table 3 summarizes the data of R. C. Hider and W. J. McCormack (personal communication). There was at least fiftyfold permeability difference between glycine and L-phenylalanine, and the permeability of individual amino acids roughly correlated with their lipid solubility. Incorporation of cholesterol into the lecithin liposomes had only a small effect on permeability. We have also calculated permeability coefficients for human red cells based on the data in Table 2. These values are included in Table 3, and are, with the exception

TABLE 3
The permeability of liposomes to amino acids

	Permeability (10^{-9} cm sec^{-1}) at 37°C		
	Liposome		
	Lecithin	Lecithin-cholesterol (3 : 4)	Human erythrocyte
Glycine	<0·5	<0·5	6·6
L-Alanine	2·7	1·4	22·4
L-Methionine	13	4·9	—
L-Valine	19	6·8	300
L-Leucine	25	21	713
L-Phenylalanine	39	36	881

Values for red cell permeability calculated by converting the initial uptake rates in Table 2 into rate constants (k) and multiplying by $1·56 \times 10^{-9}$ to obtain p in cm sec^{-1} when k is in h^{-1} (V. L. Lew, personal communication).

of L-alanine, at least forty times greater than the liposome permeabilities. Similar relative neutral amino acid permeability sequences have been obtained by Klein et al. (1971) and Wilson and Wheeler (1973). The former group also demonstrated that alterations in the degree of lecithin saturation caused small but significant changes in permeability and that liposomes could not differentiate between D- and L-alanine. Recently, Hider and McCormack (personal communication) have found that substituting sphingomyelin for lecithin causes a dramatic (fiftyfold) reduction in amino acid permeability.

Although liposomes do show specificity with respect to amino acid structure, this selectivity does not correlate with that seen in red cells (e.g.

stereospecificity, and the relative permeabilities of L-alanine and L-phenylalanine in ruminant red cells). This, together with the much higher permeability rates seen in red cells compared with liposomes of comparable lipid composition, emphasize the likelihood of specific amino acid transport systems in red cells. It is interesting to speculate that the very low amino acid permeability of GSH-deficient sheep red cells may represent the ground-state permeability of the lipid membrane. In any case it is likely that the ground-state permeability of sphingomyelin-containing cells (e.g. sheep) is much lower than that of lecithin-containing cells (e.g. human) (De Gier et al., 1960).

3 Na dependence of red cell amino acid transport

Since a number of tissues can accumulate amino acids in a Na-dependent manner, this section considers the evidence for active amino acid transport in mammalian red cells. None of the neutral amino acids studied by Winter and Christensen (1964) gave equilibrium distribution ratios (concentration of amino acid in cell water : concentration in extracellular medium) significantly greater than 1, with the possible exception of glycine (distribution ratio 1·3). These distribution ratios were obtained by isotope distribution measurements rather than by direct amino acid analyses, and it is probable that intracellular metabolism contributed to the high glycine distribution ratio since this amino acid is incorporated into GSH both by *de novo* peptide synthesis and by exchange (see e.g. Snoke and Bloch, 1955; Minnich et al., 1971). Similar neutral amino acid equilibrium distribution ratios have been obtained in other species (Winter and Christensen, 1965; Yunis and Arimura, 1965; McCormick, 1970; Young et al., 1975b; Wise, 1976; Young and Ellory, unpublished observations). Yunis and Arimura (1965) reported ^{14}C-lysine distribution ratios of between 1·7 and 2·0 for human red cells. Gardner and Levy (1972), however, demonstrated that this amino acid was also significantly metabolized by human red cells, and when this was taken into consideration, they found no significant accumulation of the amino acid.

The effect of Na on neutral and dibasic amino acid uptake has been investigated in human, rabbit, rat and sheep red cells (Winter and Christensen, 1965; Yunis and Arimura, 1965; Gardner and Levy, 1972; Wise, 1976; Young et al., 1976). With the possible exceptions of glycine and L-alanine transport by both human and rabbit cells, and L-2,4-diamino-*n*-butyrate uptake by rabbit red cells, no Na dependence has been observed. The Na dependence in these exceptional cases was only partial, and has not been subjected to even minimal kinetic analysis, so that effects other than a direct Na dependence of amino acid transport may have been involved.

4 Kinetic analysis of amino acid transport in red cells

A kinetic approach has been applied to amino acid transport in mammalian red cells in two distinct ways. Most studies have been concerned with the number and specificity of amino acid transport systems present in a given situation, and have therefore concentrated on the interaction of different amino acids in both competition and exchange experiments. In other investigations a detailed kinetic analysis of one transport system has been carried out in an attempt to gain a better understanding of the mechanism

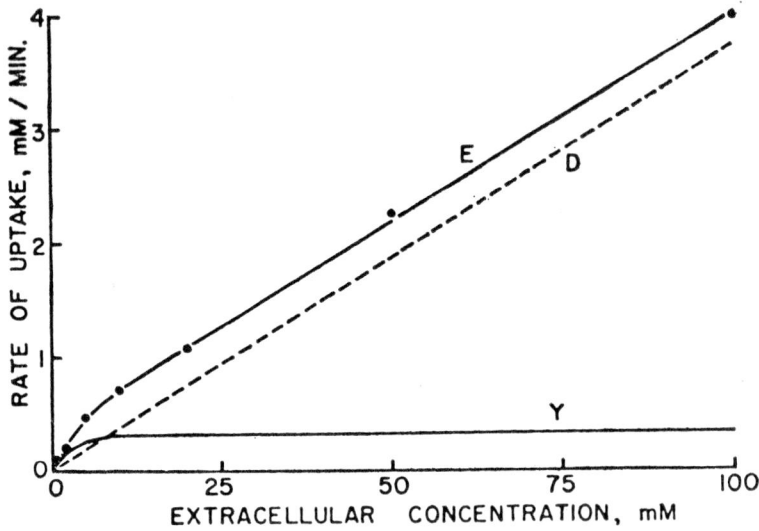

FIG. 1. Concentration dependence of L-methionine uptake by human erythrocytes. The experimentally derived curve (E) is resolved into saturable (Y) and non-saturable (D) components of uptake. Incubation temperature 37°C. Reproduced with permission from Winter and Christensen (1964).

by which translocation occurs. Each of these approaches will be considered in turn.

Winter and Christensen (1964) proposed that human red cells possess three distinct neutral amino acid transport routes: (*a*) a low-capacity saturable system for glycine and L-alanine; (*b*) a saturable system for amino acids with large hydrocarbon side chains; (*c*) a high-capacity, non-saturable route with a preference for amino acids with large side chains. These conclusions were based on the following evidence. All the amino acids studied gave concentration dependence curves similar to that shown for L-methionine in Fig. 1. These curves were analysed in terms of two components of uptake; a low-capacity, high-affinity system, and a contrasting high-capacity, non-saturable route. Kinetic constants for a number of neutral amino acids are shown in Table 4. On the basis of these analyses and additional inhibition studies it was proposed that the saturable route for glycine and L-alanine entry was distinct from the saturable uptake of larger amino acids. However, approximately half of the L-alanine, but not glycine, low-affinity component represented uptake via the saturable system for large neutral amino acids. Similar results were obtained for rabbit red cells, except that the glycine/L-alanine saturable system was usually absent (Table 4) (Winter and Christensen, 1965).

TABLE 4
Kinetic constants for amino acid uptake by mammalian red cells

	Human[a]			Rabbit[b]		
	K_m (mM)	V_{max} (μmol min^{-1} 1. cell water)$^{-1}$)	K_D (min^{-1})	K_m (mM)	V_{max} (μmol min^{-1} (l cell water)$^{-1}$)	K_D (min^{-1})
Glycine	0·3	1·2	0·004			0·033
L-Alanine	0·3	6·8	0·007			0·052
L-Valine	7·0	1000	0·050	2·8*	1300*	0·087*
L-Methionine	5·2	560	0·042			
L-Leucine	1·8	520	0·100	1·1*	1050*	0·043*
	8·7[e]	3120[e]				
	5·8[f]	3390[f]	0·002[f]			
L-Phenylalanine	4·3	1500	0·048			
L-Lysine I	0·02[d]	2·2[d]		0·1[c]	100[c]	0·012–0·020[c]
II	1·3[d]	16[d]				

* 20°C.

Saturable components of amino acid uptake are described by K_m and V_{max}, and nonsaturable uptake by apparent diffusion constants (K_D). Data from (a) Winter and Christensen (1964), (b) Winter and Christensen (1965), (c) Antonioli and Christensen (1969), (d) Gardner and Levy (1972), (e) Hoare (1972b) and (f) Young and Ellory (unpublished observations). All estimations at 37°C unless otherwise stated. For comparison with these data, the K_m and V_{max} for L-alanine uptake by high-GSH sheep red cells were 13·4 mM and 360 μmol min^{-1} (1 cell water)$^{-1}$, respectively at 37°C. L-alanine uptake by low-GSH cells was linear with a K_D of $1\cdot6\ 10^{-4}$ min^{-1} (Young et al., 1976).

A possible limitation of these analyses was revealed by the studies of Hoare (1972a,b), who found that L-leucine transport by human red cells was entirely consistent with simple Michaelis-Menten kinetics over the temperature range 5–40°C, with no evidence for the presence of an additional high-capacity, non-saturable route as proposed by Winter and

Christensen. Data from this laboratory (Young and Ellory, unpublished observations) confirm the results of Hoare (Fig. 2 and Table 4), for although we find some indication of a nonsaturable uptake component at very high L-leucine concentrations, its magnitude is small compared with the flux through the saturable system. The discrepancy between the analyses of Winter and Christensen on the one hand and Hoare and ourselves on the other is large (Fig. 2), particularly since similar methods were used in all

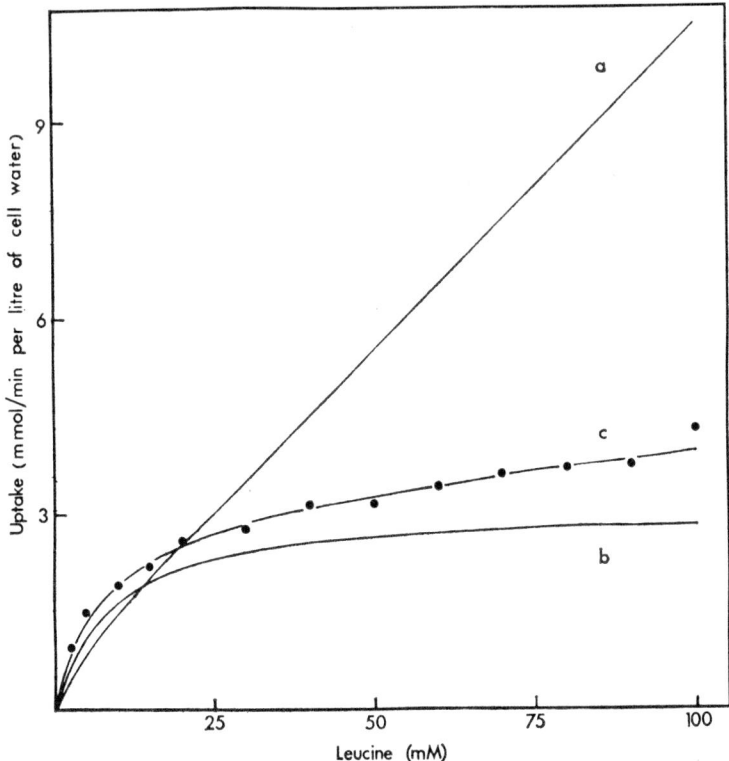

FIG. 2. Concentration dependence of L-leucine uptake by human erythrocytes. Curve c represents the concentration dependence of L-leucine uptake by human erythrocytes as determined in our laboratory by the method of Young et al. (1976). This curve is compared with those derived from the kinetic data of Winter and Christensen (1964) (a) and Hoare (1972b) (b) presented in Table 4.

three studies. Some of the experiments reported by Winter and Christensen were performed on outdated bank blood, and it has been suggested that the low-affinity component may represent an artifact resulting from the use of stored erythrocytes (H. N. Christensen, personal communication). According to Winter and Christensen, L-leucine had the largest non-saturable uptake component of all the amino acids tested. It is therefore probable that only one route exists in human red cells for the translocation of large neutral amino acids. In this context it may be worth while re-examining the non-saturable amino acid uptake also seen in rabbit cells.

By a similar method of analysis to that employed by Winter and Christensen, Gardner and Levy (1972) suggested that human red cells have two distinct routes for dibasic amino acid transport. The kinetic constants for L-lysine uptake are summarized in Table 4. The usefulness of this study is limited because no attempt was made to relate dibasic amino acid transport to the transport of other amino acids. It is therefore not certain whether human red cells have one or more distinct dibasic amino acid transport systems or whether these amino acids share one of the neutral amino acid transport systems discussed earlier.

The transport of dibasic amino acids by rabbit red cells was investigated by Christensen and Antonioli (1969) and Antonioli and Christensen (1969). Saturable and non-saturable components of uptake were observed (see Table 4 for kinetic constants), and on the basis of competition and reticulocyte maturation studies it was proposed that the saturable component of uptake represented a distinct dibasic amino acid transport system.

As mentioned in the previous section, red cells from certain sheep show a genetically controlled low permeability to a number of amino acids which is the result of a membrane transport defect. An examination of the permeability characteristics of normal (high GSH) and GSH-deficient (low GSH) cells (Table 1) suggests that the high-GSH cells possess a transport system for neutral amino acids of intermediate size which is lacking in the deficient red cells. The relative uptake rates of D- and L-alanine indicate that this system (the cysteine system) is highly stereospecific, and it is striking that whereas L-alanine uptake was thirtyfold greater than D-alanine uptake in high-GSH cells, both isomers entered the low-GSH cell at the same slow rate. Further, while L-alanine uptake in high-GSH cells was saturable, it was linear in low-GSH cells (Fig. 3), suggesting that the cysteine transport system is completely inoperative in low-GSH cells. These data also indicate that the cysteine transport system is the major amino acid transport system in sheep red cells. L-Ornithine and L-lysine, but not L-arginine, showed significant differences in uptake rate between high- and low-GSH cells. Since L-lysine uptake was markedly inhibited by both L-alanine and L-α-amino-n-butyrate, but not by D-alanine, it was proposed that the cysteine system has a significant affinity for these dibasic amino acids.

Neutral and dibasic amino acid transport in sheep red cells was further characterized by competition and exchange studies (Ellory et al., 1976;

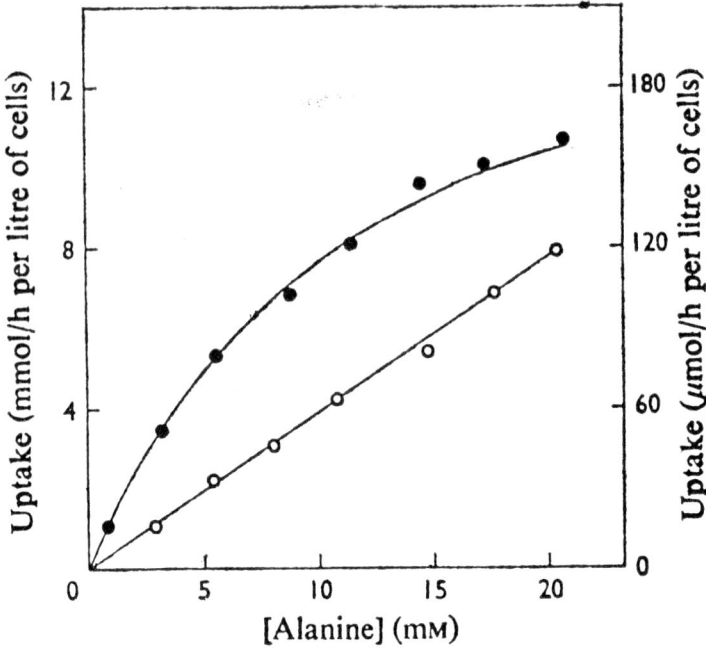

FIG. 3. Concentration dependence of L-alanine uptake by high- and low-GSH sheep erythrocytes. Incubation temperature 37°C. ● = high-GSH cells, left-hand ordinate; ○ = low-GSH cells, right-hand ordinate. Reproduced with permission from Young et al. (1976).

Young and Ellory, 1977). In one series of experiments, the ability of amino acids to inhibit L-alanine influx into high-GSH cells was investigated. Figure 4 shows the effect of L-α-amino-n-butyrate on L-alanine uptake, and demonstrates that the inhibition was competitive. Apparent K_i values for a series of neutral and dibasic amino acids are listed in Table 5. Competition experiments suffer from the limitation that an analogue which inhibits the transport of another is not necessarily transported by the same system (e.g. Christensen, 1975a). It was therefore interesting to find that L-alanine transport in high-GSH cells showed the phenomenon of accelerative exchange diffusion (Fig. 5), an effect which is attributed to the ability of an occupied carrier to reorientate more rapidly than an empty one (Stein, 1967; Hoare, 1972a,b). Thus the presence of an amino acid on one side of the membrane will stimulate the transport of another in the opposite direction if they are both transported by the same system. The ability of the same series of amino acids to stimulate L-alanine efflux from preloaded cells is also shown in Table 5. These two sets of data are entirely consistent with the permeability studies in high- and low-GSH cells, and further permit several detailed conclusions to be made regarding the structural specificity of the cysteine system. The optimal substrates are small neutral amino acids of intermediate size such as L-alanine, L-α-amino-n-butyrate, L-norvaline and L-cysteine. Decreasing or increasing the length of the amino acid side chain, branching of the side chain or the presence of an aromatic ring all result in a decrease in affinity. The inability of D-alanine, D-α-amino-n-butyrate or α-aminoisobutyrate to interact with the system stresses the structural requirements at the α-carbon atom, and the results with γ-amino-n-butyrate, butyrate and cadavarine emphasize the importance of both the α-amino and carboxyl groups. Furthermore, the transport system has the ability to distinguish between L-cysteine and L-serine on the

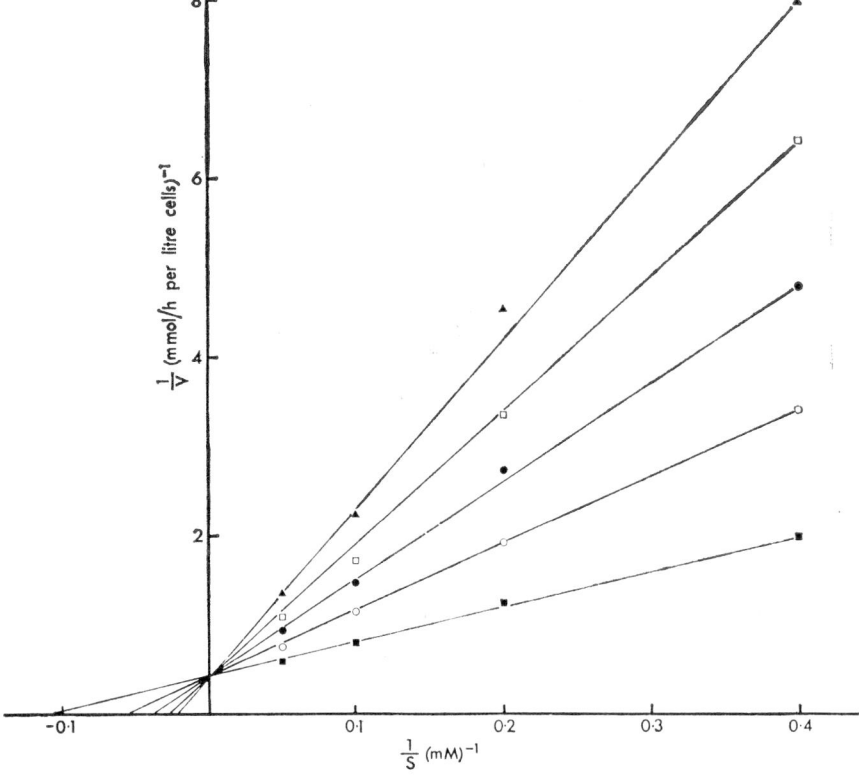

Fig. 4. Effect of L-α-amino-n-butyrate on L-alanine uptake by high-GSH sheep erythrocytes. The L-α-amino-n-butyrate concentrations employed were 0 (■), 5 (○), 10 (●), 15 (□) and 25 (▲) mM. Analysis of these data by the Dixon (1953) procedure gave an apparent K_i value for L-α-amino-n-butyrate of 6·5 mM. Incubation temperature 25°C. Reproduced with permission from Young and Ellory (1977).

TABLE 5

Effects of amino acids on L-alanine influx and efflux in high-GSH sheep red cells

	Apparent K_i value (mM)	Stimulation of L-alanine efflux (%)
Glycine	*	*
Proline	*	*
L-Alanine	†	167
D-Alanine	*	13
L-α-Amino-n-butyrate	6·5	125
D-α-Amino-n-butyrate	*	19
γ-Amino-n-butyrate	*	*
α-Aminoisobutyrate	*	*
Sodium butyrate	*	*
L-Norvaline	8·5	140
L-Valine	41·5	69
L-Norleucine	40·0	22
L-Leucine	*	*
L-Isoleucine	*	*
L-Cycloleucine	*	*
L-Phenylalanine	*	*
L-Cysteine	7·0	143
L-Serine	38·0	89
L-Threonine	*	23
L-Methionine	*	*
L-Asparagine	*	*
L-Glutamine	*	*
L-α,β-Diaminopropionate	*	60
L-2,4-Diamino-n-butyrate	23·0	116
L-Ornithine	*	57
L-Lysine	*	42
D-Lysine	*	*
S-2-Aminoethyl-L-cysteine	*	54
L-Arginine	*	*
Cadaverine	*	*

* No inhibition of influx or stimulation of efflux measurable.
† Under these experimental conditions the apparent K_m value for L-alanine influx was 6·0 mM. Temperature 25 °C; data from Young & Ellory (1977).

one hand, and L-methionine and L-norleucine on the other, demonstrating a high degree of selectivity at two positions along the amino acid side chain. In contrast, the system accepts the presence of a terminal amino group on the side chain. The bulkier guanidinium group of L-arginine is not, however, tolerated. For a system with such a high substrate selectivity in other respects, it is perhaps surprising that the cysteine system accepts dibasic amino acids. This, however, is not an unusual feature of so-called neutral amino acid transport systems (Christensen, 1975a), and Christensen has developed the idea that (Na + neutral amino acid) may be functionally equivalent to a dibasic amino acid in some systems (Christensen *et al.*, 1969; Thomas *et al.*, 1971). This, however, is not the case in the present system, since no Na dependence of L-alanine uptake can be demonstrated.

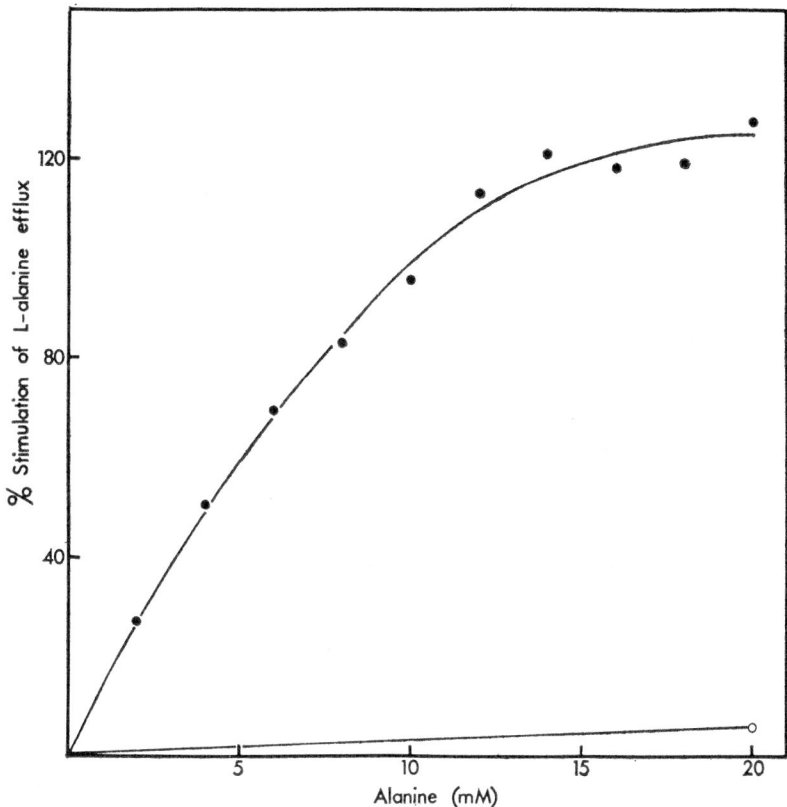

FIG. 5. Stimulation of L-alanine efflux from high-GSH sheep erythrocytes by extracellular D- and L-alanine. Initial L-alanine efflux rates from preloaded cells were measured in the presence of extracellular L-alanine (●) and D-alanine (○) at 25°C. The initial intracellular L-alanine concentration was 10·6 mmol (l cells)$^{-1}$. Data from Young and Ellory (1977).

Furthermore, inhibition of L-lysine transport by L-alanine does not require the presence of Na (Young and Ellory, 1977). Another possibility to be considered is the transport of dibasic amino acids as neutral species. However, the high pK of, for example, the ε-amino group of lysine makes only a very small percentage of the amino acid available in the uncharged form. Therefore, unless the amino acid binding site has the ability to dramatically suppress protonation of the terminal amino group, dibasic amino acids must be transported in the ionized form.

The specificity of the cysteine system, which appears to be the major route for amino acid transport in sheep red cells, is unlike that previously described for other mammalian red cells. However, in this respect it does resemble the ASC system which has been found in rabbit reticulocytes but not in mature mammalian red cells (see next section). The ASC system, unlike the cysteine system, is Na dependent, and seems to be limited to transport by exchange. The absence of the cysteine system from GSH-deficient sheep red cells is responsible for the low intracellular GSH concentration, and may also account for the high concentration of dibasic amino acids in these cells, since a comparison of the permeability characteristics of high- and low-GSH erythrocytes suggests that the cysteine system is an important route for dibasic amino acid transport in normal sheep red cells (Young et al., 1976).

Although kinetic models have been applied extensively to other red cell transport systems, only two serious attempts have been made to analyse the transport kinetics of a specific amino acid in depth (Gardner and Levy, 1972; Hoare, 1972a,b). Both L-leucine and L-lysine transport by human red cells were consistent with Michaelis-Menten kinetics, and simple models involving translocation of a membrane carrier, either alone or complexed with amino acid, have been proposed. Hoare found that carrier re-orientation was the rate-limiting step of L-leucine translocation in human red cells, and that binding of amino acid to the carrier markedly increased the re-orientation rate, giving rise to the phenomenon of accelerative exchange diffusion. Although the kinetic parameters (i.e. K_m and V_{max}) of leucine influx and efflux were similar at 37°C, a marked kinetic asymmetry developed at low temperatures. Hoare interpreted this in terms of an unequal equilibrium distribution of carriers between inward and outward orientations, arising from changes in the activation energies of individual translocation steps.

5 Amino acid transport in reticulocytes

Unlike mature mammalian red cells, reticulocytes and earlier red cell precursors have the facility for a wide range of biochemical operations. There is therefore a greater requirement for amino acid uptake, and it is not surprising that reticulocytes show differences in amino acid transport systems from mature cells. Unfortunately, it has proved difficult to define the various routes of amino acid entry into reticulocytes since transport is rapid and several overlapping systems seem to be involved. Furthermore, most of the published work on reticulocytes has been aimed at testing for transport systems found in other cells rather than exploring the characteristics of amino acid entry in depth. The nomenclature and properties of amino acid transport systems found in other cell types has recently been reviewed by Christensen (1975a,b) and LeFevre (1975).

Following the initial study of Riggs et al. (1952) with glycine, Winter and Christensen (1965) compared the transport of glycine, L-alanine, L-valine and L-leucine by mature rabbit red cells with a reticulocyte-rich cell population produced by treating animals with phenylhydrazine. While L-leucine and L-valine fluxes were the same in both cell populations, glycine and L-alanine transport in reticulocytes seemed to involve three additional concentrative, Na-dependent components not present in mature red cells. Two of these systems appeared specific for glycine, and the third specific for L-alanine (kinetic constants given in Table 6). The study of Na-dependent glycine and L-alanine transport in Ehrlich ascites-tumour cells and avian red cells has attracted much detailed attention over the last decade, and results particularly from the laboratories of Eddy, Vidaver and Christensen have confirmed the complexity of the systems, for example, variable Na:amino acid coupling ratios (see e.g. Eddy et al., 1967; Vidaver and Shepherd, 1968; Schultz and Curran, 1970; Kregenow, this volume). In the present context it seems that glycine and L-alanine transport in reticulocytes shares many common features with their transport in other, nucleated cells, and the Na-dependent L-alanine system has been proposed to be identical to the ASC system defined by Christensen and coworkers in other cell types (Thomas and Christensen, 1970).

Dibasic amino acids were found to be more rapidly transported into rabbit reticulocytes than mature cells (Christensen and Antonioli, 1969). Transport was nonconcentrative, and, with the exception of L-2,4-diamino-n-butyrate, was largely Na independent. Uptake was resolved into saturable (Ly^+ system) and nonsaturable components (Table 6). In the case of L-2,4-diamino-n-butyrate, the presence of an additional Na-dependent saturable system was suggested, although the possibility of a single L-2,4-diamino-n-butyrate saturable system with a partial Na dependence was not ruled out. Cross-inhibition studies indicated that the Na-dependent L-2,4-diamino-n-butyrate uptake was not mediated by the Na-dependent glycine or L-alanine systems. Certain neutral amino acids, particularly L-cysteine and L-homoserine, were found to inhibit the uptake of dibasic amino acids if Na was present. This interaction, functionally equating (Na + neutral amino acid) with a dibasic amino acid, has been pursued in some detail by Christensen's group. It seems that certain dibasic amino acids can act as inhibitors of the Na-dependent ASC system by interaction of the side chain amino group with the Na binding site, and conversely, neutral amino acids, especially with —OH or —SH groups, can act together with Na or certain other cations (K or guanidinium) as inhibitors of the Ly+ system. Thomas and Christensen (1970, 1971) go further in defining the relationship between the Na and amino acid binding sites for the ASC system. Using various hydroxyproline isomers and the alkali metal cation series in conjuction with different chain length neutral amino acids, they concluded that Na and the amino acid bind in juxtaposition, so that a hydroxyl or other polar group on the side chain, if suitably located (on carbons 3 or 4, and *trans* with respect to the α-carboxyl group), can participate in a bond between the two co-substrates.

TABLE 6

Kinetic constants for amino acid uptake by rabbit reticulocytes

	K_m (mM)	V_{max} (μmol min^{-1} (1 cell water)$^{-1}$)	K_D (min^{-1})
Glycine I	0·039	85	0·060
II	6·1	1200	
L-Alanine	0·22	1200	0·054
L-Valine	2·8*	830*	0·054*
L-Leucine	0·99*	960*	0·042*
L-Lysine	0·08–0·19	80–560	0·012–0·020
L-Ornithine	0·18	510	0·091
L-Arginine	0·07	460	0·131
L-2,4-Diamino-*n*-butyrate +Na	0·50–1·11	200–530	0·028–0·058
−Na	1·02–1·25	130–540	0·028–0·058
Difference	0·26–0·17	50–160	—

Data for cell populations containing approximately 60 per cent reticulocytes (Winter and Christensen, 1965; Christensen and Antonioli, 1969). Kinetic constants are defined in the legend to Table 4. Incubation temperature 37°C, or *20°C.

Antonioli and Christensen (1969) attempted to follow the change in amino acid transport properties of rabbit reticulocytes during maturation. One surprising feature of their study was that the nonsaturable components of uptake remained constant for all amino acids during maturation. For the saturable systems, as one would expect, changes in V_{max} rather than K_m were the principal effects, and the authors suggested that there were differences in the rate of regression of the various amino acid transport systems. It was proposed that the L-alanine (ASC) and Na-dependent L-2,4-diamino-*n*-butyrate systems were most rapidly lost, followed by the Ly+ system and finally by the two glycine systems which apparently regressed at the same rate. Unfortunately, the data presented are limited and we feel that further studies are necessary before it can be definitively concluded that significant differences exist in the maturation schedules of the various amino acid transport systems.

Wise (1976) compared the uptake of L-alanine, α-aminoisobutyrate and N-methyl-α-aminoisobutyrate by mature rat red cells, reticulocytes (induced by phenylhydrazine) and erythroblastic leukaemic cells (a model immature erythroid cell). On the basis of cross-inhibition studies, it was proposed that the erythroblastic leukaemic cell possessed three distinct concentrative, Na-dependent systems for these amino acids: one specific for L-alanine and α-aminoisobutyrate (suggested to be the ASC system); one which transports all three amino acids (system A); and one specific for N-methyl-α-aminoisobutyrate. The second of these systems (system A) was absent from reticulocytes, and mature red cells showed no detectable Na-dependent transport. Na-independent amino acid transport was similar in all three cell types.

To summarize, it seems clear that the maturation of the blast cell to the mature red cell is characterized by the systematic loss of a number of transport systems. It is possible that in certain species some of these systems may persist sufficiently long to be detected in mature red cell preparations. Thus, these systems may be responsible for the partial Na dependence of glycine and L-alanine transport in human red cells, and glycine, L-alanine and L-2,4-diamino-n-butyrate uptake by rabbit red cells. Similarly, the reticulocyte Ly$^+$ system may account for some of the dibasic amino acid transport seen in mature mammalian red cells. In contrast to these systems, other amino acid transport systems seem to remain unaltered during the maturation sequence.

6 The role of thiol groups in red cell amino acid transport

The enzymes of GSH biosynthesis and degradation form what has been termed the γ-glutamyl cycle. The reactions catalysed by two of these enzymes, γ-glutamyltransferase and γ-glutamylcyclotransferase, involve the uptake and release of free amino acids, and it has been suggested that the γ-glutamyl cycle may participate in amino acid transport by a number of tissues, notably the kidney (see Meister, 1973, 1976, for details of the proposed mechanism). The finding that both γ-glutamyltransferase and γ-glutamylcyclotransferase were present in high activity in rabbit red cells prompted the proposal that GSH may also be involved in red cell amino acid transport (Palekar et al., 1974). Indeed, Agar et al. (1974) have suggested that this may represent a major role of GSH in the red cell. An unattractive feature of the γ-glutamyl cycle hypothesis is that it implies active transport, since ATP is required by the cycle, whereas the available evidence suggests that mammalian red cells are incapable of active amino acid transport. The hypothesis also predicts that 1 mol of GSH is degraded for each mol of amino acid entering the cell. To test this, we measured the GSH concentration rabbit red cells, incubated in the absence of glucose, during large net transport of L-alanine, L-phenylalanine and L-lysine (Young et al., 1975b). In no case was there any evidence of GSH degradation, suggesting that the γ-glutamyl cycle does not participate in amino acid transport by these cells. Similar results have been obtained with sheep red cells (Young, unpublished observations), and the recent studies of Srivastava et al. (1976) suggest that the high γ-glutamyltransferase activity found by Palekar et al. (1974) in rabbit red cells represented leucocyte contamination of the cell preparation. Previous investigations have demonstrated that the diminished amino acid permeability of GSH-deficient Finnish Landrace sheep red cells was not a secondary consequence of the low intracellular GSH concentration because a second type of GSH-deficient sheep red cell (found in Tasmanian Merino sheep and associated with a diminished activity of the first enzyme of GSH biosynthesis) gave normal amino acid uptake values (Young et al., 1975a).

The possible involvement of thiol groups in red cell amino acid transport has also been investigated by the use of thiol-reactive agents (Young, 1976). L-Alanine transport by the sheep cysteine system was inhibited by p-chloromercuriphenyl sulphonate (PCMBS), N-ethyl maleimide (NEM) and azodicarboxylic acid-bis-dimethylamide (diamide), but not by 5,5'-dithiobis-(2-nitrobenzoate) (DTNB) or iodoacetamide. PCMBS and diamide inhibition were reversed by treatment with dithioerythritol, and diamide was found to protect the cell against NEM inhibition whereas PCMBS did not, indicating that PCMBS acts at a different site from NEM and diamide. NEM and diamide considerably reduced the red cell GSH concentration, but their inhibitory action was not a consequence of this, since L-alanine uptake was only slightly inhibited by concentrations of t-butyl hydroperoxide sufficient to reduce the intracellular GSH concentration to less than 2 per cent of its initial value, again suggesting that GSH is not directly involved in the transport process. PCMBS inhibition was not associated with any significant decrease in the red cell GSH concentration, and the transport system was protected against reaction with PCMBS by extracellular L-alanine but not by D-alanine. These results indicate that PCMBS reacts with thiol groups on the outer surface of the cell membrane in the region of the transport site.

7 The physiological and biochemical significance of red cell amino acid transport systems

In a review of red cell amino acid transport mechanisms it is relevant to discuss the possible reasons for their existence. In contrast to typical nucleated cells from other tissues, the metabolic capacity of the mature mammalian red cell is limited. These cells do not contain nuclei, ribosomes or m-RNA and are therefore incapable of protein synthesis. Nor do they possess mitochondria or a functional urea cycle (Nishibe, 1974; Owczarczyk and Barej, 1975). This absence of an obvious amino requirement may have contributed to the reluctance of investigators to study red cell amino acid transport, and has given rise to a widely held view that these systems may simply be nonfunctional relics from the reticulocyte stage.

Red cells contain high concentrations of GSH, where its major role is the protection of the cell against oxidative damage, the GSH:GSSG couple acting as a redox buffering system. The vital importance of this protective mechanism to red cell function and integrity is readily apparent from the numerous studies of red cell congenital defects in man in which the metabolism of GSH is perturbed (see e.g. Beutler, 1972). GSH is continuously synthesized in the red cell from its constituent amino acids (L-glutamate, L-cysteine and glycine) in two ATP-dependent steps catalysed by γ-glutamyl cysteine synthetase and GSH synthetase (Majerus et al., 1971; Minnich et al., 1971) and removed from the cell by a GSSG transport system (Srivastava, this volume). The possibility of an enzymic system for GSH degradation has also been investigated (see previous section). In rat red cells GSH turns over with a half-life of approximately 3 days (Elder and Mortensen, 1956), and in sheep red cells the half-life has been estimated to be 11 days (Smith, 1974). There is therefore a continuous requirement for the constituent amino acids of GSH, and it is of interest that the major amino acid transport system in sheep red cells has a high affinity for L-cysteine. As discussed earlier, the absence of this transport system from certain sheep red cells results in a considerable reduction in the intracellular GSH concentration. Some L-cysteine may also enter the red cell as L-cystine (Miller and Horiuchi, 1962). Red cells also require glycine and L-glutamate for GSH biosynthesis. Although they are permeable to glycine, they appear virtually impermeable to L-glutamate. It is possible that glutamate enters the cell as L-glutamine (Miller and Horiuchi, 1962; Hochberg et al., 1964; Prins et al., 1966) or even as α-keto glutarate (Sass, 1963).

Amino acids are released endogenously by the intracellular degradation of cell protein during reticulocyte maturation (Rapoport et al., 1974). This may represent the source of the amino acids found in high concentrations in transport-deficient sheep red cells, and suggests another possible function for red cell amino acid transport systems. In this context it is noteworthy that sheep red cells contain arginase (Owczarczyk and Barej, 1975) so that the L-ornithine present in transport-deficient cells may have arisen from L-arginine.

It is generally believed that plasma rather than the red cell is the vehicle of amino acid transport between tissues (Munro, 1970). However, it has recently been proposed that red cells may play a highly significant role in interorgan transport of various amino acids, particularly L-alanine, which is an important substrate for liver gluconeogenesis and which may also participate in the transfer of ammonia from peripheral tissues to the liver (Aoki et al., 1972; Elwyn et al., 1972; Felig et al., 1973). One difficulty with this proposal is that the permeability of red cells to amino acids as determined in vitro appears to be too low to allow red cells to function in this way (Felig et al., 1973).

Conclusions

The data presented in this review provide convincing evidence that mature mammalian red cells possess specific, but not concentrative, amino acid transport systems. Thus red cells exhibit stereospecificity and selectivity patterns and permeation rates which do not correlate with lipid solubility or lipsome permeability data. Furthermore, transport is inhibited by thiol-reactive agents. Red cells also show saturation kinetics and accelerative exchange diffusion, and where the kinetics of amino acid entry and efflux have been investigated in sufficient detail, transport has been found to be consistent with a simple facilitated-diffusion type mechanism, although it has been suggested that a number of amino acids may have additional, nonsaturable uptake routes. It remains to be established whether these additional routes represent simple diffusion through the lipid bilayer or transport via a system with a low affinity for the amino acid. Some may represent artifacts resulting from the use of stored cells. Studies of carrier-mediated L-leucine transport by human red cells suggest that carrier re-orientation is the rate-limiting step of translocation.

It is unfortunate that there have been few attempts to define the number and specificity of red cell amino acid transport systems. As a result the data which is available is often fragmentary and, in some cases, conflicting. Nevertheless, present evidence suggests that mammalian red cells have a number of distinct amino acid transport systems with differing specificities and translocation capacities, but the characteristics of most of these systems have not been investigated in any depth. In our study of amino acid transport in sheep red cells we were fortunate enough to have a mutant lacking a single transport component and this has allowed us to go further towards defining the properties of a single amino acid transport system in detail. This system (the cysteine system) exhibits a high degree of substrate specificity and appears to have a major role in the transport of cysteine for GSH biosynthesis. The importance of GSH to red cell metabolism raises the question of whether the cysteine system is present in all mammalian red cells, since one might expect a certain ubiquity of functional amino acid transport systems. Although there are large differences between species with regard to the uptake of certain amino acids (Table 2), it is striking that the uptake of L-alanine is relatively uniform, and if the stereospecific alanine flux (i.e. the difference between L- and D-alanine uptake rates) is considered, the uptake rate becomes virtually the same for all species. This is consistent with the cysteine system being present in all red cells, but with additional components (e.g. the system for large neutral amino acids) present in some species. Against this interpretation are the kinetic analyses of L-alanine uptake by human red cells (Winter and Christensen, 1964) (see also Table 4). A reinvestigation of the kinetics of L-alanine (and L-cysteine) transport in human cells is clearly desirable, particularly in view of the conflicting data for L-leucine uptake.

It is interesting that reticulocytes have different amino acid transport characteristics from mature red cells. These differences can be attributed to the presence of several additional transport components which are lost during reticulocyte maturation and it will be interesting to establish whether species show differences in reticulocyte amino acid transport or whether the species variations seen in mature cells only develop after maturation. Similarly, it will be important to find out if the amino acid transport defect in sheep red cells is present in reticulocytes or whether the lesion only develops on cell maturation. A certain structural correlation in terms of substrate reactivities exists between the concentrative, Na-dependent ASC system and the nonconcentrative, Na-independent sheep cysteine system. The ASC system has been found in reticulocytes, but not in mature red cells, and a fascinating proposition would be that the ASC system loses its concentrating ability and Na dependence during reticulocyte maturation and is converted into the sheep cysteine system.

Clearly this field has considerable scope and further work on the maturation of reticulocytes, together with detailed kinetic analyses and species comparisons, coupled with modern techniques of membrane biochemistry, promise to provide further insights into the mechanism of red cell amino acid transport. We hope that this review has helped to stimulate interest in what has been a rather neglected area of membrane transport research.

References

ABDERHALDEN, E. and KÜRTEN, H. (1921). *Pflügers Archiv.* **189**, 311.
AGAR, N. S., GRUCA, M. and HARLEY, J. D. (1974). *Anim. Blood Groups Biochem. Genet.* **5**, 63–64.
ANTONIOLI, J. A., and CHRISTENSEN, H. N. (1969). *J. Biol. Chem.* **244**, 1505–1509.

Aoki, T. T., Brennan, M. F., Muller, W. A., Moore, F. D. and Cahill, G. F. Jr. (1972). *J. Clin. Invest.* **51**, 2889-2894.
Beutler, E. (1972). *Advan. Metab. Disord.* **6**, 131-160.
Christensen, H. N. (1975a). "Biological Transport", 2nd edn. W. A. Benjamin, Massachusetts.
Christensen, H. N. (1975b). *Curr. Top. Membr. Transp.* **5**, 227-258.
Christensen, H. N. and Antonioli, J. A. (1969). *J. Biol. Chem.* **244**, 1497-1504.
Christensen, H. N., Cooper, P. F., Johnston, R. D. and Lynch, E. L. (1947). *J. Biol. Chem.* **168**, 191.
Christensen, H. N., Handlogten, M. E. and Thomas, E. L. (1969). *Proc. Nat. Acad. Sci. USA*, **63**, 948-955.
Christensen, H. N., Riggs, T. R. and Ray, N. E. (1952). *J. Biol. Chem.* **194**, 41-51.
Constantino, A. (1913). *Biochem. Z.* **55**, 411.
Danielson, I. S. (1933). *J. Biol. Chem.* **101**, 505-522.
De Gier, J., Mulder, I. and van Deenen, L. L. M. (1960). *Naturwissenschaften*, **48**, 54.
Dixon, M. (1953). *Biochem. J.* **55**, 170.
Eddy, A. A., Mulcatry, M. F. and Thompson, P. J. (1967). *Biochem. J.* **103**, 863-876.
Elder, H. A. and Mortensen, R. A. (1956). *J. Biol. Chem.* **218**, 261-268.
Ellory, J. C., Tucker, E. M. and Deverson, E. V. (1972). *Biochim. Biophys. Acta*, **279**, 481-483.
Ellory, J. C., Tucker, E. M. and Young, J. D. (1976). *J. Physiol.* **256**, 12-13P.
Elwyn, D. H., Launder, W. J., Parikh, H. C. and Wise, E. M. Jr. (1972). *Amer. J. Physiol.* **222**, 1333-1342.
Felig, P., Wahren, J. and Raf, L. (1973). *Proc. Nat. Acad. Sci. USA*, **70**, 1775-1779.
Gardner, J. D. and Levy, A. G. (1972). *Metab. Clin. Exp.* **21**, 413-431.
Gryns, G. (1896). *Pflügers Archiv.* **63**, 86.
Hedin, S. G. (1897). *Pflügers Archiv.* **68**, 229.
Hoare, D. G. (1972a). *J. Physiol.* **221**, 311-329.
Hoare, D. G. (1972b). *J. Physiol.* **221**, 331-348.
Hochberg, A., Rigbi, M. and Dimant, E. (1964). *Biochim. Biophys. Acta*, **90**, 464-471.
Klein, R. A., Moore, M. J. and Smith, M. W. (1971). *Biochim. Biophys. Acta*, **233**, 420-433.
LeFevre, P. G. (1975). *Curr. Top. Membr. Transp.* **5**, 109-215.
Majerus, P. W., Brauner, M. J., Smith, M. B. and Minnich, V. (1971). *J. Clin. Invest.* **50**, 1637-1643.
McCormick, G. J. (1970). *Exp. Paristol.* **27**, 143-149.
Meister, A. (1973). *Science*, **180**, 33-39.
Meister, A. (1976). *In* "The Structural Basis of Membrane Function" (Y. Hatefi and L. Djavadi-Ohaniance, eds), pp. 95-104. Adademic Press, New York and London.
Miller, A. and Horiuchi, M. (1962). *J. Lab. Clin. Med.* **60**, 756-764.
Minnich, V., Smith, M. B., Brauner, M. J. and Majerus, P. W. (1971). *J. Clin. Invest.* **50**, 507-513.
Munro, H. N. (1970). *In* "Mammalian Protein Metabolism" (H. N. Munro, ed), vol. IV, pp. 299-386. Academic Press, New York and London.
Nishibe, H. (1974). *Clin. Chim. Acta*, **50**, 305-310.

OWCZARCZYK, B. and BAREJ, W. (1975). *Comp. Biochem. Physiol.* **50B**, 555–558.
PALEKAR, A. G., TATE, S. S. and MEISTER, A. (1974). *Proc. Nat. Acad. Sci. USA*, **71**, 293–297.
PRINS, H. K., OORT, M., LOOS, J. A., ZURCHER, C. and BECKERS, T. (1966). *Blood*, **27**, 145–166.
RAPOPORT, S. M., ROSENTHAL, S., SCHEWE, T., SCHULTZE, M. and MILLER, M. (1974). *In* "Cellular and Molecular Biology of the Reticulocyte" (H. Yoshikawa and S. M. Rapoport, eds), pp. 93–141. University Park Press, Tokyo.
RIGGS, T. R., CHRISTENSEN, H. N. and PALATINE, I. M. (1952). *J. Biol. Chem.* **194**, 53–55.
ROHRS, H. C. and ARCHDEACON, J. W. (1967). *Proc. Soc. Exp. Biol. Med.* **124**, 645–650.
SASS, M. D. (1963). *Nature (Lond.)*, **200**, 1209–1210.
SBARSKY, B. (1941). *Enzymologia*, **9**, 302.
SCHULTZ, S. G. and CURRAN, P. F. (1970). *Physiol. Rev.* **50**, 637–718.
SMITH, J. E. (1974). *J. Lab. Clin. Med.* **83**, 444–450.
SNOKE, J. E. and BLOCH, K. (1955). *J. Biol. Chem.* **213**, 825–835.
SRIVASTAVA, S. K., AWASTHI, Y. C., MILLER, S. P., YOSHIDA, A. and BEUTLER, E. (1976). *Blood*, **47**, 645–650.
STEIN, W. D. (1967). "The Movement of Molecules Across Cell Membranes", pp. 126–176. Academic Press, New York and London.
THOMAS, E. L. and CHRISTENSEN, H. N. (1970). *Biochem. Biophys. Res. Commun.* **40**, 277–283.
THOMAS, E. L. and CHRISTENSEN, H. N. (1971). *J. Biol. Chem.* **246**, 1682–1688.
THOMAS, E. L., SHAO, T. C. and CHRISTENSEN, H. N. (1971). *J. Biol. Chem.* **246**, 1677–1681.
TUCKER, E. M. and KILGOUR, L. (1970). *Experientia*, **26**, 203–204.
USSING, H. H. (1943). *Acta Physiol. Scand.* **5**, 335–351.
VIDAVER, G. A. and SHEPHERD, S. L. (1968). *J. Biol. Chem.* **243**, 6140–6150.
WILSON, P. D. and WHEELER, K. P. (1973). *Biochem. Soc. Trans.* **1**, 369–372.
WINTER, C. G. and CHRISTENSEN, H. N. (1964). *J. Biol. Chem.* **239**, 872–878.
WINTER, C. G. and CHRISTENSEN, H. N. (1965). *J. Biol. Chem.* **240**, 3594–3600.
WISE, W. C. (1976). *J. Cell. Physiol.* **87**, 199–212.
YOUNG, J. D. (1976). Abstract presented at FEBS Symposium on The Biochemistry of Membrane Transport, Zurich.
YOUNG, J. D. and ELLORY, J. C. (1977). *Biochem. J.* **162**, 33–38.
YOUNG, J. D., ELLORY, J. C. and TUCKER, E. M. (1975a). *Nature (Lond.)*, **254**, 156–157.
YOUNG, J. D., ELLORY, J. C. and TUCKER, E. M. (1976). *Biochem. J.* **154**, 43–48.
YOUNG, J. D., ELLORY, J. C. and WRIGHT, P. C. (1975b). *Biochem. J.* **152**, 713–715.
YUNIS, A. A. and ARIMURA, G. K. (1965). *J. Lab. Clin. Med.* **66**, 177–186.

Glutathione movements

S. K. SRIVASTAVA

Department of Human Biological Chemistry and Genetics, The University of Texas Medical Branch, Galveston, Texas

1 Introduction	327
2 Transport of GSSG against a concentration gradient	328
3 Requirement of energy for the transport of GSSG	331
4 Sensitivity of GSSG transport to temperature and metabolic inhibitors	333
5 Kinetics of GSSG transport	333
6 Physiological significance of GSSG transport	334
References	335

1 Introduction

Glutathione is a tripeptide of glutamate, cysteine and glycine (γ-glutamylcysteinylglycine). Due to the presence of the γ-peptide bond, red cell peptidases which are specific for α-peptide bonds do not cleave this tripeptide. It is synthesized in the red cell with a turnover rate of about 2–3 days (Hochberg *et al.*, 1964; Boivin and Galand, 1965). Glutathione has a highly reactive sulfhydryl group and can neither enter nor leave the red cell (Srivastava and Beutler, 1969a). γ-Glutamyl transpeptidase which can transfer the γ-glutamyl moiety from glutathione to an accepter amino acid was found to be present in human and rabbit erythrocytes (Jackson, 1969; Palekar *et al.*, 1974; Azzopardi and Jayle, 1975). However, the presence of this enzyme in erythrocytes has been disputed (Srivastava, 1971; Srivastava *et al.*, 1976). Srivastava *et al.* (1976) have, in fact, demonstrated that small amounts of enzyme activity observed by previous workers could have been due to the contamination of the red cell preparation with leukocytes. Thus there is no known degradative pathway to account for the turnover rate of glutathione.

Various investigators (Szeinberg and Chari-Bitron, 1957; Jocelyn, 1960; Güntherberg and Rost, 1966) have reported that 2·5–15 per cent of total GSH (2–2·5 mM) in red cells exists as GSSG. However, when N-ethylmaleimide was used to alkylate all the GSH in the hemolysate before protein precipitation to prevent auto-oxidation (Srivastava and Beutler, 1968), less than 0·25 per cent of total red cell GSH was found to be present as GSSG. Red cell GSH can be readily oxidized to GSSG by glutathione peroxidase in the presence of oxidants, such as H_2O_2 and lipid peroxides. The GSSG formed in the red cell can be reduced to GSH by glutathione reductase and NADPH. The GSSG can also form mixed disulfides with hemoglobin and other proteins in the red cell (Srivastava and Beutler, 1970; Birchmeir et al., 1973), which can be cleaved by glutathione reductase and NADPH (Srivastava and Beutler, 1970). When red cells are challenged with oxidants, such as H_2O_2, methylphenyldiazine carboxylate (azoester), or diazene-dicarboxylic acid bis-(N,N'-dimethylamide) (diamide), substantial amounts of oxidized glutathione were found in the medium of incubation (Srivastava and Beutler, 1967, 1969a,b). Evidence is presented in this chapter that the diffusion of GSSG from the red cell into the medium is due to an active transport system.

The transport of GSSG from red cells was achieved by subjecting a 25 per cent washed red cell suspension in phosphate-saline (phosphate buffer, 0·1 M, pH 7·4, 1 part + NaCl, 0·15 M, 9 parts) to oxidative stress by H_2O_2 diffusion in a Warburg flask according to the method described by Cohen and Hochstein (1961). The red cell GSH could also be oxidized nonenzymatically by azoester or diamide or enzymatically by t-butyl hydroperoxide or cumene hydroperoxide (Srivastava et al., 1974). When the red cells in which GSH has been oxidized are suspended in phosphate-saline with 0·014 mM glucose in the case of glucose-6-P dehydrogenase-deficient red cells, or without glucose in the case of normal red cells, a substantial amount of GSSG was found to be present in the incubation medium (Fig. 1). The diffusion of GSSG from the normal and glucose-6-P dehydrogenase-deficient red cell was found to be linear with respect to time for about 4 h (Fig. 2). Incubation of washed erythrocytes with 3 mM GSSG did not increase the red cell GSH or GSSG (Table 1). Identical results were obtained when ^{35}S labeled GSSG was used in the medium of incubation. The diffusion of GSSG from erythrocytes was found to be unidirectional (Srivastava and Beutler, 1969a), i.e. it could only leave the red cells, but not enter.

2 Transport of GSSG against a concentration gradient

The diffusion of GSSG from the red cell exposed to H_2O_2 was found to be against a concentration gradient (Srivastava and Beutler, 1969). In the case of glucose-6-P dehydrogenase-deficient red cells incubated in the medium containing glucose and GSSG, and subjected to H_2O_2 diffusion, the ratio of GSSG in the red cell water to GSSG in the medium of incubation dropped to about 0·09, without affecting the rate of GSSG transport (Table 2). In the case of erythrocytes from normal subjects, the ratio of GSSG in the red cell water to GSSG in the medium of incubation could be lowered to 0·76 without affecting the rate of GSSG transport. The movement, or diffusion, of GSSG from the red cell against a concentration gradient is a very strong evidence in support of an active transport of GSSG rather than a passive diffusion.

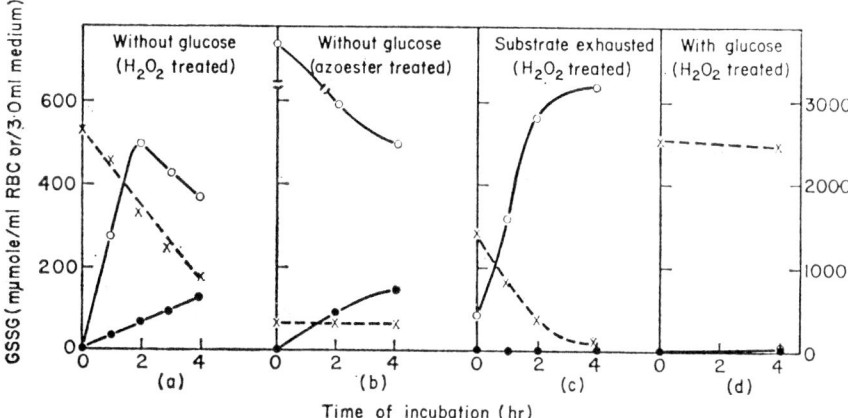

FIG. 1. Transport of GSSG from normal erythrocytes. The red cells were either subjected to H_2O_2 diffusion or treated with methyl phenylazoformate (azoester). H_2O_2 diffusion was carried out by incubating 1 ml of packed washed red cells with 3 ml of phosphate-NaCl solution, pH 7·4, at 37°C with or without glucose, in a Warburg flask with 0·2 ml of 30 per cent H_2O_2 in the center well. The flasks were shaken in a Dubnoff shaker at 100 oscillations per minute. Azoester treatment was carried out by incubating equal amounts of a 1:125 dilution of azoester in glycylglycine-phosphate buffer, pH 7·4, and an 80 per cent suspension of red cells in glycylglycine phosphate buffer, pH 7·4, for 10 min at 4°C and washing two times in phosphate-NaCl solution. 1 ml of the packed washed red cells was incubated in 3 ml of phosphate-NaCl solution, pH 7·4. GSH determinations were carried out with the 5,5′-dithio-bis(2-nitrobenzoic acid) method: GSSG determinations were carried out enzymically after alkylation of GSH with NEM. (a) subjected to H_2O_2 diffusion, incubated without glucose; (b) treated with azoester, incubated without glucose; (c) washed red cells incubated in 2 vol of phosphate-NaCl solution without glucose for 8 h at 37°C and then subjected to H_2O_2 diffusion in the absence of glucose; (d) subjected to H_2O_2 diffusion, 0·014 M glucose present in the incubation medium. ●——● = GSSG medium; ○——○ = GSSG RBC; X---X = GSH RBC. (From Srivastava and Beutler, 1969a.)

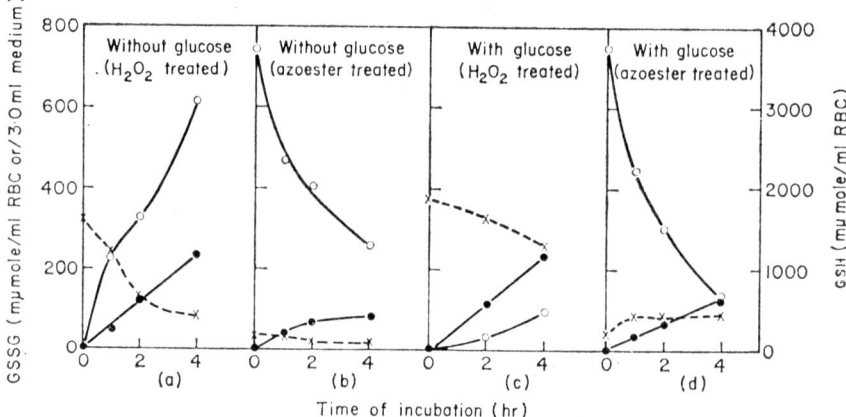

FIG. 2. The transport of GSSG from Glc-6-PD-deficient erythrocytes. Conditions of the experiment are identical with those given in legend of Fig. 1. (a) Subjected to H_2O_2 diffusion, incubated without glucose; (b) treated with azoester, incubated without glucose; (c) subjected to H_2O_2 diffusion, 0·014 M glucose present in the incubation medium; (d) treated with azoester, 0·014 M glucose present in the incubation medium.
●——● = GSSG medium; ○——○ = GSSG RBC; X---X = GSH RBC.
(From Srivastava and Beutler, 1969a.)

TABLE 1

Outward transport of GSSG from normal and Glc-6-PD-deficient red cells against a concentration gradient in presence of peroxide

Sample	Addition to medium	Transport of GSSG	Ratio
Normal (10)	None	191 ± 11	10·55 ± 0·99
	GSSG	221 ± 28	0·76 ± 0·04
Glc-6-PD-deficient (5)	None	283 ± 20	0·55 ± 0·16
	GSSG	323 ± 41	0·09 ± 0·03

1 ml of washed red blood cells from normal blood was added to 3·0 ml of phosphate-NaCl solution (1 part phosphate buffer, pH 7·4, 0·15 M + 9 parts NaCl, 0·145 M) with or without the addition of GSSG in the main compartment of the Warburg flask. H_2O_2, 0·2 ml (30 per cent), was placed in the center well of the flask. The contents of the stoppered flask were agitated at 37°C in a Dubnoff shaker at 100 oscillations per minute for 4 h. The red cells from the Glc-6-PD-deficient blood were incubated in the same way as normal red cells except that 0·014 M glucose was incorporated in the incubation medium. At the end of the incubation period the contents of each flask were centrifuged and GSH and GSSG were determined. (From Srivastava and Beutler, (1969a.)

TABLE 2

Role of ATP in outward transport of GSSG from substrate-exhausted normal and Glc-6-PD-deficient erythrocytes

Blood sample	Post-exhaustion treatment	No. of samples	Red blood cell ATP (mM)			Transport of GSSG (mμmol/ ml red blood cells/4 h)
			Post-exhaustion	After H_2O_2 2 h treatment	After H_2O_2 diffusion for 4 h	
Normal (pre-exhaustion GSSG transport rate, 195 mμmol/ml red blood cells/4 h)	None	7	0.21 ±0.12			15 ±9
	Glucose	3	0.31 ±0.11	0.82 ±0.14	0.31 ±0.05	53 ±6
	Inosine + adenine	7	0.21 ±0.12	1.10 ±0.12	1.11 ±0.32	65 ±02
Glc-6-PD-deficient (pre-exhaustion GSSG transport rate, 240 mμmol/ml red blood cells/4 h)	None	1	0.27		0.16	30
	Glucose	2	0.20			137
			0.27		0.71	106
	Inosine + adenine	2	0.20	1.27	1.31	64
			0.27	1.56	1.54	62

Washed red blood cells from normal and Glc-6-PD-deficient blood were suspended in 2 vol of phosphate-NaCl solution and incubated for 8 h at 37°C. The contents of the tube were centrifuged for 30 min at 1000 g at 4°C and red cells were washed once with phosphate-NaCl solution and ATP levels determined. Red cells from normal and Glc-6-PD-deficient blood were subjected to H_2O_2 diffusion for 4 h in the absence of glucose and Glc-6-PD-deficient cells in the presence of glucose also. Red cells from both normal and Glc-6-PD-deficient blood were incubated with 3 vol of phosphate-NaCl solution containing 1 mM adenine + 10 mM inosine, and normal cells were incubated also in the presence of phosphate-NaCl solution containing 0.014 M glucose for 2 h at 37°C. The red cells were washed two times with phosphate-NaCl solution and subjected to H_2O_2 diffusion for 4 h. The results in the case of normal blood samples are given as mean ± S.D. (From Srivastava and Beutler, 1969a.)

3 Requirement of energy for the transport of GSSG

Transport of GSSG practically halted after about 7 h of H_2O_2 diffusion in normal red cells incubated in the absence of glucose (Fig. 3). There was a simultaneous decrease in the level of ATP (Fig. 3) indicating a correlation of GSSG transport and ATP levels in the red cell (Srivastava and Beutler, 1969a). More direct evidence for the requirement of energy for GSSG

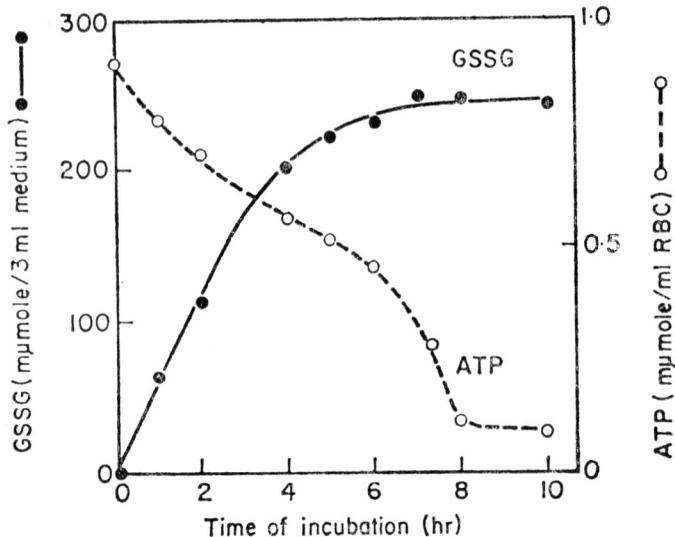

FIG. 3. The relationship between GSSG transport and red cell ATP levels. Washed normal human erythrocytes were suspended in 3 vol of phosphate-NaCl solution and exposed to H_2O_2 by diffusion for 10 h. The content of GSSG in the medium and ATP in the red cells was estimated at intervals. (From Srivastava, 1971.)

transport was obtained when washed red cells were incubated for 8 h at 37°C in phosphate-saline to exhaust the endogenous glucose and high-energy compounds, and subjected to H_2O_2 diffusion (Srivastava and Beutler, 1969a). The transport of GSSG was practically halted (Fig. 1c). However, incubation of these red cells, prior to H_2O_2 diffusion, with glucose or a mixture of 1 mM adenine and 10 mM inosine for 2 h, followed by washing, partially regenerated the transport of GSSG from the red cells (Table 2). Similar results were obtained when glucose-6-P dehydrogenase-deficient red cells were incubated for 8 h at 37°C in phosphate-saline, prior to H_2O_2 diffusion. Incubation of these red cells with glucose or inosine plus adenine regenerated ATP levels in the red cells as well as GSSG transport. Thus, it was established that the transport of GSSG from red cells required energy, probably in the form of ATP (Srivastava and Beutler, 1969a). Prchal et al. (1975) have demonstrated the requirement of ATP for GSSG transport from the reconstituted red cell ghosts. The red cell ghosts were prepared as described by Bodemann and Passow (1972) and GSSG or ATP, or both, were incorporated in the swelling solution. This enabled the radioactive GSSG as well as ATP to enter into the red cell. When the reconstituted red cell ghosts were incubated with phosphate-saline, it was found that in those ghosts without ATP the efflux of GSSG was very small. However, the red cell ghosts which contained both GSSG and ATP had a significantly higher efflux of GSSG.

4 Sensitivity of GSSG transport to temperature and metabolic inhibitors

The transport of GSSG from normal and glucose-6-P dehydrogenase-deficient erythrocytes was found to be sensitive to changes in temperature (Fig. 4). The transport of GSSG was inhibited by fluoride, whereas cyanide and ouabain had no effect (Fig. 5).

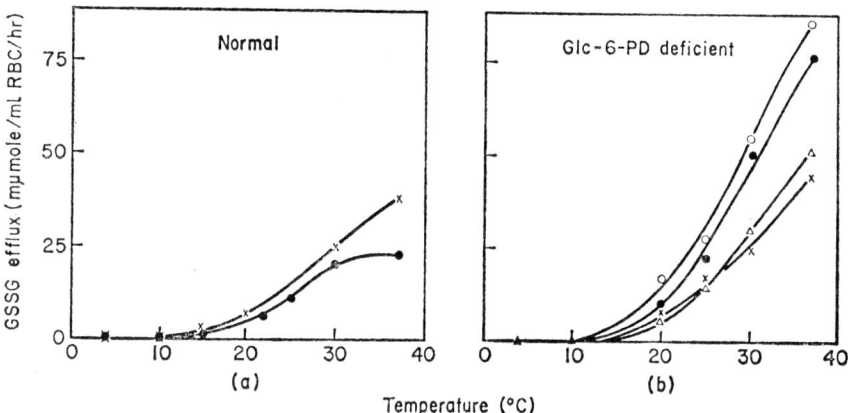

FIG. 4. The effect of temperature on the transport of GSSG from normal (a) and Glc-6-PD-deficient (b) erythrocytes. GSSG was permitted to accumulate in the red cells by subjecting them to H_2O_2 diffusion for 2 h or treatment with azoester as described in the legend of Fig. 1. The cells were washed twice with phosphate-NaCl solution. 1 ml of the treated red cells was suspended in 3 ml of phosphate-NaCl solution with or without 0·014 M glucose. The GSSG levels of the medium were estimated after 2 h (b) or 4 h (a) incubation at various temperatures. The efflux rate has been expressed as millimicromoles of GSSG per milliliter of red cells per hour.
● = H_2O_2 without glucose; ○ = H_2O_2 with glucose; X = azoester without glucose; △ = azoester with glucose.
(From Srivastava and Beutler, 1969a.)

5 Kinetics of GSSG transport

The kinetics of GSSG transport from erythrocytes were studied at various GSSG concentrations (Prchal et al., 1975) by using reconstituted human red cell ghosts in which radioactive GSSG and ATP were incorporated. At lower concentrations of GSSG, the rate of efflux was very low, whereas at higher concentrations of GSSG in the red cell ghosts, the efflux was significantly faster.

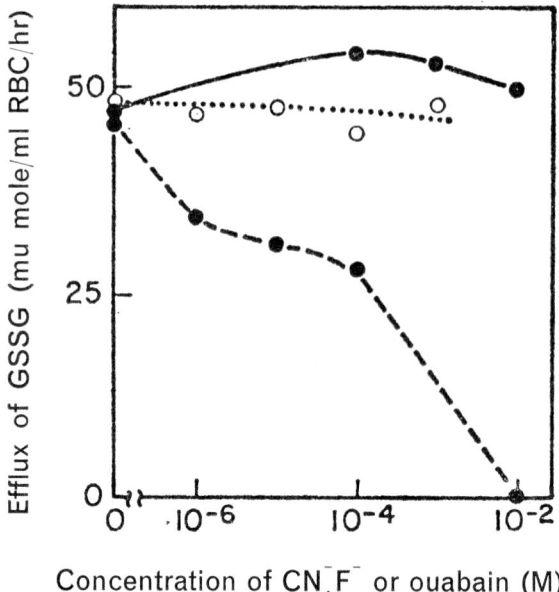

FIG. 5. The effect of metabolic inhibitors on GSSG efflux from red blood cells treated with H_2O_2. The effect of cyanide (○---○), ouabain (●——●), and fluoride (●---●) on outward transport of GSSG from human erythrocytes. The washed red cells were suspended in 3 vol of a phosphate-NaCl solution containing the indicated concentration of cyanide, or fluoride. The suspensions were exposed to H_2O_2 by diffusion and the quantity of GSSG appearing in the medium after 4 h was measured. (From Srivastava, 1971.)

6 Physiological significance of GSSG transport

Glutathione probably acts in the red cell as the first line of defense against oxidants such as H_2O_2. Its highly reactive —SH group may function to protect the membrane, hemoglobin and enzyme protein —SH groups. The GSSG formed in the presence of oxidants, either enzymatically or nonenzymatically, is fairly toxic to red cells. GSSG may combine with the —SH groups of the proteins to form a mixed disulfide. Mixed disulfide formation with the membrane proteins may alter their permeability properties and with hemoglobin may lead to unfolding of the β-chain of globin. Mixed disulfide formation with enzyme proteins may inhibit their activity. Thus, the GSSG transport system may protect the erythrocyte from the toxic effects of GSSG. Kinetic studies of GSSG transport using red cell ghosts indicated that at physiological concentrations of GSSG, the transport is extremely slow. This would indicate that the GSSG transport system in the red cell probably plays a major role only when GSSG levels are significantly higher. However, a definitive conclusion regarding the physiological role of GSSG transport cannot be drawn based upon this system because the red cell ghost is not an ideal system to study the kinetic parameters of GSSG transport. The transport of GSSG may explain the turnover rate of GSH, especially in the absence of any known degradative pathway. Smith (1974) has, in fact, demonstrated an excellent correlation between GSH turnover and GSSG transport in sheep red cells.

References

AZZOPARDI, O. and JAYLE, M. F. (1975). *Biochim. Biophys. Acta*, **389**, 339.
BIRCHMEIR, W., TUCHSCHMID, P. E. and WINTERHALTER, K. H. (1973). *Biochemistry*, **12**, 3667.
BODEMANN, H. and PASSOW, H. (1972). *J. Membrane Biol.* **8**, 1.
BOIVIN, P. and GALAND, C. (1965). *Nouv. Rev. Franc. Hemat.* **5**, 707.
COHEN, G. and HOCHSTEIN, P. (1961). *Science*, **134**, 1756.
GÜNTHERBERG, H. and ROST, J. (1966). *Anal. Biochem.* **15**, 205.
HOCHBERG, A., RIGBI, M. and DIMONT, E. (1964). *Biochim. Biophys. Acta*, **90**, 464.
JACKSON, R. C. (1969). *Biochem. J.* **111**, 309.
JOCELYN, P. C. (1960). *Biochem. J.* **77**, 363.
PALEKAR, A. G., TATE, S. S. and MEISTER, A. (1974). *Proc. Nat. Acad. Sci. USA*, **71**, 293.
PRCHAL, J., SRIVASTAVA, S. K. and BEUTLER, E. (1975). *Blood*, **46**, 111.
SMITH, J. E. (1974). *J. Lab. Clin. Med.* **83**, 444.
SRIVASTAVA, S. K. (1971). *Exp. Eye Res.* **11**, 294.
SRIVASTAVA, S. K., AWASTHI, Y. C. and BEUTLER, E. (1974). *Biochem. J.* **139**, 289.
SRIVASTAVA, S. K., AWASTHI, Y. C., MILLER, S. P., YOSHIDA, A. and BEUTLER, E. (1976). *Blood*, **47**, 645.
SRIVASTAVA, S. K. and BEUTLER, E. (1967). *Biochem. Biophys. Res. Commun.* **28**, 659.
SRIVASTAVA, S. K. and BEUTLER, E. (1968). *Anal. Biochem.* **25**, 70.
SRIVASTAVA, S. K. and BEUTLER, E. (1969a). *J. Biol. Chem.* **244**, 9.
SRIVASTAVA, S. K. and BEUTLER, E. (1969b). *Biochem. J.* **114**, 833.
SRIVASTAVA, S. K. and BEUTLER, E. (1970). *Biochem. J.* **119**, 353.
SZEINBERG, A. and CHARI-BITRON, A. (1957). *Acta Haemat.* **18**, 229.

Genetic abnormalities of cation transport in the human erythrocyte

J. S. WILEY

Department of Medicine, University of Melbourne Austin Hospital, Heidelberg, Victoria 3084, Australia

1 Introduction	337
2 Hereditary stomatocytosis	339
2.1 Diagnosis	339
2.2 Intracellular cation content	341
2.3 Na^+ and K^+ permeability	342
2.4 Active cation pumps	346
2.5 Role of calcium	349
3 Hereditary spherocytosis	350
3.1 Concept of a membrane defect	350
3.2 Lipid loss from the membrane	350
3.3 Cation content and permeability	351
3.4 Coordinate increase of pump and leak	352
3.5 Summary of membrane defects	354
4 Red cell calcium leak in a congenital haemolytic anaemia	354
4.1 A new syndrome	354
4.2 Calcium influx	355
4.3 Calcium concentration	357
4.4 Calcium efflux	357
4.5 Significance of membrane Ca^{2+}	359
References	359

1 Introduction

The mechanisms controlling the cation content of the human erythrocyte have generally been considered within the framework of the "pump-leak" hypothesis. Uphill pumping of monovalent cations against their electrochemical concentration gradient is known to be mediated by a membrane (Na + K)-stimulated ATPase and red cells are unique in having very few pumps—of the order of 500 sites per cell (Ellory and Keynes, 1969; Hoffman and Ingram, 1969; Gardner and Conlon, 1972). Pump rate, however, matches the rate of downhill leaks of both Na^+ and K^+, which are slow compared with other tissues. Moreover, these passive Na^+ and K^+ fluxes show anomalous features which cannot be explained on the basis of simple diffusion through an aqueous pore (Glynn, 1956). There is now good evidence that passive cation influxes are partly mediated by a facilitated diffusion pathway which mediates the inward fluxes of Na^+ plus K^+ ions in equimolar amounts (Wiley and Cooper, 1974). These mutually dependent inward movements of Na^+ and K^+ may be analysed as a cotransport process (Fig. 1) analogous to the Na^+-amino acid or Na^+-

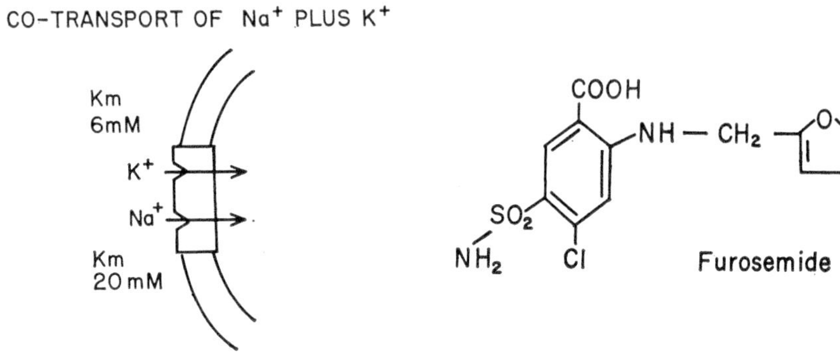

FIG. 1a. The inward cotransport system for $Na^+ + K^+$ in the human red cell. Michaelis-Menten constants (K_m) for each of the cosubstrates is shown.
FIG. 1b. Structure of the diuretic, furosemide which at 1 mM concentration completely inhibits cotransport.

glucose cotransport observed in kidney or gut. Under physiological conditions the cotransport process produces a 1 : 1 exchange of Na^+ and K^+ ions. Nonphysiological conditions cause a net movement of cations through the cotransport pathway so that cotransport is in no way equivalent to exchange diffusion as defined by Ussing (1949). Furosemide (see Fig. 1) has been found to inhibit $Na^+ + K^+$ cotransport in the human red cell and the magnitude of inhibition by this diuretic can be taken as a convenient measure of the cotransport component of the total flux (Table 1).

Some of the hereditary haemolytic anaemias show alterations in the passive fluxes of Na^+, K^+ and Ca^{2+} ions. In two anaemias, hereditary stomatocytosis and hereditary spherocytosis, there is a large increase in passive Na^+ and K^+ fluxes and it is clear that the mutation affects some aspect of membrane structure which is intimately concerned in regulating monovalent cation permeability. Moreover, one patient with hereditary stomatocytosis also showed an interesting kinetic abnormality in the active

TABLE 1

Passive (ouabain-insensitive) Na^+ and K^+ influxes in human erythrocytes

	Furosemide-sensitive components (cotransport component)	Furosemide-insensitive components (linear leak)
Dependence on cation concentration	Influx saturates at high external concentration	Influx shows linear dependence on external concentration
Mutual dependence (synergism) of Na^+ and K^+	Na^+ influx stimulated by K^+_o K^+ influx stimulated by Na^+_o	Influx of each ion is independent of concentration of other
Analysis by Michaelis-Menten kinetics	K_m for Na^+ 20–35 mM K_m for K^+ 5–8 mM	Inapplicable
Effect of enriching membrane with cholesterol*	Inhibits Na^+ and K^+ influx equally	No effect
GENETIC MUTATIONS		
(a) Dehydrated hereditary stomatocytosis	Increased	Increased
(b) Overhydrated hereditary stomatocytosis (patient R.Y.)	Absent	Increased

* Red cell cholesterol was doubled to give a cholesterol:phospholipid mol ratio of 1·8 (Wiley and Cooper, 1975).

cation pump. Another patient has now been described with increased red cell permeability to Ca^{2+} ions, but with normal fluxes of monovalent cations. It is clear that study of such genetic mutants will tell us much about the normal regulation of cation permeability in the red cell.

2 Hereditary stomatocytosis

2.1 DIAGNOSIS

The original description of hereditary stomatocytosis by Lock *et al.* (1961) drew attention to the occurrence of stomatocytic* red cells in a family with

* Stomatocye defines cells showing a narrow slit or stoma on dry morphology.

hereditary haemolytic anaemia of unknown aetiology. Microscopy of a wet preparation of blood showed bowl forms and these are now accepted as a necessary but nonspecific finding for the diagnosis. Later investigators showed an association of stomatocytosis with abnormal cell Na^+ and K^+ content and a consistent finding has been the great increase in Na^+ and K^+ permeability (Zarkowsky et al., 1968; Oski et al., 1969). Their early descriptions of stomatocytes emphasized the swollen overhydrated red cells with an increased mean corpuscular volume. Other families with normal or low cell water have been described and it is clear that there are wide variations in red cell hydration within the spectrum of this disease (Miller et al., 1971; Glader et al., 1974; Wiley et al., 1975).

In general, two varieties of hereditary stomatocytosis have been recognized, one with cell overhydration and stomatocytes on blood smear (Fig. 2a) while the other with cell dehydration shows mainly target cells on smear (Fig. 2b). In families with normal cell water both stomatocytes and some targets are seen (e.g. Miller et al., 1971). Interconversion of targets and stomatocytes has been reported *in vitro* merely by osmotic swelling or shrinking of cells, so it is likely that the cell water content in this disease influences the cell morphology during the drying of blood on a glass slide (Wiley et al., 1975).

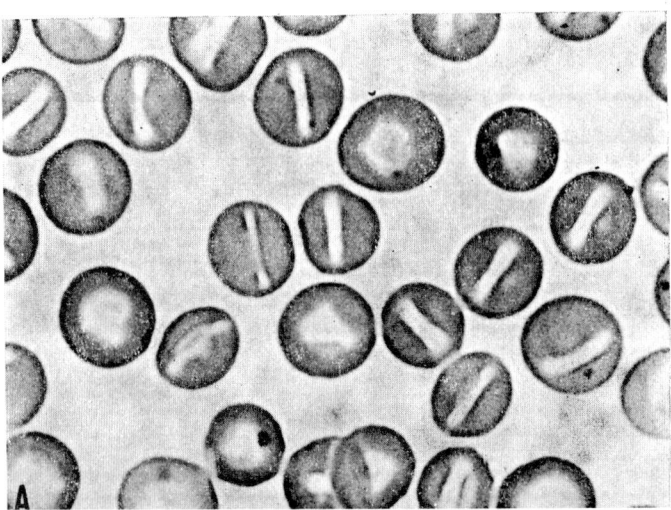

FIG. 2a. Peripheral blood smear, stained by Wright-Giemsa, from patient R.Y. showing overhydrated stomatocytes, i.e. cells with slit-like central pallor. Reticulocyte count 8 per cent.

2.2 INTRACELLULAR CATION CONTENT

The cation and water content of red cells from two representative patients are shown in Table 2. Patient R.Y., first reported by Zarkowsky et al. (1968), showed reversal of the usual cell K^+ : Na^+ ratio and had "high Na^+ low K^+" red cells. The sum of red cell monovalent cations ($Na^+ + K^+$) was 125 μequiv (ml cells)$^{-1}$, which is substantially above the normal $Na^+ + K^+$ of 107 μequiv (ml cells)$^{-1}$. Red cells from R.Y. showed a corresponding overhydration (697 mg water (g wet wt red blood cells)$^{-1}$) compared with normal (658 mg g^{-1}) and this change was also reflected by the reciprocal decrease in mean cell haemoglobin concentration (MCHC). The dehydrated variety is illustrated by patient N.S. who had the typical

TABLE 2

Cation and water content in two varieties of hereditary stomatocytosis

Blood smear	Na^+	K^+	$Na^+ + K^+$	Cell water (mg (g wet wt)$^{-1}$)	MCHC (g Hb dl^{-1})
	(μequiv (ml cells)$^{-1}$)				
Stomatocytes (R.Y.)	87·0	38	125	697	27
Targets (N.S.)	15·1	79·5	95	622	37
Normals	7·9	99	107	658	33
±S.D.	1·5	5·2	5	6	2

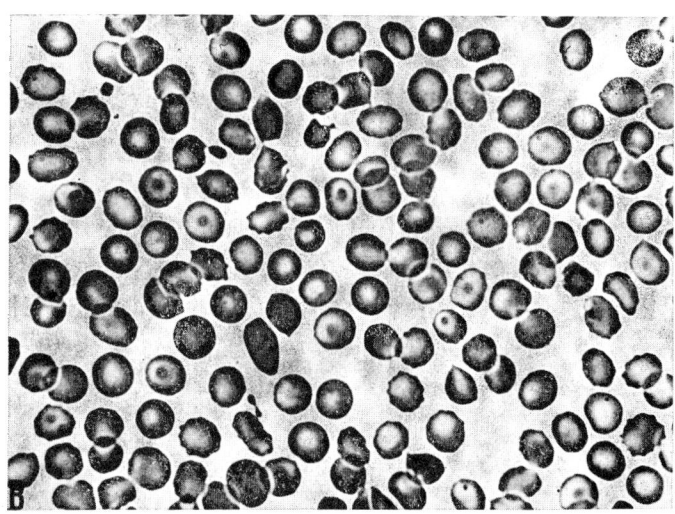

FIG. 2b. Blood smear from patient N.S. showing dehydrated target cells. Reticulocyte count 6·5 per cent.

cation changes of this condition (Wiley et al., 1975). Cell Na^+ was slightly increased (by 7 μequiv (ml cells)$^{-1}$) whereas cell K^+ was substantially reduced below normal (by 20 μequiv (ml cells)$^{-1}$), so that the total sum of $Na^+ + K^+$ was 95 μequiv (ml cells)$^{-1}$, or 12 per cent below normal. Red cell water in N.S. was low (622 mg (g wet wt red blood cells)$^{-1}$) and again there was a reciprocal increase in MCHC. The monovalent cation content of the normal red cell determines its water content (Beilin et al., 1966) and this data in hereditary stomatocytosis suggests the same is true in disease states. The diagnostic importance of the MCHC estimation in hereditary haemolytic anaemias is readily apparent since a high MCHC may be the first clue to the presence of red cell dehydration, i.e. hereditary stomatocytosis or hereditary spherocytosis.

2.3 PASSIVE Na^+ AND K^+ PERMEABILITY

The most consistent finding in hereditary stomatocytosis is an increased permeability to Na^+ and K^+, and since the Na^+ influx is reproducible in the same patient on different days, this measurement is probably of diagnostic value. Na^+ influx ranged between 6 and 12 μequiv (ml cells)$^{-1}$ h^{-1} in the dehydrated variety compared with a normal of $2\cdot0\pm0\cdot2$ μequiv (ml cells)$^{-1}$ h^{-1}, while two patients with overhydrated hereditary stomatocytosis had Na^+ fluxes of 107 and 6 μequiv (ml cells)$^{-1}$ h^{-1}, respectively (Zarkowsky et al., 1968; Oski et al., 1969; Honig et al., 1971; Miller et al., 1971; Shohet et al., 1973; Glader et al., 1974; Wiley et al., 1975). Sodium efflux was also increased in hereditary stomatocytes and both the active (ouabain-sensitive) and passive (ouabain-insensitive) components were raised in equal proportion. Potassium fluxes were raised in hereditary stomatocytes and again the active and passive components of K^+ influx were present in the same proportion as normal.

This greatly increased passive permeability to Na^+ and K^+ may be analysed in another way. Normal red cells show two components of their passive Na^+ or K^+ influx; a "cotransport component" which shows saturation kinetics with respect to the transported ion and a "linear leak" which shows linear dependence on external ion concentration. The diuretic furosemide may be used to distinguish the two components since cotransport of $Na^+ + K^+$ is inhibited by 1 mM furosemide while the linear leak is unaffected. In the dehydrated variety of hereditary stomatocytosis both Na^+ and K^+ influx (in the presence of ouabain) show a nonlinear or saturating dependence on external concentration (Figs 3a, 4a). Moreover, just as in normal red cells, furosemide inhibits a saturable component while leaving unaffected a component with linear dependence on concentration. This furosemide-sensitive component is amenable to a Michaelis-Menten analysis, which shows that both V_{max} and K_m for this system are greatly increased above values for normal red cells (Figs 3b, 4b). Thus in this mutation both the "linear leak" and the "cotransport component" of Na^+ and K^+ fluxes are increased in parallel. Contrasting results are obtained for a patient (R.Y.) with the overhydrated form of hereditary stomatocytosis. In these cells both Na^+ and K^+ influx (in the presence of ouabain) show a linear dependence on the external concentration of the cation. In addition, Na^+ influx is unaffected by K^+_o, the K^+ influx is unaffected by Na^+_o and furosemide has no effect on either flux (Fig. 5). Clearly in this patient the linear leak is greatly increased while at the same time the cotransport pathway for passive Na^+ and K^+ fluxes has disappeared (Table 1). The contrasting effect of these different mutations on the nature of Na^+ and K^+ leaks also highlights the utility of describing passive cation movements in terms of these two components.

Ethacrynic acid has been used as another probe for transport mechanisms in the red cell since it inhibits a large fraction of the ouabain-insensitive Na^+ efflux (Hoffman and Kregenow, 1966). In the dehydrated variety of hereditary stomatocytosis the ouabain-insensitive Na^+ efflux is increased several-fold and ethacrynic acid largely inhibits this flux (J. C. Parker, unpublished data). The effect of ethacrynic acid on ouabain-insensitive K^+ influx is more complex. In normal cells ethacrynic acid (1 mM) increases K^+ influx, while in dehydrated hereditary stomatocytes ethacrynic acid decreases K^+ influx (J. S. Wiley, unpublished data). It seems likely that this diuretic inhibits the "cotransport component" of Na^+ and K^+ fluxes at least in some partial way, but this action seems to be obscured by some nonspecific effect to make cells leaky and cause haemolysis.

Recently it was found that exposure of cells to the protein cross-linking reagent, dimethyl adipidate, markedly reduces the Na^+ and K^+ movements in hereditary stomatocytes while only slightly reducing Na^+ and K^+ permeability in normal cells (Mentzer et al., 1976). Cross-linking reagents thus offer an approach to the chemical isolation of membrane components associated with cation leaks and suggest that an unusual mobility of some membrane component is necessary for the high Na^+ and K^+ permeability of stomatocytes.

2.4 ACTIVE CATION PUMPS

Na^+ efflux is consistently increased in hereditary stomatocytosis and in several patients the active Na^+ efflux was disproportionately high for the observed level of internal Na^+ ions. The basis for this increased flux was

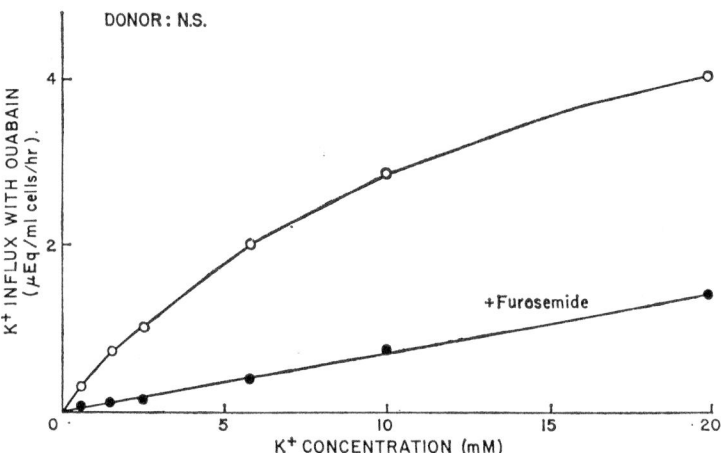

Fig. 3a. Dependence of K^+ influx on external K^+ concentration in dehydrated hereditary stomatocytes (donor N.S.). Ouabain (0·1 mM) was always present either with or without 1 mM furosemide.

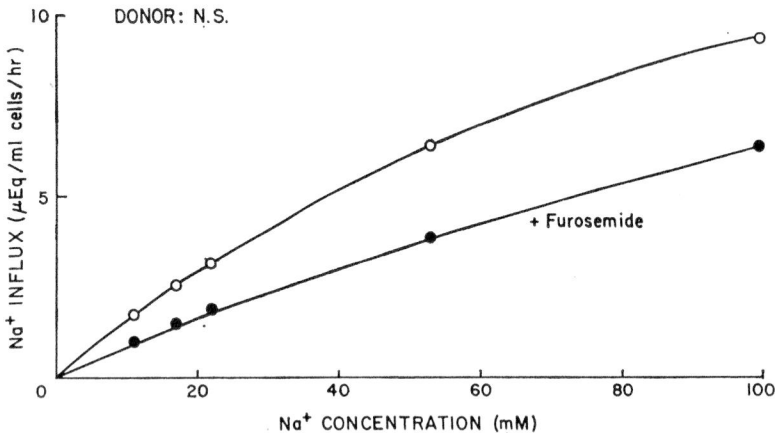

Fig. 4a. Dependence of Na^+ influx on external Na^+ concentration in dehydrated hereditary stomatocytes (donor N.S.). All media contained KCl (50 mM) and ouabain (0·1 mM) either in the presence or absence of 1 mM furosemide.

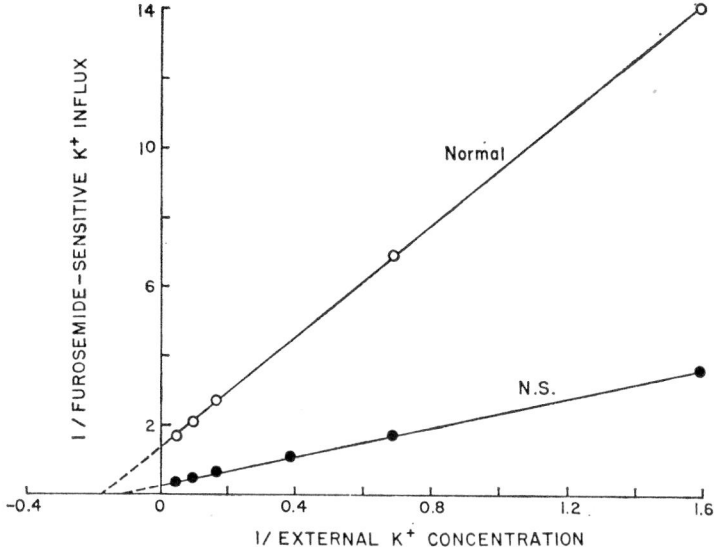

Fig. 3b. Michaelis-Menten plot between reciprocals of the furosemide-sensitive K^+ influx and the external K^+ concentration; for N.S. V_{max} 3·3 and K_m 9 mM K^+. Plot of normal cells is shown for comparison; V_{max} 0·8 and K_m 6 mM Na^+.

studied by measurements of ^{3}H-ouabain binding which showed that cells of the dehydrated variety bound on average 2·5-fold more ouabain than normal. Moreover, overhydrated stomatocytes from two other patients (E.S. and R.Y.) bound 1·5- and 12-fold more ouabain than normal (Wiley et al., 1975). Clearly, hereditary stomatocytes have more cation pump sites than normal and this conclusion is supported by the finding of a higher stromal ATPase in these cells (Oski et al., 1969). The increased number of pumps in this condition seems to be closely connected with the increase in passive Na^+ leak, since there is a positive correlation between Na^+ influx and numbers of ouabain-binding sites per cell (Fig. 6) (Wiley and Cooper, unpublished data). Two factors, cell surface area and mean cell age, must now be considered as possible explanations for the increase in both pump and leak.

Many studies have shown that hereditary stomatocytes often contain excessive amounts of lipid, which in the mature cell is localized to the cell membrane (Jaffe and Gottfried, 1968; Oski et al., 1969; Zarkowsky et al., 1968). In one study a linear relation existed between the median osmotic fragility and the amount of cholesterol or phospholipid per cell, suggesting that the excess lipid contributed directly to the surface area of these cells (Wiley et al., 1975). Red cell lipids of seven patients with hereditary

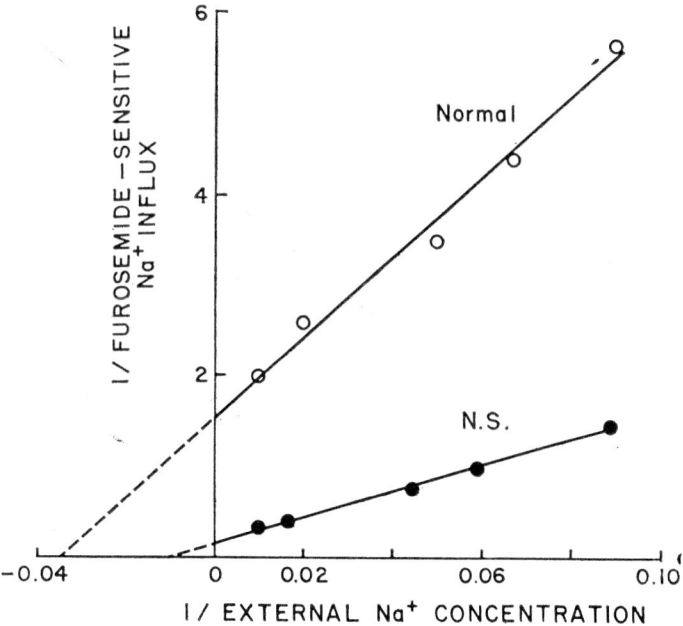

FIG. 4b. Michaelis-Menten plot between reciprocals of the furosemide-sensitive Na^+ influx and external Na^+ concentration; for N.S. V_{max} 5·0 and K_m 100 mM Na^+. Plot of normal cells under the same conditions is shown for comparison; V_{max} 0·7 and K_m 36 mM Na^+.

stomatocytosis ranged from 100 to 135 per cent of normal, although cholesterol : phospholipid ratios (C : P) remained around the normal value of 0·9. The increase in Na^+ leak and pump was far greater than expected from the increment in surface area revealed by the lipid analyses. Sodium influx and ouabain-binding sites were twenty-five- and twelve-fold normal in one patient (R.Y.) but his lipids were only increased by +35 per cent. Likewise, another patient (N.S.) had a 6- and 3·5-fold increase in leak and pump but only a +12 per cent increment in cell lipids (Wiley and Cooper, unpublished data). A second factor affecting both leak and pump is the red cell age, since both active and passive cation fluxes are increased in reticulocytes. Although reticulocytes have increased Na^+ influx, the data of Bernstein (1959) indicate that passive Na^+ movements are only increased by 20–30 per cent in cells with a 5 per cent reticulocytosis. It seems probable that the two- to twenty-fivefold increase in Na^+ turnover of hereditary stomatocytes (reticulocytes 2–12 per cent) was not due to the younger mean cell age of these cells. Although reticulocytes possess increased amounts of cation pump ATPase (Yunis and Arimura, 1966) the

GENETIC ABNORMALITIES OF CATION TRANSPORT 347

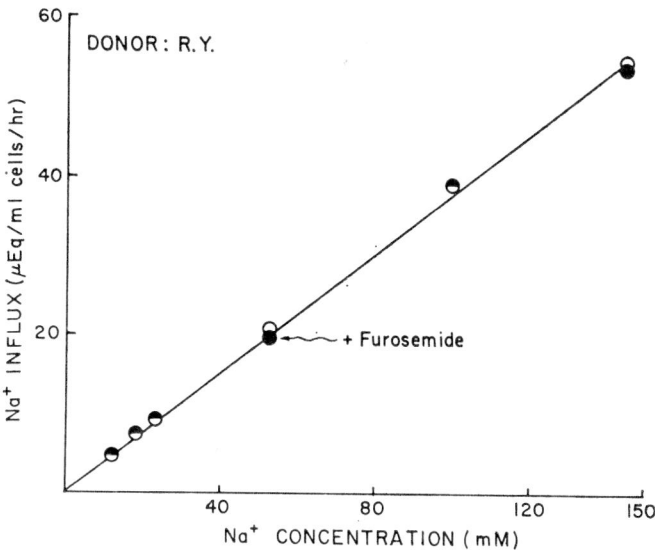

FIG. 5. Dependence of Na$^+$ influx on external Na$^+$ concentration in overhydrated hereditary stomatocytes (donor R.Y.). Isotonicity was maintained with KCl. Ouabain (0·1 mM) was always present either with or without 1 mM furosemide.

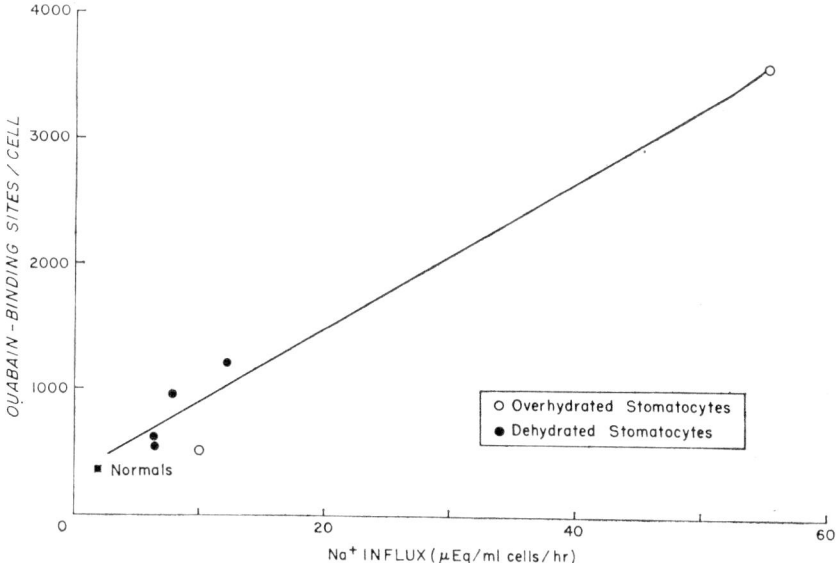

FIG. 6. Correlation of Na$^+$ influx and numbers of ouabain-binding sites per cell (i.e. cation pumps) in six patients with hereditary stomatocytosis.

elevated reticulocytes in hereditary stomatocytosis cannot entirely account for the increase in cation pumps. In one study, the active fluxes of Na^+ and K^+ differed only slightly between a reticulocyte-rich and reticulocyte-poor fraction of hereditary stomatocytic blood (Oski et al., 1969).

Neither cell surface area nor mean cell age can account for the large and parallel increase in cation leak and pumps, so other explanations must be considered for this finding. One hypothesis assumes some defect in the process of membrane degradation which occurs during the maturation of the reticulocyte. Such a defect could lead to a selective sparing of those parts of the membrane containing pumps and leak elements while overall reduction in membrane mass (as shown by the lipid data) would be only slightly affected. An alternative hypothesis assumes that the underlying mutation leads to a variable increase in the passive Na^+ leak. Inward movement of Na^+ would occur in the developing erythroblast and increase the cell Na^+ concentration, which in turn would induce a compensatory synthesis of more cation pump molecules. Such a compensatory synthesis of more cation pump molecules is well documented in a remaining kidney following unilateral nephrectomy (Katz and Epstein, 1967) as well as in HeLa cells which have been exposed to low concentrations of ouabain causing partial but irreversible inhibition of the cation pumps (Boardman et al., 1974). An increased cell Na^+ in the erythroblast might also interfere with membrane lipid turnover in such a way as to increase the lipid content of these cells.

Several studies have investigated the functional properties of the active cation pump. Kinetic parameters such as activation by K^+ and Na^+ have been generally normal while the coupling ratio of active Na^+ efflux to active K^+ influx does not differ greatly from the normal value of 3 : 2. Measurement of active cation fluxes in one patient (J.M.), however, yielded a coupling ratio of 26 : 1 (Miller et al., 1971). When active cation movements were studied both by flame photometry (i.e. net movements) as well as isotope fluxes it became apparent that the high ouabain-sensitive Na^+ efflux resulted from considerable Na^+-Na^+ exchange through the pump and that the $Na^+ : K^+$ coupling ratio estimated by net movements was normal (Table 3) (Dutcher et al., 1975). A further finding in stomatocytic cells from J.M. was that ouabain-insensitive Na^+-Na^+ exchange was greatly elevated when compared either to normal or other stomatocytic cells. Ouabain-insensitive Na^+-Na^+ exchange is carrier-mediated and is inhibited by furosemide in normal cells (Wiley and Cooper, 1974) so that a study of the cotransport system in cells from J.M. would be of interest. The mutation in hereditary stomatocytosis affects a single gene locus so this finding (in J.M.) does suggest that cation pump and carrier-mediated portion of the cation leak may share some common structural element.

TABLE 3

Increased Na^+–Na^+ exchange in unusual stomatocytic cells (J.M.) compared with typical stomatocytes (J.C.)

	Patient J.M.[a]		Patient J.C.[b]	
	$^{22}Na^+$ efflux	$^{42}K^+$ influx	$^{22}Na^+$ efflux	$^{42}K^+$ influx
	(μequiv (ml cells)$^{-1}$ h^{-1})		(μequiv (ml cells)$^{-1}$ h^{-1})	
(A) No ouabain	60	7·5	8·0	5·4
(B) Ouabain	20	1·0	1·9	1·1
(C) = (A) − (B) or ouabain-sensitive isotope flux	40	6·5	6·1	4·3
(D) Net active movements by flame photometry[c]	7·3	6·3	4·8	3·8
(E) = (C) − (D) or inhibition by ouabain of Na^+–Na^+ exchange	32	—	1·3	—

(a) From Dutcher et al. (1976).
(b) From Wiley et al. (1975) Tables 3 and 4.
(c) Uphill net movements of Na^+ and K^+ were derived from separate experiments in which cells were incubated with glucose either with or without ouabain and analysed for Na^+ and K^+ after 3 or 6 h at 37°C. The difference in cation concentration with and without ouabain represented a net movement by the active cation pump.

2.5 ROLE OF CALCIUM

The role of Ca^{2+} in governing the monovalent cation permeability of stomatocytes is unclear. Entry of Ca^{2+} into human red cells has been shown to mediate a rapid outward K^+ movement with little change in the Na^+ content (Gardos, 1968; Lew, 1971). On the one hand the low cell K^+ concentration (mean deficit 14 μequiv (ml cells)$^{-1}$) with normal or near-normal cell Na^+ concentration might suggest an increased Ca^{2+} permeability in the dehydrated variety of hereditary stomatocytosis. However, the Ca^{2+} concentration of hereditary stomatocytes, 4·0 ± 1·9 (S.D.) nmol (ml cells)$^{-1}$, was not different from normal values, 5·4 ± 2·4 nmol (ml cells)$^{-1}$. Moreover, the Ca^{2+} permeability measured in ATP-depleted cells was increased only to the same values as found with control cells with comparable reticulocytosis. Finally, the Ca^{2+} pump seems to be fully functional in these cells since the maximal rate of Ca^{2+} extrusion is normal (Wiley et al., 1975). Despite the impressive evidence against any role of Ca^{2+} in the K^+ deficit of dehydrated stomatocytes, it should be remembered that only minute amounts of Ca^{2+} will cause an outward K^+ leak (Kregenow and Hoffman, 1972) and that current techniques may not detect such an increment.

3 Hereditary spherocytosis

3.1 CONCEPT OF A MEMBRANE DEFECT

The first description of hereditary spherocytosis was by Vainlair and Masius (1871) and their illustrations clearly showed the microspherocytes which are characteristic of this disease. It is now recognized that spherocytes represent cells with a selective loss of membrane area, so that the cell is forced to adopt a shape with minimum surface area for its contained volume. Measurements of cation movements together with the failure to find a glycolytic defect gave the first indication that the mutation affected membrane function. Sodium influx was raised in hereditary spherocytes from nine out of ten patients (Bertles, 1957) while Na^+ efflux from red cells was likewise increased in the one patient studied by Harris and Prankerd (1953). These increased Na^+ movements were confirmed by Jacob and Jandl (1964) who postulated a primary role for the Na^+ leak in causing spherocytosis and haemolysis. While the hypothesis correctly established the cell membrane as the site of the defect it was inconsistent with a repeated finding of normal intracellular Na^+ concentration in this disease (Selwyn and Dacie, 1954; Bertles, 1957; Wiley, 1972). Furthermore, it is now established that there is no connection between the magnitude of the Na^+ leak and the rate of haemolysis *in vivo*, so the Na^+ leak is not a "primary" defect in this disorder but rather another manifestation of abnormal membrane structure (Wiley, 1970).

3.2 LIPID LOSS FROM THE MEMBRANE

Another manifestation of the abnormal membrane structure in hereditary spherocytosis is the phenomenon of lipid loss from the cell surface. Extended incubation of hereditary spherocytes gives rise to a loss of both cholesterol and phospholipid which are lost in the same proportions in which they occur in the membrane (Prankerd, 1960; Reed and Swisher, 1966; Jacob, 1967; Langley and Axell, 1968). It is now clear that no phospholipid is lost until the red cell has consumed all available glucose and ATP has fallen near zero (Cooper and Jandl, 1969b). One study has shown that lipid loss is unaccompanied by loss of either membrane protein or haemoglobin, which suggests that ATP depletion somehow reduces the affinity of an abnormal membrane protein for lipid (Langley and Axell, 1968). Irrespective of the mechanism it is clear that depletion of membrane lipid contracts the surface area and gives rise to spherocytes, which are the hallmark of this disease.

3.3 CATION CONTENT AND PERMEABILITY

Cation and water abnormalities in hereditary spherocytosis are well recognized and consist of a normal cell Na^+, low cell K^+ concentration and both a reduced sum of $Na^+ + K^+$ and low cell water content (Selwyn and Dacie, 1954; Bertles, 1957; Wiley, 1972). This low cell water content is also reflected by the higher MCHC which has been noted by many authors and may be useful in the diagnosis (Erslev and Atwater, 1963; Murphy, 1967). Sodium influx is consistently increased up to threefold normal and this measurement in a large group of patients showed twenty-eight out of thirty had a $^{22}Na^+$ influx above the normal range (Wiley, 1972). The majority of patients with hereditary spherocytosis have a Na^+ influx which is only 30–40 per cent above normal, but since some have a very high influx the mean for all patients, $3 \cdot 9 \pm 1 \cdot 1$ (S.D.) μequiv (ml cells)$^{-1}$ h^{-1}, is almost double the normal mean, $2 \cdot 0 \pm 0 \cdot 2$ μequiv (ml cells)$^{-1}$ h^{-1} (Fig. 7). Some families show a strong tendency for all affected members to have a high $^{22}Na^+$ influx ("high-flux families"). The frequency of this "high-flux" mutation is low: three out of fifteen families in Sydney, none out of eight families in London and one out of five families in Philadelphia had members with a Na^+ influx greater than $4 \cdot 0$ μequiv (ml cells)$^{-1}$ h^{-1}, giving an overall prevalence of about 15 per cent (Wiley, unpublished data). The finding of these "high-flux families" makes it probable that the mutation producing hereditary spherocytosis is not identical in all families, but whether each family represents a unique mutation or the disorder is made up of a limited number of sub-groups cannot be decided at present.

Can the reticulocytosis in hereditary spherocytic blood account for the raised Na^+ influx? Influx has been measured in five patients both before and after splenectomy, an operation which cures the anaemia and invariably increases the lifespan of the cell by a factor up to fivefold. No consistent change in influx was found after operation and this result excludes the younger mean cell age of hereditary spherocytes as a cause for their higher Na^+ leak (Wiley, 1972).

The K^+ permeability of hereditary spherocytes has been reported to be normal and this conclusion is based on the net leak of intracellular K^+ from cells incubated under conditions which inhibit active cation transport (Jacob and Jandl, 1964). Isotopic K^+ influx into cells in the presence of ouabain is also a passive process and values for this flux allow accurate measurement of passive permeability. This passive K^+ influx was greater in ten patients with hereditary spherocytosis than normals (0·70 compared with 0·46 μequiv (ml cells)$^{-1}$ h^{-1} at K^+_o of 5 mM) and the difference between the two means was significant (Ellory and Wiley, unpublished data). The permeability defect thus involves both Na^+ and K^+ fluxes and this conclusion is consistent with the finding of a low cell K^+ concentration noted above.

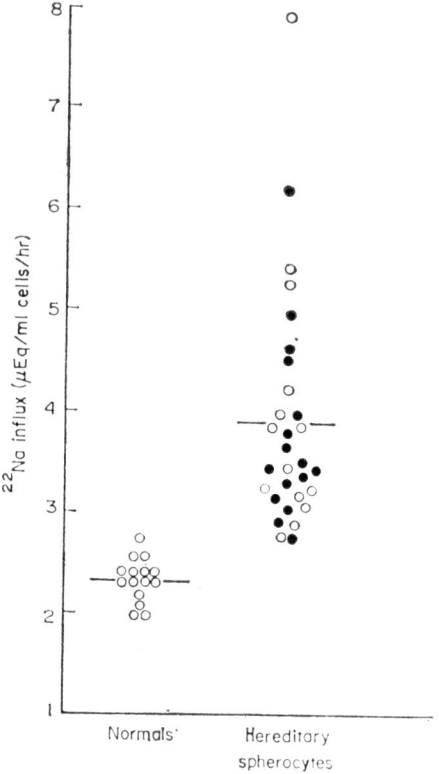

FIG. 7. $^{22}Na^+$ influx into red cells of fifteen normal individuals and thirty patients with hereditary spherocytosis. The mean of each group is shown by a horizontal bar. Patients with intact spleens are shown by the closed circles, while patients with spleens removed are shown by the open circles.

3.4 COORDINATE INCREASE OF PUMP AND LEAK

Hereditary spherocytes allow a greater inward leak of Na^+ ions, which must be balanced by supra-normal rates of Na^+ extrusion to maintain a steady state (Harris and Prankerd, 1953; Jacob and Jandl, 1964). Sodium extrusion is mediated by the cation pump, which will only extrude Na^+ at increased rates when the intracellular concentration of Na^+ is raised. However, Na^+ concentration in freshly drawn hereditary spherocytes is identical to that in normal red cells (Bertles, 1957). This apparent contradiction has been explained by the finding of a greater maximal activity of cation pump ATPase in hereditary spherocytes, when this enzyme is assayed in haemoglobin-free ("white") stroma incubated under optimal conditions of cofactors (Wiley, 1972). Since V_{max} of this enzyme measures the concentration of pump molecules in the membrane it is clear that hereditary spherocytes possess more cation pumps than normal. When Na^+ leak and V_{max} of cation pump ATPase were compared in nine patients with hereditary spherocytosis, a significant correlation was obtained (Fig. 8). Thus patients with a Na^+ leak near normal show a normal cation pump ATPase. In contrast, red cells from members of "high-flux families" show the highest values for cation-pump ATPase. The coordinate increase in Na^+ leak and Na^+ pumps is thus analogous to that found in hereditary stomatocytosis (see Fig. 6).

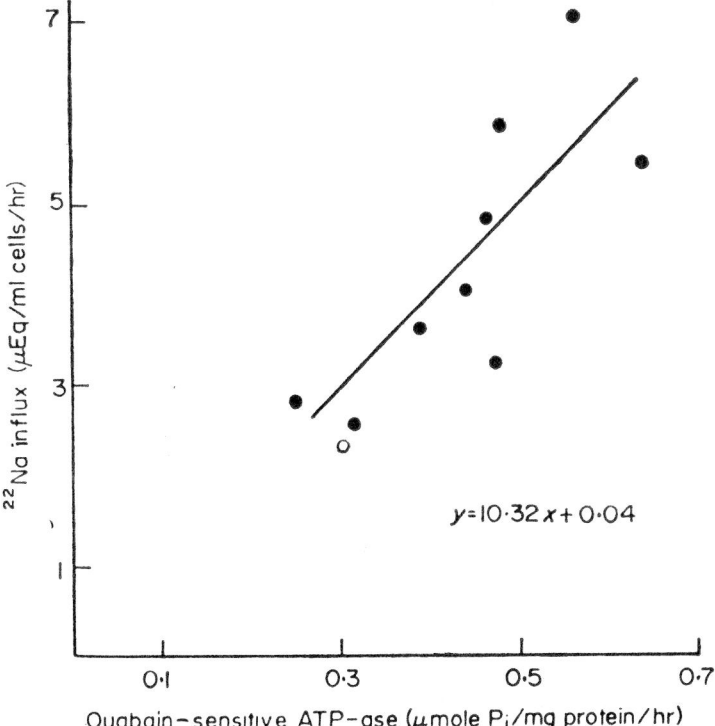

Fig. 8. Correlation between $^{22}Na^+$ influx and maximum activity of cation pump ATPase in hereditary spherocytes. Cation pump ATPase was taken as the ouabain-sensitive component of ATPase in the washed stroma. All patients had been splenectomized. The open circle represents the mean value for twelve normals.
The regression line has been fitted by the method of least squares.

3.5 SUMMARY OF MEMBRANE DEFECTS

It is striking that the mutation in this disease can change both Na^+ leak and pump parameters in these abnormal cells. Moreover, the fluxes of K^+ ions appear to be affected to the same extent as for Na^+ ions. Second, the stability of membrane lipid is reduced in hereditary spherocytic cells, since they show a lower total amount of membrane lipid as well as an increased loss of lipid on prolonged *in vitro* incubation (Reed and Swisher, 1966; Weed and Reed, 1966; Jacob, 1967; Cooper and Jandl, 1969a). Another manifestation of this lipid instability is the greater incorporation of inorganic ^{32}P into membrane phospholipid of hereditary spherocytes compared with normal red cells (Reed, 1968). Both filterability and deformability of hereditary spherocytes is impaired (Jandl *et al.*, 1961; Murphy, 1967; LaCelle and Weed, 1969) and the abnormal membranes show an elevated microviscosity (Aloni *et al.*, 1975).

Whatever the underlying defect in the hereditary spherocyte, its rapid destruction requires a functioning spleen since red cell survival is prolonged to 80 per cent of the normal life span following splenectomy (Chapman, 1968). Understanding of the mechanism by which the spleen destroys these cells is based on the "erythrostasis" theory of Ham and Castle (1940). Hereditary spherocytes become sequestered in the spleen and deprived of glucose by the active metabolism of adjacent cells. Such metabolic depletion leads to loss of lipid and further increases the osmotic fragility by analogy with the autohaemolysis studies. Ultimately these membrane changes predispose the cell to phagocytosis by the splenic macrophages.

4 Red cell calcium leak in a congenital haemolytic anaemia

4.1 A NEW SYNDROME

Fragmentation and distortion of red cell shape is an unusual finding in the hereditary haemolytic anaemias, although it has been described in isolated cases of thalassaemia, pyruvate kinase deficiency and unstable haemoglobin haemolytic anaemia, e.g. haemoglobin Hammersmith (Oski *et al.*, 1964; Nathan and Gunn, 1966; White and Dacie, 1971; Friedman *et al.*, 1973). Anisocytosis, microcytosis and fragmentation have also been reported in several families, thought to be variants of hereditary elliptocytosis, although this diagnosis has been based on red cell morphology (Lipton, 1955; Dacie, 1960). A recent study described a child with congenital haemolytic anaemia, extreme microcytosis and striking distortion of red cell shape in whom there was no evidence for any of the above disorders (Wiley and

Gill, 1976). The peripheral blood film is shown in Fig. 9 and is similar to these rare cases of "hereditary elliptocytosis" and to three other patients recently described with haemolytic anaemia and an abnormal sensitivity of red cells to thermal fragmentation (Zarkowsky *et al.*, 1975). The cases studied by Wiley and Gill (1976) and by Zarkowsky *et al.*, (1975) show unique haematological features which suggests they form a new syndrome or distinct entity. Microcytes are prominent and the mean corpuscular volume was as low as 25 fl (normal 82–98 fl) in one case. MCHC is normal or high-normal while the osmotic fragility of fresh blood is markedly increased. Autohaemolysis of blood is increased and additional glucose gives only partial or no correction. Finally, splenectomy improves the anaemia although it does not completely prevent the haemolytic process. Cation permeability studies have established that the red cell membrane is abnormal in this syndrome.

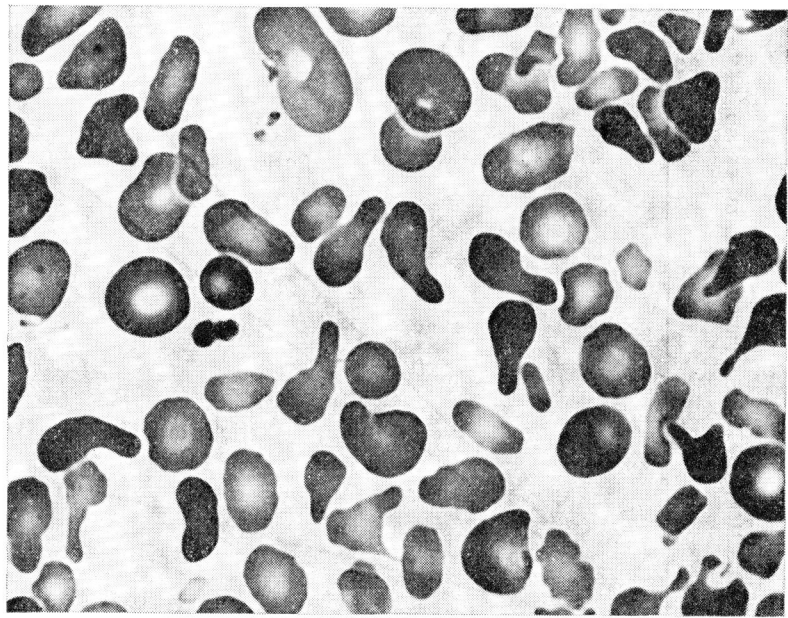

Fig. 9. Morphology of red cells on a stained smear after splenectomy. Fragmentation and microcytosis are evident. Mean corpuscular volume was 25 fl.

4.2 CALCIUM INFLUX

Measurement of Ca^{2+} influx in human red cells is complicated by the extremely low Ca^{2+} permeability of the mature cell, which is approximately a thousandfold less than the corresponding Na^+ permeability. Furthermore, the Ca^{2+} concentration of normal red cells is extremely low and is maintained by the activity of a Ca^{2+} pump which is a membrane ATPase which extrudes Ca^{2+} from the cell (Schatzmann and Vincenzi, 1969; Cha et al., 1971). The inward movement of Ca^{2+} is best studied under conditions in which the pump is inactive, such as in cells which have been depleted of ATP (Lew, 1971; Kregenow and Hoffman, 1972). ATP depletion is achieved by short incubation (2 h) of cells with inosine plus either iodoacetamide or iodoacetic acid; the cells are washed and then added to media at 37°C containing physiological levels of ionized Ca^{2+} (1·5 mM). A rapid uptake of isotopic Ca^{2+} of 2 nmol (ml cells)$^{-1}$ occurs into normal cells within several minutes followed by a slower uptake of about 1 nmol Ca^{2+} (ml cells)$^{-1}$ h^{-1} up to 4 h of incubation (Fig. 10).

The abnormal cells take up Ca^{2+} at rates almost tenfold above normal

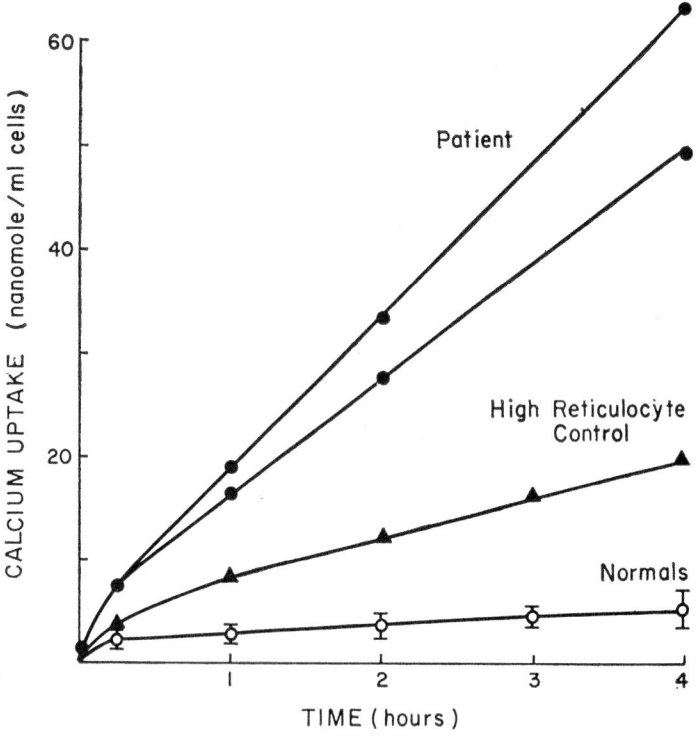

FIG. 10. Calcium uptake by patient's red cells. Patient had 2·0 per cent and 2·3 per cent reticulocytes when tested on two occasions (●), while control cells has 3·7 per cent reticulocytes (▲). Mean values for normal cells (○) show ±1 S.D. by the vertical bars.

mature cells. Reticulocytes also have an increased Ca^{2+} permeability but the abnormal cells still show a two- to threefold greater Ca^{2+} influx than control cells with the same percentage reticulocytes (Fig. 10). In contrast to this increased Ca^{2+} permeability, the abnormal cells in this syndrome exhibit a completely normal Na^+ and K^+ influx. Cell water content and the intracellular concentration of Na^+ and K^+ ions is also normal, so the defect seems to be selective for Ca^{2+} ions (Wiley and Gill, 1976).

4.3 CALCIUM CONCENTRATION

Measurement of red cell Ca^{2+} by atomic absorption spectroscopy shows that the abnormal cells contain increased amounts of this cation. Normal red cells contain 5.4 ± 2.4 nmol Ca^{2+} (ml cells)$^{-1}$ (n = 11). On four separate occasions, the patient's red cells contained 13·5, 10·0, 16·4 and 16·9 nmol Ca^{2+} (ml cells)$^{-1}$ so that the mean cell Ca^{2+} of 14.2 ± 3.1 nmol (ml cells) is significantly higher than normal (Wiley and Gill, 1976). The slight reticulocytosis in the patient's red cells cannot explain their higher Ca^{2+} levels, since reticulocyte-rich red cells have a normal Ca^{2+} concentration (Wiley and Shaller, unpublished). Mean values of 16 and 15 nmol Ca^{2+} (ml cells)$^{-1}$ have been obtained for normal red cells by Harrison and Long (1968) and Lichtman and Weed (1972). However, the concept of a "true" red cell Ca^{2+} concentration is probably inappropriate since cell Ca^{2+} depends on many factors such as ambient Ca^{2+} levels and the number of saline washes prior to dry ashing of red cells. Despite the lower values for normal cell Ca^{2+} obtained by Wiley and Gill (1976) their analyses were performed by the same method with paired observations, which validates the major conclusion that the patient's red cells have a higher Ca^{2+} concentration relative to normals.

The location of the red cell Ca^{2+} was established by haemolysing washed red cells in 10 vol of 5 mM Tris-HCl buffer, pH 7·4, and separating the stroma by centrifugation. Stroma from the patient contain 55 per cent of the total cell Ca^{2+}; normal stroma contain 35 per cent.

4.4 CALCIUM EFFLUX

The above results show that membrane Ca^{2+} content is increased in this syndrome. Supporting evidence for this conclusion comes from measurements of Ca^{2+} efflux (Wiley and Gill, 1976). When red cells are loaded with 0·6–0·7 µmol Ca^{2+} (ml cells)$^{-1}$ at 0°C and subsequently reincubated at 37°C, a rapid extrusion of Ca^{2+} occurs. This efflux consists of at least two kinetic components. An initial component of about 20 per cent of cell Ca^{2+} is lost within the first 30 sec with kinetics which are too rapid to study by standard pipetting techniques. Extrusion of the major fraction of cell Ca^{2+} is less rapid and follows first-order kinetics with a half-time of 2·1 min (Fig. 11). This second component probably represents the efflux mediated by the Ca^{2+} pump.

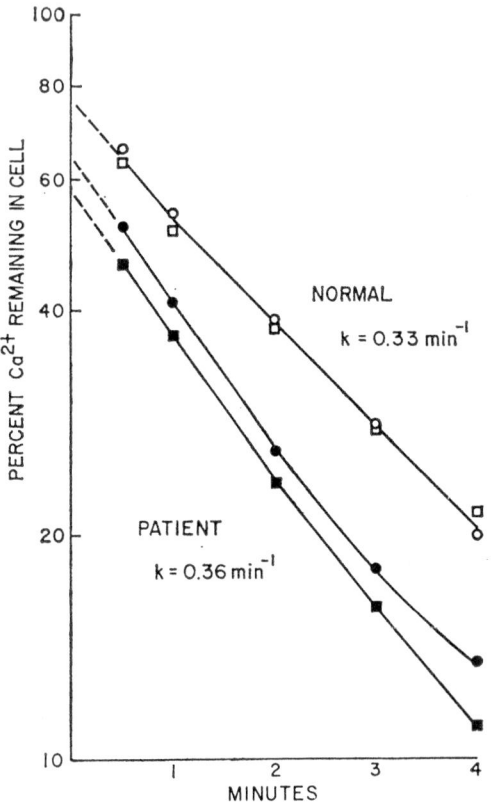

FIG. 11. Calcium extrusion from red cells. Cells were preloaded with Ca^{2+} at 0°C and reincubated at 37°C in media containing no Ca^{2+} (○, ●) or 1·5 mM Ca^{2+} (□, ■). Initial cell calcium was 0·7 and 0·6 μmol (ml cells)$^{-1}$ for normal and patient, respectively.

Calcium extrusion from the patient's red cells show one important difference from normal—the rapid initial Ca^{2+} loss is increased about double to 40 per cent of the initial cell Ca^{2+} concentration (Fig. 11). The magnitude of this rapid initial loss is estimated graphically by extrapolating the time-course of Ca^{2+} extrusion back beyond the 0·5 min point to zero time (dotted lines in Fig. 11). The value of cell Ca^{2+} where this extrapolation intersects zero time is then subtracted from initial cell Ca^{2+} to give the amount of rapidly extruded Ca^{2+}. Rapid initial Ca^{2+} loss for the patient is 35–42 per cent of initial cell Ca^{2+} (20 per cent for normals) then the major fraction of cell Ca^{2+} is extruded with kinetics almost identical to normal. It appears that the rapid initial loss of cell Ca^{2+} represents a fraction of cell Ca^{2+} which is bound to the plasma membrane in a superficial and readily exchangeable location. This intramembranous Ca^{2+} seems to be increased about double in the abnormal cells and this conclusion is consistent with the direct analysis of stromal Ca^{2+}.

4.5 SIGNIFICANCE OF MEMBRANE Ca^{2+}

The association of haemolytic anaemia with increased cell Ca^{2+} content may suggest a deleterious effect of this cation on the survival of the cell. Accumulation of intracellular Ca^{2+} markedly reduces filterability and increases viscosity of the human red cell. Since the same effect is apparent in haemoglobin-poor ghosts, it appears that Ca^{2+} reduces the deformability of the cell membrane (Weed et al., 1969). Red cells from the patient studied by Wiley and Gill (1976) failed to pass through polycarbonate filters with 3 μm nominal pores. This reduced filterability is consistent with the increased membrane Ca^{2+} content and suggests membrane rigidity as a cause of the haemolysis. It may be inferred from the beneficial effect of splenectomy that this organ is the major site of cell destruction. Marked distortion of the red cell must occur as it passes from splenic cord into splenic sinus through gaps between endothelial cells. Clearly the abnormal cells are less able to traverse these narrow segments of the microvasculature. The finding of mutant red cells with increased membrane Ca^{2+} and reduced deformability both *in vitro* and *in vivo* (i.e. splenic destruction) confirms the significance of membrane Ca^{2+} which has been proposed by Weed *et al.* (1969) as one determinant of red cell lifespan.

References

ALONI, B., SHINITZKY, M., MOSES, S. and LIVNE, A. (1975). *Brit. J. Haemat.* **31**, 117.
BEILIN, L. J., KNIGHT, G. J., MUNRO-FAURE, A. D. and ANDERSON, J. (1966). *J. Clin. Invest.* **45**, 1817.
BERNSTEIN, R. E. (1959). *J. Clin. Invest.* **38**, 1572.
BERTLES, J. F. (1957). *J. Clin. Invest.* **36**, 816.
BOARDMAN, L., HUETT, M., LAMB, J. F., NEWTON, J. P. and POLSON, J. M. (1974). *J. Physiol.* **241**, 771
CHA, Y. N., SHIN, B. C. and LEE, K. S. (1971). *J. Gen. Physiol.* **57**, 202.
CHAPMAN, R. G. (1968). *J. Clin. Invest.* **47**, 2263.
COOPER, R. A. and JANDL, J. H. (1969a). *J. Clin. Invest.* **48**, 736.
COOPER, R. A. and JANDL, J. H. (1969b). *J. Clin. Invest.* **48**, 906.

DACIE, J. V. (1960). "The Haemolytic Anaemias Congenital and Acquired. Part 1. The Congenital Anaemias", 2nd edit., p. 160. Crune and Stratton, New York.
DUTCHER, P. O., SEGEL, G. B., FEIG, S. A., MILLER, D. R. and KLEMPERER, M. R. (1975). *Paediat. Res.* **9**, 924.
ELLORY, J. C. and KEYNES, R. D. (1969). *Nature*, **221**, 776.
ERSLEV, A. J. and ATWATER, J. (1963). *J. Lab. Clin. Med.* **62**, 401.
FRIEDMAN, S., OZSOYLU, S., LUDDY, R. and SCHWARTZ, E. (1976). *Brit. J. Haemat.* **32**, 65.
GARDNER, J. D. and CONLON, T. P. (1972). *J. Gen. Physiol.* **60**, 609.
GARDOS, G. (1968). *Biochim. Biophys. Acta*, **30**, 653.
GLADER, B. E., FORTIER, N., ALBALA, M. M. and NATHAN, D. G. (1974). *New Engl. J. Med.* **291**, 491.
GLYNN, I. M. (1956). *J. Physiol.* **134**, 278.
HAM, T. H. and CASTLE, W. M. (1940). *Trans. Assoc. Am. Physns.* **55**, 127.
HARRIS, E. J. and PRANKERD, T. A. J. (1953). *J. Physiol.* **121**, 470.
HARRIS, D. G. and LONG, C. (1968). *J. Physiol.* **199**, 367.
HOFFMAN, J. F. and INGRAM, C. J. (1969). *In* "Proceedings of the First International Symposium on Metabolism and Membrane Permeability of Erythrocytes and Thrombocytes", p. 420. Georg Thieme, Stuttgart.
HOFFMAN, J. F. and KREGENOW, F. M. (1966). *Ann. N.Y. Acad. Sci.* **137**, 566.
HONIG, G. R., LACSOW, P. S. and MAURER, H. S. (1971). *Pediat. Res.* **5**, 159.
JACOB, H. S. (1967). *J. Clin. Invest.* **46**, 2083.
JACOB, H. S. and JANDL, J. H. (1964). *J. Clin. Invest.* **43**, 1704.
JAFFE, E. R. and GOTTFRIED, E. L. (1968). *J. Clin. Invest.* **47**, 1375.
JANDL, J. H., SIMMONS, R. S. and CASTLE, W. B. (1961). *Blood*, **18**, 133.
KATZ, A. I. and EPSTEIN, F. H. (1967). *J. Clin. Invest.* **46**, 1999.
KREGENOW, F. M. and HOFFMAN, J. F. (1972). *J. Gen. Physiol.* **60**, 406.
LACELLE, P. L. and WEED, R. I. (1969). *J. Clin. Invest.* **48**, 48a.
LANGLEY, G. R. and AXELL, M. (1968). *Brit. J. Haemat.* **14**, 593.
LEW, V. L. (1971). *Biochim. Biophys. Acta*, **233**, 827.
LICHTMAN, M. A. and WEED, R. I. (1972). *Nouv. Rev. Franc. Hemat.* **12**, 79.
LIPTON, E. L. (1955). *Pediatrics*, **15**, 67.
LOCK, S. P., SEPHTON SMITH, R. and HARDISTY, R. M. (1961). *Brit. J. Haemat.* **7**, 303.
MENTZER, W. C., LUBIN, B. H. and EMMONS, S. (1976). *New Engl. J. Med.* **294**, 1200.
MILLER, D. R., RICKLES, F. R., LICHTMAN, M. A., LACELLE, P. L., BATES, J. and WEED, R. I. (1971). *Blood*, **38**, 184.
MURPHY, J. R. (1967). *J. Lab. Clin. Med.* **69**, 758.
NATHAN, D. G. and GUNN, R. B. (1966). *Amer. J. Med.* **41**, 815.
OSKI, F. A., NAIMAN, J. L., BLUM, S. F., ZARKOWSKY, H. S., WHAUN, J., SHOHET, S. B., GREEN, A. and NATHAN, D. G. (1969). *New Engl. J. Med.* **280**, 909.
OSKI, F. A., NATHAN, D. G., SIDEL, V. W. and DIAMOND, L. K. (1964). *New Engl. J. Med.* **270**, 1023.
PRANKERD, T. A. J. (1960). *Q. J. Med.* **29**, 199.
REED, C. F. (1968). *J. Clin. Invest.* **47**, 2630.
REED, C. F. and SWISHER, S. N. (1966). *J. Clin. Invest.* **45**, 777.
SCHATZMANN, H. J. and VINCENZI, F. F. (1969). *J. Physiol.* **201**, 369.
SELWYN, J. G. and DACIE, J. V. (1954). *Blood*, **9**, 414.
SHOHET, S. B., NATHAN, D. G., LIVERMORE, B. M., FEIG, S. A. and JAFFE, E. R. (1973). *Blood*, **41**, 1.

USSING, H. H. (1949). *Physiol. Rev.* **29**, 127.
VANLAIR, C. and MASIUS, P. (1871). *Bull. Acad. r. Med. Belg.* **5** (3rd series), 515.
WEED, R. I., LACELLE, P. L. and MERRILL, E. W. (1969). *J. Clin. Invest.* **48**, 795.
WEED, R. I. and REED, C. F. (1966). *Amer. J. Med.* **41**, 795.
WHITE, J. M. and DACIE, J. V. (1971). *Progress in Hematology*, **7**, 69.
WILEY, J. S. (1970). *J. Clin. Invest.* **49**, 666.
WILEY, J. S. (1972). *Brit. J. Haemat.* **22**, 529.
WILEY, J. S. and COOPER, R. A. (1974). *J. Clin. Invest.* **53**, 745.
WILEY, J. S. and COOPER, R. A. (1975). *Biochim. Biophys. Acta*, **413**, 425.
WILEY, J. S., ELLORY, J. C., SHUMAN, M. A., SHALLER, C. C. and COOPER, R. A. (1975). *Blood*, **46**, 337.
WILEY, J. S. and GILL, F. M. (1976). *Blood*, **47**, 197.
YUNIS, A. S. and ARIMURA, G. N. (1966). *Proc. Soc. Exp. Biol. Med.* **121**, 327.
ZARKOWSKY, H. S., MOHANDAS, N., SPEAKER, C. B. and SHOHET, S. B. (1975). *Brit. J. Haemat.* **29**, 537.
ZARKOWSKY, H. S., OSKI, F. A., SHA'AFI, R., SHOHET, S. B. and NATHAN, D. G. (1968). *New Engl. J. Med.* **278**, 573.

The sodium pump in ruminant red cells

J. C. ELLORY

Physiological Laboratory, Cambridge University, UK

1 Introduction	363
2 Kinetic properties of the sodium pump in HK and LK cells	365
3 Ouabain-binding studies	371
4 Partial reactions of the Na pump	371
5 The sodium pump in lamb red cells and reticulocytes	372
6 Properties of the L and M antigens	375
7 The nature of the anti-L antibody	377
8 Differences in K polymorphism in sheep, goats and cattle	378
References	380

1 Introduction

One rather surprising conclusion that can be drawn from the contents of this book is that red cells from different species can have very different transport properties. This chapter considers the polymorphism of the sodium pump in red cells from ruminants. Inevitably I shall emphasize some topics and neglect others. As a starting point to correct my inadequacies or amplify certain points readers are referred to the excellent reviews of Tucker (1971) and Lauf (1975). Historically, Abderhalden (1898) and Kerr (1937) first demonstrated that sheep red cells can have very low potassium concentrations. The situation was finally defined by Evans and his coworkers (Evans, 1954; Evans and King, 1955; Evans *et al.*, 1956) who confirmed genetically the division of sheep into two populations, one having "normal" high red cell potassium concentrations (HK) and the other having low (about 25 per cent of normal K) levels (LK). The LK type was dominant, and the inheritance conformed to a simple Mendelian pattern. Other ruminants, including goats (Evans and Phillipson, 1957), cattle (Ellory and Tucker, 1970a) and buffaloes (Pandey and Roy, 1968) have also been shown to have this polymorphism, although the distributions in these species is not so clear-cut and is discussed in some detail later.

The classic transport studies of Tosteson and Hoffman (1960) resolved the difference in intracellular K levels in HK and LK sheep by measuring pump and leak fluxes in the two cell types. They showed that HK cells had higher active and lower passive Na and K fluxes, whilst the sodium pump was only operating at about a quarter of the rate in LK cells. This finding was subsequently reinforced by (Na–K)-activated ATPase measurements (Tosteson, 1963). The question of whether LK cells had fewer, normal Na pumps, or whether their Na pumps showed some kinetic modification, was still open. Binding studies with tritiated ouabain should have provided the answer, but in fact the situation was experimentally complicated and it is only recently that more systematic studies have been undertaken (see below). Sheep red cell workers have been denied the resealed ghost technique exploited so successfully by those working with human red cells (Hoffman, 1962). This is due to their small volume:surface area ratio and high sphingomyelin content. However, the PCMBS (Garrahan and Rega, 1967) and nystatin (Cass and Dalmark, 1973) methods have been successfully employed to vary intracellular cations in ruminant red cells. The first exciting experiments with the PCMBS technique revealed that the sodium pump in LK sheep red cells had different kinetic properties from HK cells with regard to the internal cation affinities (Hoffman and Tosteson, 1971). These results were extended by more systematic studies using goat red cells (Sachs *et al.*, 1974a) and finally, data from ATPase experiments with broken membranes from goat red cells defined the kinetic situation exactly (Cavieres and Ellory, 1975).

The property which made transport in sheep red cells uniquely interesting was the discovery of a blood group antigen system linked to K type. Thus the M antigen is associated with HK (MM) and heterozygous LK (ML) cells (Rasmusen *et al.*, 1960; Rasmusen and Hall, 1966) and the L antigen with homozygous (LL) and heterozygous (ML) LK cells (Ellory and Tucker, 1969a; Rasmusen, 1969). The associated isoantibodies are raised by immunizing MM sheep with LL cells or vice versa (e.g. see Tucker and Ellory, 1970), and the cells from HK or LK sheep show complement lysis following sensitization with the appropriate antibody. A further exciting property of the anti-L antibody was that it stimulated the Na pump five- to eightfold when added to LK cells (Ellory and Tucker, 1969a). In contrast, the anti-M antibody has no effect on active transport in HK or ML LK cells.

There are two situations in which an LK sheep can have HK cells. The first is at birth, and the other is after severe haemorrhage. It is therefore of interest to follow the development of the LK trait, and the L antigen, during red cell maturation. Finally, since the L antigen is unique in being the only blood group antigen with a function, the limited data on its

2 Kinetic properties of the sodium pump in HK and LK cells

The sodium pump in human red cells has been the subject of extensive investigation over the last 25 years. Its normal function is now established as exchanging three internal Na ions for two external K ions with the hydrolysis of 1 molecule of ATP. The data available for HK and LK sheep indicate a similar ratio of 1–1·5 Na:K (Tosteson and Hoffman, 1960; Hoffman and Tosteson, 1971) although the experimental measurement is complicated by the presence of a very large ouabain-insensitive exchange component in ruminant red cells. This makes a very large background against which to measure Na pump fluxes (e.g. see Motais and Sola, 1973).

The first data suggesting that the sodium pump in LK sheep red cells may differ from HK cells in its kinetic properties came from the experiments of Hoffman and Tosteson (1971). Using the PCMBS method they varied the ratio of Na and K in the cells, whilst keeping the total constant at 150 mM. The ouabain-sensitive K influx was much smaller in LK cells with high internal K and low internal Na. This effect was probably due to a higher internal affinity for K than Na, but this experiment was difficult to interpret since Na and K were varied in a reciprocal way. In a more systematic investigation, choline was introduced as a replacement ion, with Na and K varied independently (Sachs *et al.*, 1974a). Figure 1 shows the effect in LK goat cells of increasing internal K at a constant Na concentration. It is clear that raising the cell K progressively inhibits the pump, and the concave shape of the curve implies that the affinity for K is greater than Na (see also Ellory *et al.*, 1971). When the cells are treated with the anti-L antibody, the inhibitory effect of K is less, and on the basis of these experiments it was proposed that the anti-L effect could be completely explained by a change in the internal affinities for Na and K. In fact, rigorous kinetic analysis is difficult using PCMBS-loaded cells, since each data point means preparing a separate batch of cells, and hence the labour involved in making an experiment to solve for three unknown parameters is enormous. Sachs *et al.* (1974a) did attempt to fit the data by Michaelis-Menten kinetics, but were largely unsuccessful. An alternative approach, which allows more experimental manipulation but introduces another parameter (the external K site), is the measurement of ouabain-sensitive ATPase activity in broken membranes. One problem here is the destruction of membrane asymmetry, involving the exposure of both inside and outside sites to the same ionic conditions. The early approach to this (Ellory *et al.*, 1971; Glynn and Ellory, 1972) was to limit conditions to K concen-

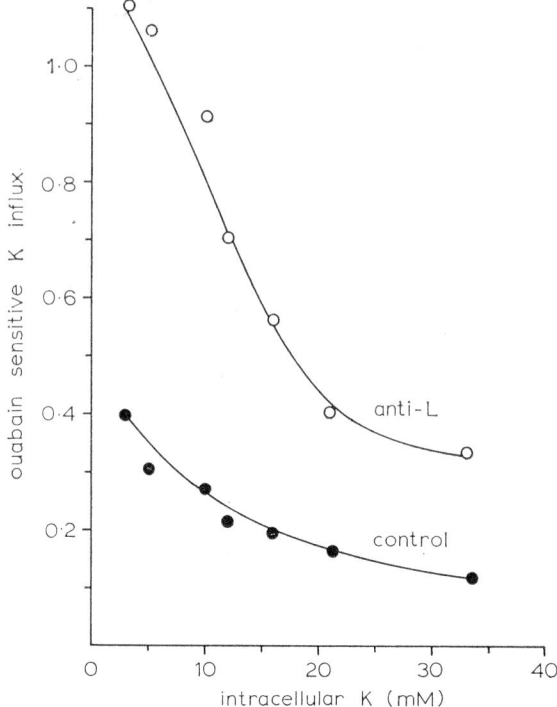

FIG. 1. The effect of anti-L on the ouabain-sensitive K influx into LK goat red cells with varying intracellular K levels. Cell Na is constant at 80 ± 2 mM. Cations altered by the PCMBS method, with partial choline replacement. ○—○ = anti-L; ●—● = control.

trations greater than 10 mM, where the external site is near saturation. In later experiments over a wider range of Na and K concentrations the effect of the external site was corrected for at each concentration, using data obtained in parallel influx studies in intact cells. Figure 2 shows the ouabain-sensitive ATPase activity in LK goat ghosts as a function of K concentration. The initial rise represents the external site saturating with K, whilst the fall represents K inhibition at the internal site. Again, anti-L alters the sensitivity to K. If the system obeys Michaelis-Menten kinetics, the curve should be represented by the function (Cavieres, 1975; Cavieres and Ellory, 1975)

$$V = \frac{V_{\max}}{\left(1 + \frac{K_m{}^o}{K}\right)^m \left(1 + \frac{K_m}{\text{Na}}\left(1 + \frac{K}{K_i}\right)\right)^n}$$

Where K_m, K_i and K_m^o represent the internal affinities for Na and K and the external affinity for K, respectively, and the indices m and n reflect the number of sites involved. In LK goats as in human cells (Garay and Garrahan, 1973; see also Chap. 1, pp23 –27), the best fit to the data is obtained with $m = 2$ and $n = 3$. Having corrected for the external site using data obtained from influx experiments, a plot of $1/\sqrt[3]{v}$ against $1/\text{Na}$ is made (Fig. 3). The y intercept gives $1/\sqrt[3]{V_{\max}}$ directly, and replotting the slopes of the lines against K gives K_m and K_i. The fact that the data fit the plot reasonably well implies that Na and K compete at the same sites, with affinities of 18 mM and 3 mM, respectively. The measured $V_{\max}$ is 1·4 mmol (l cells)$^{-1}$ h^{-1} for these cells, which compares well with values for HK cells. The same Figure shows the effect of anti-L. Again the data give a good fit to a straight line, and significantly the y intercept

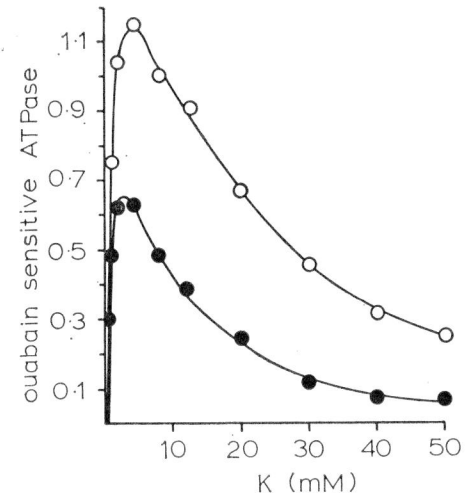

FIG. 2. The effect of anti-L on the ouabain-sensitive ATPase activity measured at different K concentrations in broken membranes from LK goat red cells. Na is constant at 100 mM. ○—○ = anti-L; ●—● = control.

is identical. This proves that the antibody acts entirely by altering the internal affinities and does not increase the $V_{\max}$, e.g. by unmasking new pump sites. The Na and K affinities after anti-L treatment were 2 mM and 1 mM, respectively, thus the antibody alters the ratio of affinities from 6:1 in favour of K to 2:1. An obvious way to investigate this internal site in more detail is to use the various alkali metal cations. Cavieres and Ellory (1977) determined that the relative affinities for K:Rb:Na:Cs were

1:1·8:6:14·6 in LK goat red cells, whilst treating them with anti-L produced the sequence 1:1·8:2:5·9.

As discussed by Cavieres (this volume), the equivalent sequence for human cells is Na > K, Rb > Cs > Li. Cavieres (1975 and in this

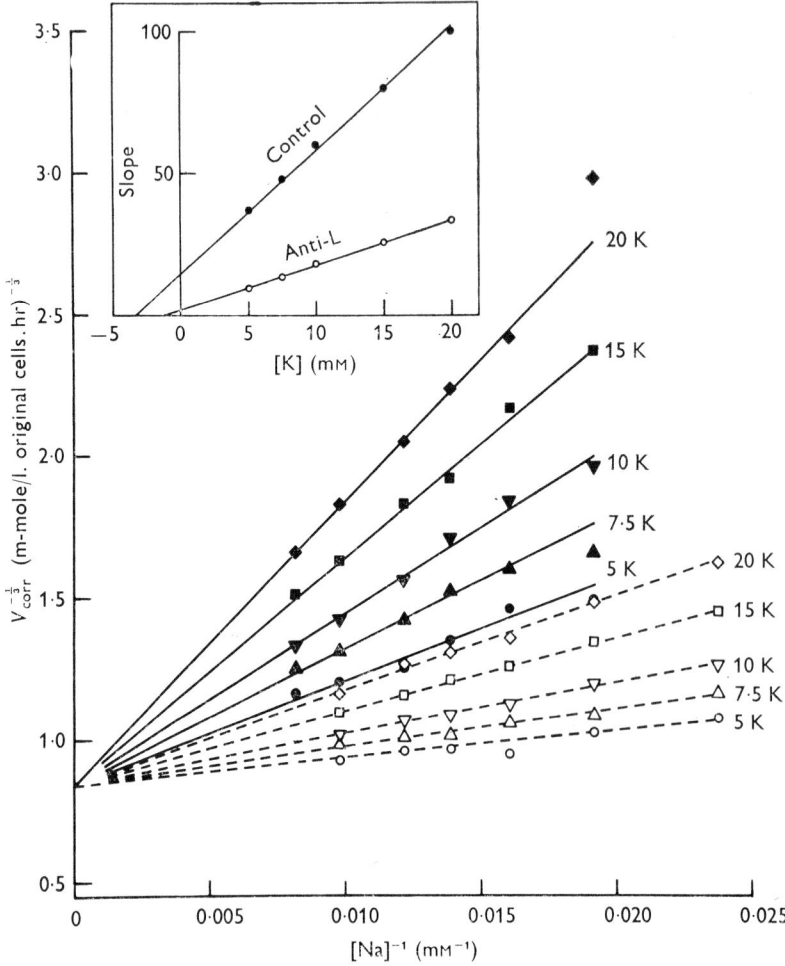

FIG. 3. Cubic double-reciprocal plot of LK goat ouabain-sensitive ATPase against Na concentration at various K concentrations. Activities have been corrected for the external site by the expression $(1 + 0·45/[K])^2$. Closed symbols and continuous lines = untreated membranes; open symbols and discontinuous lines = anti-L sensitized membranes. Inset is the slope replots against [K] to extract K_i and K_m values. Reproduced with permission from Cavieres and Ellory (1975).

volume) has combined the data on the affinity sequences of the external and internal sites to propose a conical model for the operation of the sodium pump. Using Eisenman's (1960) interpretation of the various sequences, Cavieres proposes that the intersite spacing between the three internal sites is less than for the external sites increasing the effective field strength, and altering the selectivity. On this model, the L antigen could be effective by preventing the sodium pump from fully completing its transformation, thus retaining an intermediate affinity sequence between the inside and outside sites. Anti-L would move the antigen enough to allow the sodium pump to move further towards the HK situation (see Fig. 4 and cf. Fig. 6, Cavieres, this volume). In this context it is interesting to compare the situation in HK goat red cells with human cells. Sachs *et al.* (1974a) presented data for HK cells with altered intracellular Na and K concentrations. Although compared with LK cells HK goat cells obviously show a higher internal affinity for Na and lower affinity for K (Fig. 5a), their kinetic characteristics are quite distinct from human cells (Fig. 5b), showing a lower Na affinity reminiscent of the anti-L treated LK cells.

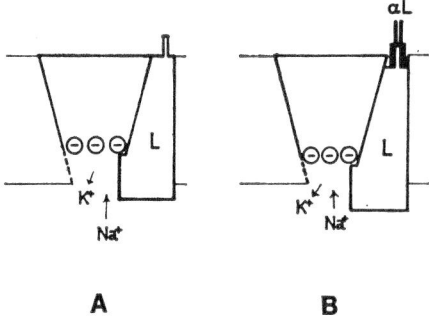

FIG. 4. A model for the proposed change in selectivity of the internal Na and K binding sites following anti-L sensitization by changing the inter-site spacing. Taken with permission from Cavieres (1975).

Quantitative analysis of Fig. 5a has been unsuccessful, since the K influx data do not conform to Michaelis-Menten kinetics. This was due in part to an activatory effect of K at low K concentrations (see Ellory *et al.*, 1972a; Garay and Garrahan, 1973) and also to the participation of ouabain-sensitive K–K exchange in the measured K influx. Recently, Dunham and Blostein (1976) have also seen this activatory effect of internal K in HK sheep red cells, although these cells showed very little subsequent inhibition by internal K (cf. Sachs *et al.*, 1974a, Fig. 2).

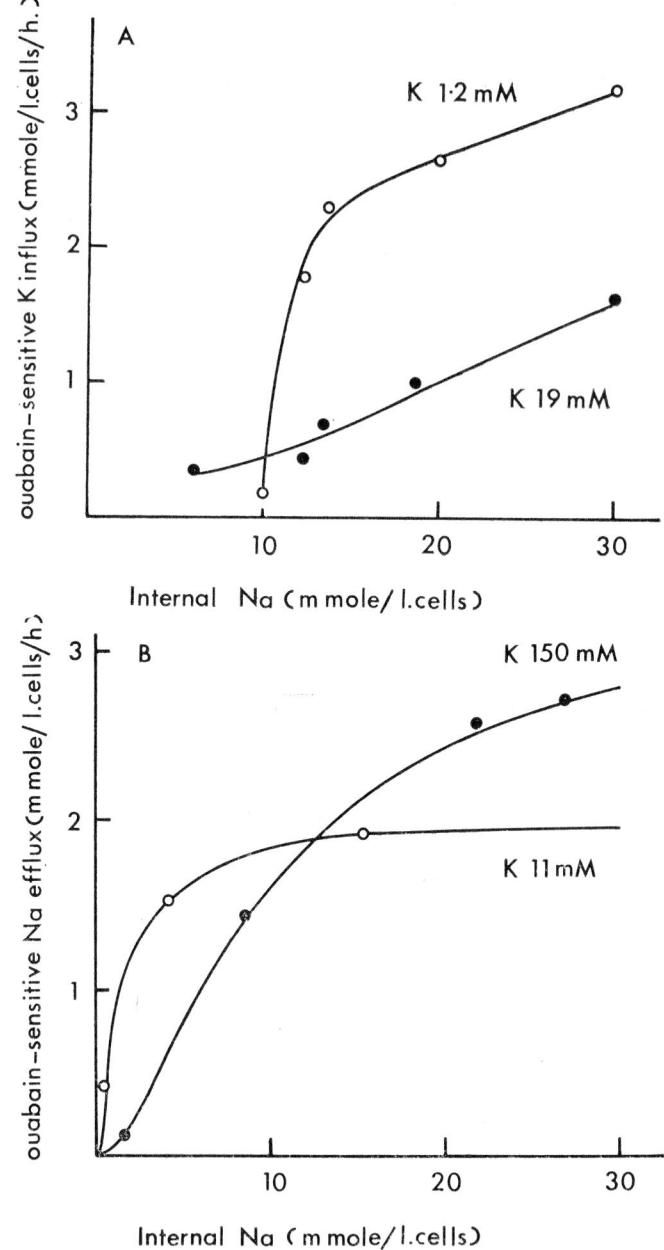

Fig. 5. The operation of the sodium pump measured as ouabain-sensitive K influx or Na efflux in HK goat (A) or human (B) red cells as a function of intracellular Na at two different K levels. Data are redrawn from Garay and Garrahan (1973) (B) and Sachs *et al.* (1974a) (A).

3 Ouabain-binding studies

As specific inhibitors of the sodium pump with a high affinity and slow reversibility, radioactive cardiac glycosides should offer the ideal system for measuring the number of pump sites on different types of cells. In practice, several difficulties and anomalies exist, with estimates for the human red cell varying from 10^2–10^3 sites per cell (Hoffman, 1969; Baker and Willis, 1972; Gardner and Conlon, 1972; Bodemann and Hoffman, 1976). One criterion emphasized by most workers is the measurement of number of molecules bound as a function of fractional inhibition of the ouabain-sensitive K influx. The relationship should be linear and ideally pass through the origin. Hoffman's group have used the presence of Cs or K externally as a means to reduce the nonspecific binding component, although this has been questioned (e.g. see Gardner and Frantz, 1974).

For sheep red cells the initial studies of Dunham and Hoffman (1971a) produced values of 42 sites per cell for HK animals, and 8 sites for LK individuals. Our early estimates for HK and LK sheep cells were 71 and 37 sites per cell respectively (Ellory and Tucker, 1970b) and Lauf et al. (1970) found 30 sites per LK cell. Both these studies also showed an increase in the number of sites up to twofold after treatment with anti-L. These results gave rise to the idea of unmasking new sites as the mechanism for antibody action. Recently, two more comprehensive studies on LK and HK cells have at least partially clarified the situation. Joiner and Lauf (1975) have measured ouabain binding to sheep cells. They found 110–140 sites per HK cell, 30–40 on heterozygous LK cells, and 50–80 on homozygous LK cells. Interestingly, the rate of ouabain binding was slowest on LL cells and fastest on MM cells. Treatment with anti-L increased the *rate* of ouabain binding, but not the equilibrium level.

In a parallel study on goat red cells, Sachs et al. (1974b) found about the same number of sites per cell (50–60) on both HK and LK types. The rate of ouabain binding was faster to HK than LK cells, and was increased by exposure to anti-L, or by lowering the intracellular K concentration. There was a considerable heterogeneity in the population of pumps as assessed from the plot of number of ouabain molecules bound versus fractional inhibition of the pump. Indeed, the experiments do not show a linear function, which lead to the suggestion that a fraction of the pumps in LK cells have a very small turnover number and rate of ouabain binding. It is this fraction which is sensitive to lowering internal K or treatment with the antibody.

4 Partial reactions of the Na pump

The fact that the sodium pump can be regarded as a multireaction sequence enzyme, in which the substrate ATP initially gives a Na-dependent phosphorylation and then a K-dependent dephosphorylation, has been extensively used to try and probe the reaction mechanism. A series of studies by Blostein and coworkers (Blostein *et al.*, 1971; Whittington and Blostein, 1971; Blostein and Whittington, 1973; Blostein *et al.*, 1974) have shown kinetic differences between HK and LK sheep red cells by measuring the Na-ATPase activity and Na-dependent ADP–ATP exchange in the presence of oligomycin, with a broken membrane preparation. These experiments are done at low substrate concentrations (0·2 μM ATP) and 0°C. Although there are several unresolved effects, the results are in general consistent with the K_m value for Na being much higher in LK cells, as emerged from the (Na–K)-activated ATPase study. Another partial reaction investigated was the K-dependent p-nitrophenyl phosphatase activity (Ellory and Lew, 1974). K-dependent PNPPase activity is barely detectable in LK cells, but is stimulated by treatment with anti-L, and also with Na + ATP (see Nagai and Yoshida, 1966).

In the presence of Na + ATP, the PNPPase activity in LK membranes is inhibited by increasing K in a manner reminiscent of the (Na–K)-activated ATPase. However, the K inhibition seems to show exactly the same characteristics, with no change in the apparent affinity for K following anti-L treatment. Similarly, Lauf *et al.* (1971) found that the Na-ATPase in anti-L treated LK sheep membranes still showed LK rather than HK characteristics (see also Lauf, 1975). Ellory and Lew (1974) concluded that the PNPPase may involve a different class of sites from those involved in normal operation of the pump, and it seems fair to conclude that although these studies on partial reactions emphasize that there are kinetic differences between HK and LK sodium pumps, we do not know enough about the sodium pump to use these observations for making detailed distinctions between the cell types.

5 The sodium pump in lamb red cells and reticulocytes

The two situations in which an LK-type sheep can have HK-type red cells are at birth and during anaemia, when reticulocytosis is occurring. To consider lamb red cells first, at birth even an LL LK type sheep would have high intracellular K levels and a large ouabain-sensitive K influx. These parameters both decline during development to reach adult levels at about 45 days (Hallman and Karvonen, 1949; Drury and Tucker, 1963; Ellory and Tucker, 1969b). Simultaneously, the L antigen, which is only weakly developed at birth, increases its level over the same time period. Figure 6 shows the time-course of the fall in intracellular K and active K transport with the simultaneous rise in L whether measured serologically

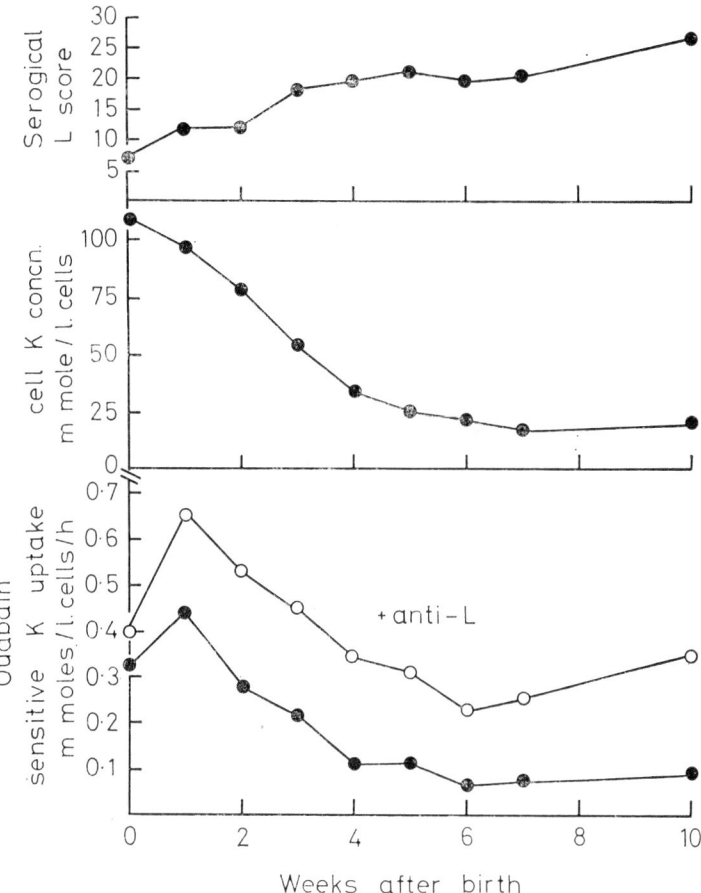

FIG. 6. Development of serological L activity, low intracellular K levels and anti-L sensitive fluxes in red cells from a newborn LK-type lamb. Redrawn from Ellory and Tucker (1969b).

(the L score) or by its ability to stimulate active transport. That this change was due to a new population of cells appearing rather than the L antigen gradually being expressed on circulating cells was shown by treating cells from a 2-week-old lamb with anti-L, adding complement and collecting the unlysed cells. It was found that these L-negative cells had only foetal haemoglobin, and a high intracellular K and low Na concentration (Tucker and Ellory, 1970). Later experiments revealed that the (Na–K)-activated ATPase activity measured in newborn lamb red cell membranes showed HK characteristics. From ouabain-binding studies, Dunham and Hoffman (1971b) concluded that there was no difference in the number of pump sites between lamb and HK adult cells, while there was a two to three times greater number of sites on LK lambs than adults. Therefore the cells in all newborn lambs seem to be "normal" HK type, while LK cells carrying the L antigen are put into the circulation to replace them from birth onwards.

The situation with regard to reticulocytes is more interesting. It has been known for a long time that following haemorrhage LK sheep produce cells with a high internal K (Drury and Tucker, 1963; Evans, 1963) and raised active transport (Lee et al., 1966). A typical experiment is shown in Fig. 7. Following heavy bleeding on days 0, 1 and 2 the animal produces a peak reticulocyte response on day 5. The cell K is raised from 20 to 70 mM, and the ouabain-sensitive K influx increased from 0·1 to 2·5 mmol (l cells)$^{-1}$ h^{-1}. Preliminary ouabain-binding experiments indicated a twentyfold increase in the number of pump sites on reticulocytes (Ellory and Tucker,

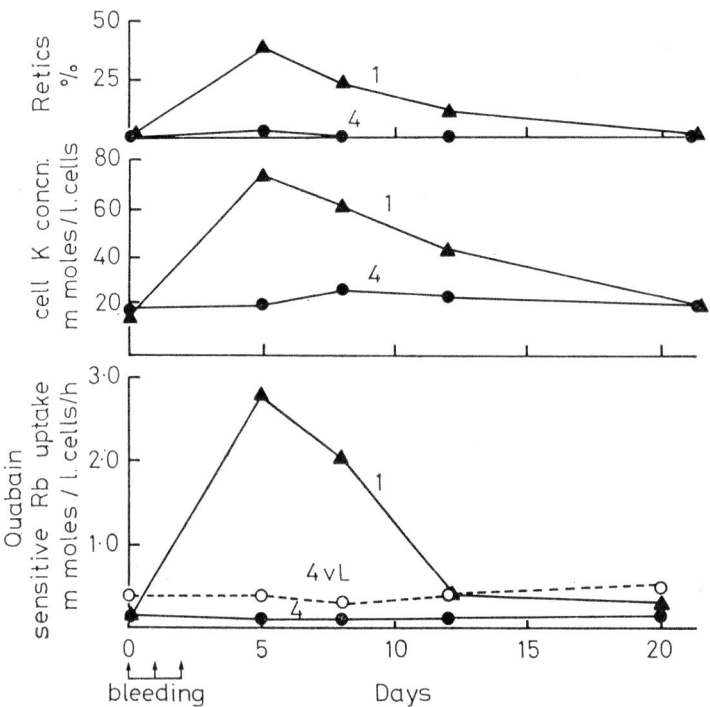

FIG. 7. The changes in intracellular K levels, sodium pump activity (measured as ouabain-sensitive Rb uptake) and anti-L sensitivity of the pump during reticulocytosis induced by phlebotomy in an LK-type sheep. Fractions 1 and 4 represent reticulocyte-rich and old cell rich fractions achieved by differential centrifugation. Redrawn from Tucker and Ellory (1970).

1970c), and (Na–K)-activated ATPase measurements indicated HK kinetics. Similarly, Blostein et al. (1974) found kinetic differences between HK and LK reticulocytes and mature cells, measuring ATPase activity at very low ATP levels. Recently, Dunham and Blostein (1976) have used nystatin treatment to alter the intracellular cation levels in reticulocyte-rich fractions derived from anaemic LK sheep, and have shown that the internal affinities are similar to those of HK type cells. An important difference between their results and ours is that they were able to get a large stimulation of active transport in the reticulocyte preparation following sensitization with anti-L.

We were unable to show any stimulation of transport in the peak reticulocyte response cells following anti-L treatment, and serologically the cells also showed less sensitivity to lysis with complement following anti-L treatment. However, absorption studies showed that the cells were capable of binding just as much antibody as normal LK cells (Tucker and Ellory, 1971). We concluded that LK type reticulocytes clearly possessed the L antigen, but that either it was not expressing its role in inhibiting transport or that its effect was masked by a large excess of HK pumps which were subsequently lost on maturation. Both these effects are probably significant and the difference between our results and those of Dunham and Blostein probably indicate different periods in the schedule of reticulocyte maturation. Since reticulocytes are known to have a larger surface area and smaller surface charge than mature cells (Ellory et al., 1970), and are known to lose specific membrane lipids (Kemp et al., 1975) and amino acid transport systems on maturation (e.g. see pp. 316–319), it seems likely that the cell loses some of its HK type pumps, revealing the underlying LK pump activity left in the membrane and possibly relocating some of the L antigen molecules in the membrane on to HK type pumps. This is clearly a fascinating situation which will merit further investigation.

6 Properties of the L and M antigens

The expression of the antigen on LK cells can be measured functionally in two main ways: by the lysis of the cells subsequent to the addition of complement, or by the stimulation of a sodium pump parameter, e.g. ouabain-sensitive K influx or ATPase. Quite early on two separate pieces of work suggested that these components might be discrete. Lauf et al. (1971) showed that treating sheep cells with trypsin destroyed the pump-stimulating capacity of anti-L but not the serological activity. Ellory and Tucker (1970c) showed that LK goat red cells absorbed only a fraction of anti-L activity against sheep cells, and would not lyse with anti-L plus complement. Further, anti-L eluted from LK goat red cells stimulated transport in both sheep and goat cells, but was nonlytic against goat and only weakly lytic against sheep cells. Comparing pump-stimulating activity with serological activity for different batches of anti-L revealed a negative correlation (Ellory and Tucker, 1970a). Recently, Lauf (1975) has questioned the separation of activity into these two entities, whilst Dunham has confirmed and extended these findings (Dunham, 1976). We have also prepared a goat anti-goat anti-L, which is completely nonlytic against LK goat cells. Anti-L can therefore be divided into two separate antibodies: anti-L_p and anti-L_{ly} representing the transport-stimulating and serological activities, respectively. This division is probably not exact, but represents the extreme ends of a spectrum of overlapping activities. A further idea proposed and pursued by Dunham (Dunham and Hoffman, 1971b; Dunham, 1976) is that part of the leak or ouabain-insensitive K influx is convertible into a pump flux by treatment with the anti-L_{ly} but not anti-L_p antibody. Although this appears to be in conflict with the ATPase and ouabain-binding experiments of Cavieres and Ellory (1975) and Joiner and Lauf (1975) giving the same V_{max} or number of pump sites after anti-L treatment, it is undeniable that there is a *decrease* in the ouabain-insensitive K influx following treatment with anti-L for certain sheep and certain batches of antibody (e.g. see Lauf et al., 1970, Table 3; Ellory et al., 1972a; Dunham, 1976). It is also clear that the ouabain-insensitive K influx is not entirely a passive diffusion since it shows some saturation kinetics (Dunham and Hoffman, 1971b; Dunham, 1976). This fascinating point must await further studies to be finally resolved.

It is obviously of interest to try and measure the number of antigen sites on an LK cell directly, to see if they correlate with the number of ouabain-binding sites. Three studies have been performed so far, two using sheep cells and one on LK goats. Using iodine-labelled anti-L, Kropp and Sachs (1974) found 60 binding sites on an LK goat red cell, compared with 55 ouabain sites. Obviously this suggests a 1:1 correspondence. Using the same radioiodine technique, Lauf and Sun (1975) found between 100 and 1000 anti-L binding sites on an LK sheep red cell, suggesting a much higher number of antigens than pumps.

A different technique was adopted by Tucker et al. (1976). They used a pig anti-sheep IgG conjugated with haemocyanin to directly visualize sites by electronmicroscopy. This uses a single reagent to allow several different antibodies to be followed, and was used to measure the number and topographical distribution of both L_p, L_{ly} and M antigens on MM, ML and LL cells. Using a pure anti-L_p prepared by absorbing anti-L with newborn LL cells gave 340 sites per cell for LL cells and 120 for ML cells, while the unabsorbed anti-L_p + L_{ly} gave numbers of 900 sites on LL cells. For comparison, anti-M gave 2000 sites on an MM cell and 1300 on an ML type. On the heterozygote anti-M and anti-L were completely additive. The number of M sites agrees well with the data of Sun and Lauf (1975) who found 2000–5000 sites per MM and 40 per cent less per ML.

It seems clear that there are more L antigen sites than Na pumps, and that the antigen is distributed randomly over the cell surface (Tucker et al., 1976). Perhaps even the anti-L_p used in this study contained some anti-L_{ly} component, and there are about ten times as many lytic sites as pump inhibiting sites for L on a sheep cell.

The L antigen has proved very refractory to chemical isolation and analysis. Although a limited success has been achieved with detergent solubilization of the M antigen (see Lauf, 1975), any treatment so far tried for extracting L leads to inactivation. The only technique to yield any information so far has been irradiation inactivation analysis. This method, which enjoyed a fashionable period in the 1950s, was first applied to membrane-bound enzymes systematically by Kepner and Macey (1968). When applied to freeze-dried LK goat red cells, this method yielded very interesting results. It seemed that the target size measured depended on the assay conditions chosen. Thus the enzyme activity assayed at 5 mM K gave a much larger apparent target size than when assayed at 25 mM K. We finally interpreted this result as the product of an inhibitor (the L antigen) being more radiation-sensitive than the ATPase, and hence showing a smaller apparent target when assayed under inhibiting conditions (high K concentrations). In fact, measuring L_p binding by absorptions following irradiation gave a target size equivalent to a spherical protein of 7×10^5 daltons, suggesting that the antigen is a large hydrophobic membrane-bound protein.

7 The nature of the anti-L antibody

Since the anti-L antibody is directly altering a membrane transport component, it may be of interest to examine the properties of the antigen-antibody interaction in terms of antibody structure, particularly since bivalency of antibody binding has been interpreted as involving cross-linking. Anti-L is normally a sheep IgG antibody. Treatment with papain causes degradation to give monovalent F(ab) fragments (Porter, 1959). While Snyder et al. (1971) found that anti-L F(ab) fragments were inactive in stimulating the pump in LK cells, Ellory et al. (1973) found that they were about half as effective as IgG or F(ab')$_2$. However, since the monovalent fragment was equally effective on both LL and ML cells, we concluded that double attachment probably is necessary.

8 Differences in K polymorphism in sheep, goats and cattle

So far experimental results with sheep and goats have been used almost interchangeably, and the impression has been given of a simple polymorphism with cells of either high or low K type. In fact, within a single category considerable variation can exist in K levels. For example, LK type means 7 mM for an Australian Merino ram and 35 mM for an LK Finnish Landrace sheep (Turner and Koch, 1961; Tucker and Kilgour, 1970). This kind of difference also exists in goats (Ellory and Tucker, 1970b), but is most exaggerated with cattle, where within a single breed individuals with any intracellular K between 15 and 110 mM can be found (Ellory and Tucker, 1970d). Although, as in sheep, newborn calves are HK type, developing LK characteristics during the first 6 weeks after birth (e.g. see Israel et al., 1972), when an adult has achieved a steady K concentration this remains constant over several years. If ouabain-sensitive ATPase activity is measured at constant high Na and varying K in washed broken red cell ghosts from cattle, a family of curves is obtained (Fig. 8) in which the degree of K inhibition correlates with the resting K level of that individual animal's red cells (Ellory and Carleton, 1974). This implies that intracellular K is modulated by altering the apparent affinities for K and Na inside the cell, rather than increasing the number of standard pump units inserted in the membrane. Attempts to analyse the cattle red cell ATPase data in detail kinetically have so far been unsuccessful, in contrast with the situation for LK goats and sheep. However, cattle cells do react with anti-L to give a stimulation of active transport, even when their intracellular K is high (60 mM). Whether cattle have a mixed population of HK and LK cells, a mixed population of HK and LK pumps within each cell, or individually preset K_m and K_i values for homogeneous pumps has yet to be determined. Perhaps some of the complex results described earlier, e.g. the ouabain-binding data, and some of the apparent conflicts between results from different laboratories could be a reflection of different mixtures of pump types even in sheep red cells.

Microprobe analysis would be an obvious way to test the mixed cell hypothesis. Kinetic analysis of the ATPase data as described earlier should allow resolution of HK and LK type pumps if they are as extremely different as human and LK goat cells. In fact, our experiments designed to test this possibility have failed to give satisfactory results.

The third suggestion, of individually designed sodium pumps, seems very complex in terms of cell biology. If the analogy of Cavieres's conical model is pursued, variations in the position which the L antigen takes up will result in the internal sites having different separations, and would provide a way of producing differences in individual internal affinities.

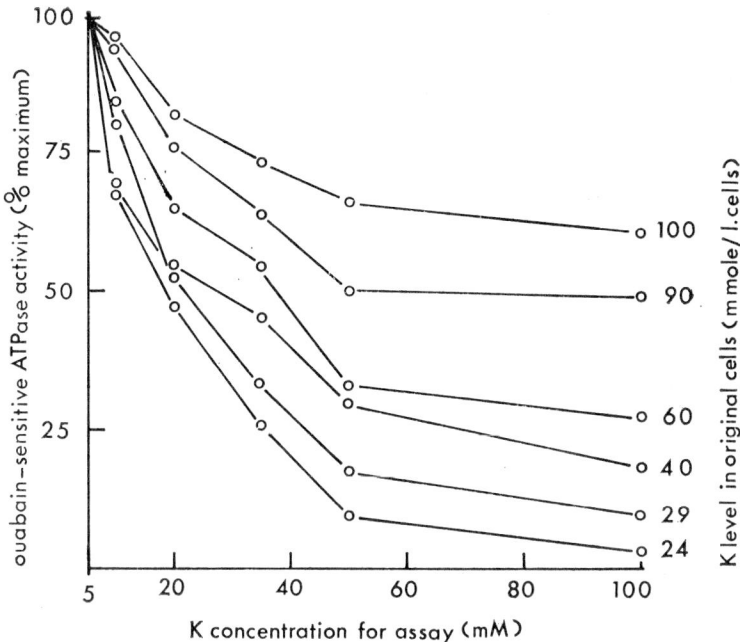

FIG. 8. Variations in the K-sensitivity of ouabain-sensitive ATPase activity measured in broken red cell membranes from individual cows with varying original K levels. Redrawn from Ellory and Carleton (1974).

Whichever possibility is correct, the cell must decide early on what kind of pumps it is going to produce. In sheep there is another genetically determined transport defect, for certain amino acids, which results in the cell accumulating high concentrations (20 mM) of cationic amino acids. This results in a lowering of the cell K and Na. For example, LK Finnish Landrace sheep which normally have 35 mM K intracellularly only have 16 mM K if they accumulate cationic amino acids (Ellory et al., 1972b). If we look at ATPase activity as a function of K in broken ghosts from these cells we find that, as in the cattle, the cells with low cell K show a greater K inhibition than the normal cells. In other words, the cell has apparently adjusted to the new intracellular K by adjusting its internal Na/K affinities, a subtle variation on the pump/leak hypothesis.

Bearing in mind that mature red cells are dead, or at least sleeping in terms of protein synthesis and membrane mobility, it is clearly during the maturation of a potentially LK type reticulocyte that its affinities are set. Hopefully, studies with cultured reticulocytes will allow us to discover the way in which ruminant red cells achieve this versatility in their sodium pumps.

References

ABDERHALDEN, E. (1898). *Hoppe-Seyler's Z. Physiol. Chem.* **25**, 65.
BAKER, P. B. and WILLIS, J. S. (1972). *J. Physiol.* **224**, 441.
BLOSTEIN, R., LAUF, P. K. and TOSTESON, D. C. (1971). *Biochim. Biophys. Acta,* **249**, 623.
BLOSTEIN, R. and WHITTINGTON, E. S. (1973). *J. Biol. Chem.* **248**, 1772.
BLOSTEIN, R., WHITTINGTON, E. S. and KUEBLER, E. S. (1974). *Ann. N.Y. Acad. Sci.* **242**, 305.
BODEMANN, H. H. and HOFFMAN, J. F. (1976). *J. Gen. Physiol.* **58**, 94.
CASS, A. and DALMARK, M. (1973). *Nature New Biol.* **244**, 47.
CAVIERES, J. D. (1975). Ph.D. Thesis, Cambridge University.
CAVIERES, J. D. and ELLORY, J. C. (1975). *J. Physiol.* **245**, 93P.
CAVIERES, J. D. and ELLORY, J. C. (1977). *J. Physiol.* in press.
DRURY, A. N. and TUCKER, E. M. (1963). *Res. Vet. Sci.* **4**, 568.
DUNHAM, P. B. (1976). *Biochim. Biophys. Acta,* **443**, 219.
DUNHAM, P. B. (1976). *J. Gen. Physiol.* **68**, 567.
DUNHAM, P. B. and BLOSTEIN, R. (1976). *Biochim. Biophys. Acta,* **455**, 749
DUNHAM, P. B. and HOFFMAN, J. F. (1971a). *J. Gen. Physiol.* **58**, 94.
DUNHAM, P. B. and HOFFMAN, J. F. (1971b). *Biochim. Biophys. Acta,* **241**, 399.
EISENMAN, G. (1960). *In* "Membrane Transport and Metabolism" (A. Kleinzeller and A. Kotyk, eds), p. 163. Academic Press, New York and London.
ELLORY, J. C. and CARLETON, J. S. (1974). *Biochim. Biophys. Acta,* **363**, 397.
ELLORY, J. C. and LEW, V. L. (1974). *Biochim. Biophys. Acta,* **332**, 215.
ELLORY, J. C. and TUCKER, E. M. (1969a). *Nature,* **222**, 477.
ELLORY, J. C. and TUCKER, E. M. (1969b). *J. Physiol.* **204**, 101P.
ELLORY, J. C. and TUCKER, E. M. (1970a). *Biochim. Biophys. Acta,* **219**, 160.
ELLORY, J. C. and TUCKER, E. M. (1970b). *In* "Permeability and Function of Biological Membranes" (L. Bolis, A. Katchalsky, R. D. Keynes, W. R. Loewenstein and B. A. Pethica, eds), p. 120. North-Holland, Amsterdam.
ELLORY, J. C. and TUCKER, E. M. (1970c). *J. Physiol.* **208**, 18P.
ELLORY, J. C. and TUCKER, E. M. (1970d). *J. Agric. Sci.* **74**, 595.
ELLORY, J. C., FEINSTEIN, A. and HERBERT, J. (1973). *Immunochem.* **10**, 785.
ELLORY, J. C., GLYNN, I. M., LEW, V. L. and TUCKER, E. M. (1971). *J. Physiol.* **217**, 61P.
ELLORY, J. C., O'DONNELL, J. M. and TUCKER, E. M. (1970). *J. Physiol.* **210**, 111P.
ELLORY, J. C., SACHS, J. R., DUNHAM, P. B. and HOFFMAN, J. F. (1972a). *In* "Biomembranes 3" (F. Kreuzer and J. F. G. Slegers, eds), p. 237. Plenum Publishing, New York.
ELLORY, J. C., TUCKER, E. M. and DEVERSON, E. V. (1972b). *Biochim. Biophys. Acta,* **279**, 481.
EVANS, J. V. (1954). *Nature,* **174**, 931.
EVANS, J. V. (1963). *Aust. J. Agric. Res.* **14**, 540.
EVANS, J. V. and KING, J. W. B. (1955). *Nature,* **176**, 171.
EVANS, J. V. and PHILLIPSON, A. T. (1957). *J. Physiol.* **139**, 87.
EVANS, J. V., KING, J. W. B., COHEN, B. L., HARRIS, H. and WARREN, F. L. (1956). *Nature,* **178**, 849.
GARAY, R. P. and GARRAHAN, P. J. (1973). *J. Physiol.* **231**, 297.
GARDNER, J. D. and CONLON, T. R. (1972). *J. Gen. Physiol.* **60**, 609.
GARDNER, J. D. and FRANTZ, C. (1974). *J. Membrane Biol.* **16**, 43.

GARRAHAN, P. J. and REGA, A. F. (1967). *J. Physiol.* **193**, 459.
GLYNN, I. M. and ELLORY, J. C. (1972). In "Role of Membranes in Secretory Processes" (L. Bolis, R. D. Keynes and W. Wilbrandt, eds), p. 224. North-Holland, Amsterdam.
GLYNN, I. M. and KARLISH, S. J. D. (1975). *Ann. Rev. Physiol.* **37**, 13.
HALLMAN, N. and KARVONEN, M. J. (1949). *Annals Med. Exp. Biol. Fenn.* **27**, 221.
HOFFMAN, J. F. (1962). *J. Gen. Physiol.* **45**, 837.
HOFFMAN, J. F. (1969). *J. Gen. Physiol.* **54**, 343s.
HOFFMAN, P. G. and TOSTESON, D. C. (1971). *J. Gen. Physiol.* **58**, 438.
ISRAEL, Y., MACDONALD, A., BERNSTEIN, J. and ROSENMANN, E. (1972). *J. Gen. Physiol.* **59**, 270.
JOINER, C. H. and LAUF, P. K. (1975). *J. Membrane Biol.* **21**, 99.
KEMP, P., ELLORY, J. C. and MUNN, E. A. (1975). *Biochem. Soc. Trans.* **3**, 749.
KEPNER, G. R. and MACEY, R. I. (1968). *Biochim. Biophys. Acta*, **163**, 188.
KERR, S. E. (1937). *J. Biol. Chem.* **117**, 227.
KROPP, D. L. and SACHS, J. R. (1974). *Nature*, **252**, 244.
LAUF, P. K. (1975). *Biochim. Biophys. Acta*, **415**, 173.
LAUF, P. K., PARMALEE, M. L., SNYDER, J. J. and TOSTESON, D. C. (1971). *J. Membrane Biol.* **4**, 52.
LAUF, P. K., RASMUSEN, B. A., HOFFMAN, P. G., DUNHAM, P. B., COOK, P., PARMALEE, M. L. and TOSTESON, D. C. (1970). *J. Membrane Biol.* **3**, 1.
LAUF, P. K. and SUN, W. W. (1975). *Soc. Gen. Physiologists 29th Meeting Abstr.* **29**.
MOTAIS, R. and SOLA, F. (1973). *J. Physiol.* **233**, 423.
NAGAI, K. and YOSHIDA, H. (1966). *Biochim. Biophys. Acta*, **128**, 410.
PANDEY, M. D. and ROY, A. (1968). *Curr. Sci.* **37**, 256.
PORTER, R. R. (1959). *Biochim. J.* **73**, 119.
RASMUSEN, B. A. (1969). *Genetics*, 549.
RASMUSEN, B. A. and HALL, J. G. (1966). *Science*, **151**, 1551.
RASMUSEN, B. A., STORMONT, C. and SUZUKI, Y. (1960). *Genetics*, **45**, 1595.
SACHS, J. R., ELLORY, J. C., KROPP, D. L., DUNHAM, P. B. and HOFFMAN, J. F. (1974a). *J. Gen. Physiol.* **63**, 389.
SACHS, J. R., DUNHAM, P. B., KROPP, D. L., ELLORY, J. C. and HOFFMAN, J. F. (1974b). *J. Gen. Physiol.* **64**, 536.
SNYDER, J. J., RASMUSEN, B. A. and LAUF, P. K. (1971). *J. Immunol.* **107**, 623.
TOSTESON, D. C. (1963). *Fed. Proc. Fed. Am. Socs. Exp. Biol.* **22**, 19.
TOSTESON, D. C. and HOFFMAN, J. F. (1960). *J. Gen. Physiol.* **44**, 169.
TUCKER, E. M. (1971). *Biol. Rev.* **46**, 341.
TUCKER, E. M. and ELLORY, J. C. (1970). *Anim. Blood Gps. Biochem. Genet.* **1**, 101.
TUCKER, E. M. and ELLORY, J. C. (1971). *Anim. Blood Gps. Biochem. Genet.* **2**, 77.
TUCKER, E. M. and KILGOUR, L. (1970). *Experientia*, **26**, 203.
TUCKER, E. M., ELLORY, J. C., WOODING, F. B. P., MORGAN, G. and HERBERT, J. (1976). *Proc. Roy. Soc. B*, **194**, 271.
TURNER, H. W. and KOCH, J. H. (1961). *Aust. J. Biol. Sci.* **14**, 260.
WHITTINGTON, E. S. and BLOSTEIN, R. (1971). *J. Biol. Chem.* **246**, 3518.

Transport in avian red cells

F. M. KREGENOW

Laboratory of Kidney and Electrolyte Metabolism, National Heart and Lung Institute, National Institutes of Health, Bethesda, Maryland, USA

1 Introduction	383
2 Characteristics of avian red cells	384
2.1 Appearance (light and electron microscopic observations)	384
2.2 Plasma membrane	385
2.3 Metabolism	386
3 Early approaches to transport study	389
4 Permeability to glucose	390
5 Amino acid permeation	393
5.1 Primary glycine transport system	393
5.2 Other amino acid transport systems	395
6 Other	396
6.1 Permeability to water	396
6.2 Oxidized glutathione transport	397
7 Cation transport	397
7.1 General	397
7.2 Volume regulation	399
References	421

1 Introduction

Avian erythrocytes were used in the first systematic study of animal cell permeability. Since then, investigators interested in membrane transport have continued to use avian erythrocytes more often than other non-mammalian red cells. Avian red cells, besides possessing characteristics common to all mature erythrocytes, have properties that make them especially useful for certain transport problems. This chapter focuses on studies which have capitalized on some of these properties. We also point out, whenever possible, similarities between avian and mammalian red cells. Of necessity and with regrets, the choice of studies has been selective. Recent findings involving cation transport and volume regulation have been emphasized, while an extensive literature dealing with the transport of malaria-infected avian cells has been omitted.

2 Characteristics of avian red cells

2.1 APPEARANCE (LIGHT AND ELECTRON MICROSCOPIC OBSERVATIONS)

The appearance of mature avian erythrocytes is similar to other non-mammalian red cells. They are flattened oval cells with an oval nucleus. Most avaian cells used experimentally are somewhat larger than the human red cell. Table 1 gives the average length and width of pigeon and

TABLE 1

Measurements on pigeon and duck red cells

	Long diameter	Short diameter	Source
Pigeon	12·9 μm	4·7 μm	(Kennedy and Clemenko, 1928)
Duck	11·2 μm	6·7 μm	(Magath and Higgins, 1934)

duck red cells. In a study of some fifty North American species, Bartsch et al. (1937) found that length varied from 6 μm in the Carolina Chickadee to 16 μm in Osprey. The following references provide observations on other avian species or a bibliography to the early morphological literature (Gulliver, 1875; Cullen, 1903; Goodall, 1910, Lucas and Jamroy, 1961; Sturkie, 1965a).

The nucleus is the most prominent sub-cellular structure in avian red cells. It has condensed chromosomes and no nucleoli. When viewed with the light microscope, the nuclear outline is not quite concentric with the contour of the cell. Estimates of nuclear volume as a percentage of total cell volume range from 10 to 30 per cent (Luyet and Frei, 1935; Melampy, 1948; Ponder, 1948). Electron microscopic studies demonstrate that the nucleus is surrounded by an inner and outer membrane, both of which contain pores (Davis, 1961). Observations on freeze-etched preparations reveal, besides nuclear pores, "membrane-associated particles" (Koehler, 1968).

Avian erythrocytes contain mitochondria. They were first recognized by Forkner (1929) when he stained chicken red cells with the vital dye, Janus green. Both position and number vary with cell age. In mature erythrocytes they are sparse and randomly oriented within the cytoplasm; younger cells have more, and these remain in close proximity to the nucleus in apparent association with "nuclear pores" (Rudzinska and Trager, 1957; Schjeide et al., 1964).

By using supravital staining, one can visualize microtubules in amphibian erythrocytes with the light microscope. They appear as a bundle of filaments that encircle the erythrocyte just beneath the plasma membrane (Ranvier, 1875; Meves, 1903, 1906, 1911). (Amphibian erythrocytes are, in general, much larger cells than avian erythrocytes). Avian red cells also contain microtubules (Dehler, 1895), but they cannot be visualized as easily with the light microscope. For an account of the discovery and rediscovery of this sub-cellular structure in erythrocytes, one should consult the article by Fawcett and Witebsky (1964). Microtubules are best visualized with the electron microscope when cross-sectional views are taken at either erythrocyte pole. Numerous tubules clustered in a band and lying beneath the plasma membrane have been seen in several avian species (Maser and Philpott, 1964; Simpson, 1967; Behnke, 1970). It has been suggested that microtubules serve as cytoskeletal elements and thereby determine cell shape. This role has been questioned by Behnke (1970) and Barrett and Dawson (1974).

Fibrillar structures have been reported in association with nuclei, mitochrondria and the plasma membrane (Harris and Brown, 1971b; Zentgraf et al., 1971). Whether the fibers represent real sub-cellular structures is unclear. Harris and Brown (1971b) have postulated that they either aid in positioning the nucleus and mitochrondria or assist in maintaining cell shape.

2.2 PLASMA MEMBRANE

Workers have used several approaches to isolate avian plasma membranes. Harris and Brown (1971a,b) produced ghosts by using a modified version of the Dodge et al. (1963) technique, and then subjected the ghosts to controlled ultrasonification. Cells have also been disrupted by using pressure homogenization (Davoren and Sutherland, 1963b) or homogenization with high-speed rotary knives (Zentgraf et al., 1971). Membranes, isolated by these procedures, are usually fractionated further. At present the procedure of Zentgraf et al. (1971), which subjects membranes to centrifugation in a continuous sucrose density gradient, results in the purest membrane fraction.

The similarity between human and avian plasma membrane is most apparent when one compares their composition (Kleinig et al., 1971; Zentgraf et al., 1971). For instance, the electrophoretic pattern of acidic proteins from avian membranes, which have been separated on sodium dodecyl sulfate polyacrylamide gels, shows a close correspondence to their human counterpart (Shelton, 1973; Blanchet, 1974; Rudolph and Greengard, 1974). The plasmalemma of chicken erythrocytes also contains sialic acid and, like human red cells, neuraminadase treatment cleaves an α-glycosidic linkage at the membrane interface, releasing N-acetylneuraminic acid. As with human red cells, such treatment produces a cell which has a slower electrophoretic mobility (Klenk and Uhlenbruck, 1958; Eylar et al., 1962; Seaman and Uhlenbruck, 1963).

Our limited knowledge about the enzymatic activity of avian membranes also suggests a qualitative but not quantitative parallelism with the activity of mammalian red cell membranes. Zentgraf et al. (1971) demonstrated ouabain-inhibitable, (Na + K)-activated, Mg-dependent ATPase activity (see also Hamilton (1966) and Blanchet (1974)). Interestingly, studies by Brown et al. (1968) suggest that the ouabain-inhibited ATPase activity of membranes from the red cells of myopathic Pekin ducks is abnormal. Weckstein and Engelhardt (1959) have reported the presence of an active Mg-stimulated "Ecto" ATPase, which is incapable of acting on intracellular ATP but cleaves ATP in the medium. And finally, avian erythrocyte membranes contain adenyl cyclase activity (Davoren and Sutherland, 1963a,b).

Antigens responsible for the different blood groups in birds are located in the membrane. Chicken erythrocytes contain at least eleven separate blood groups, each of which is determined by a separate genetic locus. Eight are classified as simple, while three are considered complex (Gilmore, 1971).

2.3 METABOLISM

2.3.1 *Protein synthesis*

Autoradiographic studies have shown a progressive loss of RNA synthesizing capability and protein synthetic activity with maturation of the avian erythrocyte (Cameron and Prescott, 1963; Scherrer et al., 1966; Cameron and Kustberg, 1969). Fully mature erythrocytes lack both abilities. However, persistent reports of minor quantities of RNA, slight but continuous RNA synthesis and low template activity in the mature erythrocyte, have raised the possibility that protein synthesis is not zero, but a very much reduced "smoldering" level. See Zentgraf et al. (1975) for a bibliography on this controversial subject.

2.3.2 Glycolysis

The available evidence indicates that avian erythrocytes can degrade glucose to lactic acid (Warburg, 1909; Rüter, 1923) via the Emden-Meyerhof pathway. Meyerhof (1932) demonstrated that goose red cells contain all of the glycolytic enzymes, and Dische and Ashwell (1955) showed that a membrane-free hemolysate from pigeon erythrocytes can glycolyse anaerobically. Furthermore, duck red cells under anaerobic conditions produce approximately two molecules of lactate for every molecule of glucose consumed (Tosteson and Johnson, 1957a; Allen and McManus, 1967). Also, fluoride, iodoacetic acid and arsenate, inhibitors of specific steps in the Emden-Meyerhof pathway, produce the predicted effect on glucose consumption and lactate production (Bornstein and Ascher, 1926; Tosteson and Johnson, 1957a).

2.3.3 Hexose-monophosphate shunt

Avian erythrocytes also metabolize glucose via the hexose-monophosphate shunt. The studies of Barron and Harrop (1928) and Harrop and Barron (1928) precede an explicit description of this pathway but provide the first indication of its existence in avian red cells. They showed that small amounts of methylene blue simultaneously increased glucose degradation and diminished lactic acid formation in goose erythrocytes undergoing glycolysis. Coincident with this metabolic shift there was an increase in oxygen consumption and CO_2 production that was insensitive to cyanide (see also Dische, 1946). Much later, several workers (Buhler and Ihler, 1963; Shields et al., 1964) using ^{14}C-glucose, labeled in the 1 and 6 positions, provided direct evidence for glucose oxidation through the pentose phosphate pathway. Glucose-6-phosphate dehydrogenase and 6-phosphogluconic dehydrogenase activities have been measured in several species (Salvidio et al., 1963; Ghosh and Swarup, 1966; Narasimhan and Nair, 1973). Isoenzymes, responsible for this enzymatic activity, have also been isolated from several avian species (Cooper et al., 1969; Nóbrega et al., 1970; Leung and Haley, 1974).

2.3.4 Organic phosphate

Our understanding of the role played by organic acids in cell metabolism is not extensive. "Phytic acid"* and ATP have been the most thoroughly studied. Avian erythrocytes contain more organic phosphate than human cells. Most of this additional phosphate is nuclear in origin (Rapoport et

---

* "Phytic acid" (myoinosital hexaphosphate) has been placed in quotes because improved chromotographic techniques have recently established that, in at least pigeons and chickens, the "phytic acid" fraction is primarily 1, 3, 4, 5, 6-myoinositol pentaphosphate (Johnson and Tate, 1969; Steward and Tate, 1969).

al., 1941). Accordingly, the acid-soluble fraction in birds constitutes only 34 per cent (34·8 per cent, Heller *et al.*, 1932; 34·1 per cent ± 0·7 per cent, Spears and Kregnow, 1975*) of the total cellular phosphate. Rapoport (1940) and Rapoport and Guest (1941) first showed that "phytic acid", not 2,3-diphosphoglyceric acid as in human erythrocytes, was the major component of the acid-soluble fraction; ATP was the next most prevalent compound, accounting for 27 per cent of the acid-soluble fraction (Gerlach *et al.*, 1957). Other nucleotides were present in much smaller amounts (Gerlach *et al.*, 1957; Bartlett, 1970; Whitfield and Morgan, 1973).

The finding that bird cells contain "phytic acid" was revolutionary at the time, for although this compound was known to occur ubiquitously in plants, it had not been found previously in animals. Studies with radioactive phosphorous showed it to be much more stable than ATP (Rapoport *et al.*, 1941; Gerlach *et al.*, 1957).

Benesch and Benesch (1967) and Chanutin and Curnish (1967) showed that organic phosphates of the acid-soluble fraction lower the oxygen affinity of hemoglobin and thus could regulate oxygen unloading in tissues. "Phytic acid", because of its prevalence, should serve this function in avian erythrocytes. It has been confirmed that inositol hexophosphate and pentaphosphate do actually lower the oxygen affinity of hemoglobin (Benesch and Benesch, 1969; Ochiai *et al.*, 1972; Coates, 1975; Vandecasserie *et al.*, 1975). "Phytic acid" is also a significant osmotic constituent within cells, behaving, in part, as a charged nondiffusable anion.

2.3.5 *Citric acid cycle*

Warburg (1909) showed that avian erythrocytes consume oxygen. Their oxygen uptake, however, is less than that of most somatic cells (Tipton, 1933). The oxygen consumption is linked to the tricarboxylic acid cycle. Early studies had suggested that avian red cells contain the cycle (Severin, 1937; Ashwell and Dische, 1950; Hunter *et al.*, 1954); two subsequent studies established its presence. First, Rubinstein and Denstedt (1953, 1954) showed that chicken hemolysates contain all of the Krebs cycle enzymes except oxalacetic decarboxylase (see also Hunter and Hunter, 1957). Secondly, Dajani and Orten (1958, 1959) demonstrated directly a functioning tricarboxylic acid cycle. Using column chromatography, they showed that all the metabolites involved in the citric acid cycle were present in chicken red cells and that the amount of each increased when cells were incubated with the following substrates: acetate, citrate, α-ketoglutarate or malate. Also, they demonstrated labeling of all the Krebs cycle intermediates following incubation of the cells with ^{14}C-acetate or ^{14}C-glycine.

* Unpublished findings: mean ± S.E. ($n = 4$).

3 Early approaches to transport study

Chicken erythrocytes were one of the types of cells used in the earliest systematic study of animal cell permeability (Grjins, 1896). What was asked in this and other early studies was whether certain solutes entered the cells, as judged by their ability to cause osmotic lysis. Numerous solutes were classified on this basis. Jacobs (1931) summarized studies that indicated red cells were very permeable to water, O_2 and CO_2 and anions, such as chloride and bicarbonate. Köeppe (1897) had originally proposed that red cells were permeable to chloride and bicarbonate; this view was confirmed by the finding that the "chloride shift" occurs in the erythrocytes of many animals (Henderson, 1928), including birds (Mond, 1930).

Jacobs et al. (1950) extended the earlier studies on permeating substances, using a refined version of the hemolysis method. He and his coworkers in an extensive study that lasted nearly two decades showed that by comparing the relative permeability of erythrocytes to water and four selected solutes—ethylene glycol, glycerol, urea and thiourea—one could properly place most erythrocytes in their appropriate zoological class. Thus, they were able to classify animals not only morphologically but on the basis of species-related transport characteristics of their red blood cells. Striking similarities were observed between ten of the eleven species of avian red cells studied, including pigeon. They had a low permeability to urea and thiourea, but a high permeability to glycerol and the homologous compound, ethylene glycol. Only the chicken erythrocyte was atypical (see also Höber and Ørskov, 1933).

Interest in these four solutes has continued. Hunter studied their permeation and also that of erythritol in chicken (Hunter, 1960, 1961; Hunter et al., 1965) and pigeon (Hunter, 1970) erythrocytes and tried to determine whether permeation was carrier-mediated. His criteria for carrier involvement was based on the differential effect tannic acid and n-butanol have on nonelectrolyte and electrolyte permeability; inhibition of permeation indicated the involvement of carriers. Hunter and coworkers used a photoelectric method to measure the permeability of chicken red cells, which were atypical in Jacob's study, and concluded that none of the four solutes studied utilized a carrier in this species. In contrast, Hunter (1970) did find carrier kinetics for the permeation of pigeon red cells by glycerol, erythritol and urea, and also suggestive evidence for carrier in-involvement in permeation by ethylene glycol and thiourea. The more rapid penetration by nonelectrolytes in pigeon red cells made it necessary to measure permeability with a different technique, one modeled after that of Widdas (1954). The permeability to erythritol of goose erythrocytes had previously been studied by Mond (1930) and was found to be rapid.

Kaplan et al (1974), using the hemolysis method, studied permeability to urea from a comparative viewpoint and asked whether urea permeation differed in the various vertebrate classes. They accepted the following criteria as evidence that urea enters cells via a facilitated diffusion system: (1) inhibition by phloretin (see Macey and Farmer, 1973) and (2) more rapid penetration than its lipid soluble analog, acetamide. By these criteria they identified facilitated diffusion of urea in amphibian, reptilian and mammalian erythrocytes, but not in fish and avian red cells. Thus, the facilitated diffusion system developed with emergence to terrestial life, but was lost, for unknown reasons, in birds. They speculated that this loss in birds was associated with the shift in nitrogen excretion from urea to uric acid.

Wieth et al. (1974) had studied efflux of ^{14}C-urea from chicken red cells previously and had shown the efflux was slow and unresponsive to changes in the extracellular urea concentration—characteristics which were compatible with a process of simple diffusion.

4 Permeability to glucose

Pasteur first recognized that consumption of glucose varies depending on whether metabolism is anaerobic or oxidative. He observed that glycolysis decreased when yeast was switched from an anaerobic to an aerobic environment (Pasteur effect). It was not recognized, however, that changes in respiration could alter glucose transport and thereby control glycolysis until the studies of Randel and Smith (1958a,b) on diaphragm muscle, Morgan et al. (1959) on heart muscle, and Kleinzeller and Kotyk (1965) on yeast. The possible importance of altered transport in the changes that occur during anoxia is still frequently overlooked.

Morgan and Whitfield (1973) pointed out that avian erythrocytes are especially useful for studying the interrelationship between respiration, glucose transport and the cell's energy levels. The work of early investigators had suggested their applicability. Grjins (1896), Hedin (1897) and Masing (1912) noted that the glucose permeability of avian erythrocytes was low and much less than that of human red cells (Mond, 1930; Höber and Ørskov, 1933). The slow rate of entry made it easy to evaluate transport with radioactive sugars (Wood and Morgan, 1969). It was also known that glucose uptake increased when avian red cells were made anaerobic, either by gassing in a nitrogen atmosphere (Negelein, 1925), or carbon monoxide (Bornstein and Ascher, 1926). Finally, several studies indicated that the concentration of glucose in cells remained much lower than in plasma (Masing, 1912; Bell, 1953).

Morgan and coworkers studied the respiratory control of glucose transport in goose erythrocytes. Figure 1 (Wood and Morgan, 1969) demonstrates that glucose uptake increased when oxidative metabolism was inhibited by treatment with 1 mM sodium cyanide in a nitrogen atmosphere. Despite the presence of glucose in the bath, there was none measurable in either the aerobic or cyanide-treated cells. Thus, glucose utilization (phosphorylation and subsequent metabolism) outpaced glucose uptake in both conditions so that glucose transport was the rate-limiting step for glucose consumption.

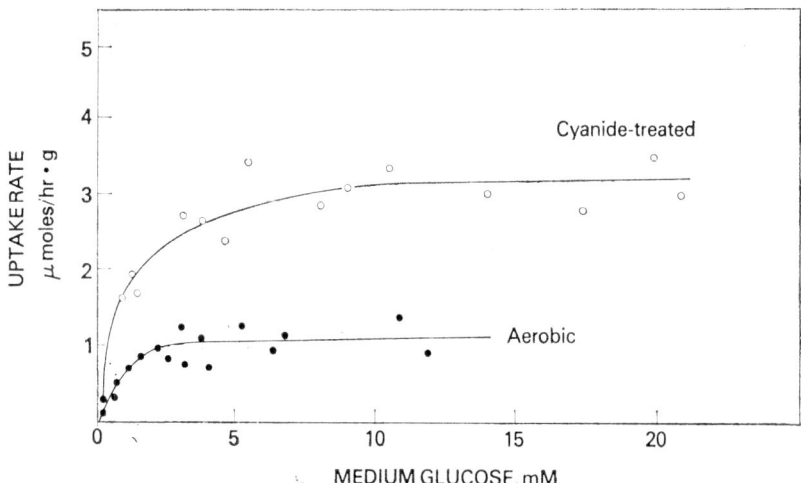

FIG. 1. Glucose uptake by goose erythrocytes in the aerobic and anoxic state. Suspensions of goose erythrocytes were incubated at 37°C in stoppered flasks which had been flushed with either oxygen or nitrogen. The nitrogen-exposed suspensions also contained 1 mM NaCN. Cellular glucose uptake was determined by measuring glucose loss from the medium after a 15–20 min preliminary incubation period. (From Wood and Morgan, 1969.)

By studying the influx and efflux of a nonmetabolizable sugar (3-O-methyl glucose) it was possible to measure more directly the anoxic stimulation of sugar transport. Figure 2 shows that anoxia caused the uptake of 3-O-methyl glucose to increase. The experimental conditions were similar to those used in the study described in Fig. 1. Sugar uptake increased because of an acceleration of a carrier-mediated process. Evidence for carrier involvement included the fit to Michaelis-Menten kinetics, substrate specificity, competition between related sugars, and countertransport. Flux measurements showed that anoxia increased the carrier's maximal transport rate (Wood and Morgan, 1969). There was also a change in K_m, but to a lesser extent (Wood and Morgan, 1969; Cheung et al., 1976).

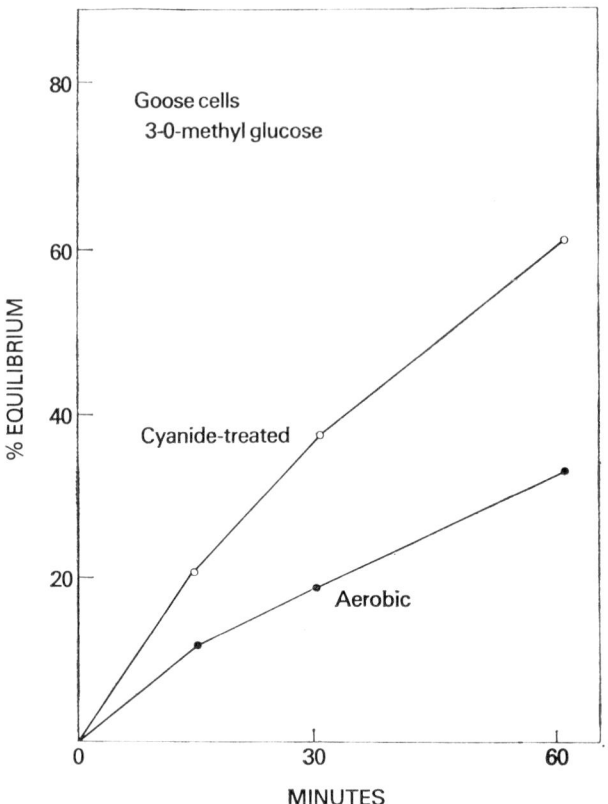

FIG. 2. 3-O-methyl glucose entry into goose erythrocytes. Suspensions of goose erythrocytes were prepared according to procedures described in the legend of Fig. 1, using sugar-free media. After the 15–20 min preliminary incubation period ^{14}C-3-O-methyl glucose was added to each flask and the cellular uptake of labeled sugar followed. After determining the equilibrium value for ^{14}C-3-O-methyl glucose content, the rates of entry were expressed as per cent equilibrium per minute using the initial slope of the entry curve. (From Wood and Morgan, 1969.)

Carrier-mediated sugar transport also increased when cells were made anoxic by treatment with dinitrophenol (Wood and Morgan, 1969) or prolonged incubation in a nitrogen atmosphere (Whitfield and Morgan, 1973). Using a nitrogen atmosphere to induce anoxia, Whitfield and Morgan (1973) correlated changes in the cellular levels of high-energy phosphate with the onset of the increase in sugar transport.

It is not understood how respiratory changes alter carrier-mediated transport. Sulfhydryl groups may be involved, since $HgCl_2$ and other sulfhydryl blocking agents produce an increase in 3-O-methyl glucose transport similar to anoxia (Wood and Morgan, 1969). In addition, studies of hemolysed and restored ghosts are suggestive that an intracellular substance which escapes during hemolysis normally immobilizes the carrier in aerobic cells (Wood and Morgan, 1969).

Whitfield and Morgan (1973) and Whitfield et al. (1974) observed that addition of ATP or catecholamines to the bathing medium also accelerated carrier-mediated 3-O-methyl glucose transport. (The catecholamines, however, did not increase glucose transport.) The externally applied ATP was rapidly hydrolysed to AMP and phosphate (Whitfield and Morgan, 1973). Catecholamines also affect cation transport (see section 7), but the effect differs in several ways from that on 3-O-methyl glucose transport (Whitfield et al., 1974) and the two responses are presumed to be unrelated.

5 Amino acid permeation

5.1 PRIMARY GLYCINE TRANSPORT SYSTEM

Studies by Vidaver and coworkers on glycine transport in pigeon red cells have provided one of the most detailed examinations of how sodium interacts with an amino acid transport system. Under ordinary conditions,* glycine entry into pigeon red cells was separated into two components (Vidaver, 1964a). A small quantity entered by a nonspecific Na-independent pathway with diffusion-like characteristics (Vidaver, 1964a,c), while the bulk entered by a Na-dependent process that actively accumulates glycine and is highly specific. Only two amino acids (N-methylglycine and N-ethylglycine) out of a total of thirty-three examined showed significant competition with glycine for entry via the specific route (Vidaver et al., 1964).

Vidaver and coworkers distinguished the primary glycine transport system experimentally by using, whenever possible, low glycine concentrations, adding L-threonine to prevent glycine transport with endogenous amino acids (Terry and Vidaver, 1973), and subtracting that portion of the flux utilizing the Na-independent route. The sodium-dependent system was identified and studied in intact cells (Vidaver, 1964a,c,d; Vidaver et al., 1964; Kittams and Vidaver, 1969; Terry and Vidaver, 1973), hemolysed and restored ghosts (Vidaver, 1964b,d; Vidaver and Shepherd, 1968; Vidaver, 1971) and membrane vesicles, prepared by sonicating intact cells (Lee et al., 1973).

---

* Wheeler et al. (1965) and Eavenson and Christensen (1967) showed that under other conditions (high glycine concentration or sodium concentration less than 20 mM), glycine also enters by another route, the ASCP system of Christensen (for alanine-serine-cysteine-proline).

The major characteristics of the system are:

a. The effect of sodium is specific. Potassium, lithium, choline or Tris hydroxymethyl aminomethane) do not substitute for sodium (Vidaver, 1964a). Michaelis-Menten type analysis reveals that sodium primarily affects K_m, not V_{max} (Vidaver, 1964a).

b. ^{22}Na is taken up along with glycine. The average ratio of sodium to glycine uptake is approximately 2 (Vidaver, 1964d), suggestive that two molecules of sodium and one molecule of glycine are transported together on a carrier. Consistent with this view, a double reciprocal plot of glycine entry is linear if plotted against the square of the sodium concentration.

c. Glycine uptake also obeys Michaelis-Menten kinetics when plotted against the external glycine concentration (Vidaver, 1964a) or chloride concentration (Vidaver, 1964c).

d. At high external sodium concentrations, glycine efflux from preloaded ghosts, which contained more sodium than normal cells, decreased (Vidaver and Shepherd, 1968). This transinhibition by Na depends upon a power of the sodium concentration greater than one, and is counteracted by extracellular glycine. There is a similar transinhibitory effect of sodium on glycine influx, but in other respects glycine influx and efflux are kinetically dissimilar (Vidaver and Shepherd, 1968).

Vidaver and Shepherd (1968) formulated a transition transport model incorporating these features. In this model, glycine transport occurs via a quaternary complex involving E (the carrier), two sodium ions and glycine (ENa_2G). Translocation rates for ENa or ENa_2 are negligible compared to the rates for E or ENa_2G. The complete complex (ENa_2G) is formed by the binding to the sodium ions, followed by the glycine. In order to explain the kinetic dissimilarities between influx and efflux, they supposed that either the association-dissociation constants for the reactions differ on the two sides of the membrane or that the rate constants for the translocation of ENa_2G and E across the membrane are not the same in both directions.

Vidaver and coworkers also investigated whether the Na electrochemical gradient provides the energy source for active glycine transport. They varied the sodium concentration in hemolysed and restored ghosts and showed that net glycine transport only occurred down the apparent Na gradient (Vidaver, 1964b,d; Vidaver and Shepherd, 1968). Neither the external nor internal Na concentration alone was important. These studies, insofar as they apply to ghosts of pigeon erythrocytes, are a convincing demonstration that a sodium gradient can provide energy for the transport of a nonelectrolyte.

The question remained, however, whether there is another energy source in addition to the Na gradient that drives part of the net glycine transport. This question arose because of uncertainty about the sodium activity within intact cells (Terry and Vidaver, 1973) and because of studies of amino acid transport in other cells which appeared to show additional energy sources for transport (Johnstone, 1972; Kimmich, 1972; Pietrzyk and Heinz, 1972; Christensen et al., 1974). In order to test whether the sodium gradient was adequate to explain completely the active glycine transport, Vidaver (1971) calculated glycine accumulation and expulsion ratios for the Na electrochemical gradient using the previously described transition model. Although the calculated values agreed, in general, with the experimental values for hemolysed and restored ghosts, there were some discrepancies. Along the same lines, Terry and Vidaver (1973) eliminated the sodium gradient by treating cells with gramicidin. Na-dependent glycine accumulation was largely abolished, but a small amount remained.

5.2 OTHER AMINO ACID TRANSPORT SYSTEMS

Eavenson and Christensen (1967) postulated that pigeon erythrocytes have at least four systems for handling neutral amino acids other than the glycine system described by Vidaver. Two of the additional systems are sodium-independent and two are sodium-dependent. The two sodium-independent systems are: (1) a nonsaturable system which shows a similar rate constant for all amino acids examined, independent of their structure, and (2) a system reactive with amino acids which have branches or rings on their side chain (like leucine and phenylalanine), called the LP system. A synthetic amino acid, BCH (b-2-aminobicyclo [2,2,1] heptane-2-carboxylic acid), serves as a model substrate for this system (Christensen et al., 1969). The two sodium-dependent systems are: (1) the β system which transports β-alanine and taurine, but not α-amino acids, and (2) the ASCP system, a system which transports alanine, serine, cysteine and proline. The ASCP system is the only one that shows significant counter-transport. It has not been possible to demonstrate unequivocally that any of the four systems can transport amino acids uphill (Eavenson and Christensen, 1967).

These transport systems are defined operationally and lack specificity. Many amino acids are carried by more than one system. Classification was established by competitive inhibition (Christensen, 1969). For a discussion of how these systems relate to similar ones in other cells, especially Ehrlich ascites tumor cells, one should consult the reviews by Christensen (1969, 1973).

Christensen and coworkers extended Vidaver's studies on the interaction of sodium and amino acids in pigeon red cells. Their major findings are:

1. Only amino acids transported by a Na-dependent system cause Na influx to increase (Wheeler and Christensen, 1967). These amino acids also stimulate a component of Na efflux other than the cation pump (Wheeler and Christensen, 1967).
2. Sodium can affect V_{max} in addition to its effect on the K_m of the primary glycine system. In the ASCP system Na affects the V_{max} and K_m nearly equally, whereas V_{max} is primarily altered in the β-amino acid system (Wheeler et al., 1965; Eavenson and Christensen, 1967).
3. A poor correlation exists between the way $[Na]_o$ affects amino acid influx, as determined by a double reciprocal plot, and the experimentally determined coupling coefficient for all sodium-dependent systems except the primary glycine system. For instance, a double reciprocal plot of serine influx is linear if plotted against the first order of $[Na]_o$, whereas the coupling coefficient is 4·0 (Eavenson and Christensen, 1967).
4. Amino acid structure is important in determining the coupling coefficient of the ASCP system. Previous studies indicated this system included receptor sites which could recognize sodium and the α-amino and carboxyl group of a suitable amino acid. Additional studies showed that other features of amino acid structure, besides the α-amino and carboxyl group, influenced the avidity with which sodium was bound and transported (Christensen, 1973). Amino acids with a methyl group on the side chain (alanine) interacted with sodium. A hydroxyl, mercapto or carboxamide group, located on carbon 3 or 4 of the amino acid and situated so that it was *trans* to the carboxylate group, caused a stronger interaction with sodium (Koser and Christensen, 1971; Thomas and Christensen, 1971). To explain the latter interaction, Thomas and Christensen (1971) suggested that the oxygen atom in the hydroxyl group actually formed an alkali metal complex with sodium.

6 Other

6.1 PERMEABILITY TO WATER

Blum and Forster (1970) and Farmer and Macey (1970) measured the permeability to water (P_w) of chicken red cells by using photometric methods that follow the rapid volume changes that develop when these cells are subjected to a sudden osmotic pressure gradient. Since both studies focused on mammalian erythrocytes, the measurements on avian cells are not extensive. Nevertheless, both laboratories found that the values for chicken red cells, although high, were less than those for the human erythrocytes.

6.2 OXIDIZED GLUTATHIONE TRANSPORT

Beutler and Srivastava (1968) and Srivastava and Beutler (1969a,b) described a transport system for oxidized glutathione (GSSG) in red cells. This system, studied most extensively in human erythrocytes, transports GSSG only out of cells against concentration gradients. Since normal erythrocytes do not contain appreciable quantities of GSSG, the transport system can only be demonstrated by artificially elevating cellular GSSG levels. In order to elevate GSSG, Srivastava and Beutler (1969a) oxidized cellular glutathione with H_2O_2 or methyl phenylazoformate. In normal cells, it was also necessary to inhibit intracellular GSSG reduction via glutathione reductase by adding chromate to the medium (Srivastava and Beutler, 1969b).

Erythrocytes from nine avian and nonavian species were examined for GSSG transport after such treatment (Srivastava and Beutler, 1969b). Of all nine species, transport was fastest in pigeons and slowest in chickens. It has been suggested that this system functions as a secondary defense mechanism against the accumulation of deleterious levels of GSSG (Srivastava, 1971; Smith, 1974).

7 Cation transport

7.1 GENERAL

Avian erythrocytes (Maizels, 1954; Ørskov, 1956; Tosteson and Robertson, 1956; Banaschak, 1959; Sturkie, 1965b; Gardner et al., 1973) contain a high concentration of potassium and a low concentration of sodium. The membrane potential in avian erythrocytes has not been measured directly, but has been estimated from the chloride ratio.* In duck red cells it is approximately 14 mv, inside negative (Kregenow, 1971a). Since avian plasma has a high concentration of Na and a low concentration of K, both sodium and potassium are maintained far from equilibrium under steady-state conditions. To maintain this disequilibrium, the cell must expend energy since it is permeable to both ions (Maizels, 1954; Tosteson and

* The response of cellular chloride to changes in pH (Allen and McManus, 1967), along with the rapid way ^{36}Cl crosses the membrane (Tosteson and Robertson, 1956; Allen and McManus, 1967; Vidaver, 1971; Kregenow, unpublished observations), indicates that chloride is distributed passively and that the distribution of chloride across the membrane can be used to estimate the membrane potential.

Robertson, 1956; Allen and McManus, 1967; Kregenow, 1971a,b, 1974, 1976b).

Tosteson and Hoffman (1960) first formulated an explicit model utilizing the pump-leak hypothesis to explain the cation composition and steady-state volume of a cell. In this model, active sodium and potassium transport balanced the leak for these ions. Figure 3 is a schematic drawing in which similar properties are attributed to an avian red cell. The cell is shown as having a high K and low Na concentration while incubating in a medium with a high Na and low K concentration. According to the model, the cell's cation composition and steady-state volume result from the continued action of a cation pump (labeled A in the drawing) balancing diffusional leaks for Na and K (labeled B in the drawing). The cation pump has been pictured as a coupled mechanism, moving Na out of and K into cells. Both movements occur against their respective electrochemical gradients and require the expenditure of energy.

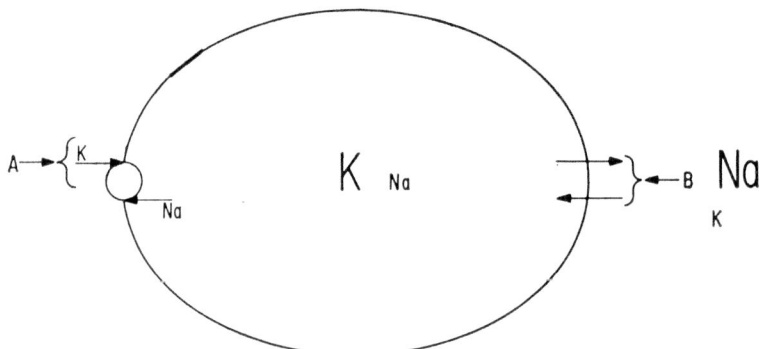

FIG. 3. Schematic drawing of a typical avian erythrocyte maintaining a steady-state cation composition and content.

The limited information indicates that the cation pump is similar in avian and human erythrocytes. The similarities are:

1. Pump activity increases as internal Na rises (Clarkson and Maizels, 1955; Kregenow, 1971b, 1974).
2. External potassium is required (Kregenow, 1971a,b; Gardner et al., 1973) and transport is a saturable function of external K concentration (Clarkson and Maizels, 1955; Tosteson and Robertson, 1956; Gardner et al., 1975b).
3. Ouabain blocks the pump, thereby preventing the net uptake of K and loss of Na, and inhibiting K influx and Na efflux (Kregenow, 1971a,b; Gardner et al., 1974; Gardner et al., 1975a).

Although Maizels (1954) originally suggested that energy for operating the pump was produced only aerobically, Tosteson and coworkers (Tosteson and Robertson, 1956; Tosteson and Johnson, 1957a,b) and Allen and McManus (1967) subsequently showed that the pump also functions under anaerobic conditions. This discrepancy is resolvable if: (1) ATP is the proximate energy source for the pump, and (2) the conditions used by Maizels to raise internal sodium before assessing pump activity eliminated all of the cell's ATP. The findings of Banaschak (1959), Allen and McManus (1967) and Whitfield and Morgan (1973) that ouabain has an "ATP sparing" effect support the notion that ATP is the proximate energy source.

7.2 VOLUME REGULATION

Duck erythrocytes proved to be a valuable model for studying the regulation of cell volume. When duck erythrocytes were added to a hypotonic solution, they swelled initially; when added to a hypertonic solution, they shrank. This initial response is expected from osmosis. Upon continued incubation, however, the duck red cells returned to their original isotonic volume even though they remained in the anisotonic media. This response to *continued* incubation in anisotonic media represents volume regulation. It is caused by changes in cation transport that lead to shifts in cell water.

The ability of duck red cells to regulate their volume in anisotonic media bears a resemblance to a form of volume regulation common to euryhaline invertebrates (Potts and Parry, 1964). This special adaptation of invertebrate cells to alterations in the osmolarity of the bathing media has been labeled "isosmotic intracellular regulation" by Florkin and coworkers (Jeuniaux *et al.*, 1961; Florkin and Schoffeniels, 1969). As in the duck erythrocytes, volume regulation in the invertebrate cells involves shifts in cell water. The adjustments result from alterations in the number of osmotic particles within cells, so that the cells change volume while remaining isosmolar with their surroundings. The adjustable cellular constituents are primarily organic acids (usually nonessential amino acids), not electrolytes as in the duck erythrocytes. Although changes in electrolytes occur, they are smaller and vary in the different species of invertebrates. Measurements of the osmolarity of duck red cells incubating in anisotonic media confirmed that they remained isosmolar with their surroundings despite changes in volume (Kregenow, 1973). Within the error of measurement ($\sim$2 milliosmoles per litre), duck red cells remained in osmotic equilibrium with their environment before, during and after they readjusted their volume.

The regulatory process in duck red cells principally involves the controlled movement of potassium into or out of the cell. The potassium in turn is followed by diffusable anion, primarily chloride, and finally osmotically obliged water. Duck erythrocytes contain, therefore, a system which regulates the total number of osomotic particles, specifically the total content of Na plus K. We labeled the cellular elements of this system a "volume controlling mechanism".

Although ouabain inhibited the classical sodium and potassium pump in duck erythrocytes, and caused sodium and potassium concentrations to change reciprocally, it did not inhibit the "volume controlling mechanism" (Kregenow, 1971a,b). Thus, within the pump-leak concept the "volume controlling mechanism" is a system which is functionally separate from the usual cation pump. We will see in this section that although the macromolecular elements that comprise the "volume controlling mechanism" are independent of the pump, they have a transport capacity and precision of control nearly comparable to the pump.

The process that causes cells to shrink and lose K (volume regulatory decrease) differs from the process that causes enlargement and gain of K (volume regulatory increase). For this reason, the two phenomena will be discussed separately.

7.2.1 Shrinkage (volume regulatory decrease)

(a) *General.* Figure 4 shows schematically what happens when cells shrink. The small dark ellipse represents a cell with a normal volume, and the larger ellipse a swollen cell. Volume regulatory decrease (VRD) occurs not only in hypotonic media (Kregenow, 1971a) but also in isotonic media (Kregenow, 1973), provided the cells are previously swollen. (Cells may be swollen in isotonic media either because a catecholamine, such as norepinephrine, has caused accumulation of cations or because the cells have been loaded with salts by a special experimental procedure.)

The swollen state triggers VRD, provided conditions are appropriate. The nature of the triggering mechanism is unknown, but could involve the stretching of an elastic membrane protein (Kregenow, 1971a). The increase in cell size which triggers the response can be as small as 4 per cent or as large as 50 per cent. The only apparent upper limit is hemolysis that results when the solution becomes too dilute. To initiate VRD in isotonic media, one removes from the bathing medium the norepinephrine which had caused cell swelling. Once the cells are free of hormone, they shrink in volume by 7–15 per cent, provided the concentration of potassium in the medium is normal.

The cells shrink rapidly, returning to near their original isotonic volume within 15–45 min. The response of norepinephrine-swollen cells incubating in an isotonic medium of 320 mosmol l^{-1} is comparable in all respects to the response of untreated cells in a hypotonic medium which has an osmolarity 70 mosmol less. *Controlled* loss of potassium characterizes the response. Chloride, and to a lesser extent bicarbonate, follow the potassium so that electroneutrality is maintained. Changes in sodium content and permeability are not significant. In fact, sodium permeability may actually be reduced (Kregenow, 1971a, 1973).

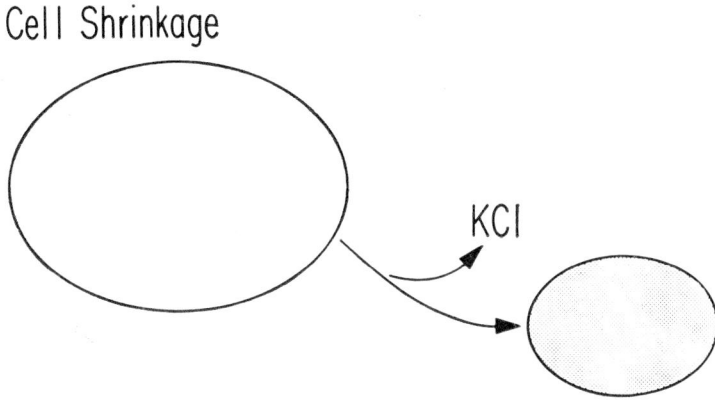

FIG. 4. Schematic representation of the process of cell shrinkage (volume regulatory decrease).

Figure 5 illustrates the fine control of K loss. The cells were initially swollen 25 per cent by introducing them to a hypotonic medium. The figure shows cellular changes in the K content (Part A), K efflux (Part B) and cell volume (Part C) during successive 15 min intervals. As the cells shrink, they lose K. The loss is the result of a temporary increase in K efflux. Note that K efflux was initially very high in the swollen cells, but returned to normal value as cell K content decreased and cell volume was corrected. We infer that K efflux is constantly monitored by the degree of cell swelling.

The increase in K efflux is presumably caused by an increase in a diffusional process similar to the leak. The following evidence supports this hypothesis (Kregenow, 1971a, 1973). The net movement of K is downhill. Eliminating the K electrochemical gradient by raising the extracellular K concentration (at constant extracellular chloride concentration) blocks both net K loss and volume changes. As would be expected a higher concentration of extracellular K is required to block the response with isotonic cells, because of their higher intracellular potassium concentration, than with swollen hypotonic cells. The major change in permeability is an increase in K efflux—a finding consistent with the potassium leak hypothesis. Ouabain, which specifically inhibits the pump, does not alter volume changes, net K loss or increase in K efflux.

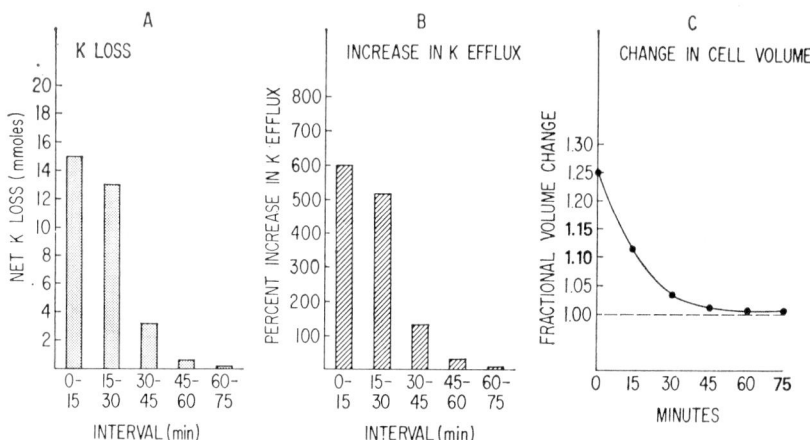

FIG. 5. The temporal changes in potassium content, potassium efflux and cell volume as duck erythrocytes regulate their volume in a hypotonic medium. The changes in K content are measured in millimoles; the changes in K efflux are presented as the per cent increase in K efflux above the value of control cells incubating in an isotonic medium. Changes in cell volume are expressed as fractional volume change—isotonic control cells have a value of 1·00 on this scale.

Figure 6 demonstrates this latter point. As in Fig. 5, the bath was sufficiently hypotonic to produce an initial 25 per cent enlargement. The ordinate is fractional volume change. The dashed lines represent cells incubated with 10^{-4} ouabain, and the solid lines untreated cells. Ouabain had no appreciable effect on either the size of control cells in isotonic media or the response of experimental cells in hypotonic media. Ouabain, however, did block the pump and alter the Na and K concentration, but not the total Na and K content of both groups of cells. Both lost about 3 mmol of K and gained 3 mmol of Na per 30 min interval. For the cells undergoing VRD in hypotonic media, this small K loss added to the much larger 35–40 mmol K loss produced by the "volume controlling mechanism".

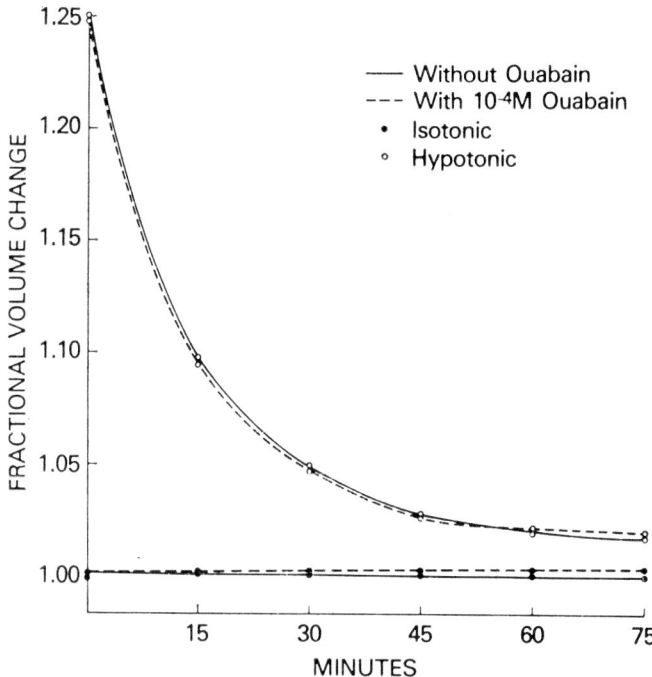

FIG. 6. Ouabain's lack of effect on changes in cell volume during volume regulatory decrease.

(b) *Cation-substituted cells.* To increase our understanding of VRD and to study the role played by cellular Na and K, we enlarged cells by loading them with salts and studied their response in isotonic media (Kregenow, 1974). To increase the NaCl or KCl content of cells, we subjected them to a modified version of the procedure of Garrahan and Rega (1967). This procedure involves treatment with *p*-chloromercuriphenyl sulfuric acid (PCMBS), a sulfhydryl blocking agent, followed by incubation with dithiothreitol (DTT), a reducing agent. During PCMBS treatment, the cells become leaky and acquire the ionic composition of their bathing media. By controlling the bathing media, one can set the ionic composition of the cells. Removal of the PCMBS and incubation with DTT eliminates the membrane injury. If, as a control, cells are processed in this way so as to have an ionic composition and volume identical to untreated cells, they retain normal cation permeability characteristics. Four populations of cells were produced—high K cells, high Na cells and two kinds of intermediate cells. The four populations all contained as much as twice the normal quantity of cation; the intermediate cells differed in that they contained both K and Na rather than all K or all Na.

Figure 7 shows schematically what happened when these experimentally enlarged cells were incubated in isotonic media. Consider the high K cells first. Enlarged high K cells reacquired and then maintained their original volume (represented by the schematic drawing of a smaller cell). The same "volume controlling mechanism" considered earlier was responsible for regulating their volume. The high K cells shrank rapidly at first, then more slowly, as the cells approached their original volume. Shrinkage resulted from the controlled loss of K, Cl and water (Kregenow, 1974). The K loss, in turn, resulted from a temporary increase in K efflux (Kregenow, 1974). Ouabain had no effect on the volume changes, but the response was blocked by raising the external potassium concentration high enough to eliminate the electrochemical gradient (Kregenow, 1974).

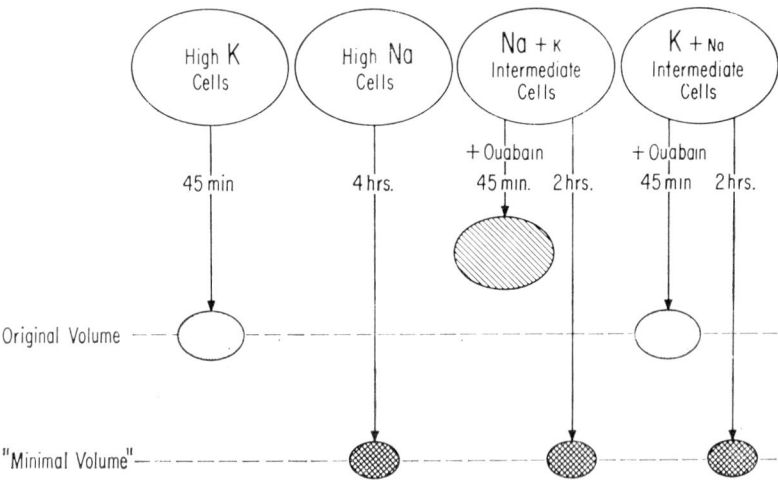

FIG. 7. Schematic representation of the response of experimentally enlarged (cation-loaded) cells to incubation in isotonic media. Four kinds of enlarged cells are shown; all contained twice the normal quantity of cations. High K cells contained almost all potassium; high Na cells contained almost all sodium. Intermediate Na + K cells contained more sodium than potassium, whereas intermediate K + Na cells contained more potassium than sodium. Both kinds of intermediate cells were incubated with and without 10^{-4} M ouabain.

The high Na cells also shrank, but the mechanism differed. First, they shrank at a lower rate. Whereas high K cells required 45 min to reach their original volume, high Na cells of comparable size required nearly 4 h. Secondly, the high Na cells shrank to four-fifths of their original volume and stabilized at that smaller size. We have labeled this latter volume the "minimal volume" and have represented it in Fig. 7 by the drawing of the smallest cell. Shrinkage resulted from the loss of Na, Cl and water. The mechanism responsible for removing the Na was the pump rather than the "volume controlling mechanism". Inhibiting the pump by removing all extracellular potassium or adding ouabain prevented the Na loss and shrinkage (Kregenow, 1974). Further, Na left the cell against its electrochemical gradient. Thus, the Na pump removed the excess Na from these cells without them regulating to normal volume.

Figure 7 shows two kinds of intermediate cells. Intermediate cells containing slightly more Na than K have been labeled Na + K cells, whereas cells containing more K than Na have been labeled K + Na cells. We incubated both cell types in the presence and absence of ouabain. Note first the response of ouabain-treated cells. Since ouabain blocks the cation pump, ouabain-treated cells cannot use this mechanism to remove Na. Under these conditions, the cells re-established their original volume by using the "volume controlling mechanism" only when they contained sufficient potassium. The quantity of K was limited in Na + K cells, so that even when K was completely lost via the "volume controlling mechanism" the resultant water loss was too small to return the cells to their original volume. These cells shrank rapidly at first, but stopped before reaching their original volume. In contrast, K + Na cells contained sufficient K and regulated to their original volume.

Without ouabain, on the other hand, the pump remained operative and both types of intermediate cells shrank until they reached either "minimal volume" or a volume limited by return of the internal sodium concentration to normal. Each group lost both sodium and potassium and shrank faster than high Na cells and slower than high K cells. Evidently the pump and the "volume controlling mechanism" operated simultaneously, the pump removing sodium and the "volume controlling mechanism" removing potassium.

Using intermediate cells and this experimental system, we asked whether the pathway taken by a K ion as it left the cell through the "volume controlling mechanism" was different from that taken by a Na ion expelled by the pump. If both mechanisms shared the same pathway, competition for the route was expected. The presence of Na exiting through the pump should alter the rate at which K leaves via the "volume controlling mechanism" and vice versa.

Two types of experiments were performed to answer this question (Kregenow, 1974). In the first, we examined the rate of K loss via the "volume controlling mechanism" in K + Na cells. These cells rapidly lose both Na and K through the respective mechanisms. Blocking the Na loss through the pump by incubating the cells with ouabain did not affect K loss through the "volume controlling mechanism" as measured by K efflux. In the second type of experiment we compared the rate of Na loss through the pump from both types of Na-rich cells, high Na cells and Na + K cells. Conditions were chosen so that pump activity was maximal in both cell types. There was negligible potassium loss in high Na cells, since they contained less than 2 mmol of K. On the other hand, Na + K cells lost appreciable quantities of K (30 mmol per half hour). Desite this marked difference in potassium loss, sodium loss through the pump was similar in both groups of cells (Kregenow, 1974).

Both experimental approaches suggest that the pathways are separate. Figure 8 illustrates this point. This schematic drawing represents a cell that is regulating its volume by shrinking. Under these *unsteady state* conditions, unlike the *steady state* conditions of Fig. 3, membrane pathway C becomes apparent in duck erythrocytes. It is through this potassium selective pathway that the "volume controlling mechanism", labeled D, controls K loss from enlarged cells. It is possible that pathway C is identical to the diffusional pathway for potassium, labeled B in the drawing.

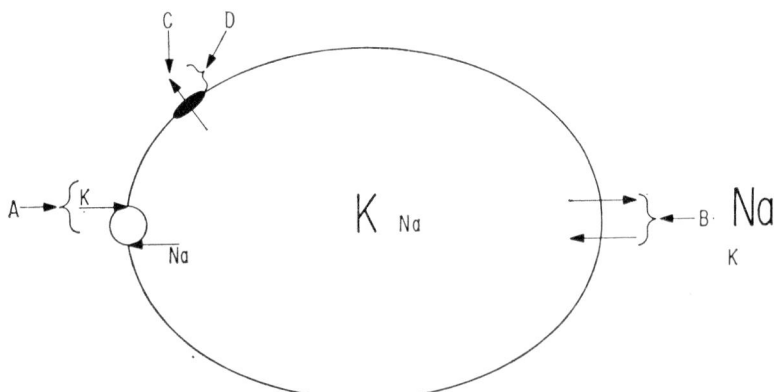

FIG. 8. Schematic drawing of a duck erythrocyte undergoing cell shrinkage (volume regulatory decrease).

(c) *Anion-substituted cells.* There is no specific anion requirement for VRD (Kregenow, 1976b), in contrast to the specific requirement for K. Figure 9 compares the volume changes of cells containing chloride with those of cells containing bromide or sulfate, when each is incubated in appropriate hypotonic media.* The ordinate is fractional volume change and the abscissa time in hours. The response of cells containing chloride

* Since cells containing sulfate are shrunken in isosmotic sulfate media (fractional volume 0·94), a more hypotonic solution is needed with these cells (25 mosmol l^{-1} less) to produce a comparable initial osmotic swelling. (The isosmotic volume of cells containing sulfate is smaller because they need contain only half as many anions as cells containing chloride to maintain electroneutrality within the cell.)

(circle) was similar to that of cells containing bromide (triangle), despite the fact that a different anion accompanies the exiting potassium. Cells containing sulfate (square) also regulated their volume; however, the readjustment took four times as long and the final regulated volume was slightly larger than the original.

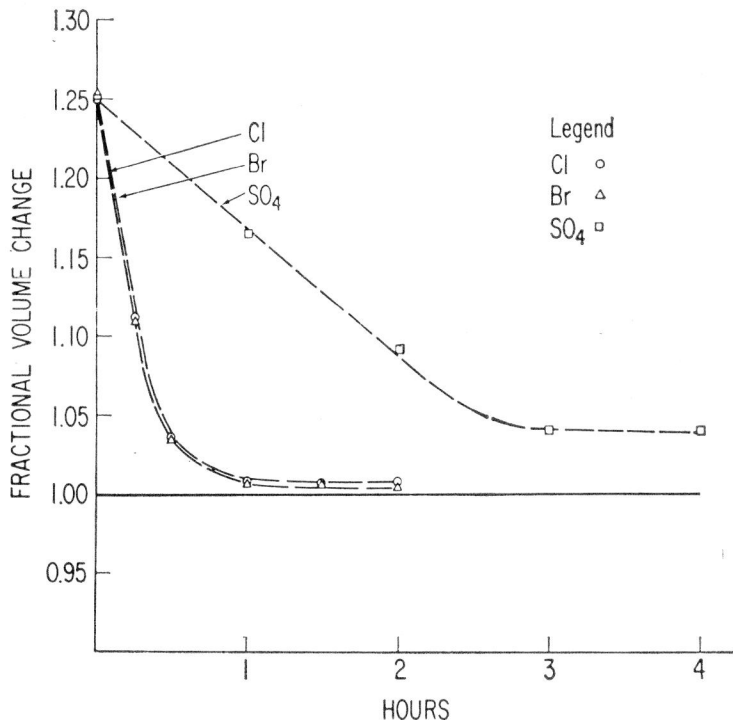

FIG. 9. Response of anion-substituted cells to incubation in hypotonic media. We produced bromide (△) or sulfate (□) cells by first washing normal chloride cells (○) with bromide or sulfate media, isosmotic to the standard isotonic chloride medium and then incubating them in this medium during the usual 90 min preincubation period.

7.2.2 Enlargement (volume regulatory increase)

(a) *General.* Figure 10 is a schematic drawing which illustrates cell enlargement, or volume regulatory increase (VRI). The phenomenon develops not only in hypertonic media where the initial osmotic shrinkage seems to trigger the response (Kregenow, 1971b), but also in isotonic media to which norepinephrine in concentrations as low as 5×10^{-9} M is added (Riddick et al., 1971; Kregenow, 1973). The cells enlarge 4–15 per cent in volume by accumulating potassium, chloride and H_2O. The potassium accumulates against an electrochemical gradient. The response requires an external potassium concentration above 2·5 mM in order for the cells to enlarge (but not for the typical permeability changes to occur). This effect of external potassium on cell enlargement plateaus at 15 mM.

Cell Enlargement

Volume Regulation occurs in:
(1) Hypertonic Media, containing an elevated $[K]_o$ (2.5 ⟶ 15mM)

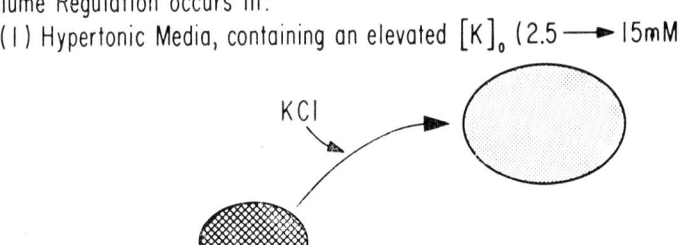

(2) Isotonic Media, containing both norepinephrine and an elevated $[K]_o$ (2.5 ⟶ 15mM)

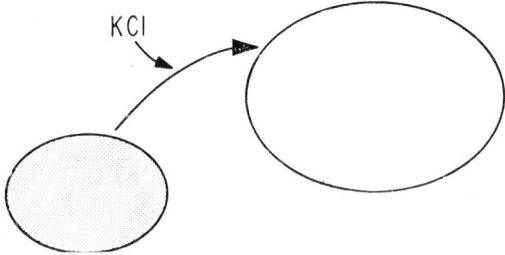

FIG. 10. Schematic representation of the process of cell enlargement (volume regulatory increase).

Part of the gain in cell K results from the following sequence. The permeability to Na increases, bringing sodium into the cell down its electrochemical gradient. The cation exchange pump, stimulated by the additional sodium, exchanges it for K. Removing Na from the medium prevents the cells from enlarging (Kregenow, 1971b, 1973). Also, the additional Na entry, which results from an increase in Na influx, was dependent on the external K concentration being above 2·5 mM (Kregenow, 1971b, 1973). The process described above accounts for nearly half of the K taken up by cells during VRI. The rest of the uphill accumulation of K occurs by a process which is independent of the pump. If the pump is inhibited by ouabain, K still accumulates in the cells in addition to sodium. This K uptake is especially prominent in the early stages of the response (Kregenow, 1971b, 1973). Subsequent work has focused on analysing the change in cation fluxes that is responsible for both this uphill K transport and the increase in Na permeation (Kregenow, 1971b, 1973).

Dramatic increases in permeability to both sodium and potassium occur when cells are stimulated with norepinephrine or hypertonicity (Kregenow, 1971b, 1973). Figure 11 demonstrates how great the changes are. Influx and efflux of K and Na in the control condition (open column) are compared to those after the addition of cells to either hypertonic media (solid column) or an isotonic solution containing norepinephrine (slashed

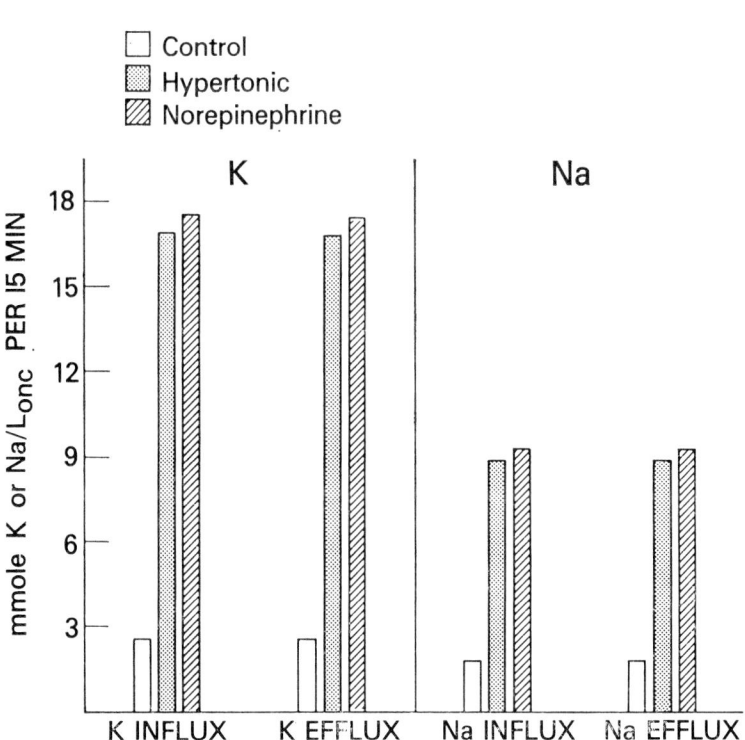

FIG. 11. The increase in sodium and potassium fluxes produced by norepinephrine or hypertonicity. Flux measurements were determined for a 15 min interval beginning with either (1) the introduction of 10^{-6} M norepinephrine to a suspension of cells in an isotonic medium or (2) the addition of cells to a hypertonic medium (475 mosmol l^{-1}). All media had a $[K]_o$ of 2·5 mM.

column). The ordinate is the flux measurement at 15 min. Since the external potassium concentration was 2·5 mM, the change occurred without net cation movement or swelling of the cells. Both hypertonicity and norepinephrine increased all four fluxes above control values by a factor of 5 to 10. (By way of comparison, the K influx value of norepinephrine-treated cells is nearly fifty times larger than the K influx of normal human red cells.)

The following evidence indicates that this generalized increase in permeability is an intrinsic part of the process by which cells enlarge (Kregenow, 1971b, 1973, 1977). First, identical increases in permeability develop irrespective of whether the stimulus is hypertonicity or catecholamines. Secondly, almost all of the increase in permeability is ouabain-insensitive, as is the process of cell enlargement. Thirdly, the increase in permeability shows the following relationship to cell enlargement. If the external potassium is 2·5 mM and the cells fail to enlarge, the increase in permeability persists. In contrast, if the external potassium is greater than 2·5 mM and cells enlarge, the increase in permeability gradually subsides as the cells approach their final volume. Finally, three of the four fluxes that result from the increase in permeation, K influx and efflux and Na influx, decrease upon removing both external sodium and potassium. The decreases in fluxes provide an explanation for the inhibition of VRI when both extracellular K and Na are lowered.

The following picture of VRI emerges. Both stimuli, norepinephrine and hypertonicity, activate an ouabain-insensitive transport process (s) whose salient feature is the rapid movement of sodium and potassium in and out of the cell. When the $[K]_o$ is greater than 2·5 mM, Na and K influx exceed already elevated effluxes, causing the cells to accumulate both Na and K. This additional Na and K, followed by anions and water, is responsible for cell enlargement. Any newly acquired Na is ordinarily extruded by the pump in exchange for extracellular K. The final result is an enlarged cell, containing more K, Cl and water. Thus, potassium is actively transported into the cell through two mechanisms, one associated with the rapid bidirectional K fluxes, the other the classical Na–K exchange pump. Ouabain inhibits only the latter.

(b) *Membrane potential.* Before proceeding to a description of experiments examining the nature of the rapid bidirectional fluxes, let us consider what happens to the membrane potential during the generalized increase in permeability. Knowledge about this parameter is essential to a basic understanding of the mechanism.

Estimates of the membrane potential made using either the chloride ratio or the carbocyanine dye (Di-S-C_3) indicate that it does not change by more than a few millivolts during VRI (Kregenow, 1971b, 1973, 1977). Figure 12 shows an experiment in which Dr. J. Goldinger and I used Di-S-C_3 to estimate the potential. This dye is one of several used by Hoffman and Laris (1974) to measure changes in the membrane potential of mammalian and nonmammalian erythrocytes. Red cells quantitatively take up Di-S-C_3 when hyperpolarized or release it when depolarized (measured as a decrease or increase in medium fluorescence respectively).

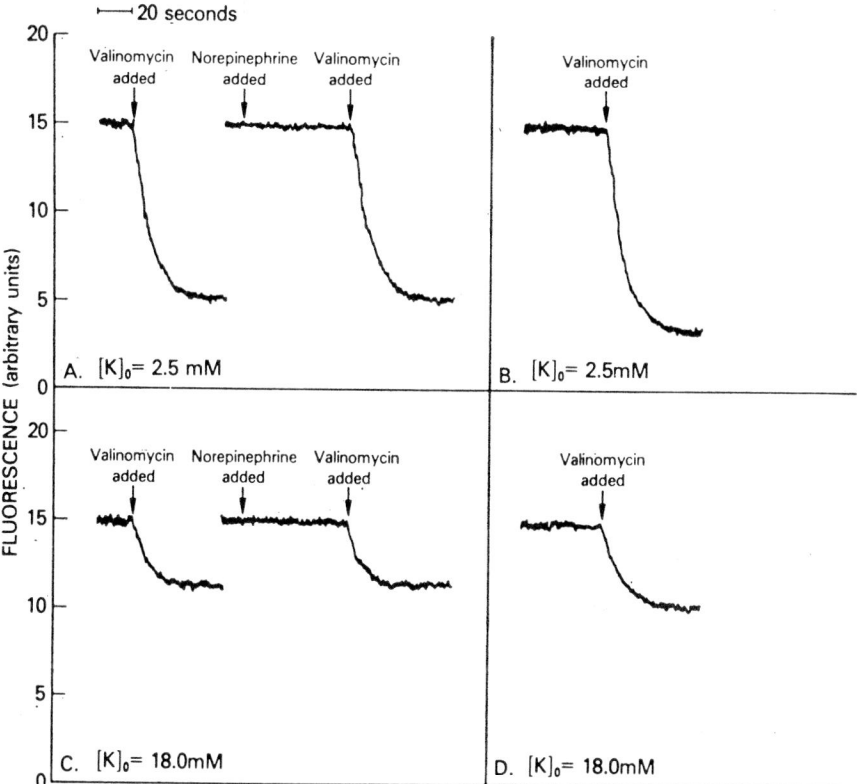

FIG. 12. Estimates of the membrane potential during the generalized increase in cation permeability using the carbocyanine dye, DI-S-C_3. The generalized increase in cation permeability was initiated by either introducing norepinephrine (10^{-6} M) to a suspension of cells in an isotonic medium (Parts A and C), or adding cells to a hypertonic medium (420 mosmol l^{-1}) (Parts B and D). The $[K_o]$ of the media was either 2·5 mM (Part A and B) or 18·0 mM (Part C and D). Approximately 1 min after initiating the generalized increase in permeability, control (far left) and experimental cells were hyperpolarized by adding 10^{-6} M valinomycin. A decrease in fluorescence indicates that the membrane potential has become more negative (hyperpolarized).

This change in fluorescence is used to estimate alterations in potential. If norepinephrine is added to cells incubating in isotonic media (A and C), medium fluorescence does not change despite the generalized increase in permeability. In addition, if cells stimulated previously either with norepinephrine (A and C) or by placement in hypertonic media (B and D) are hyperpolarized, they sequester the same amount of dye and show the same decrease in medium fluorescence as control cells. (Cells were hyperpolarized by adding valinomycin, which selectively increases potassium permeation.) Comparable fluorescence changes indicate that the cells were hyperpolarized to the same extent; this, in turn, implies that their membrane potentials were similar before hyperpolarization. Evidently the rapid cation movements are not associated with any major change in membrane potential.

(c) *Replacement of extracellular sodium and potassium.* Figures 13–15 examine the relationship between extracellular sodium or potassium and the increased cation flux. Figures 13 and 14 show the effect of extracellular K on Na and K fluxes. Figure 15 demonstrates the effect of altering extracellular Na on K fluxes. Only norepinephrine or hypertonicity-induced, ouabain-insensitive fluxes which are most pertinent are shown. We have subtracted the much smaller ouabain-insensitive control fluxes. The response to norepinephrine is on the left and hypertonicity on the right. Influx and efflux measurements, which represent uptake or loss during the initial 4 min, have been plotted together, permitting simultaneous examination of both flux values and determination of cation gain or loss by cells.

These three figures show that three of the fluxes, K influx and efflux (Figs 13 and 15) and Na influx (Fig. 14*), require the presence of both extracellular Na and K. If either is absent, movement ceases. For two of the three fluxes (K influx and Na influx) the combined effect of Na and K acts on the *cis* side of the transport process, while in the third, K influx, the effect originates on the *trans* side.

The findings with $[K]_o$ of 2·5 mM were unexpected for a transport process consisting of simple diffusion, and suggested that there is some coupling of the fluxes as in cotransport (Kregenow 1971b, 1977). A mobile carrier shuttling across the membrane only when combined with Na and K, and not if combined with only one of the cations, is more compatible with the findings. Then, Na entering the cell would be driven by its electrochemical gradient and would drag K along against its gradient. Similarly, the driving force for K exit from cells would be the K electrochemical gradient and Na would be carried out of the cell against its

* Not shown is the obvious effect of removing extracellular Na on Na influx.

gradient. Transport systems with similar features have been described previously for Na and nonelectrolytes in this (Vidaver and Shepherd, 1968) and other tissues (Schultz and Curran, 1970).

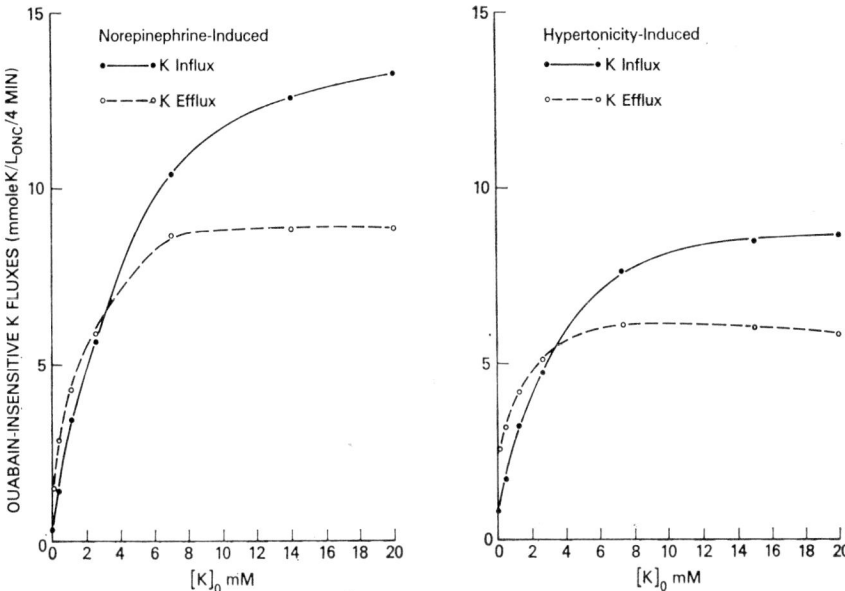

FIG. 13. The effect of varying the extracellular K concentration on the norepinephrine and hypertonicity-induced (ouabain-insensitive) K fluxes of duck erythrocytes. K influx and efflux were determined immediately after either (1) introducing norepinephrine (10^{-6} M) to a suspension of cells in an isotonic medium containing 10^{-4} M ouabain, or (2) adding cells to a hypertonic medium (420 mosmol l^{-1}) containing 10^{-4} M ouabain. Ouabain-insensitive increments have been obtained by subtracting the much smaller values for the corresponding K fluxes of control cells incubating in an isotonic medium containing ouabain (10^{-4} M). The extracellular K concentration was varied by isosmotically replacing some of the NaCl with KCl.

The following findings also support this idea. First, the response of these three fluxes to $[Na]_o$ or $[K]_o$ is curvilinear and approximates, in some cases, Michaelis-Menten kinetics. Secondly, at a $[K]_o$ of 2·5 mM, the calculated K electrochemical potential is approximately equal ($+96$ mV) and opposite to the Na electrochemical potential (-94 mV). Thus at this $[K]_o$, despite the rapid bidirectional cation movements, there should be no net cation flux, since there is no net force. Under these conditions, then, the system would be acting passively.

On the other hand, there were other observations that are not explained by this scheme. For instance, Na efflux did not decrease when

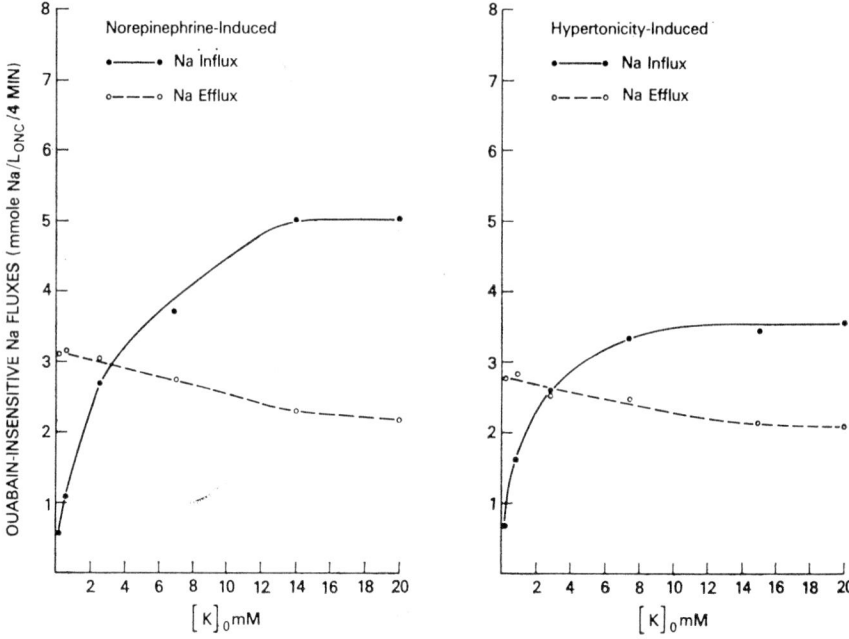

FIG. 14. The effect of varying the extracellular K concentration on the norepinephrine and hypertonicity-induced (ouabain-insensitive) Na fluxes of duck erythrocytes. The experimental protocol for measuring Na influx and efflux was similar to that described in Fig. 13 except for differences related to the use of ^{24}Na.

extracellular K was removed (Fig. 14) despite the observed decrease in K efflux (Fig. 13). Under these conditions, the enhanced Na efflux was evidently not obligatorily coupled to K efflux. In addition, Na efflux seemed to represent a form of active transport that could be explained only in part by the cotransport hypothesis but one that utilized a mechanism other than the classic cation pump. Inspection of Fig. 14 shows that when the $[K]_o$ is near zero, a large Na efflux exists in the absence of a similar increase in Na influx. This arrangement should result in the net loss of sodium from the cell. The predicted sodium loss would occur against a large electrochemical gradient at a time when the pump is blocked both because ouabain is present and external potassium is absent. Indeed, under these conditions norepinephrine produces a net Na loss of 1·2 mmol in 5 min. Cells treated without norepinephrine but with ouabain gain, as expected, 0·3 mmol. Thus, norepinephrine causes a net Na loss of 1·5 mmol in 5 min (Kregenow, 1977). Also unexplained is why cation accumulation plateaus when $[K]_o$ exceeds 15 mM. It is difficult to conceive of a simple cotransport system which encompasses all the findings.

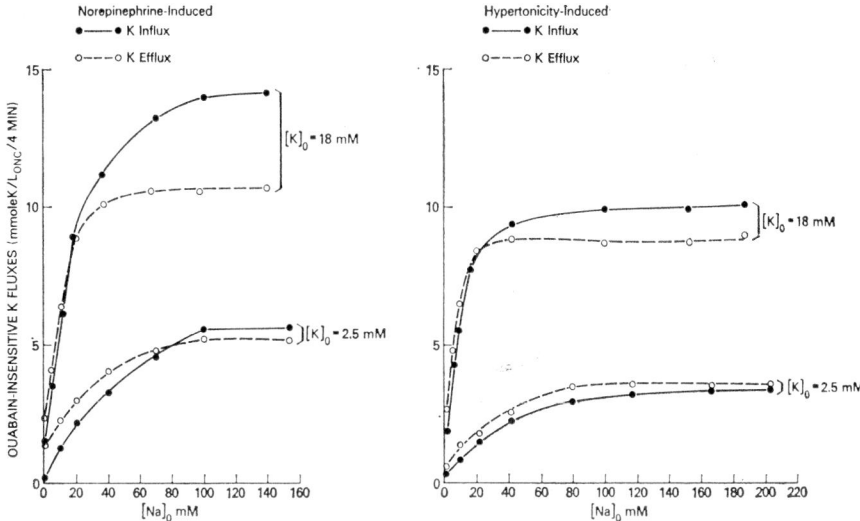

FIG. 15. The effect of varying the extracellular Na concentration on the norepinephrine and hypertonicity-induced (ouabain-insensitive) K fluxes at two extracellular K concentrations (2·5 and 18·0 mM). The experimental protocol was similar to that in Fig. 13 except that the extracellular K concentration was either 2·5 or 18·0 mM and the extracellular Na concentration was varied by isosmotically replacing some of the NaCl with choline Cl.

(d) *Relationship to transport by the cation pump.* Although many questions about VRI remain unanswered, the following study established that transport by the pump and the generalized increase in permeability are independent (Kregenow, 1976b). We took cells exhibiting both mechanisms and selectively inhibited the generalized increase in permeability rather than the pump. Table 2 shows that replacing all extra- and intracellular chloride with sulfate and treating isotonic chloride cells with 1 mM furosemide eliminated the generalized increase in permeability, but left the pump unaltered.

Figure 16 illustrates this point and pictures the cation pump and "volume controlling mechanism" as functionally distinct entities. The cell shown here is enlarging and is therefore in an *unsteady state*. This figure resembles Fig. 8 and differs only in that a double-headed arrow has been drawn to represent the pathway(s) through which the rapid bidirectional cation movements characteristic of cell enlargement take place.

TABLE 2

Comparison of the activity of the cation pump and that aspect of the volume controlling mechanism concerned with cell enlargement

Cell type	Cation pump	Increase in cation permeability associated with cell enlargement
Cl cells (control)	+	+
SO₄ cells	+	−
Cl cells treated with furosemide (1 mM)	+	−

The pump was assayed by noting ouabain's ability to inhibit K influx while we tested for the generalized increase in permeability by stimulating cells with 10^{-6} M norepinephrine and noting the increase in K influx. Untreated chloride cells served as controls. (Furosemide, at the concentration used, has a slight inhibiting effect on the pump.)

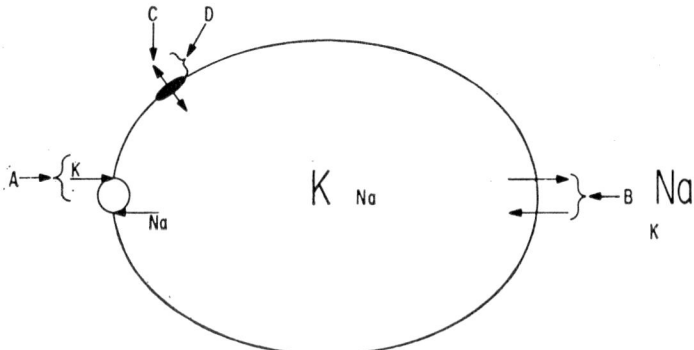

FIG. 16. Schematic drawing of duck erythrocyte undergoing cell enlargement (volume regulatory increase).

(e) *Cyclic AMP and hormonal response.* Interest in avian erythrocytes as a system for studying how hormones act began with the pioneering studies of Ørskov and of Sutherland. In 1956, Ørskov reported that pigeon erythrocytes, incubated with norepinephrine, lowered the plasma potassium concentration. This important finding was ignored for many years, in part because of the presence of unexplained hemolysis. Then in 1962 Sutherland and coworkers (Klainer et al., 1962; Davoren and Sutherland, 1963a) showed that catecholamines produce an elevation of cyclic AMP in pigeon erythrocytes. This finding served as part of the basis for their general hypothesis that a variety of hormones exert their characteristic effect in receptor cells via the intermediacy of cyclic AMP (Sutherland and Robinson, 1966). Subsequently, Davoren and Sutherland (1966) established that avian red cell membranes contain a catecholamine-sensitive adenyl cyclase system. Others have since confirmed both findings by Sutherland and coworkers (Shaw et al., 1971; Schramm et al., 1972; Bilezikian and Aurbach, 1973; Gardner et al., 1973). The studies of Riddick et al. (1971) connected the transport process of Ørskov with the postulated role for cyclic AMP by showing that dibutyryl cyclic AMP, when added to the bathing medium, mimicked the action of norepinephrine on transport. (See also Gardner et al. (1973, 1975a) for the effects of cyclic AMP alone.)

In the experiments shown in Fig. 17 we tested the effect of norepine-

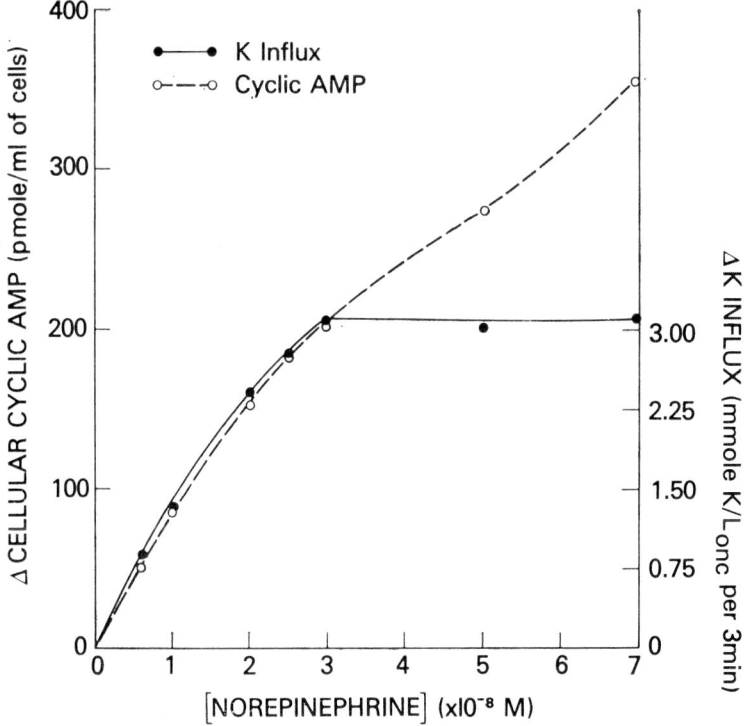

FIG. 17. Comparison of transport and cyclic AMP accumulation in norepinephrine-treated cells. K influx was determined for a 3 min interval immediately after adding norepinephrine. Cyclic AMP levels are values at the midpoint of this 3 min interval. Hormone-dependent increments were obtained by subtracting the appropriate values for paired control cells incubated without norepinephrine. All flasks contained an isotonic solution with a $[K]_o$ of 2·5 mM. (From Kregenow et al., 1976.)

phrine on the cellular level of cyclic AMP and on K influx, and found a correlation between the two responses. The change in each at different concentrations of norepinephrine is shown. The left ordinate shows hormone-sensitive increases in cyclic AMP, and the right, hormone-sensitive increases in K influx. At concentrations of hormone up to 3×10^{-8} M both cyclic AMP and K influx increase in parallel. However, at higher levels of norepinephrine, above the point at which transport saturates, cyclic AMP continues to increase. Besides this parallelism at low hormone concentrations, further evidence that the increase in cyclic AMP is necessary for the increase in K transport can be found in other experiments in which propranolol, a β-adrenergic blocking agent, prevented both norepinephrine-induced transport and the elevation in cyclic AMP content (Riddick et al., 1971; Kregenow, 1973; Gardner et al., 1974; Kregenow et al., 1976).

The response to hypertonicity, in contrast, is not mediated by cyclic AMP. Figure 18 compares cellular cyclic AMP levels, corrected for changes in cell volume, in control cells (open column), hypertonicity-stimulated cells (dark column) and norepinephrine-stimulated cells (slashed column). The response to norepinephrine has been included for comparison. Note cyclic AMP levels were not elevated in the hypertonicity-stimulated cells despite a similar increase in K flux. Thus, although both stimuli cause the same effect on transport, cyclic AMP is not an intermediate when the stimulus is hypertonicity. One can picture the two stimuli (norepinephrine and hypertonicity) as initiating events which are at first dissimilar, but which eventually impinge upon a common pathway leading to cation translocation (Kregenow et al., 1976). Consequently, the hypertonicity-stimulated transport process represents a useful system for examining, independent of any cyclic AMP effects, those events that develop beyond the point at which cyclic AMP acts.

To better define these unknown events, Rudolph and Greengard (1974) have examined the interrelationship between transport and the metabolism of membrane proteins. They reported the phosphorylation of a 240 000 Mw membrane protein from turkey erythrocytes, and discussed the possibility that this protein phosphorylation was associated with the change in Na transport. However, the causal relationship between increased phosphorylation and cyclic AMP-mediated transport remains problematical. Cholera enterotoxin, which acts via cyclic AMP (Field, 1974) to cause cell enlargement (Rudolph et al., 1976), does not affect the phosphorylation of this protein.

7.2.3 Elements of both VRD and VRI

(a) *Receptor and effector properties.* We presume that the "volume con-

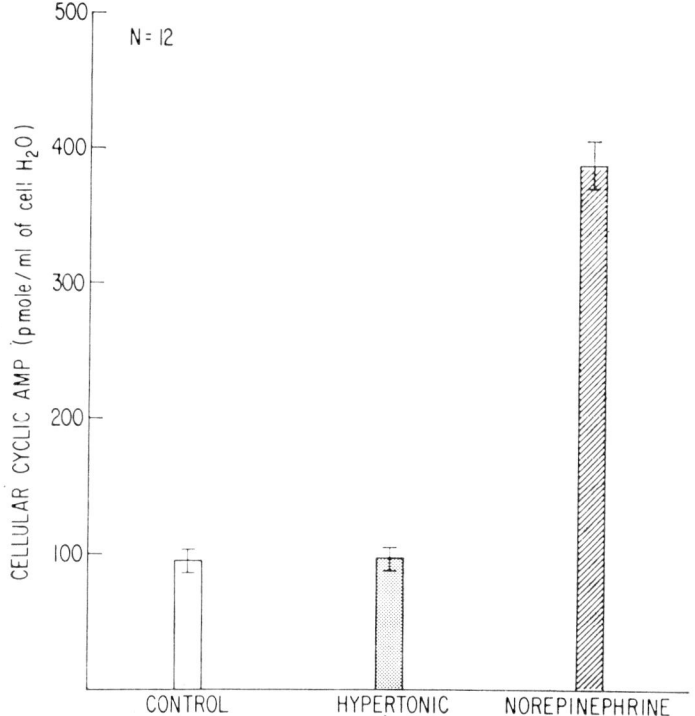

FIG. 18. Effect of hypertonicity and norepinephrine on cyclic AMP accumulation. The experimental protocol was similar to that described in the legend of Fig. 17 and differs only in that the addition of cells to the hypertonic solution (427 mosmol l^{-1}) coincided with the addition of norepinephrine ($2 \cdot 5 \times 10^{-8}$ M) to the isotonic solution. Both solutions had a $[K]_o$ of 2·5 mM. Cyclic AMP levels represent values taken at 3 min. Brackets represent S.E. (From Kregenow et al., 1976.)

trolling mechanism" contains both a receptor and effector. Very little is known about the receptor. It is even unclear whether the same receptor serves swollen and shrunken cells. Since the receptor responds to small changes in cell size (<5 per cent), it is unlikely that a change in the concentration of a metabolite, created by shrinking or swelling the cell by this amount, could serve as the sensitive variable. Also excluded are the cellular Na and K concentrations or content and intracellular osmolarity since they either fail to vary or vary inappropriately. More can be said about the effector. The many differences between transport associated with VRD and VRI reported in the preceding sections suggest that the effector (that portion of the "volume controlling mechanism" responsible for transport) is composed of more than one element. Probably two pathways exist, depending on whether the cells are initially enlarged or shrunken.

Additional observations support this hypothesis. When one measures that part of transport common to both VRI and VRD (elevated K efflux), it is found that agents which inhibit VRI affect VRD differently. For instance, removing K from the bathing medium has no effect on the increased K efflux associated with VRD (Nordan and Kregenow, unpublished observations) whereas it inhibits the increased K efflux associated with VRI (Fig. 13). Nevertheless, one must be cautious about concluding that there are two pathways, since no agent has yet been found that inhibits the K efflux component of VRD and not that of VRI.

(b) Relation between the cation pump and "volume controlling mechanism". As already emphasized, transport by the "volume controlling mechanism" and pump are separate processes. The two mechanisms are related, however, in that the Na and K gradients maintained by the pump are utilized by the "volume controlling mechanism" and appear essential to its operation. Thus, the separation between all aspects of both mechanisms may not be complete.

(c) Presence in other cells. It is not clear how prevalent the "volume controlling mechanism" is among vertebrate cells. The essential feature of this particular mechanism is that it re-establishes and then maintains the cell's original volume and that the volume changes are associated with large changes in cation permeability. In evaluating other cells for the presence of this mechanism, consideration must be limited to cells which control their volume and also show the relevant permeability changes. Care must be taken to exclude experiments in anisotonic media in which there is no purposeful change in volume or in which the changes in permeability result from membrane injury. Other avian erythrocytes, pigeon (Ørskov, 1954, 1956; Kregenow, unpublished observations) and turkey (Gardner, 1973, 1975a,b,c; Rudolph *et al.*, 1976) demonstrate the hormonal aspect of cell enlargement. Nucleated fish erythrocytes probably also contain the mechanism (Fugelli, 1967; Cala, 1973). Giant red cells from the salamander (*Amphiuma means*) demonstrate VRD in response to hypotonicity (Kregenow, unpublished observations). Also Parker (1973, 1975) found that dog red cells, which are not nucleated and contain a high concentration of sodium, control their size in anisotonic media; however, it is unclear whether the same mechanism is involved.

Roti Roti and Rothstein (1973) first demonstrated the mechanism in cells other than erythrocytes. They reached a similar explanation for how mammalian lymphoblasts undergo VRD. Chicken lymphocytes also regulate their size in hypotonic media by this mechanism (Doljanski *et al.*, 1974). Ehrlich cells use the mechanism to control their volume in hypotonic media (Hendel and Hoffman, 1974), but these cells lose nearly equivalent amounts of K and ninhydren positive substances and only small amount of chloride. Grantham and coworkers (Dellasega and Grantham, 1973; Grantham et al., 1974) provided evidence that mammalian kidney cells also contain the mechanism.

(d) *Future research.* Studies of volume regulation in avian erythrocytes and other cells have important implications for understanding how cells control their volume under both physiological and pathological conditions. Many important questions are unanswered. Does the "volume controlling mechanism" function normally to control the steady-state volume of cells? Is it responsible for the change in size associated with cell division and differentiation? The importance of volume regulation for clinical medicine has been considered by Whittembury and Grantham (1976).

(e) *Evolutionary significance.* From a theoretical standpoint, the emergence of the "volume controlling mechanism" or its functional counterpart could have represented a crucial evolutionary step. This mechanism allows cells to regulate their volume dynamically, a capability which is a prerequisite for development of plastic cell surfaces and elimination of the rigid cell wall which plant cells use to stabilize their volume. A plastic cell surface was essential for the evolution of many of the cell functions in moving animals, such as muscle contraction.

References

ALLEN, D. W. and MCMANUS, T. J. (1967). PhD Thesis, Duke University, Durham, North Carolina.
ASHWELL, G. and DISCHE, Z. (1950). *Biochim. Biophys. Acta*, **4**, 276–292.
BANASCHAK, H. (1959). *Acta Biol. Med. Germ.* **2**, 278–283.
BARRETT, L. A. and DAWSON, R. B. (1974). *Dev. Biol.* **36**, 72–81.
BARRON, E. S. G. and HARROP, G. A. (1928). *J. Biol. Chem.* **79**, 65–87.
BARTLETT, G. R. (1970). In "Advances in Experimental Medicine" (G. J. Brewer, ed), vol. 6, pp. 245–256. Plenum Press, New York.
BARTSCH, P. W., BALL, W. H., ROSENZWEIG, W. and SALMAN, S. (1937). **Auk, 54**, 516–519.
BEHNKE, O. (1970). *J. Ultrastruct. Res.* **31**, 61–75.
BELL, D. J. (1953). *Q. J. Exp. Physiol.* **42**, 410–416.
BENESCH, R. and BENESCH, R. E. (1967). *Biochem. Biophys. Res. Commun.* **26**, 162.
BENESCH, R. and BENESCH, R. E. (1969). *Nature*, **221**, 618–622.
BEUTLER, E. and SRIVASTAVA, S. K. (1968). In "Metabolism and Membrane Permeability of Erythrocytes and Thrombocytes" (E. Deutsch, E. Gerlach and K. Moser, eds), pp. 91–95. Georg Thieme, Stuttgart.
BILEZIKIAN, J. P. and AURBACH, G. D. (1973). *J. Biol. Chem.* **248**, 5575–5583.
BLANCHET, J. P. (1974). *Exp. Cell. Res.* **84**, 159–166.
BLUM, R. M. and FORSTER, R. E. (1970). *Biochim. Biophys. Acta*, **203**, 410–423.

BORNSTEIN, A. and ASCHER, O. (1926). *Z. Ges. Exp. Med.* **52**, 607–614.
BROWN, H. D., RIGDON, R. H., CHATTOPADHYAY, S. K. and PATEL, A. B. (1968). *Enzym. Biol. Clin.* **9**, 433–446.
BUHLER, D. R. and IHLER, G. S. (1963). *J. Lab. Clin. Med.* **62**, 306–318.
CALA, P. M. (1973). *Bull. Mt. Desert Isl. Biol. Lab.* **13**, 20–25.
CAMERON, I. L. and KUSTBERG, M. L. (1969). *Cytobios*, **1**, 229.
CAMERON, I. L. and PRESCOTT, D. M. (1963). *Exp. Cell. Res.* **30**, 609–612.
CHANUTIN, A. and CURNISH, R. R. (1967). *Arch. Biochem. Biophys.* **121**, 96–102.
CHEUNG, J. F., WHITFIELD, C. F., REGEN, D. M. and MORGAN, H. E. (1976). *Fed. Proc.* **35**, 780.
CHRISTENSEN, H. N. (1969). *Adv. Enzymol.* **31**, 1–20.
CHRISTENSEN, H. N. (1973). *J. Bioenergetics.* **4**, 31–61.
CHRISTENSEN, H. N., DE CESPEDES, C., HANDLOGTEN, M. E. and RONQUIST, G. (1974). *Ann. N.Y. Acad. Sci.* **227**, 355–379.
CHRISTENSEN, H. N., HANDLOGTEN, M. E., LAM, I., TAGER, H. S. and ZAND, R. (1969). *J. Biol. Chem.* **244**, 1510–1520.
CLARKSON, E. M. and MAIZELS, M. (1955). *J. Physiol. (Lond.)*, **128**, 476–503.
COATES, M. L. (1975). *J. Mol. Evol.* **6**, 285–307.
COOPER, D. W., IRWIN, M. R. and STONE, W. H. (1969). *Genetics*, **62**, 597–606.
CULLEN, E. K. (1903). *Bull. Johns Hopkins Hosp.* **14**, 352–356.
DAJANI, R. M. and ORTEN, J. M. (1958). *J. Biol. Chem.* **231**, 913–924.
DAJANI, R. M. and ORTEN, J. M. (1959). *J. Biol. Chem.* **234**, 877–879.
DAVIS, H. G. (1961). *J. Biophys. Biochem. Cytol.* **9**, 671–687.
DAVOREN, P. R. and SUTHERLAND, E. W. (1963a). *J. Biol. Chem.* **238**, 3009–3015.
DAVOREN, P. R. and SUTHERLAND, E. W. (1963b). *J. Biol. Chem.* **238**, 3016–3023.
DEHLER, A. (1895). *Arch. Mikrosk. Anat.* **46**, 414–430.
DELLASEGA, M. and GRANTHAM, J. J. (1973). *Amer. J. Physiol.* **224**, 1288–1294.
DISCHE, Z. (1946). *J. Biol. Chem.* **163**, 575–576.
DISCHE, Z. and ASHWELL, G. (1955). *Biochim. Biophys. Acta*, **17**, 56–66.
DODGE, J. T., MITCHELL, C. D. and HANAHAN, D. S. (1963). *Arch. Biochem. Biophys.* **100**, 119–130.
DOLJANSKI, F., BEN-SASSON, S., REICH, M. and GROVER, N. B. (1974). *J. Cell. Physiol.* **84**, 215–224.
EAVENSON, E. and CHRISTENSEN, H. N. (1967). *J. Biol. Chem.* **242**, 5386–5396.
EYLAR, E. A., MADOFF, M. A., BRODY, O. V. and ONCLEY, J. L. (1962). *J. Biol. Chem.* **237**, 1992–2000.
FARMER, R. E. L. and MACEY, R. I. (1970). *Biochim. Biophys. Acta*, **196**, 53–56.
FAWCETT, D. W. and WITEBSKY, F. (1964). *Z. Zellforsch Mikrosk. Anat.* **62**, 785–806.
FIELD, M. (1974). *Proc. Nat. Acad. Sci. USA*, **71**, 3299–3303.
FLORKIN, M. and SCHOFFENIELS, E. (1969). *In* "Molecular Approaches to Ecology", p. 89. Academic Press, New York and London.
FORKNER, C. E. (1929). *J. Exp. Med.* **50**, 121–142.
FUGELLI, K. (1967). *Comp. Biochem. Physiol.* **22**, 253–260.
GARDNER, J. D., MENSH, R. S., KIINO, D. R. and AURBACH, G. D. (1975a). *J. Biol. Chem.* **250**, 1155–1163.
GARDNER, J. D., KIINO, D. R. (1975b). *J. Biol. Chem.* **250**, 1164–1175.
GARDNER, J. D., JOW, N. and KIINO, D. R. (1975c). *J. Biol. Chem.* **250**, 1176–1185.
GARDNER, J. D., KLAEVEMAN, H. L., BILEZIKIAN, J. P. and AURBACH, G. D. (1973). *J. Biol. Chem.* **248**, 5590–5597.

GARDNER, J. D., KLAEVEMAN, H. L., BILEZIKIAN, J. P. and AURBACH, G. D. (1974). *J. Biol. Chem.* **249**, 516–520.
GARRAHAN, P. J. and REGA, A. F. (1967). *J. Physiol. (Lond.)*, **193**, 459–466.
GERLACH, E., FLECKENSTEIN, A. and FREUNDT, K. J. (1957). *Pflügers Archiv.* **263**, 682–703.
GHOSH, S. K. and SWARUP, S. (1966). *Bull. Calcutta Sch. Trop. Med. Hyg.* **14**, 31–33.
GILMORE, D. G. (1971). In "Physiology and Biochemistry of the Domestic Fowl" (D. J. Bell and B. M. Freeman, eds), vol. 2, pp. 884–896. Academic Press, New York and London.
GOODALL, A. (1910). *J. Path. Bact.* **14**, 195–199.
GRANTHAM, J. J., LOWE, C., DELLASEGA, M. (1974). *Fed. Proc.* **33**, 387.
GRJINS, G. (1896). *Pflügers Archiv.* **63**, 86–119.
GULLIVER, G. (1875). *Proc. Zool. Soc. Lond.* **43**, 474–495.
HAMILTON, B. B. (1966). *Fed. Proc.* **25**, 622.
HARRIS, J. R. and BROWN, J. N. (1971a). *Br. Poult. Sci.* **12**, 95–99.
HARRIS, J. R. and BROWN, J. N. (1971b). *J. Ultrastruct. Res.* **36**, 8–23.
HARROP, G. A. and BARRON, E. S. G. (1928). *J. Exp. Med.* **48**, 207–223.
HEDIN, S. G. (1897). *Pflügers Archiv.* **68**, 229–338.
HELLER, V. G., HUNTER, K. R. and THOMPSON, R. B. (1932). *J. Biol. Chem.* **97**, 127–132.
HENDEL, K. B. and HOFFMAN, E. K. (1974). *J. Physiol. (Lond.)*, **84**, 115–126.
HENDERSON, L. J. (1928). In "Blood: A study in General Physiology", pp. 309–329. Yale University Press, New Haven, Connecticut.
HÖBER, R. and ØRSKOV, S. L. (1933). *Pflügers Archiv.* **231**, 599–615.
HOFFMAN, J. F. and LARIS, P. C. (1974). *J. Physiol. (Lond.)*, **239**, 519–552.
HUNTER, A. S. and HUNTER, F. R. (1957). *J. Cell. Comp. Physiol.* **49**, 479–502.
HUNTER, F. R. (1960). *J. Cell. Comp. Physiol.* **55**, 175–188.
HUNTER, F. R. (1961). *J. Cell. Comp. Physiol.* **58**, 203–216.
HUNTER, F. R. (1970). *Amer. J. Physiol.* **218**, 1765–1772.
HUNTER, F. R., BAKER, A. S. and BURR, M. J. (1954). *Fed. Proc.* **13**, 73.
HUNTER, F. R., GEORGE, J. and OSPINA, B. (1965). *J. Cell. Comp. Physiol.* **65**, 299–312.
JACOBS, M. H. (1931). *Ergebn. Biol.* **7**, 1–55.
JACOBS, M. H., GLASSMAN, H. N. and PARPART, A. K. (1950). *J. Exp. Zool.* **113**, 277–300.
JEUNIAUX, C. H., BRICTEUX-GREGOIRE, S. and FLORKIN, M. (1961). *Cah. Biol. Mar.* **2**, 373.
JOHNSON, L. F. and TATE, M. E. (1969). *Can. J. Chem.* **47**, 63–73.
JOHNSTONE, R. M. (1972). In "Na^+-linked Transport of Organic Solutes" (E. Heinz, ed), pp. 51–67. Springer-Verlag, Berlin.
KAPLAN, M. A., HAYS, L. and HAYS, R. M. (1974). *Amer. J. Physiol.* **226**, 1327–1332.
KENNEDY, W. P. and CLEMENKO, D. P. (1928). *Q. J. Exp. Physiol.* **19**, 43–49.
KIMMICH, G. A. (1972). In "Na^+-linked Transport of Organic Solutes" (E. Heinz, ed), pp. 116–129. Springer-Verlag, Berlin.
KITTAMS, D. W. and VIDAVER, G. A. (1969). *Biochim. Biophys. Acta*, **173**, 540–547.
KLAINER, L. M., CHI, Y. M., FREIDBERG, S. L., RALL, T. W. and SUTHERLAND, E. W. (1962). *J. Biol. Chem.* **237**, 1239–1243.
KLEINIG, H., ZENTGRAF, H., COMES, P. and STADLER, J. (1971). *J. Biol. Chem.* **246**, 2996–3000.

KLEINZELLER, A. and KOTYK, A. (1965). *Colloq. Int. Cent. Nat. Rech. Sci.* p. 372.
KLENK, E. and UHLENBRUCK, G. (1958). *Hoppe-Seyler's Z. Physiol. Chem.* **311**, 227–233.
KOEHLER, J. K. (1968). *Z. Zellforsch Mikrosk. Anat.* **85**, 1–17.
KÖEPPE, H. (1897). *Pflügers Archiv.* **67**, 189–206.
KOSER, B. H. and CHRISTENSEN, H. N. (1971). *Biochim. Biophys. Acta*, **241**, 9–19.
KREGENOW, F. M. (1971a). *J. Gen. Physiol.* **58**, 372–395.
KREGENOW, F. M. (1971b). *J. Gen. Physiol.* **58**, 396–412.
KREGENOW, F. M. (1973). *J. Gen. Physiol.* **61**, 509–527.
KREGENOW, F. M. (1974). *J. Gen. Physiol.* **64**, 393–412.
KREGENOW, F. M., ROBBIE, D. E. and ORLOFF, J. (1976). *Amer. J. Physiol.* **231**, 306–312.
KREGENOW, F. M. (1977). *In* "Osmotic and Volume Regulation" (C. B. Jørgensen and E. Skadhauge, eds). Alfred Benzon Symposium XI, Munksgaard, Copenhagen and Academic Press, New York. In press.
LEE, J. W., BEYGU-FARBER, S. and VIDAVER, G. A. (1973). *Biochim. Biophys. Acta*, **298**, 446–459.
LEUNG, E. S. and HALEY, L. E. (1974). *Biochem. Genet.* **11**, 221–230.
LUCAS, A. M. and JAMROY, C. (1961). *In* "Atlas of Avian Hematology". US Department of Agriculture, Washington, D.C.
LUYET, B. J. and FREI, C. F. (1935). *Biodynamica*, **1**, 1–8.
MACEY, R. I. and FARMER, R. E. L. (1973). *Amer. J. Physiol.* **224**, 1109–1115.
MAGATH, T. B. and HIGGINS, G. M. (1934). *Folia Haemat.* **51**, 230–241.
MAIZELS, M. (1954). *J. Physiol. (Lond.)*, **125**, 263–277.
MASER, M. D. and PHILPOTT, C. W. (1964). *Anat. Rec.* **150**, 365–382.
MASING, E. (1912). *Pflügers Archiv.* **149**, 227–249.
MELAMPY, R. M. (1948). *J. Biol. Chem.* **175**, 589–593.
MEVES, F. (1903). *Anat. Anz.* **23**, 212–213.
MEVES, F. (1906). *Anat. Anz.* **28**, 444–446.
MEVES, F. (1911). *Arch. Mikrosk. Anat. EntwMech*, **77**, 465–540.
MEYERHOF, O. (1932). *Biochem. Z.* **246**, 249–284.
MOND, R. (1930). *Pflügers Archiv.* **224**, 161–166.
MORGAN, H. E., RANDLE, P. J. and REGEN, D. M. (1959). *Biochem. J.* **73**, 573–579.
MORGAN, H. E. and WHITFIELD, C. F. (1973). *In* "Current Topics in Membranes and Transport" (F. Bronner and A. Kleinzeller, eds), vol. IV. Academic Press, New York and London.
NARASIMHAN, T. R. and NAIR, S. G. (1973). *Comp. Biochem. Physiol.* **45B**, 791–796.
NEGELEIN, E. (1925). *Biochem. Z.* **158**, 121–135.
NÓBREGA, F. G., MAIA, J. C. C., COLI, W. and SALDANHA, P. H. (1970). *Comp. Biochem. Physiol.* **33**, 191–199.
OCHIAI, T., GOTOH, T. and SHIKIMA, K. (1972). *Arch. Biochem. Biophys.* **149**, 316–322.
ØRSKOV, S. L. (1954). *Acta Physiol. Scand.* **31**, 221–229.
ØRSKOV, S. L. (1956). *Acta Physiol. Scand.* **37**, 299–306.
ØYE, I. and SUTHERLAND, E. W. (1966). *Biochim. Biophys. Acta*, **127**, 347–354.
PARKER, J. C. (1973). *J. Gen. Physiol.* **62**, 147–156.
PARKER, J. C., GITELMAN, H. J., GLOSSEM, P. S. and LEONARD, D. S. (1975). *J. Gen. Physiol.* **65**, 84–96.
PIETRZYK, C. and HEINZ, E. (1972). *In* "Na^+-linked Transport of Organic Solutes' (E. Heinz, ed), pp. 84–90. Springer-Verlag, Berlin.

PONDER, E. (1948). In "Hemolysis and Related Phenomena", pp. 348–353. Grune and Stratton, New York.
POTTS, W. T. W. and PARRY, G. (1964). In "Osmotic and Ionic Regulation in Animals". Pergamon Press, Oxford.
RANDEL, P. J. and SMITH, G. H. (1958a). *Biochem. J.* **70**, 490–500.
RANDEL, P. J. and SMITH, G. H. (1958b). *Biochem. J.* **70**, 501–508.
RANVIER, L. (1875). *Arch. Physiol.* **2**, 1–15.
RAPOPORT, S. (1940). *J. Biol. Chem.* **135**, 403–406.
RAPOPORT, S. and GUEST, G. M. (1941). *J. Biol. Chem.* **138**, 269–282.
RAPOPORT, S., LEVA, E. and GUEST, G. M. (1941). *J. Biol. Chem.* **139**, 633–639.
RIDDICK, D. H., KREGENOW, F. M. and ORLOFF, J. (1971). *J. Gen. Physiol.* **57**, 752–766.
ROTI ROTI, L. W. and ROTHSTEIN, A. (1973). *Exp. Cell. Res.* **79**, 295–310.
RUBINSTEIN, D. and DENSTEDT, O. F. (1953). *J. Biol. Chem.* **204**, 623–637.
RUBINSTEIN, D. and DENSTEDT, O. F. (1954). *Can. J. Biol. Chem. Physiol.* **32**, 548–552.
RUDOLPH, S. A. and GREENGARD, P. (1974). *J. Biol. Chem.* **249**, 5684–5687.
RUDOLPH, S. A., SCHAFER, D. E. and GREENGARD, P. (1976). *Biophys. J.* **16**, 171a.
RUDZINSKA, M. A. and TRAGER, W. (1957). *J. Protozool.* **4**, 190–199.
RÜTER, E. (1923). *Z. Ges. Exp. Med.* **37**, 151–153.
SALVIDIO, E., PANNACCIULLI, I. and TIZIANELLO, A. (1963). *Nature*, **200**, 372–373.
SCHERRER, K. L., MARCUAD, L., ZAJDELA, F., LONDON, I. M. and GROS, F. (1966). *Proc. Nat. Acad. Sci. USA*, **56**, 1571–1578.
SCHJEIDE, O. A., MCCANDLESS, R. G. and MUMM, R. J. (1964). *Growth*, **28**, 29–39.
SCHRAMM, M., FEINSTEIN, H., NAIM, E., LANG, M. and LASSER, M. (1972). *Proc. Nat. Acad. Sci. USA*, **69**, 523–527.
SCHULTZ, S. G. and CURRAN, P. F. (1970). *Physiol. Rev.* **50**, 637–718.
SEAMAN, G. V. F. and UHLENBRUCK, G. (1963). *Arch. Biochem. Biophys.* **100**, 493–502.
SEVERIN, W. A. (1937). *Chem. Abstr.* **31**, 5418.
SHAW, J., GIBSON, W., JESSUP, S. and RAMWELL, P. (1971). *Ann. N.Y. Acad. Sci.* **180**, 241–266.
SHELTON, K. R. (1973). *Can. J. Biochem.* **51**, 1442–1447.
SHIELDS, C. E., HERMAN, Y. F. and HERMAN, R. H. (1964). *Nature*, **203**, 935–936.
SIMPSON, C. F. (1967). *Cornell Vet.* **57**, 390–397.
SMITH, J. E. (1974). *J. Lab. Clin. Med.* **83**, 444–450.
SRIVASTAVA, S. K. (1971). *Exp. Eye Res.* **11**, 294–305.
SRIVASTAVA, S. K. and BEUTLER, E. (1969a). *J. Biol. Chem.* **244**, 9–16.
SRIVASTAVA, S. K. and BEUTLER, E. (1969b). *Biochem. J.* **114**, 833–837.
STEWARD, J. H. and TATE, M. E. (1969). *J. Chromat.* **45**, 400–406.
STURKIE, P. D. (1965a). In "Avian Physiology", p. 2. Cornell University Press, New York.
STURKIE, P. D. (1965b). In "Avian Physiology", p. 39. Cornell University Press, New York.
SUTHERLAND, E. W. and ROBINSON, G. A. (1966). *Pharmacol. Rev.* **18**, 145–161.
TERRY, P. M. and VIDAVER, G. A. (1973). *Biochim. Biophys. Acta*, **323**, 441–455.
THOMAS, E. L. and CHRISTENSEN, H. N. (1971). *J. Biol. Chem.* **246**, 1682–1688.
TIPTON, S. R. (1933). *J. Cell. Comp. Physiol.* **3**, 313–340.
TOSTESON, D. C. and HOFFMAN, J. F. (1960). *J. Gen. Physiol.* **44**, 169–194.
TOSTESON, D. C. and JOHNSON, J. (1957a). *J. Cell. Comp. Physiol.* **50**, 169–184.

TOSTESON, D. C. and JOHNSON, J. (1957b). *J. Cell. Comp. Physiol.* **50**, 185–197.
TOSTESON, D. C. and ROBERTSON, J. S. (1956). *J. Cell. Comp. Physiol.* **47**, 147–165.
VANDECASSERIE, C., LORKIN, P. A., SCHNEK, A. G. and LEONIS, J. (1975). *Arch. Int. Physiol. Biochim.* **83**, 409–410.
VIDAVER, G. A. (1964a). *Biochemistry*, **3**, 662–667.
VIDAVER, G. A. (1964b). *Biochemistry*, **3**, 795–799.
VIDAVER, G. A. (1964c). *Biochemistry*, **3**, 799–803.
VIDAVER, G. A. (1964d). *Biochemistry*, **3**, 803–808.
VIDAVER, G. A. (1971). *Biochim Biophys. Acta*, **233**, 231–234.
VIDAVER, G. A., ROMAIN, L. F. and HAUROWITZ, F. (1964). *Arch. Biochem.* **107**, 82–87.
VIDAVER, G. A. and SHEPHERD, S. L. (1968). *J. Biol. Chem.* **243**, 6140–6150.
WARBURG, O. (1909). *Hoppe-Seyler's Z. Physiol. Chem.* **59**, 112–121.
WECKSTEIN, T. W. and ENGELHARDT, W. A. (1959). *Folia Haemat.* **76**, 422–431.
WHEELER, K. P. and CHRISTENSEN, H. N. (1967). *J. Biol. Chem.* **242**, 3782–3788.
WHEELER, K. P., INUI, Y., HOLLENBERG, P. F., EAVENSON, E. and CHRISTENSEN, H. N. (1965). *Biochim. Biophys. Acta*, **109**, 620–622.
WHITFIELD, C. F. and MORGAN, H. E. (1973). *Biochim. Biophys. Acta*, **307**, 181–196.
WHITFIELD, C. F., RANNELS, S. R. and MORGAN, H. E. (1974). *J. Biol. Chem.* **249**, 4181–4188.
WHITTEMBURY, G. and GRANTHAM, J. J. (1976). *Kidney Int.* **9**, 103–120.
WIDDAS, W. F. (1954). *J. Physiol.* (Lond.), **125**, 163–180.
WIETH, J. O., FUNDER, J., GUNN, R. B. and BRAHM, J. (1974). In "Comparative Biochemistry and Physiology of Transport" (L. Bolis, K. Bloch, S. E. Luria and F. Lynen, eds), pp. 317–336. North-Holland, Amsterdam.
WOOD, R. E. and MORGAN, H. E. (1969). *J. Biol. Chem.* **244**, 1451–1460.
ZENTGRAF, H., DEUMLING, B., JARASCH, E. D. and FRANKE, W. W. (1971). *J. Biol. Chem.* **246**, 2986–2995.
ZENTGRAF, H., SCHEER, U., FRANKE, W. W. (1975). *Exp. Cell. Res.* **96**, 81–95.

Solute and water transport in dog and cat red blood cells

J. C. PARKER

Division of Hematology, Department of Medicine, University of North Carolina School of Medicine, Chapel Hill, North Carolina, USA

1 Introduction	427
2 Composition of dog and cat RBC	428
3 Water permeability	431
4 Movements of anions and nonelectrolytes	433
5 Transport of metabolic substrates and intermediates	436
6 Passive cation movements	436
6.1 Cell volume	439
6.2 Metabolic perturbations	442
6.3 Lyotropic effects	443
6.4 Alkaline earths and heavy metals	445
6.5 Narcotics and phloretin	446
6.6 pH and temperature	446
6.7 Miscellaneous effects	447
6.8 Conclusions	448
7 Active cation transport	448
8 Cell volume control	454
9 Dog and cat RBC *in vivo*	455
References	457

1 Introduction

The early history of red cell (RBC) transport physiology is written in the blood of dogs and cats. Observations on these species brought into question the old belief in the cation-impermeability of the plasma membrane (Kerr, 1926a,b; Yannet *et al.*, 1935–6; Hegnauer and Robinson, 1936; Robinson and Hegnauer, 1936). Dog RBC were used in the first investigations of radioactive Na transport (Cohn and Cohn, 1939). The pump-leak model for cation movements was enunciated by Dean in a public discussion with Davson (1940a) about cat RBC. It is ironic that with the development of knowledge of cation transport in many tissues, dog and cat RBC have emerged as highly exceptional and atypical: they are among the few cells of any type in the animal kingdom that lack a Na–K exchange pump. The RBC of other carnivores, such as the seal (Robin et al., 1971), are probably similar in this respect but have not been as extensively studied.

There are many differences between dog and cat RBC. The shared characteristic that distinguishes them from the cells of most other species is the way they transport Na ions. This review will therefore concentrate on that topic. Water and other solute permeabilities will be discussed to provide a context for the information about Na.

2 Composition of dog and cat RBC

Ion and water contents of dog and cat RBC are given in Table 1. In preparing these Na-leaky cells for flame photometry it is a mistake to wash them in media free of Na. This often results in cell shrinkage or lysis for reasons detailed in the section on passive cation movements. It is preferable to use a buffered, isotonic NaCl wash solution with an extracellular space marker. The cells may be spun directly out of whole blood with no wash, in which case the correction required for 1–2 per cent trapping is very small, since the Na, K and Cl concentrations in cells and plasma are so similar (DeMendonca et al., 1970). The values in Table 1 are for mature RBC from adult animals. Table 2 shows that in the case of dogs (I cannot find comparable data for cats) the composition of the cells varies with the age of the dog and the age of the cell in the circulation. Newborn puppies' RBC are larger in volume and have more total cation (Na + K) than cells from adult dogs (Lee and Miles, 1972, 1973; Miles and Lee, 1972). The transition takes place over the first 12–16 weeks of life and is explained both by alterations in the fetal cells present at birth and by the proliferation of a new population of low K adult cells. Similar changes of RBC ion content with animal age occur in cattle (Israel et al., 1972).

Induction of a brisk hemolytic anemia in dogs results in an outpouring of reticulocytes with a K concentration (100 mequiv (l cells)$^{-1}$) close to that of human RBC (Henriques and Ørskov, 1936; Parker, 1973c). This suggests that in their nucleated, precursor state, dog RBC sustain a high K gradient between cytoplasm and plasma. Lubin (1967) has pointed out that many of the steps in RNA and protein synthesis require or are favored by a high K environment. In the case of dog RBC the fall in cytoplasmic K as the reticulocyte matures can be viewed as a kind of adaptation to the loss of protein synthetic capacity. The glycolytic enzyme, pyruvate kinase, which in most tissues is activated by K (Suelter, 1970) has no requirement for this cation in mature dog RBC (Bashan et al., 1975).

Although an early report (Villegas et al., 1958) suggested that dog RBC might be perfect osmometers, subsequent investigations have shown that,

TABLE 1

Surface area, volume, ion and water content, and ion distribution ratios of dog and cat RBC

	Dog	Cat
Surface area (μm^2)	117[i]	83[i]
Volume (μm^3)	67[i]	48[i]
Water (% wet weight)	63·6[f]	62·5[g]
Cell Na (mequiv (kg cell water)$^{-1}$)	135[a]	142[a]
	170[b]	
	162[f]	
	156[d]	
Cell Na (mequiv (l cells)$^{-1}$)	106[h]	104[c]
	87–106[e]	
	99[d]	
Cell K (mequiv (kg cell water)$^{-1}$)	10[a]	8·6[a]
	10[b]	
	8[f]	
	6·7[d]	
Cell K (mequiv (l cells)$^{-1}$)	5·5[h]	8[c]
	4·2[d]	
Cell Cl (mequiv (kg cell water)$^{-1}$)	87[a]	84[a]
	80[f]	
Ion concentration ratios in cell and plasma water		
Na (plasma per cells)	1·03[d]	1·11[a]
	1·02[a]	
	1·13[f]	
K (plasma per cells)	0·70[d]	0·58[a]
	0·48[a]	
	0·59[f]	
Cl (cells per plasma)	0·78[a]	0·75[a]
	0·65[f]	

(a) Bernstein, 1954; (b) Davson, 1942; (c) Davson and Reiner, 1942; (d) De-Mendonca et al., 1970; (e) Elford, 1975a; (f) Parker, 1973a; (g) Sha'afi, 1965; (h) Sheppard et al., 1951; (i) Wieth et al., 1974.

as in other mammals, only 80 per cent of RBC water appears to participate in the volume changes induced by varying the tonicity of the surrounding medium (Rich et al., 1967). The notion that this "anomalous" osmotic behavior arises from concentration-dependent changes in the ionization constant of hemoglobin (Gary-Bobo and Solomon, 1968) has some support from recent observations on the pattern of ion movements in dog RBC during volume regulation (Parker, 1973b).

Compared with human cells, dog and cat RBC are relatively low in ATP

TABLE 2

Cation concentrations in puppy RBC and in adult dog reticulocytes

	(mmol K (l cells)$^{-1}$)	K : Na ratio
Puppy age		
1 day	21·4	0·20
3 weeks	15·5	0·15
Adult	7·4	0·05
Adult reticulocyte	100	—

Data from Miles and Lee (1972) and Parker (1973c).

content (Table 3), but this is true of other species like the horse and guinea-pig, which maintain a high cellular K:Na ratio (Prankerd, 1961; McManus, 1974). Dogs are like rats and rabbits in having 2,3-diphosphoglycerate levels higher than those of human cells, but cats are in the very low 2,3-DPG group along with sheep and cows (Torrance, 1973).

TABLE 3

Levels of ATP and 2,3-diphosphoglycerate in dog, cat and human RBC

	Dog	Cat	Man
ATP (mmol (l cells)$^{-1}$)	0·25[d]	0·21[d]	1·3[f,g]
	0·57[c]	0·53[j]	
	0·40[a]	0·40[a]	
	0·5[e]		
	0·6[h]		
2,3-DPG (mmol (l cells)$^{-1}$)	4·27[d]	0·50[d]	5[f,h]
	4·23[i]	1·70[j]	
	5·00[a]	0·60[a]	
	6·90[b]	0·70[b]	
	6[h]		

(a) Bartlett, 1970; (b) Bunn, 1971; (c) Burr, 1972; (d) Harkness et al., 1969; (e) McManus, 1974; (f) Parker, 1969; (g) Parker, 1971; (h) Parker and Snow, 1972; (i) Passo et al., 1971; (j) Robin et al., 1971; (k) Torrance, 1973; see also Kaneko, 1974.

Review of the data on membrane lipid content of mammalian RBC (Rouser et al., 1968) shows no characteristics which set dogs and cats together apart from other species. Dog cells are high in phosphatidyl cholines and unsaturated fatty acids, but so are rats. Cats and humans have intermediate amounts of these compounds, while sheep and goats have almost none.

A comparative study of RBC membrane proteins in mammals was reported by Kobylka et al. (1972), who used three different methods of hypotonic hemolysis to prepare ghosts. The membranes were solubilized in sodium dodecyl sulfate and electrophoresed on acrylamide gel. The species showed remarkable homology in that all had nine major protein bands of comparable molecular weight distribution. There were no features which were peculiar to dogs and cats. Dog RBC, however, were of interest because the electrophoretic pattern varied greatly with the method of ghost preparation. With Tris-EDTA hemolysis major changes occurred which were thought by the authors to be due to proteolytic digestion of the membrane. A lesson from this work is that studies with ghosts—particularly from dogs—may be subject to the complication that the protein-mediated functions sought (e.g. ATPases) may be destroyed, changed or eluted by inappropriate preparative methods.

3 Water permeability

Movements of water and small, hydrophilic organic molecules in dog, cat and human RBC have been extensively studied in Solomon's laboratory, where the results have been interpreted in terms of a theory of "equivalent pores" or structures in the membrane which permit the bulk flow of water and solutes between cytoplasm and extracellular fluid (Solomon, 1968; see also Redwood et al., 1974).

Part of the evidence for equivalent pores comes from studies in which net water movements in response to an imposed osmotic pressure gradient are compared with the diffusion of tritiated water (THO) across the membrane. Table 4 summarizes data for measurements of net cell volume

TABLE 4

Species	P_f (cm^4 (sec osmol)$^{-1}$)
Man	0·22
Beef	0·28
Dog	0·36
Cat	0·61

Data from Rich et al., 1967.

change in response to an osmotic stress. Dog and cat RBC have a higher hydraulic (or filtration) permeability coefficient (P_f) than do human or beef cells (Rich et al., 1967, 1968).

The finding that P_f was greater than P_d (the THO diffusion permeability coefficient expressed in the same units as P_f) in all species of RBC studied was taken as an indication that the membranes possess channels through which viscous, bulk flow of water can occur. The radius of these equivalent pores was calculated from the ratio P_f/P_d and is given in Table 5.

TABLE 5

Method of estimation	Equivalent pore radius Å		
	Dog	Man	Beef
P_f/P_d	5·9	4·5	4·1
Reflection coefficients (urea, ethylene glycol, various amides, glycerol, arabinose)	6·2	4·3	—
Diffusion method (ethylene glycol, glycerol, erythritol, dicarboxylic acids, hexoses, pentoses)	>4·2	>3·5	3·8–4·2

Data from Solomon, 1968.

Other deductions about pore size based on the reflection coefficient (Goldstein and Solomon, 1961) or the diffusion permeability of various hydrophilic solutes are shown in Table 5.

Dog RBC have by all these estimates equivalent pores which are 40 per cent greater in radius and therefore twice as large in cross-sectional area as the pores in human RBC membranes (Vieira et al., 1970). In measuring the temperature dependence of water movement in both species, Vieira et al. (1970) found that the apparent activation energy for THO diffusion (kcal mol^{-1}) was 6·0 for human and 4·9 for dog RBC. The latter value is almost the same as that for self-diffusion of water (4·6–4·8), suggesting that water diffusion in the human RBC is constrained by membrane-water interactions while in dog RBC the larger equivalent pores allow water to diffuse through the membrane as if it were in bulk solution.

Forster (1971), in a critical overview of the work on water transport, considers the evidence for bulk flow ambiguous and joins the authors of the equivalent pore concept in urging against an overly literal view of these as continuous, water-filled channels through the membrane. Furthermore, the notion that small, hydrophilic solutes cross the membrane through aqueous channels (Sha'afi et al., 1971) has been challenged by recent evidence: it is possible to reduce the hydraulic permeability of human RBC by 90 per cent with various sulfhydryl-reactive agents while leaving the movements of inorganic anions, ethylurea and diethylene glycol unaffected (Macey and Farmer, 1970; Macey et al., 1972). Also, such often-used "pore probes" as urea, glycerol, hexoses and erythritol have been discovered in human RBC to penetrate the membrane through specific, saturable pathways (Wieth, 1971; Wieth *et al.*, 1974) which can be strongly inhibited by phloretin without at the same time influencing hydraulic water permeability. Thus the concept of equivalent pores which permit the bulk flow of water and solutes is no longer a simple or obvious explanation of the data (Brown *et al.*, 1975).

4 Movements of anions and nonelectrolytes

Many observations on RBC and other tissues are consistent with the notion that passive solute penetration can occur by two distinct types of mechanisms—simple diffusion and facilitated or "catalysed" diffusion. The movement of solutes by simple diffusion follows Fick's law (flux rate is proportional to transmembrane electrochemical gradient). Facilitated diffusion, on the other hand, is characterized by saturation kinetics, competition among structurally similar solutes and counter-transport phenomena (Stein, 1964). There are several classes of agents which non-competitively inhibit facilitated diffusion mechanisms while having either a negligible or even an accelerating action on simple diffusion.

A number of facilitated diffusion systems have been described in red blood cells, of which a partial list is given in Table 6 (nucleoside and amino acid pathways have been omitted because of lack of data on dogs and cats). Each system mediates the transfer of a group of structurally similar compounds. With the probable exception of the anion route, not all systems are present in every species.

That the systems are discrete entities is evidenced by competitive inhibition data as well as by the specificity of action of some of the non-competitive inhibitors (e.g. Cu, PCMBS—Table 6). Phloretin and its analogues appear to inhibit all of the systems.

Thus, in the cases of glycerol and acetate (which permeates in the undissociated form as acetic acid), the various mammalian species can be divided into high- and low-permeability groups depending on whether or not a facilitated diffusion system is present on their membranes (Table 7).

Among the low-permeability species there is a linear correlation between the diffusion of solutes and the degree of unsaturation of membrane lipids, whether the latter was measured directly (de Gier, 1973; Wessels and Veerkamp, 1973) or via the content of phosphatidyl cholines, which are rich in unsaturated fatty acids (Deuticke, 1974).

Within the group of species for which this correlation was seen, dogs led the list in having the highest permeability to both glycerol and acetate and also the highest proportion of membrane unsaturated fatty acids. Unfortunately, the relationship was not reported in cat RBC.

TABLE 6

Partial list of facilitated transport systems in various species of RBC, with some noncompetitive inhibitors

	Hexoses, pentoses, erythritol (k, n, p)	Glycerol (a, c, e, i, j, n, o, p, q)	Acetate (d)	Urea (f, i, j)	Inorganic anions (b, g, h, l, m, q)
Species					
Dog	+*	—	—	+	+
Cat	0	—	0	(+)	+
Man	+	+	—	+	+
Rat	0	+	+	(+)	+
Amphibians	0	0	0	+	+
Birds	0	0	0	—	(+)
Fish	0	0	0	—	(+)
Inhibitors					
Phloretin	+	+	+	+	+
Lyotropic	0	+	0	0	+
Cu	—	+	0	0	—
DNFB	+	+	0	0	+
Narcotics	+	+	0	0	+
Tannate	0	+	0	0	+
PCMBS	+	+	0	+	—

+ = facilitated diffusion present or inhibited by agent listed.
(+) = likely to be present.
— = facilitated diffusion absent or not inhibited by agent listed.
0 = not sufficient information.
* Lee, P. (1975) personal communication.
(a) Cainelli et al., 1974; (b) Dalmark and Wieth, 1972; (c) de Gier, 1973; (d) Deuticke, 1974; (e) Jacobs et al., 1935; (f) Kaplan et al., 1974; (g) Knauf and Rothstein, 1971; (h) Lassen, 1972; (i) Macey and Farmer, 1970; (j) Macey et al., 1972; (k) Park et al., 1968; (l) Passow and Schnell, 1969; (m) Sha'afi and Pascoe, 1972; (n) Stein, 1964; (o) Wessels and Veerkamp, 1973; (p) Whittam, 1964; (q) Wieth et al., 1974.

Recent information about anion permeability has led to an important conceptual distinction between "exchange" and "conductance" pathways (Tosteson et al., 1973). In the case of the exchange route, observations on saturability, competition among anions and effects of inhibitors all point to a facilitated diffusion mechanism (Gunn et al., 1973; Wieth et al., 1973), and a specific membrane protein has been strongly implicated in the process (Cabantchik and Rothstein, 1974). It is thought that mono- and divalent anions share the same carrier system (Gunn, 1972; Ho and Guidotti, 1975).

TABLE 7

Permeability of RBC to glycerol and acetate

	Glycerol (a, b)	Acetate (c)
High-permeability species	Rat Man Rabbit Guinea-pig Mouse	Rat Rabbit Guinea-pig
Low-permeability species	Cat Dog Horse Pig Ox Sheep	Dog Man Pig Ox Sheep

(a) de Gier, 1973; (b) Wessels and Veerkamp, 1973; (c) Deuticke, 1974.

In an interspecies comparison of phosphate flux with membrane phospholipid content, Deuticke and Gruber (1970, 1972) found a relationship similar to that previously described for glycerol and acetate: animals with a low percentage of phosphatidyl cholines (and hence of unsaturated fatty acids) in their RBCs showed the lowest phosphate fluxes. The high-lecithin group, which included dog, had the highest rates of phosphate transport. A similar correlation was found for chloride exchange (Wieth et al., 1974). Why this protein-mediated facilitated diffusion mechanism should be influenced by variations in the fatty acid content of membrane phospholipids is not as intuitively obvious as in the case of the simple diffusion of acetic acid and glycerol, but the correlation has some exceptions and the relationships may be coincidental.

A specific study of sulfate transport in cat RBC was reported by Sha'afi and Pascoe (1972), who used conditions which allowed them to make a direct comparison with similar experiments in human cells reported by Wieth (1970b). The rate constant for sulfate flux in cat (0·24 h^{-1}) was said to be ten times lower than that for human RBC (2·027 h^{-1}), although comparison of the published time-course figures in both papers would suggest that the difference between the two species is not that great. Unpublished work by J. Funder (1975, personal communication) showed a rate constant for sulfate flux in cat RBC at 38°C of 0·68 h^{-1}. Measurement of sulfate flux under the same conditions in dog RBC (Parker and Snow, 1972) showed a half-time of about 20 min, which is close to the value for human cells. The observation that sulfate flux in cat RBC increased with increasing cell volume (Sha'afi and Pascoe, 1972) can be explained on the basis that the cells were swollen by lowering the concentration of NaCl in the medium, thus reducing the concentration of a competing anion. Extracellular ATP, which causes a large increase in Na–K permeability in dog RBC, was without effect on sulfate movement (Parker and Snow, 1972).

5 Transport of metabolic substrates and intermediates

The high glucose permeability of primate RBC is well known, and evidence for a facilitated diffusion system for passive transport of hexoses in human RBC is abundant (Table 6). Other mammalian RBC are much less permeable to glucose. Indeed, Wilbrandt (1938) thought the permeability coefficient for this sugar in dog RBC was 0. Measurements of net glucose movements by chemical analysis led Laris (1958) to conclude that dog RBC were permeable to glucose, but he could not tell whether any mechanism other than simple diffusion was involved. Widdas (1955) found that the fetal RBC from sheep, deer, pig and guinea-pig have a much higher glucose permeability than cells from adults of the same species. Cats were the only exception to this rule. As far as I am aware there is no further published information on the mechanism of glucose penetration into dog and cat RBC. A report from the laboratory of Lee (1976) indicates that a saturable mechanism for glucose transport in adult dog RBC has been found.

Dog RBC can utilize the purine nucleoside, adenosine, in two ways: the compound can be phosphorylated to AMP, or it can be phosphorylitically cleaved into purine and ribose phosphate (McManus, 1974). These pathways are found in human RBC, but an interesting characteristic that sets dog (and guinea-pig) RBC apart from those of most other mammals is their apparent impermeability to inosine (Duhm, 1974; McManus, 1974). The substrate specificity of purine nucleoside transport in various types of mammalian RBC would be an interesting object of study, since a facilitated diffusion system appears to be involved (Cass and Paterson, 1972).

The ATP-dependent, "active" transport system whereby oxidized glutathione is excreted from RBC is present in dog RBC (Srivastava and Beutler, 1969b; Smith, 1974).

6 Passive cation movements

Passive cation movements in dog and cat RBC have received considerable attention in recent years, but hardly any information or insights have been added to the elegant studies of Davson and his colleagues in the 1930s and early 1940s—all done without radioisotopes or flame photometers (Davson, 1940a,b,c, 1942; Davson and Reiner, 1942). These investigators placed high

Na cat or dog RBC in media containing mainly K salts and measured net flux of the two ion species down their concentration gradients. Their results led them to postulate that while K moves by simple diffusion through the membrane phase, Na transport is carried out at specialized "patches" where a Na-specific, enzyme-like mechanism acts to facilitate or "catalyse" the movement of this ion. As a point of departure, Davson noted that cat RBCs are more permeable to Na than to K (Table 8), an

TABLE 8

Apparent permeabilities of cat and dog RBC to sodium (P_{Na}) and potassium (P_K)

	P_{Na}	P_K	P_{Na}/P_K
Davson and Reiner (1942) Cat, 25°C: $1\,(\mu^2)^{-1}(\min)^{-1}$ or, equally, $1\,(\mu^2)^{-1}\min^{-1}$	17×10^{-19}	8×10^{-19}	—
Davson and Reiner recalculated to dimensions cm sec^{-1}	28×10^{-10}	13×10^{-10}	2·2
"Steady-state" tracer flux in cat 37°C: cm sec^{-1}	29×10^{-10}	6×10^{-10}	5·1
"Steady-state" tracer flux in dog 37°C: cm sec^{-1}	15×10^{-10}	3×10^{-10}	4·8

Data based on cell dimensions and ion contents in Table 1. Steady-state fluxes (mmol (1 cells)$^{-1}$ h^{-1}): cat Na = 17, K = 0·18 (Sha'afi and Leib, 1967); dog Na = 10, K = 0·1 (Fig. 1).

"anomalous" situation considering that the relative mobility of the two ions in aqueous solution is in the reverse direction.

A partial summary of Davson's results is given in Table 9. Clearly, many influences and perturbations have differing effects on Na and K movements. Most of Davson's observations were made on cat RBC, but he and others have confirmed that dog RBC behave similarly. In the following sections some of these effects will be discussed in more detail.

A cautionary comment should be made concerning reports of radioactive Na and K flux measurements in dog and cat RBC. Although the entry of ^{42}K into dog RBC can be described with a single rate constant up to 94 per cent specific activity equilibrium (Sheppard et al., 1951; Frazier et al., 1954), this is not true for cat cells, in which two cellular compartments with different physiological properties have been demonstrated (Sha'afi and Leib, 1967), as will be discussed in connection with active transport. Tracer Na influx into cat cells also requires two rate constants, and these were found to vary considerably between different animals and even in samples of blood from the same cat (Sha'afi and Leib, 1967). An exhaustive compartmental analysis of Na movements in dog RBC showed that there was not only gross inhomogeneity in a given sample of cells (a result

TABLE 9

Disparate effects of various perturbations on Na and K flux in cat and dog RBC

Experimental condition or result	Na flux	K flux	Davson ref.	Confirmation ref.
Change in cell volume:			d, e, f	$g, i, j, m, n, o, p, r, s$
swell	decr.	incr.		
shrink	incr.	decr.		
pH optimum, strong acid inhibition	yes	no	f	
Temperature optimum	yes	no	f	g, h, t
Mg ion	incr.	no eff.	d, f	k, w, x, y
Cu^{++}, Pb^{++}, Zn^{++}	decr.	incr.	f	a, t
"Narcotics"	decr.	*	d, e, f	q (seal RBC)
Fatty acids				
<5 carbons	incr.	—	b	
>5 carbons	decr.	—	b	
CNS^-, I^-	decr.	incr.	b, c, f	u, v
Incubation *in vitro*	decr.	no. eff.	d, f	i, j, l, r

* Cats increase, dogs decrease.
(*a*) Castranova and Miles, 1974; (*b*) Davson, 1940a; (*c*) Davson, 1940b; (*d*) Davson, 1940c; (*e*) Davson, 1942; (*f*) Davson and Reiner, 1942; (*g*) Elford, 1975a; (*h*) Elford and Solomon, 1974a; (*i*) Elford and Solomon, 1974b; (*j*) Hoffman, 1966; (*k*) Lee and Miles, 1973; (*l*) Miles and Lee, 1972; (*m*) Parker, 1973a; (*n*) Parker *et al*., 1975; (*o*) Parker and Hoffman, 1965; (*p*) Podolsky, 1959; (*q*) Robin *et al*., 1971; (*r*) Romualdez *et al*., 1972; (*s*) Sha'afi, 1965; (*t*) Sha'afi and Hajjar, 1971; (*u*) Sha'afi and Leib, 1967; (*v*) Sha'afi and Pascoe, 1972; (*w*) Sha'afi and Pascoe, 1973; (*x*) Sha'afi and Naccache, 1975; (*y*) Sorenson *et al*., 1962.

predicted by Davson), but there was also evidence for two cell compartments. Even with these two considerations the kinetics of isotope movement could not be well described (Lange *et al*., 1970). The only author who finds a single rate constant for Na entry into dog RBC is Elford (1975a), and this is notwithstanding the fact that the cells are in an unsteady state with respect to volume and that 9 per cent of the cell Na does not exchange with the isotope. Single, unqualified values for "Na flux" in dog or cat RBC should be regarded with suspicion. The raw data showing the timecourse of isotope movement are much to be preferred.

To what extent do tracer fluxes in dog and cat RBC represent "exchange diffusion", that is, tightly coupled, one-for-one exchange of radioactive for nonradioactive ions? This is a difficult question. The classical way to demonstrate exchange diffusion is to show a slowing of isotope flux when the nonradioactive species is removed from the *trans* side of the membrane. This is not easy to do in the case of Na for dog and cat RBC because suspension of these cells in most non-Na media causes volume changes (usually shrinking) which in turn affect the flux (Sorenson et al., 1962; Sha'afi and Leib, 1967). In this connection, it is interesting to compare the permeabilities measured in net flux experiments by Davson with those computed from isotopic flux data (note caveats above). The results (Table 8) show a remarkably close correspondence, which would suggest that the isotope movements do not reflect a large exchange diffusion component. Lee and Miles (1973) looked for K exchange diffusion in puppy RBC and found none.

6.1 CELL VOLUME

The disparate effects on Na and K movements of alterations in cellular volume have been amply confirmed in both dog and cat RBC by net and tracer flux measurements (Table 9). Each method of demonstrating the effect has hazards which derive from difficulties in keeping the cells in the steady state at all volumes. Figures 1a and 1b show the influx of ^{24}Na and ^{42}K, respectively, into dog RBC in circumstances where cell volume was altered by changing the external NaCl concentration. The change in cell water content over the 4 h flux period is shown for each group of cells. The left-hand ordinates give an expression of isotope equilibration appropriate for a two-compartment system, while the right-hand ordinates simply give per cent specific activity equilibrium. It is obvious that neither isotope moves as if in a two-compartment system, but if fluxes are calculated from the initial rates of isotope entry and plotted as functions of initial cell water content (Fig. 1c), it appears that the major change in Na flux occurs below isotonic volume while the rise in K permeability occurs in swollen cells.

The qualitative response of Na and K movements to cell volume changes is independent of the medium or cellular Na and K concentration and can be demonstrated in isotonic media if the cell volume is altered by various types of preincubation (Hoffman, 1966). The rise in K permeability with cell swelling is not unique to dog and cat RBC but has been reported in many other species (Davson, 1937). Increasing Na permeability in shrunken cells may occur to a minor degree in human RBC (Poznansky and Solomon, 1972), but is easily shown in bird RBC where a requirement for external K (Na–K cotransport) appears to differentiate this response from that seen in dog and cat cells (Kregenow, 1974; Schmidt, 1975).

By what mechanisms could cellular volume influence cation movements? It is easy to show that for a solute penetrating by Fickian diffusion a change in cell volume (V) (area (A) being constant) will be accompanied by a reciprocal change in k, the rate constant, with no change in permeability

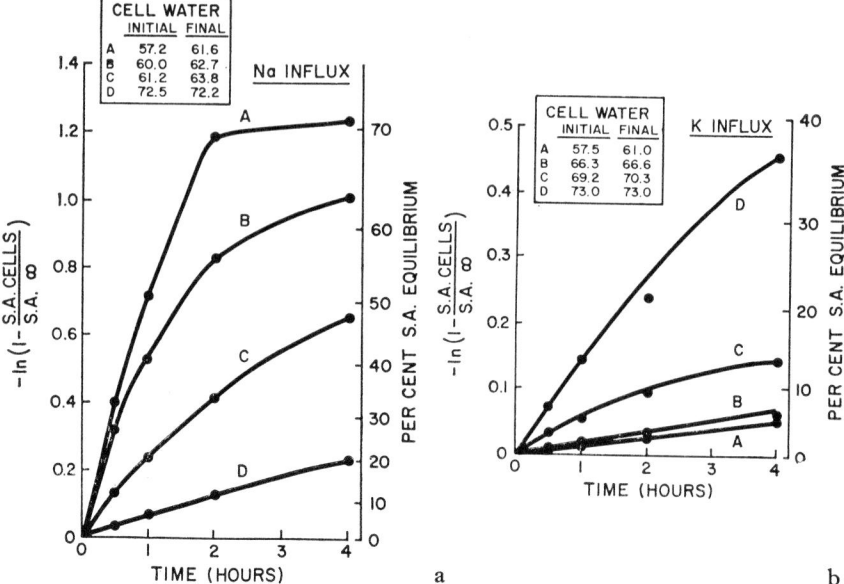

FIG. 1. Dog red blood cells. Approach of ^{24}Na (a) and ^{42}K (b) to specific activity equilibrium in solutions of differing tonicity over a 4 h incubation period at 37°C. Cells were washed and suspended in solutions with NaCl concentrations ranging from 80 to 220 mM plus (mM): KCl 5, Tris 17, glucose 10 (pH 7·5). The left ordinate shows an expression appropriate for a steady-state, two-compartment system. Specific activity (S.A.) of the cells at a given time is related to S.A. ∞, the specific activity at equilibrium. The right ordinate gives the cellular specific activity relative to the equilibrium value expressed as a percentage. The inset box shows the cell water content (per cent wet weight) at the beginning and end of the 4 h flux period. Panel (c) shows the influx of Na (left ordinate, solid line) and K (right ordinate, broken line) as functions of initial cell water content. Influx values were calculated from isotope movements during the first hour of incubation, and a correction was made to account for the changes in volume:surface ratio (Parker and Hoffman, 1976, with permission).

(P) because of the relation $k = PA/V$. If the solute is transported by a carrier which is saturated at all cell volumes, then the rate constant will be independent of cell volume. In either instance, the calculation of a *flux* (concentration × rate constant) can be misleading because of the variation in solute concentration with cell volume or with the makeup of anisotonic media. In dog and cat RBC, however, the increased rate of Na movement seen in freshly drawn cells shrunken in hypertonic media suggest a change in *permeability*. Furthermore, the effect cannot represent the activation of a tightly coupled, one-for-one Na–Na exchanger. If cells are shrunken in

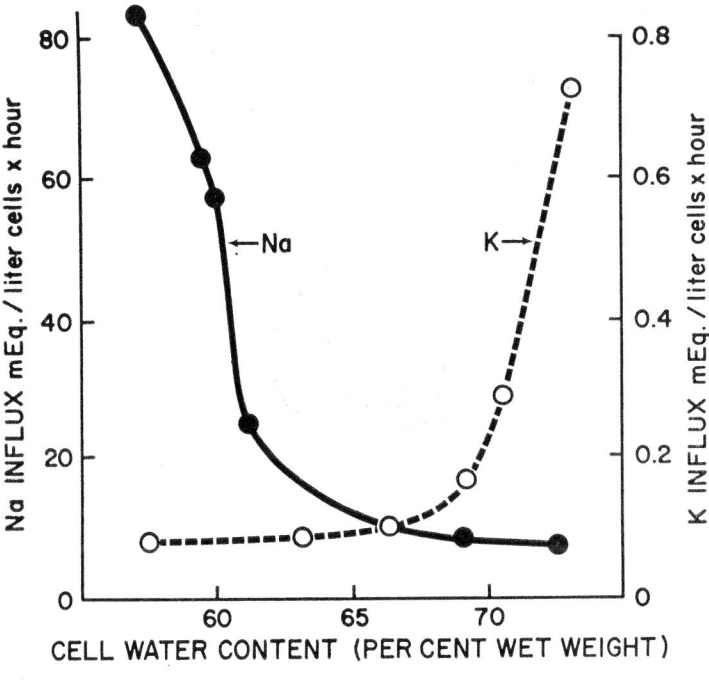

Fig. 1c.

hypertonic Na media, they gain Na (Fig. 1; Parker *et al.*, 1975); if an impermeant species like sucrose is used to shrink the cells, a net Na efflux occurs (Elford, 1975a). Indeed, the volume dependence of Na permeability was first demonstrated in studies of net ion movements (Davson, 1940c, 1942). The effect is immediately reversible on changing cell volume (Hoffman, 1966; Sha'afi and Hajjar, 1971; Romualdez *et al.*, 1972; Elford and Solomon, 1974b).

No one knows how dog and cat RBC become increasingly leaky to Na when shrunken, but there are two lines of evidence that may offer some clues. The first has to do with various inhibitors which can reduce Na permeability and abolish the volume response. The second relates to the influence on Na flux of metabolic perturbations such as cell starvation, glycolytic poisons, redox dyes and alternative substrates. The evidence will be detailed under appropriate headings below, but there are no answers to the questions: How does the cell membrane receive signals about the cell's volume (Gary-Bobo and Solomon, 1968)? How is the reversible change in permeability effected? Some speculations will be offered after a review of the evidence, but it should be kept in mind as various perturbations are discussed that cell volume is an important determinant of Na and K flux in dog and cat RBC. Any study which is not controlled for this variable should be interpreted with caution.

6.2 METABOLIC PERTURBATIONS

Davson noted that on storage in the icebox both cat (Davson, 1940c) and dog (Davson, 1942) RBC undergo as much as a two-thirds reduction in Na permeability over 2 days. It was later shown (Parker and Hoffman, 1965; Hoffman, 1966; Miles and Lee, 1972) that dog RBC incubated for 6–24 h at 37°C *in vitro* became progressively less permeable to Na, and less responsive to cell shrinkage. Although the change was observable in cells supplied with glucose during the incubation, it was most marked in cells deprived of metabolic substrate. Treatment of starved RBC with adenosine or glucose (Romualdez *et al.*, 1972; Sha'afi and Pascoe, 1973) resulted in some return of their volume responsiveness, but the incubation-starvation effect was not fully reversible by this sort of metabolic rescue. Recent studies on cat RBC suggest that Mg may be necessary for the metabolic resuscitation of the volume effect (Sha'afi and Naccache, 1975). Sha'afi and Pascoe (1973) showed that the glycolytic inhibitors iodoacetate and iodoacetamide both diminish Na influx in cat cells, and that the latter compound reduces the effect of cell shrinkage on Na influx. Fluoride did not inhibit Na movements in their hands. Redox dyes like methylene blue, which divert metabolism through the hexose monophosphate shunt, caused as much as a 60 per cent inhibition of Na flux in dog and cat RBC, but an influence on the volume effect was not reported. Elford and Solomon (1974b) studied the time-course of disappearance of glycolytic intermediates as dog RBC were incubated without glucose and found that even at 2 h, when 80–100 per cent of the triose phosphates were gone, a brisk response of Na influx to cell shrinkage could be shown. They furthermore found that bisulfite and (in contrast to the results of Sha'afi and Pascoe, 1973) fluoride inhibited the effect of shrinkage on Na flux, while sulfate and pyruvate were without effect. Elford and Solomon hypothesize that the volume effect in dog RBC may be mediated by conformational changes in the membrane-bound enzyme, phosphoglycerate kinase. They suppose that the enzyme can be prevented from changing its conformation in the direction of high Na permeability by raising the cellular 3-phosphoglycerate concentration.

These observations all suggest that changes in cellular metabolic state can affect passive Na and K movements in dog and cat RBC, but beyond this little can be said. The suggestion that phosphoglycerate kinase (or any other glycolytic enzyme) is involved is intriguing but without much support. All the evidence just cited could be interpreted as showing that some intermediate such as ATP—or even that total cell organic phosphate —is the key variable relating Na permeability to metabolic state. For example, Elford and Solomon (1974b) show that after a period of exposure to bisulfite ions (which cause a net loss of 2,3-diphosphoglycerate, the predominant organic phosphate in the cell) the Na influx has a lower "set", both in isotonic and hypertonic media.

Another way metabolism could influence membrane permeability is through some change in membrane ultrastructure or phospholipid distribution (Haest and Deuticke, 1975) associated with the spherical shape which cells assume on depletion (Nakao et al., 1960). Still another mechanism for the influence of metabolic events on the membrane could be related to the recently observed phosphorylation of spectrin by a protein kinase (Juliano et al., 1971; Guthrow et al., 1972). One approach which might be informative would be to measure the levels of all the glycolytic intermediates during prolonged incubation *in vitro* and to correlate these with the time-course of the permeability changes. An example of the success of this sort of strategy can be found in reports on the metabolic dependence of passive K permeability in human RBC (Gardos, 1966; Lew, 1971).

6.3 LYOTROPIC EFFECTS

It has been of interest for many years that the physical properties of macromolecular solutions can be modified by a variety of simple ions which also have pronounced effects on the functions of living cells and their membranes (von Hippel and Wong, 1964; Robinson and Jenks, 1965). The ions can be arranged in sequence according to the relative magnitude of their influence on, for example, protein solubility, and it is generally found that their physiologic actions follow a similar order. Such a listing of ions is called a lyotropic or Hofmeister series and includes both anions and cations. Davson (1940a,b, 1942) and Davson and Reiner (1942) found that net movements of Na and K in cat and dog RBC were greatly influenced by anions of the lyotropic series but that the pattern for K was just thee reverse of that for Na. Thus, K permeability increased as the predominant anion was changed from acetate to Cl to Br to NO_3 to I to CNS, while in the same sequence Na movements were progressively inhibited. These observations were confirmed in both dog and cat RBC with radioactive tracer techniques (Sha'afi and Leib, 1967; Sha'afi and Pascoe, 1972).

Funder and Wieth (1967) and Wieth (1970a) showed that the response of human RBC differs fundamentally from that of dogs and cats in that both Na and K follow the pattern observed by Davson for K. It was later shown that anion permeability in both human (Deuticke, 1967; Wieth,

1970b; Dalmark and Wieth, 1972) and cat (Sha'afi and Pascoe, 1972) RBC is also influenced by lyotropic anions in a sequence opposite from that of K. These findings are summarized in Table 10.

TABLE 10

Lyotropic anion	Dog and cat			Human				
	P_{Na} (b, c, d, g)	P_K (b, c, d, g)	P_{SO_3} (h)	P_{Na} (f, i)	P_K (f, i)	P_{SO_4} (j)	P_{PO_4} (e)	P_C (a, j)
Br-Cl I-NO$_3$ SCN	↑	↓	↑	↑	↓	↑	↑	↑
Salicylate					↓	↑		

Permeability increases in the direction of the arrowhead. (a) Dalmark and Wieth, 1972; (b) Davson, 1940a; (c) Davson, 1940b; (d) Davson, 1942; (e) Deuticke, 1967; (f) Funder and Wieth, 1967; (g) Sha'afi and Leib, 1967; (h) Sha'afi and Pascoe, 1972; (i) Wieth, 1970a; (j) Wieth, 1970b.

The mechanism of action of lyotropic agents is not well understood (Robinson and Jenks, 1965). Suggestions have been made that they influence water structure, or the hydration of macromolecules, or that they bind to various ionic groups on proteins or phospholipids. Davson felt that the strongest inhibitors of Na flux in cat and dog RBC (I, CNS) were the ones that were most strongly adsorbed to the membrane. In support of this he cited observations that anions with large nonpolar groups (long-chain fatty acids, phenylacetate) had marked inhibitory effects on Na permeability, due, in his view, to their association with the lipid phase of the membrane (Davson, 1940a,b; Davson and Reiner, 1942). Wieth (1970c) found that *cations* from the lyotropic series which have vastly different effects on water structure exercised no special action on anion movements and trivial influences on Na permeability in human RBC. He therefore rejected the idea that the effects of lyotropic agents were due to changes in water. He proposed instead that the lyotropic anions act to influence permeability by virtue of their adsorption to fixed positive charges in the membrane (Wieth, 1970a,b).

It seems likely that the mechanism which mediates increased Na permeability with osmotic shrinking in dog and cat RBC is also influenced by the lyotropic anions: Davson and Reiner (1942) and later Sha'afi and Pascoe

(1972) showed that SCN completely abolished the effect of hypertonic solutions on Na flux.*

Perhaps the most intriguing bit of information from the lyotropic studies is that the response of Na permeability in dog and cat RBC mimics that of an anion or of a nonelectrolyte such as erythritol, whose penetration in human RBC is reduced by CNS and salicylate (Wieth et al., 1974). In the following paragraphs this characteristic of Na permeability in dog and cat RBC will be further discussed.

6.4 ALKALINE EARTHS AND HEAVY METALS

Table 11 summarizes Davson's (1940c) findings on net Na and K move-

TABLE 11

Effects of alkaline earth and heavy metal ions on permeability to Na and K in cat RBC

Ion	Conc'n (mM)	Change in P_{Na} (%)	Change in P_K (%)
Ca	1	0	0
	5	+35	0
	10	+50	+50
Mg	10	+100	0
Sr	10	+20	−10
Ba	10	+60	−15

Data from Davson (1940c).

ments in cat RBC as affected by alkaline earth metals. The point of major interest was the difference in response of the two permeabilities. Mg and Ca were also reported to stimulate movements of radioactive Na in puppy RBC (Lee and Miles, 1973). Sha'afi and Pascoe (1973) confirmed Davson's results in cat RBC and added two interesting observations: in fresh cells Mg does not alter the volume responsiveness of the Na pathway but rather increases the flux by the same increment in both swollen and shrunken cells. In starved cells (Sha'afi and Naccache, 1975) the volume response cannot be recovered unless both Mg and glucose are present, suggesting that some metabolic process or product is necessary either for the permeation or action of Mg. Since the cells are quite leaky to Mg (Rogers, 1961) it is not clear whether the site of action on Na permeability is at the inner or outer membrane surface.

* Although not usually mentioned in the lyotropic series, bisulfite is like CNS in that it increases both Na and K permeability in human RBC (Parker, 1969). Bisulfite's ability to obliterate the volume effect on Na flux in dog RBC (Elford and Solomon, 1974b) is also analogous to that of SCN, and the two ions may therefore be acting in the same way.

Davson and Reiner (1942) reported that at concentrations between 10^{-6} and 10^{-4} M, Cu, Zn and Pb ions exert as much as a 90 per cent inhibition of Na permeability while mildly stimulating K flux, and the result for Cu has been confirmed (Sha'afi and Hajjar, 1971). Since Cu ions also inhibit glycerol penetration in human RBC, Davson and Reiner (1942) thought that the "catalysed" permeability route for Na in dog RBC and glycerol in human RBC might have similar characteristics.

6.5 NARCOTICS AND PHLORETIN

Davson was prompted to study the effects of various lipid-soluble, pharmacologically active, organic nonelectrolytes ("narcotics") because these agents were known to inhibit the rapid penetration of glycerol into the RBC of certain species, such as the rabbit (see Tables 6 and 7). He and Reiner (1942) reported a long list of compounds, including alcohols, ethers, chloroform, benzine and tannic acid which all had potent inhibitory effects on Na permeability in cat and dog RBC. In cat RBC the agents increased K flux, but in dog cells (Davson, 1942) K movements were retarded along with those of Na. (This is one of the few qualitative differences between cat and dog RBC and explains an interesting observation: in isotonic KCl media a narcotic, *n*-butyl carbamate, protects dog cells from hemolysis by inhibiting net cation uptake; in the same circumstances lysis of cat RBC is potentiated by the narcotic because Na loss is slowed while K gain is accelerated.)

Because inhibition by narcotics is such a constant feature of facilitated diffusion systems (Table 6), it seems highly likely that Na penetration in dog and cat RBC occurs by a mechanism similar in some way to that which mediates the transport of anions or (in other species) sugars, acetate or glycerol. An observation which further supports this idea is that phloretin inhibits passive Na movements in dog and cat RBC. Like butanol, phloretin completely abolishes the increase in Na flux that accompanies cell shrinkage (Romualdez et al., 1972; Sha'afi and Naccache, 1975).

6.6 pH AND TEMPERATURE

The movements of anions and water which accompany titration of intracellular buffers make it difficult to separate pH effects from those of cell volume. Davson and Reiner (1942) were aware of this and tried to deal with the problem by the rather unsatisfactory measure of working in hypertonic media so the cells would be shrunken at all levels of pH. Their curve, based on net flux of Na in exchange for K, shows an optimum for Na permeability at 7·2–7·6. At pH 6·1 net Na movements are completely inhibited. K flux is not much affected by pH over the range 6·2–8·4. I know of no studies in dog or cat RBC where the effects of pH and cell volume have been clearly dissociated.

Davson and Reiner (1942) also found that while net K flux in cat RBC increased progressively as the temperature was raised from 20°C to 50°C, Na flux showed an optimum value at around 37°C. Sha'afi and Hajjar (1971) confirmed the Na result with tracer fluxes and calculated an apparent activation energy (25–37°C) of 4·9 kcal mol^{-1}. A 22°C temperature optimum for the movement of radioactive Na was found in dog RBC at normal cell volume (Elford and Solomon, 1974a; Elford, 1975a), but in shrunken cells the Na flux increased progressively with temperature over the range studied, although the Arrhenius plot was not linear. K flux in dog RBC showed a minimum value at around 15°C (Table 12).

TABLE 12

Apparent activation energies (kcal mol^{-1}) for Na and K movements in dog RBC

	Normal cell volume	Shrunken cells
Na flux:		
5–22°C	+28·2	+35·0
22–38°C	−8·7	+14·8
K flux:		
0–15°C	−22·2	—
15–38°C	+8·5	+12·6

From Elford (1975a).

The results certainly suggest that Na and K permeate by different mechanisms, but further conclusions are difficult to make because of the likelihood that the temperature curves reflect a number of interacting processes (Wieth, 1970a).

6.7 MISCELLANEOUS EFFECTS

Dog RBC become leaky to Na and K when placed in media containing ATP in concentrations as low as 0·5 mM (Parker and Snow, 1972; Elford, 1975b; Romualdez and Sha'afi, 1975). The effect can be stopped by washing off the ATP, by adding an ATP-utilizing system (glucose + hexokinase) in the medium, or by the presence of Ca or Mg ions in concentrations equimolar with ATP. Other nucleotides (including 2-deoxy-ATP) and chelators fail to mimic the action of ATP. Along with the changes in cation permeability go a mild stimulation of glycolysis and a striking increase in viscosity of the cells when packed. The meaning of this observation is obscure but may have something to do with the common origin of RBC and platelets, which are well known to respond to external nucleotides. On the other hand, entirely similar phenomena have been reported in renal tubules and ascites tumor cells (Hempling et al., 1969; Rorive and Kleinzeller, 1972).

Various amino- and thiol-reactive chemicals are reported to increase Na flux in dog RBC, but the reports do not mention effects on the movements of other solutes, and the specificity of the effects is therefore not clear (Castranova and Miles, 1974, 1975). The actions of colchicine and vinblastine in diminishing ^{22}Na movements in cat RBC suggested to Sha'afi and Naccache (1975) that microtubular protein might be involved in permeability to this ion.

6.8 CONCLUSIONS

The evidence suggesting that passive Na movements in dog and cat RBC occur by facilitated diffusion rests largely on the effects of various noncompetitive inhibitors (lyotropic anions, copper, tannate, narcotics, phloretin). None of the other criteria (Stein, 1964) for facilitated diffusion (competition, saturation) have been examined critically. This is in part because of the massive influence of the "volume effect". Small changes in cell volume cause such large alterations in Na flux that the appropriate experiments will be formidably difficult. It is not easy to control cell volume when one is trying to make either intra- or extracellular substitutions for Na. There is some evidence that Li ions may behave like Na in dog RBC (Parker et al., 1975). Lithium–sodium exchange appears to be hastened by cell shrinkage, but for this reason lithium would not be a good ion to use as a sodium substitute in saturation experiments. Exhaustive attempts (Parker, unpublished data) to make resealed ghosts (Schwoch and Passow, 1973) from dog RBC have yielded a preparation which is fairly tight to Na and which behaves as a perfect osmometer (Kwant and Seeman, 1970). Unfortunately, Na appears to move as if by simple diffusion in these ghosts, and the volume effect is not seen even when all manner of glycolytic intermediates are included in the hemolysis medium.

Gary-Bobo and Solomon (1968) suggested that cell volume changes are accompanied by alterations of membrane voltage due to shifts in the ionization constant of hemoglobin. The idea that the volume signal is an electrical one is attractive and worthy of further testing in dog and cat RBC.

7 Active cation transport

The data on ionic equilibria in dog and cat RBC (Table 1) suggest that if all the cell ions are in solution in all the cell water, and if the activity coefficients do not differ greatly between cells and plasma, and if the chloride ratio is a valid indicator of the membrane potential, then neither cat nor dog RBC are in Donnan equilibrium with their surroundings. In each species the cell Na is lower and K higher than would be the case if these two ions were passively distributed. In other species, Na and K are kept away from equilibrium by the action of the ouabain-sensitive, ATP-driven, Na–K exchange pump. Dog and cat RBC have only a few vestiges of this apparatus.

Sha'afi and Leib (1967) found that the flux of radioactive K into a small (10 per cent of cell K), rapidly labeling (half-time less than 10 min) component of cat RBC was reduced by about 60 per cent in the presence of ouabain. Movement of tracer into the bulk of the cellular K pool was unaffected by the glycoside. Miles and Lee (1972) and Lee and Miles (1973) showed that K influx into the RBC of newborn puppies was higher than into cells from adult dogs; the difference was due to an ouabain-sensitive component in the puppies which was barely detectable in cells from older dogs. Because no ouabain-sensitive Na efflux was demonstrated in either puppy or adult dog RBC, the authors regarded the glycoside-sensitive K movements as uncoupled. The possibility of an ouabain-sensitive K–K exchange was thought unlikely (Lee and Miles, 1973). Other investigations (Sorenson et al., 1962; Hoffman, 1966; Parker, 1973a) have confirmed the absence of an ouabain-sensitive Na efflux in dog RBC, and although I can find no published data, I am assured that the same is true for cat cells. Consistent with these observations is the unanimity of reports on the absence of Na, K-ATPase activity on RBC membranes from dogs and cats (Chan et al., 1964; Greeff et al., 1964; Sha'afi, 1965; Parker, 1973a; Gupta et al., 1974).

In an earlier section of this review it was pointed out that dog reticulocytes are high in K; it is likely that these young cells and their precursors have Na–K pumps, although for technical reasons this has been difficult to demonstrate. Low K sheep manifest a fall in RBC K with increasing cell age (Blunt and Evans, 1963). In these sheep, however, the mature RBC retain a small amount of Na–K pump activity which can be augmented by treatment of the cells with certain specific antibodies (Ellory, this volume). It is possible that mature dog (and cat) RBC have "cryptic pumps" which could be unmasked by appropriate experimental maneuvers.

But how, in the absence of demonstrable pumps, are Na and K prevented from reaching equilibrium in dog and cat RBC? This question is in turn tied up with the problem of volume control. Davson and Reiner (1942) wrote:

A cell containing proteins, which is permeable to both sodium and potassium besides anions, will have a tendency for salt to penetrate continuously in accordance with the Gibbs-Donnan equilibrium; this process, unless counter-acted, would lead to haemolysis. Since this does not occur, it is possible that the cat erythrocyte actively excretes sodium in order to maintain an osmotic equilibrium in the plasma.

Evidence for active Na transport was obtained by *in vivo* studies of volume regulation in dogs (Parker, 1973a,c). A sample of RBC was drawn and incubated for 3 h in hypertonic NaCl so that the cells underwent a net accumulation of this salt. Radioactive chromium was included in the medium as a cellular label. When the salt-loaded cells were removed from the hypertonic medium and washed with isotonic ringer, their water content was now greater than it had been when freshly drawn, and for this reason their density was lower than that of normal, circulating dog RBC. The chromium-labeled, salt-and-water-loaded cells were reinjected into their owner's bloodstream. At intervals thereafter small volumes of blood were collected and centrifuged in a density gradient. In the early samples the chromium-labeled cells, because of their increased water content, were found in the least dense fractions of the gradient. At later points, however, the density of the treated cells decreased, and by 24 h the labeled cells had the same density distribution as the bulk of the animal's RBC.

Incubation of similarly salt-and-water-loaded cells *in vitro* showed no evidence for volume control, in part because of buffering problems (Parker, 1973a) and in part because the incubation media used lacked calcium. A report that volume regulation in isolated, ouabain-treated renal tubules requires calcium (Rorive et al., 1972) suggested that the influence of this cation be studied, and the experiment shown in Fig. 2 was done. It was clear that the Na and water content of preloaded dog RBC would come back to normal over the same time-course that had been seen in the *in vivo* studies, provided that calcium was included in the medium along with glucose. The calcium-dependent net Na efflux was shown to be against a Na electrochemical gradient (with the usual assumptions about the state of cell water and the membrane potential), and it was not inhibited by ouabain or by removing extracellular K (Parker, 1973b). The effect of calcium was maximal at 5 mM and half-maximal at about 2 mM (normal plasma ionized Ca is about 1·2 mM). Mg was not effective as a replacement for Ca. It is not necessary to preload the cells with Na to see the calcium-dependent net Na and water extrusion. The phenomenon can be demonstrated in fresh cells and is accentuated when the cells are swollen in hypotonic media (Parker et al., 1975). Indeed, no influence of calcium on Na or water movements can be demonstrated in osmotically shrunken cells.

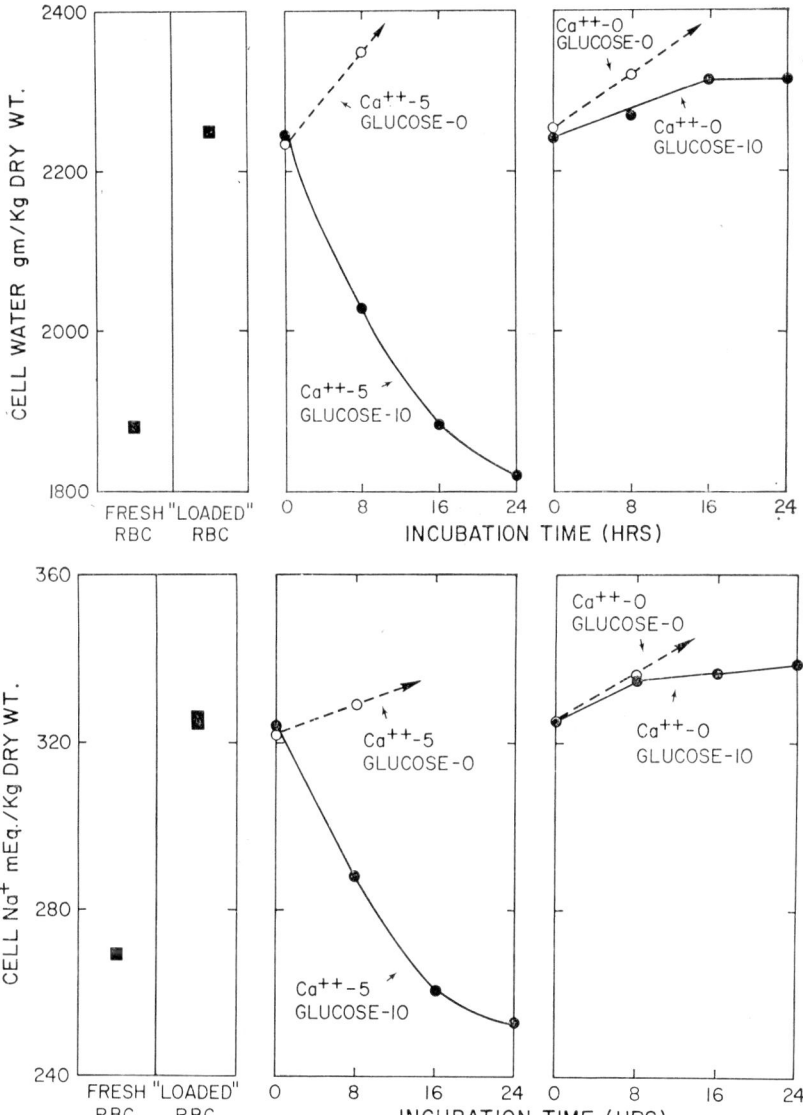

FIG. 2. Dog red blood cells. Net movements of water (a) and Na (b) in the presence and absence of Ca and glucose. Fresh cells were loaded with salt and water by preincubation for 3 h in a buffered, hypertonic (200 mM) NaCl medium. After washing with isotonic NaCl Ringer the cell water and Na were as shown at time 0. Incubation of the loaded cells in buffered, isotonic NaCl at 37°C led to alterations in water and Na content shown. Only in the presence of both Ca and glucose did the Na and water values return toward those of fresh cells.

Thus, one problem, which will be dealt with in the following section on volume control, is to explain why calcium-dependent active Na extrusion in dog RBC is so dependent on cell volume.

How does calcium work to induce active, uphill Na transport? This question was approached in an indirect way by studying net movements of calcium as a function of cell volume and of sodium concentration (Parker et al., 1975). Ca is much lower in dog RBC cytoplasm (0·020 mmol (1 cells)$^{-1}$) than in plasma (1–2 mM). The cells can be made to take on calcium from the medium, however, if they are osmotically swollen. Thus, under the very conditions in which Ca-dependent Na pumping is seen, Ca accumulates in the cells. This leads to the speculation that Ca is necessary at some intracellular site to activate the Na pump. Against this idea is the observation that treatment of cells with the ionophore A23187 or with chlorpromazine (Parker, 1974), both of which promote Ca movement from medium to cells, results in no activation of Na extrusion. Of course, it could be argued that the drugs inhibit the transport mechanism.

More germane to the question of calcium-induced Na movements is the observation, first reported by Omachi et al. (1961), that calcium accumulation in dog RBC is enhanced in low Na solutions. In pursuit of this point it was discovered (Parker et al., 1975) that calcium can be made to flow into or out of cells by manipulating the ions on either side of the membrane so that in the phase *from* which calcium is desired to move Na concentration is low, while on the opposite or "receiving" side Na is high. Put in another way, Ca tends to move away from a low Na compartment and toward a high Na one. These observations on net Ca flux gave rise to the notion that dog RBC might have a mechanism on the membrane for Ca–Na exchange (Blaustein, 1974), such as that described in cardiac muscle (Reuter and Seitz, 1968) and nervous tissue (Baker et al., 1969). The transport system, which can exchange Na for Na, Ca for Ca, or Ca for Na, is thought in excitable tissues to be responsible for maintaining a low Ca environment in the cytoplasm. Na is low in these tissues, and it is hypothesized that energy derived from passive Na entry fuels the active extrusion of calcium. A converse mechanism can be postulated for dog RBC, which have a high Na and a low Ca concentration. In these cells the Ca–Na exchanger could be using the energy from passive, inward calcium movements to drive Na out. This presumes that dog RBC have a calcium pump such as that described in human RBC by Schatzmann and Vincenzi (1969).

It is certainly possible to show a net unloading of Ca by dog RBC into a Ca-containing medium (Parker et al., 1975). Wiley (personal communication) states that this process occurs with the same kinetics seen in human RBC. Lew (personal communication) has shown that the exclusion of calcium from dog RBC is exquisitely sensitive to the cell's metabolic state.

As ATP falls in glucose-deprived cells, calcium enters at a rate which exceeds that of most species. What has been difficult to show is that dog RBC have a Ca-dependent ATPase on their membranes (Rega *et al.*, 1974). This difficulty may in part be due to the extreme lability of dog RBC membrane proteins with various methods of ghost preparation (Kobylka *et al.*, 1972). Figure 3 shows that the rate of ATP decline in dog RBC deprived of glucose is increased with increasing Ca concentration as if there were some Ca-dependent ATP catabolic mechanism in the cells.

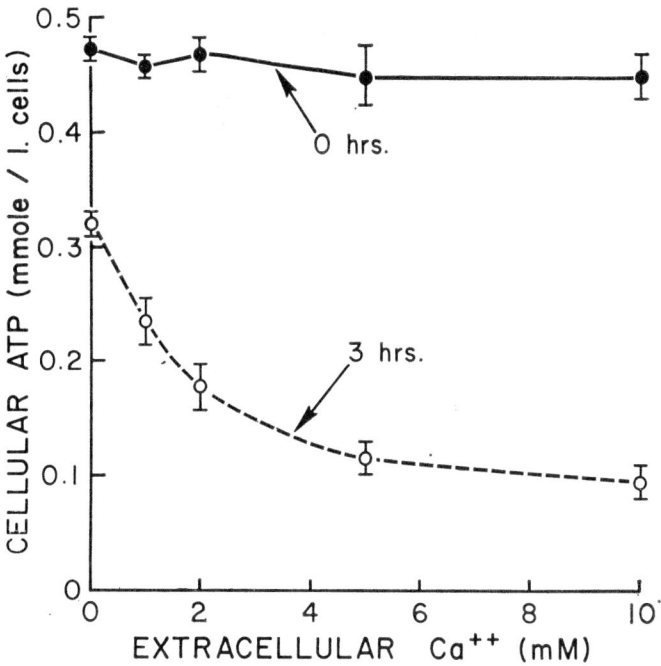

FIG. 3. Decline in ATP concentration of substrate-deprived dog red blood cells over a 3 h period, as a function of extracellular Ca. Incubation medium contained (mM): NaCl 105, NaHCO$_3$ 25, KCl 5, plus indicated concentrations of CaCl$_2$. Gassed with 95 per cent O$_2$–5 per cent CO$_2$.

An alternative suggestion about how Ca might influence cell volume and Na content is that the divalent ion can cause some muscle-like protein in the cell membrane to contract, thus raising the hydrostatic pressure inside the cell and squeezing out salt water (Kleinzeller, 1972; Rangachari *et al.*, 1973). Although no firm evidence against this notion exists, there is one observation that may be more consistent with a pump-leak model: if the Na inside dog RBC is replaced by K, Ca will no longer cause net salt and water extrusion, even when the cells are swollen (Parker et al., 1975). It would be unusual for a muscle mechanism to be incapable of function in a high K environment.

Recently, Sha'afi and Naccache (1975) found that accumulation of radioactive calcium by cat RBC is increased in hypertonic media. This result contrasts with the report in dog RBC that net calcium movements are promoted when cells are swollen (Parker et al., 1975). The two observations need not be incompatible, however, since the rate of isotope movement might not reflect changes in pool size. Indeed, it is possible that the isotopic data can be explained on the basis of Ca–Na exchange: Sha'afi and Naccache added sucrose to an isotonic NaCl medium to shrink their cat cells, thus raising the cytoplasmic Na concentration while keeping external Na constant. These conditions would be expected to increase the inward movement of calcium via a Ca–Na exchanger (Blaustein, 1974).

Long and Mouat (1971) found in an interspecies comparison of calcium adsorption versus cell neuraminic acid content that dog and cat RBC showed the highest levels of both quantities. The relevance of this to calcium metabolism in these cells is not yet clear.

8 Cell volume control

Calcium-dependent active Na transport in dog RBC is easily measurable in swollen cells, under conditions of minimal Na leak. As cells are shrunken, passive Na flux increases greatly (Fig. 1), and the effect of Ca on NaCl and water movements becomes imperceptible (Parker et al., 1975). It is a moot point whether the Ca-dependent Na pump shuts off at low cell volume or whether its detection is made impossible by the high Na leak. Whatever the behavior of the Ca–Na exchange pump, it is possible to explain volume regulation in dog RBC in terms of the response of the leak to cell volume (Fig. 4).

In the steady state there is an electrochemical gradient tending to move Na into the cell (Table 1). If too much Na should enter, the cell would swell, Na permeability would fall to a level at which Ca-dependent Na extrusion would exceed inward Na leak, and Na would be pumped out until the cell volume became normal. On the other hand, if the cell became dehydrated, Na leak permeability would rise to a level at which passive, inward Na movement would exceed Ca-dependent Na extrusion, the cell would accumulate Na, and its volume would move toward normal.

Sha'afi and Hajjar (1971) have made the intriguing suggestion that the volume-responsive Na leak in dog and cat RBC is important in protecting the kidney from blood sludging in the distal medulla where very high plasma Na concentrations may occur due to the action of the renal concentrating mechanism. When shrunken in the hypertonic environs of the renal papillary vasculature the RBCs should undergo a sudden increase in Na permeability. The resulting net entry of Na and water should protect the cells from becoming dehydrated and viscous. This would be particularly important for cat RBC, in which the solubility of hemoglobin is particularly low (Mauk *et al.*, 1974). A point against this possibility is the rather slow rate of Na accumulation by dog RBC in hypertonic saline (half-time 2–4 h) in relation to the rapid flow of blood through the kidney (Parker *et al.*, 1975). The idea is nonetheless interesting and susceptible to experimental test.

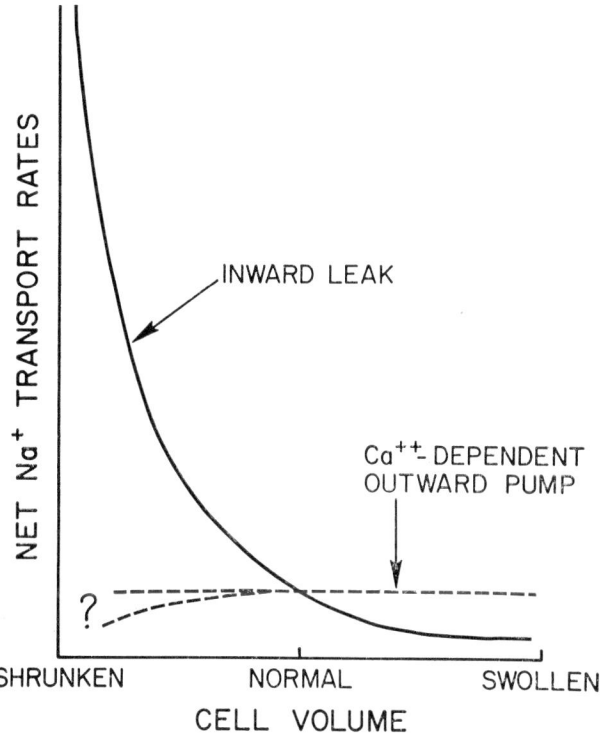

Fig. 4. Conceptual model of pump and leak transport for Na in dog red blood cells as functions of cell volume. At normal volume the two fluxes are equal.

9 Dog and cat RBC *in vivo*

The first inklings that red blood cells might be permeable to cations were based in part on early experiments showing that perturbations of plasma cation concentration are accompanied by changes in RBC electrolyte content. A summary of this work by Yannet et al. (1935–6) stated that:

> A review of the available literature on the permeability of red cells of different animals, together with the data presented, leads to the conclusion that erythrocytes containing sodium as the preponderant base are permeable to sodium. A similar permeability of erythrocytes containing potassium as the preponderant base has not been demonstrated.

While some of the findings can be explained by the high K content of dog reticulocytes (Kerr, 1926a,b), the effect of adrenalectomy in cats provides convincing evidence that the hyponatremia and hyperkaliemia wrought by that procedure is reflected by parallel changes in RBC electrolytes (Robinson and Hegnauer, 1936). Alternative methods of lowering serum Na were also found to decrease the content of RBC Na (Hegnauer and Robinson, 1936).

A modern investigation showing that the movement of radioactive Na into dog RBC *in vitro* is influenced by adrenalectomy and adrenal steroids (Spach and Streeten, 1964; Streeten and Moses, 1968) is flawed by a lack of data on cell volume and a cumbersome method of measuring influx (disappearance of extracellular radioactivity). Using different methods it has not been possible to confirm the effects (Parker and Hoffman, 1976).

A hemolytic anemia associated with ATP depletion of RBC was induced in starved dogs by infusing them with solutions of amino acids and hypertonic glucose—a procedure which leads to hypophosphatemia (Yawata et al., 1974). Although the claim was made that the RBC underwent dehydration and Na loss (Yawata et al., 1972), no data to quantitate the changes were included in the reports. *In vivo* dehydration of dog RBC was documented by Ham et al. (1973) in a study of the effects of acetyl phenylhydrazine injection. Coincident with the onset of hemolytic anemia there was a net loss from the cells of water and total cations, although separate values for Na and K were not given. The RBC showed precipitation or clumping of hemoglobin and some Heinz bodies (bits of denatured globin) were noted on special stains. Creation of Heinz bodies in human RBC also leads to cellular dehydration due to K loss (Orringer and Parker, 1973), but the mechanism in dogs must be different, since dog RBC are low in K. There is a possibility that the dehydration and K loss occurred in a high K reticulocyte fraction (Parker, 1973c).

Alkalosis (venous pH greater than 7·6) causes hemolysis in dogs, and the lability of these cells under alkaline conditions *in vitro* is well known to workers in the field (Waddell, 1956; Iampetro et al., 1967, 1969). It is possible that the mechanism has something to do with facilitation of calcium entry under conditions of slightly raised pH (Parker et al., 1975).

Two congenital hemolytic syndromes have been reported in dogs. Hereditary stomatocytosis and dwarfism (Pinkerton et al., 1974), an autosomal recessive trait in Alaskan Malamutes, is associated with mild anemia and a slight elevation in reticulocytes. The red cells are large and overhydrated, with a high Na content. The youngest cells in affected animals are more dense than older cells—exactly the opposite of the case in normal animals—suggesting that the mechanisms for Na exclusion become weaker with cell maturation. An entirely similar illness exists in humans (Oski et al., 1969).

Pyruvate kinase deficiency in Basenji dogs is associated with marked (30–50 per cent) reticulocytosis, increased osmotic fragility and hemolysis on incubation *in vitro* (Searcy et al., 1971). Like the human variants of this syndrome, cells can be protected *in vitro* with adenosine and ATP, but not with inosine (see section on metabolism). No studies are reported on ion or water content of the RBC from these dogs, but they would be expected to have very high cell K concentrations due to the reticulocytosis. Whether the mechanism of hemolysis *in vivo* involves cellular dehydration, as postulated for human pyruvate kinase deficiency (Mentzer et al., 1971), remains to be seen.

References

BAKER, P. F., BLAUSTEIN, M. P., HODGKIN, A. L. and STEINHARDT, R. A. (1969). The influence of calcium on sodium efflux in squid anons. *J. Physiol. (Lond.)*, **200**, 431.

BARTLETT, G. R. (1970). Patterns of phosphate compounds in red blood cells of man and animals. *Adv. Exp. Med. Biol.* **6**, 245.

BASHAN, N., MOSES, S., GROSS, Y. and LIVNE, A. (1975). The effect of Na and K on glycolytic enzymes: Differential response of pyruvate kinase from dog and human erythrocytes. *FEBS Lett.* **54**, 323.

BERNSTEIN, R. E. (1954). K. and Na balance in mammalian red cells. *Science*, **120**, 459.

BLAUSTEIN, M. P. (1974). The interrelationship between sodium and calcium fluxes across cell membranes. *Rev. Physiol. Biochem. Pharmacol.* **70**, 33.

BLUNT, M. H. and EVANS, J. V. (1963). Changes in the concentration of potassium in the erythrocytes and in hemoglobin type in Merino sheep under severe anemic stress. *Nature*, **200**, 1215.

BROWN, P. A., FEINSTEIN, M. B. and SHA'AFI, R. I. (1975). Membrane proteins related to water transport in human erythrocytes. *Nature*, **254**, 523.

BUNN, H. F. (1971). Differences in the interaction of 2,3-diphosphoglycerate with certain mammalian hemoglobins. *Science*, **172**, 1049.

BURR, M. J. (1972). The relationship between pH and aerobic glycolysis in human and canine erythrocytes. *Comp. Biochem. Physiol.* **41B**, 687.

CABANTCHIK, Z. I. and ROTHSTEIN, A. (1974). Membrane proteins related to anion permeability of human red blood cells. *J. Membrane Biol.* **15**, 207.

CAINELLI, S. R., CHUI, A., MCCLURE, J. D. and HUNTER, F. R. (1974). Facilitated diffusion in erythrocytes of mammals. *Comp. Biochem. Physiol.* **48A**, 815.

CASS, C. E. and PATERSON, A. R. P. (1972). Mediated transport of nucleosides in human erythrocytes. *J. Biol. Chem.* **247**, 3314.

CASTRANOVA, V. and MILES, P. R. (1974). Pharmacological modification of the Na channel in dog red blood cells. *Fed. Proc.* **33**, 265a.

CASTRANOVA, V. and MILES, P. R. (1975). Modification of amino sites which control Na permeability in dog red cells. *Fed. Proc.* **34**, 237a.

CHAN, P. C., CALABRESE, V. and THIEL, L. S. (1964). Species differences in the effect of sodium and potassium ions on the ATPase of erythrocyte membranes. *Biochim. Biophys. Acta*, **79**, 424.

COHN, W. E. and COHN, E. T. (1939). Permeability of red corpuscles of the dog to sodium ion. *Proc. Soc. Exp. Biol. Med.* **41**, 445.

DALMARK, M. and WIETH, J. O. (1972). Temperature dependence of chloride, bromide, iodide, thiocyanate, and salicylate transport in human red cells. *J. Physiol.* **224**, 583.

DAVSON, H. (1937). The loss of potassium from the erythrocyte in hypotonic saline. *J. Cell. Comp. Physiol.* **10**, 247.

DAVSON, H. (1940a). The permeability of the erythrocyte to cations. *Cold Spring Harbor Symposia on Quantitative Biology*, **8**, 255.

DAVSON, H. (1940b). The influence on the lyotropic series of anions on cation permeability. *Biochem. J.* **34**, 917.

DAVSON, H. (1940c). Ionic permeability. The comparative effects of environmental changes on the permeability of the cat erythrocyte to sodium and potassium. *J. Cell. Comp. Physiol.* **15**, 317.

DAVSON, H. (1942). The haemolytic action of potassium salts. *J. Physiol.* **101**, 265.

DAVSON, H. and REINER, J. M. (1942). Ionic permeability: An enzyme-like factor concerned in the migration of sodium through the cat erythrocyte membrane. *J. Cell. Comp. Physiol.* **20**, 325.

DE GIER, J. (1973). Comparisons between membrane model systems and erythrocyte membranes. *In* "Erythrocytes, Thrombocytes, Leukocytes" (E. Gerlach et al., eds), pp. 98–100. Georg Thieme, Stuttgart.

DEMENDONCA, M. C., SCHWARTZ, K. and TERRIER, E. (1970). Sodium, potassium and osmolality of human and canine erythrocytes—interest of trapped plasma and water and content for their full significance. *Comp. Biochem. Physiol.* **34**, 147.

DEUTICKE, B. (1967). Uber die Kinetik der Phosphat-Permeation in den Menschen-Erythrocyten bei Variation von extracellularer Phosphat-Konzentration, Anion-Mileu, und Zell-Volumen. *Pflügers Archiv.* **296**, 21.

DEUTICKE, B. (1974). Acetate transfer across mammalian red cell membranes: Evidence for two different pathways. *In* "Comparative Biochemistry and Physiology of Transport" (L. Bolis, K. Bloch, S. E. Luria and F. Lynen, eds), pp. 338–345. North-Holland, Amsterdam.

DEUTICKE, B. and GRUBER, W. (1970). Anion permeability of mammalian red blood cells: Possible relation to membrane phospholipid patterns. *Biochim. Biophys. Acta*, **211**, 369.

DEUTICKE, B. and GRUBER, W. (1972). Comparative studies on the anion permeability of mammalian red blood cells. *In* "VI Internationales Symposium über Struktur und Funktion der Erythrocyten", pp. 579–583. Akademia-Verlag, Berlin.

DUHM, J. (1974). Inosine permeability in erythrocytes of various mammalian species. *Biochim. Biophys. Acta*, **343**, 89.

ELFORD, B. C. (1975a). Interactions between temperature and tonicity on cation transport in dog red cells. *J. Physiol. (Lond.)*, **246**, 371.

ELFORD, B. C. (1975b). Independent routes for Na transport across dog red cell membranes. *Nature*, **256**, 580.

ELFORD, B. C. (1975c). Independent Na channels in the dog red cell membrane. *V. International Biophysics Congress, Copenhagen (Abstracts)*.

ELFORD, B. C. and SOLOMON, A. K. (1974a). Temperature dependence of cation permeability of dog red cells. *Nature*, **248**, 522.

ELFORD, B. C. and SOLOMON, A. K. (1974b). Factors influencing Na transport in dog cells. *Biochim. Biophys. Acta*, **373**, 253.

FORSTER, R. E. (1971). The transport of water in erythrocytes. In "Current Topics in Membranes and Transport" (F. Bronner and A. Kleinzeller, eds), vol. II, pp. 41–98. Academic Press, New York and London.

FRAZIER, H. S., SICULAR, A. and SOLOMON, A. K. (1954). Potassium uptake by the dog erythrocyte. *J. Gen. Physiol.* **37**, 631.

FUNDER, J. and WIETH, J. O. (1967). Effects of some monovalent anions on fluxes of Na and K, and on glucose metabolism of ouabain-treated human red cells. *Acta Physiol. Scand.* **71**, 168.

GÁRDOS, G. (1966). The mechanism of ion transport in human erythrocytes: The role of 2,3-Diphosphoglyceric acid in the regulation of potassium transport. *Act. Biochim. Biophys. Acad. Sci. Hung.* **1**, 139.

GARY-BOBO, C. M. and SOLOMON, A. K. (1968). Properties of hemoglobin solutions in red cells. *J. Gen. Physiol.* **52**, 825.

GOLDSTEIN, D. A. and SOLOMON, A. K. (1961). Determination of equivalent pore radius for human red cells by osmotic pressure measurement. *J. Gen. Physiol.* **44**, 1.

GREEFF, H. H., GROBECKER, H. and PEICHWOSKI, V. (1964). Membran ATPase und intrazellulärer Kationengehalt von Katzenerythrocyten. *Naturwissenschaften*, **51**, 42.

GUNN, R. B. (1972). A titrable carrier model for both mono- and di-valent anion transport in human red blood cells. In "Oxygen Affinity of Hemoglobin and Red Cell Acid-Base Status" (M. Rørth, and P. Astrup, eds), pp. 823–827. Munksgaard, Copenhagen.

GUNN, R. B., DALMARK, M., TOSTESON, D. C. and WIETH, J. O. (1973). Characteristics of chloride transport in human red blood cells. *J. Gen. Physiol.* **61**, 185.

GUPTA, J. D., PETERSON, V. J. and HARLEY, J. D. (1974). Erythrocyte ouabain-sensitive and ouabain-insensitive adenosine triphosphatase in various mammalian species. *Comp. Biochem. Physiol.* **47A**, 1123.

GUTHROW, C. E., ALLEN, J. E. and RASMUSSEN, H. (1972). Phosphorylation of an endogenous membrane protein by an endogenous, membrane-associated cyclic adenosine-3′,5′-monophosphate-dependent protein kinase in human erythrocyte ghosts. *J. Biol. Chem.* **247**, 8145.

HAEST, C. W. M. and DEUTICKE, B. (1975). Experimental alteration of phospholipid-protein interactions within the human erythrocyte membrane. Dependence on glycolytic metabolism. *Biochim. Biophys. Acta*, **401**, 468.

HAM, T. H., GRAVEL, J. A., DUNN, R. F., MURPHY, J. R., WHITE, J. G. and KELLERMEYER, R. W. (1973). Physical properties of red cells as related to effects *in vivo*: IV. Oxidant drugs producing abnormal intracellular concentration of hemoglobin (eccentrocytes) with a rigid-red-cell hemolytic syndrome. *J. Lab. Clin. Med.* **82**, 898.

HARKNESS, D. R., PONCE, J. and GRAYSON, V. (1969). A comparative study of the phosphoglyceric acid cycle in mammalian erythroctyes. *Comp. Biochem. Physiol.* **28**, 129.

HEGNAUER, A. H. and ROBINSON, E. J. (1936). The water and electrolyte distribution among plasma, red blood cells, and muscle after adrenalectomy. *J. Biol. Chem.* **116**, 769.

HEMPLING, H. G., STEWART, C. C. and GASIC, G. (1969). The effect of exogenous ATP on the electrolyte content of TA3 Ascites tumor cells. *J. Cell. Physiol.* **73**, 133.

HENRIQUES, V. and ØRSKOV, S. L. (1936). Untersuchungen über die Schwankungen des Kationgehaltes der roten Blutkörperchen. I. Die Änderung der Kaliumkonzentration in den Blutkörperchen nach einem Aderlass, nach Vergiftung mit Phenylhydrazin, und nach Einführung von destilliertem Wasser in die Blutbahn. *Skand. Archiv. Physiol.* **74**, 63.

HO, M. K. and GUIDOTTI, G. (1975). A membrane protein from human erythrocytes involved in anion exchange. *J. Biol. Chem.* **250**, 675.

HOFFMAN, J. F. (1966). The red cell membrane and the transport of sodium and potassium. *Amer. J. Med.* **41**, 666.

IAMPETRO, P. F., BURR, M. J., FIORICA, V., MCKENZIE, J. M. and HIGGINS, E. A. (1967). pH-dependent lysis of canine erythrocytes. *J. Appl. Physiol.* **23**, 505.

IAMPETRO, P. F., FIORICA, V., BURR, M. J. and MOSES, R. (1969). Hyperventilation-induced hemolysis in the dog. *Proc. Soc. Exp. Biol. Med.* **130**, 689.

ISRAEL, Y., MACDONALD, A., BERNSTEIN, J. and ROSENMANN, E. (1972). Changes from high potassium (HK) to low potassium (LK) in bovine red cells. *J. Gen. Physiol.* **59**, 270.

JACOBS, M. H., GLASSMAN, H. N. and PARPART, A. K. (1935). Osmotic properties of the erythrocyte VII. The temperature coefficients of certain hemolytic processes. *J. Cell. Comp. Physiol.* **7**, 197.

JULIANO, R. L., KIMELBERG, H. K. and PAPAHADJOPOULOS, D. (1971). Synergistic effects of a membrane protein (spectrin) and Ca on the Na permeability of phospholipid vesicles. *Biochim. Biophys. Acta*, **241**, 894.

KANEKO, J. J. (1974). Comparative erythrocyte metabolism. *Adv. Vet. Sci. Comp. Med.* **18**, 117.

KAPLAN, M. A., HAYS, L. and HAYS, R. M. (1974). Evolution of a facilitated diffusion pathway for amides in the erythrocyte. *Amer. J. Physiol.* **226**, 1327.

KERR, S. E. (1926a). Studies on the inorganic composition of blood. I. The effect of hemorrhage on the inorganic composition of serum and corpuscles. *J. Biol. Chem.* **67**, 689.

KERR, S. E. (1926b). Studies on the inorganic composition of blood. II. Changes in the potassium content of erythrocytes under certain experimental conditions. *J. Biol. Chem.* **67**, 721.

KLEINZELLER, A. (1972). Cellular transport of water. In "Metabolic Pathways. Vol. IV, Metabolic Transport" (L. E. Hokin, ed), p. 92. Academic Press, New York and London.

KNAUF, P. A. and ROTHSTEIN, A. (1971). Chemical modification of membranes. I. Effects of sulfhydryl and amino reactive reagents on anion and cation permeability of the human red blood cell. *J. Gen. Physiol.* **58**, 190.

KOBYLKA, D., KHETTRY, A., SHIN, B. C. and CARRAWAY, K. L. (1972). Proteins and glycoproteins for the erythrocyte membrane. *Arch. Biochem. Physiol.* **148**, 475.

KREGENOW, F. M. (1974). Functional separation of the Na–K exchange pump from the volume controlling mechanism in enlarged duck red cells. *J. Gen. Physiol.* **64**, 393.

KWANT, W. O. and SEEMAN, P. (1970). The erythrocyte ghost is a perfect osmometer. *J. Gen. Physiol.* **55**, 208.

LANGE, Y., LANGE, R. V. and SOLOMON, A. K. (1970). Cellular inhomogeneity in dog red cells as revealed by sodium flux. *J. Gen. Physiol.* **56**, 438.

LARIS, P. C. (1958). Permeability and utilization of glucose in mammalian erythrocytes. *J. Cell. Comp. Physiol.* **51**, 273.

LASSEN, U. V. (1972). Membrane potential and membrane resistance of red cells. *In* "Oxygen Affinity of Hemoglobin and Red Cell Acid Base Status" (M. Rørth and P. Astrup, eds), pp. 291–305. Academic Press, New York and London.

LEE, P., AUVIL, J., GREY, J. E., SMITH, M. (1976). 3-o-methyl glucose transport in new-born and adult dog red cells. *Fed. Proc.* **35**, 780.

LEE, P. and MILES, P. R. (1972). Density distribution and cation composition of red blood cells in newborn puppies. *J. Cell. Physiol.* **79**, 377.

LEE, P. and MILES, P. R. (1973). K and Na transport in erythrocytes of newborn puppies. *In* "Erythrocytes, Thrombocytes, Leukocytes" (E. Gerlach *et al.*, eds), pp. 105–108. Georg Thieme, Stuttgart.

LEW, V. L. (1971). On the ATP dependence of the Ca-induced increase in K permeability observed in human red cells. *Biochim. Biophys. Acta*, **233**, 827.

LONG, C. and MOUAT, B. (1971). The binding of calcium ions by erythrocytes and "ghost cell" membranes. *Biochem. J.* **123**, 829.

LUBIN, M. (1967). Intracellular potassium and macromolecular synthesis in mammalian cells. *Nature*, **213**, 451.

MACEY, R. I. and FARMER, R. E. L. (1970). Inhibition of water and solute permeability in human red cells. *Biochim. Biophys. Acta*, **211**, 104.

MACEY, R. I., KARAN, D. M. and FARMER, R. E. L. (1972). Properties of water channels in human red cells. *In* "Biomembranes, Vol. 3: Passive Permeability of Cell Membranes", pp. 331–340. Plenum Press, New York and London.

MAUK, A. G., WHELAN, H. T. and TAKETA, F. (1974). "Holly wreath" morphology of feline erythrocytes. The effects of cyanate and 4,4'-dipyridylsulfide. *Proc. Soc. Exp. Biol. Med.* **145**, 578.

MCMANUS, T. J. (1974). Alternate pathways for metabolism: A comparative view. *In* "The Human Red Cell in Vitro" (T. J. Greenwalt and G. A. Jamieson, eds), pp. 49–63. Grune and Stratton, New York.

MENTZER, W. C., BAEHNER, R. L., SCHMIDT-SCHÖNBEIN, H., ROBINSON, S. H. and NATHAN, D. G. (1971). Selective reticulocyte destruction in erythrocyte pyruvate kinase deficiency. *J. Clin. Invest.* **50**, 688.

MILES, P. R. and LEE, P. (1972). Sodium and potassium content and membrane transport properties in red blood cells from newborn puppies. *J. Cell. Physiol.* **79**, 367.

NAKAO, M., NAKAO, T. and YAMAZOE, S. (1960). Adenosine triphosphate and the maintenance of shape of the human red cells. *Nature*, **187**, 945.

OMACHI, A., MARKEL, R. P. and HEGARTY, H. (1961). Ca-45 uptake by dog erythrocytes suspended in sodium and potassium chloride solutions. *J. Cell. Comp. Physiol.* **57**, 95.

ORRINGER, E. O. and PARKER, J. C. (1973). Ion and water movements in red blood cells. *In* "Progress in Hematology" (E. Brown, ed), vol. VIII. Grune and Stratton, New York.

Oski, F. A., Naiman, J. L., Blum, S. F. Zarkowsky, H. S., Whaun, J., Shohet, S. B., Green, A., Nathan, D. G. (1969). Congenital hemolytic anemia with high sodium low potassium red cells. *New Eng. J. Med.* **280**, 909.

Park, C. R., Crofford, O. B. and Kono, T. (1968). Mediated (nonactive) transport of glucose in mammalian cells and its regulation. *J. Gen. Physiol.* **52**, 296s.

Parker, J. C. (1969). Influence of 2,3-diphosphoglycerate metabolism on sodium-potassium permeability in human red blood cells: Studies with bisulfite and other redox agents. *J. Clin. Invest.* **48**, 117.

Parker, J. C. (1971). Ouabain-sensitive effects of metabolism on ion and water content of red blood cells. *Amer. J. Physiol.* **221**, 338.

Parker, J. C. (1973a). Dog red blood cells: Adjustment of density *in vivo. J. Gen. Physiol.* **61**, 146.

Parker, J. C. (1973b). Dog red blood cells: Adjustment of salt and water content *in vivo. J. Gen. Physiol.* **62**, 147.

Parker, J. C. (1973c). Volume regulation in dog red blood cells. In "Erythrocytes, Thrombocytes, Leukocytes" (E. Gerlach *et al.*, eds), pp. 109–111. Georg Thieme, Stuttgart.

Parker, J. C. (1974). Calcium-dependent volume regulation by dog red blood cells. *Fed. Proc.* **33**, 266a.

Parker, J. C., Gitelman, H. J., Glosson, P. S. and Leonard, D. L. (1975). Role of calcium in volume regulation by dog red blood cells. *J. Gen. Physiol.* **65**, 84.

Parker, J. C. and Hoffman, J. F. (1965). Interdependence of cation permeability, cell volume, and metabolism in dog red blood cells. *Fed. Proc.* **24**, 589.

Parker, J. C. and Hoffman, J. F. (1976). Influences of cell volume and adrenalectomy on cation flux in dog red blood cells. *Biochim. Biophys. Acta.* **433**, 404.

Parker, J. C. and Snow, R. L. (1972). Influence of external ATP on permeability and metabolism of dog red blood cells. *Amer. J. Physiol.* **223**, 888.

Passo, T., Atkinson, K. and Manfridi, F. (1971). Effect of acute respiratory acid-base alterations and inorganic phosphate infusion on red cell 2,3-diphosphoglycerate and P50 in dogs. *J. Lab. Clin. Med.* **78**, 1010.

Passow, H. and Schnell, K. F. (1969). Chemical modifiers of passive ion permeability of the erythrocyte membrane. *Experientia (Basel)*, **25**, 460.

Pinkerton, P. H., Fletch, S. M., Bruekner, P. J. and Miller, D. R. (1974). Hereditary stomatocytosis with hemolytic anemia in the dog. *Blood*, **44**, 557.

Podolsky, R. J. (1959). Membrane geometry and sodium permeability of the cat erythrocyte. *Fed. Proc.* **18**, 121.

Poznansky, M. and Solomon, A. K. (1972). Regulation of human red cell volume by linked cation fluxes. *J. Membrane Biol.* **10**, 259.

Prankerd, T. A. J. (1961). "The Red Cell", chap. X. Blackwell, Oxford.

Rangachari, P. K., Daniel, E. E. and Paton, M. (1973). Regulation of cellular volume in rat myometrium. *Biochim. Biophys. Acta*, **323**, 297.

Redwood, W. R., Rall, E. and Perl, W. (1974). Red cell membrane permeability deduced from bulk diffusion coefficients. *J. Gen. Physiol.* **64**, 706.

Rega, A. F., Richards, D. E. and Garrahan, P. J. (1974). The effects of Ca on ATPase and phosphatase activities of erythrocyte membranes. *Ann. N.Y. Acad. Sci.* **242**, 317.

Reuter, H. and Seitz, N. (1968). Dependence of calcium efflux from cardiac muscle on temperature and external ion composition. *J. Physiol. (Lond.)*, **195**, 451.

Rich, G. T., Sha'afi, R. I., Barton, T. C. and Solomon, A. K. (1967). Permeability studies on red cell membranes of dog, cat, and beef. *J. Gen. Physiol.* **50**, 2391.

RICH, G. T., SHA'AFI, R. I., ROMUALDEZ, A. and SOLOMON, A. K. (1968). Effect of osmolality on the hydraulic permeability coefficient of red cells. *J. Gen. Physiol.* **52**, 941.

ROBIN, E. D., MURDAUGH, H. V., CROSS, C. E., SMITH, J. and THEODORE, J. (1971). Cation transport and energy metabolism in the high Na, low K erythrocyte of the harbor seal, Phoca vitulina. *Comp. Biochem. Physiol.* **39A**, 807.

ROBINSON, D. R. and JENKS, W. P. (1965). The effect of concentrated salt solutions on the activity coefficient of acetyltetraglycine ethyl ester. *J. Am. Chem. Soc.* **87**, 2470.

ROBINSON, E. J. and HEGNAUER, A. H. (1936). The water and electrolyte distribution between plasma and red blood cells following intraperitoneal injections of isotonic glucose. *J. Biol. Chem.* **116**, 779.

ROGERS, T. A. (1961). The exchange of radioactive magnesium in erythrocytes of several species. *J. Cell. Comp. Physiol.* **57**, 119.

ROMUALDEZ, A. G. and SHA'AFI, R. I. (1975). The effect of ATP on sodium and potassium transport in dog erythrocytes. *Fed. Proc.* **34**, 237a.

ROMUALDEZ, A., SHA'AFI, R. I., LANGE, Y. and SOLOMON, A. K. (1972). Cation transport in dog red cells. *J. Gen. Physiol.* **60**, 46.

RORIVE, G. and KLEINZELLER, A. (1972). The effect of ATP and Ca on the cell volume in isolated kidney tubules. *Biochim. Biophys. Acta*, **274**, 226.

RORIVE, G., NIELSEN, R. and KLEINZELLER, A. (1972). Effect of pH on the water and electrolyte content of renal cells. *Biochim. Biophys. Acta*, **266**, 376.

ROUSER, G. R., NELSON, G. J., FLEISCHER, S. and SIMON, G. (1968). Lipid composition of animal cell membranes, organelles, and organs. *In* "Biological Membranes, Physical Fact and Function" (D. Chapman, ed), pp. 5–70. Academic Press, New York and London.

SCHATZMANN, H. J. and VINCENZI, F. F. (1969). Calcium movements across the membrane of human red cells. *J. Physiol. (Lond.)*, **201**, 369.

SCHMIDT, W. (1975). Co-transport of sodium plus potassium in duck red cells. Ph.D. Thesis, Duke University, Durham, North Carolina.

SCHWOCH, G. and PASSOW, H. (1973). Preparation and properties of human erythrocyte ghosts. *Molec. and Cell. Biochem.* **2**, 197.

SEARCY, G. P., MILLER, D. R. and TASKER, J. B. (1971). Congenital hemolytic anemia in the basenji dog due to erythrocyte pyruvate kinase deficiency. *Can. J. Compar. Med.* **35**, 67.

SHA'AFI, R. I. (1965). Kinetics of ion movements across the cell membrane of cat erythrocytes and the phenomenon of active transport. PhD Thesis, University of Illinois, Urbana.

SHA'AFI, R. I., GARY-BOBO, C. M. and SOLOMON, A. K. (1971). Permeability of red cell membranes to small hydrophilic and lipophilic solutes. *J. Gen. Physiol.* **58**, 238.

SHA'AFI, R. I. and HAJJAR, J. J. (1971). Sodium movement in high sodium feline red cells. *J. Gen. Physiol.* **57**, 684.

SHA'AFI, R. I. and LEIB, W. R. (1967). Cation movements in the high sodium erythrocyte of the cat. *J. Gen. Physiol.* **50**, 1751.

SHA'AFI, R. I. and NACCACHE, P. (1975). Sodium and calcium transport in cat red cells. *J. Cell. Physiol.* **85**, 655.

SHA'AFI, R. I. and PASCOE, E. (1972). Sulfate flux in high sodium cat red cells. *J. Gen. Physiol.* **59**, 155.

SHA'AFI, R. I. and PASCOE, E. (1973). Further studies of sodium transport in feline red cells. *J. Gen. Physiol.* **61**, 709.

SHEPPARD, C. W., MARTIN, W. R. and BEYL, G. (1951). Cation exchange between cells and plasma of mammalian blood. *J. Gen. Physiol.* **34**, 411.

SMITH, J. E. (1974). Relationship of *in vivo* erythrocyte glutathione flux to the oxidized glutathione transport system. *J. Lab. Clin. Med.* **83**, 444.

SOLOMON, A. K. (1968). Characterization of biological membranes by equivalent pores. *J. Gen. Physiol.* **51**, 335s.

SORENSON, A. L., KIRSCHNER, L. B. and BARKER, J. (1962). Sodium fluxes in the erythrocytes of swine, ox, and dog. *J. Gen. Physiol.* **45**, 1031.

SPACH, C. and STREETEN, D. H. P. (1964). Retardation of sodium exchange in dog erythrocytes by physiological concentrations of aldosterone *in vitro*. *J. Clin. Invest.* **43**, 217.

SRIVASTAVA, S. K. and BEUTLER, E. (1969a). The transport of oxidized glutathione from human erythrocytes. *J. Biol. Chem.* **244**, 9.

SRIVASTAVA, S. K. and BEUTLER, E. (1969b). The transport of oxidized glutathione from the erythrocytes of various species in the presence of chromate. *Biochem. J.* **114**, 833.

STEIN, W. D. (1964). Facilitated diffusion. *In* "Recent Progress in Surface Science" (J. F. Danelli, K. G. A. Parkhurst and A. C. Riddiford, eds), vol. I, pp. 300–337. Academic Press, New York and London.

STREETEN, D. H. P. and MOSES, A. M. (1968). Action of cortisol on sodium transport in canine erythrocytes. *J. Gen. Physiol.* **52**, 356.

SUELTER, C. H. (1970). Enzymes activated by monovalent cations. *Science*, **168**, 789.

TORRANCE, J. D. (1973). Erythrocyte 2,3-DPG in various mammalian species. *In* "Erythrocytes, Thrombocytes, Leukocytes" (E. Gerlach *et al.*, eds), pp. 161–164. Georg Thieme, Stuttgart.

TOSTESON, D. C., GUNN, R. B. and WIETH, J. O. (1973). Chloride and hydroxyl ion conductance of sheep red cell membrane. *In* "Erythrocytes, Thrombocytes, Leukocytes" (E. Gerlach *et al.*, eds), pp. 62–66. Georg Thieme, Stuttgart.

VIEIRA, F. L., SHA'AFI, R. I. and SOLOMON, A. K. (1970). The state of water in human and dog red cell membranes. *J. Gen. Physiol.* **55**, 451.

VILLEGAS, R., BARTON, T. C. and SOLOMON, A. K. (1958). The entrance of water into beef and dog red cells. *J. Gen. Physiol.* **42**, 355.

VON HIPPEL, P. H. and WONG, K-Y. (1964). Neutral salts: The generality of their effects on the stability of macromolecular conformations. *Science*, **145**, 577.

WADDELL, W. J. (1956). Lysis of dog erythrocytes in mildly alkaline isotonic media. *Amer. J. Physiol.* **186**, 339.

WESSELS, J. M. C. and VEERKAMP, J. H. (1973). Some aspects of the osmotic lysis of erythrocytes. III. Comparison of glycerol permeability and lipid composition of red blood cell membranes from eight mammalian species. *Biochim. Biophys. Acta*, **291**, 190.

WHITTAM, R. (1964). "Transport and Diffusion in Red Blood Cells". Edward Arnild, London.

WIDDAS, W. F. (1955). Hexose permeability of foetal erythrocytes. *J. Physiol.* **127**, 318.

WIETH, J. O. (1970a). Paradoxical temperature dependence of sodium and potassium fluxes in human red cells. *J. Physiol.* **207**, 563.

WIETH, J. O. (1970b). Effect of some monovalent anions on chloride and sulfate permeability of human red blood cells. *J. Physiol.* **207**, 581.

WIETH, J. O. (1970c). Effects of monovalent cations on sodium permeability of human red cells. *Acta Physiol. Scand.* **79**, 76.

WIETH, J. O. (1971). Effects of hexoses and anions on the erythritol permeability of human red cells. *J. Physiol.* **213**, 435.

WIETH, J. O., DALMARK, M., GUNN, R. B. and TOSTESON, D. C. (1973). The transfer of monovalent inorganic anions through the red cell membrane. *In* "Erythrocytes, Thrombocytes, Leukocytes" (E. Gerlach *et al.*, eds), pp. 71–76. Georg Thieme, Stuttgart.

WIETH, J. O., FUNDER, J., GUNN, R. B. and BRAHM, J. (1974). Passive transport pathways for chloride and urea through the red cell membrane. *In* "Comparative Biochemistry and Physiology of Transport" (L. Bolis, K. Bloch, S. E. Luria and F. Lynen, eds), pp. 317–337. North-Holland, Amsterdam.

WILBRANDT, W. (1938). Die Permeabilität der roten Blutkörperchen für einfache Zucker. *Pflügers Archiv.* **241**, 302.

YANNET, H., DARROW, D. C. and CARY, M. K. (1935–6). The effect of changes in the composition of plasma electrolytes on the concentration of electrolytes in the red blood cells of dogs, monkeys, and rabbits. *J. Biol. Chem.* **112**, 477.

YAWATA, Y., HOWE, R., HEBBEL, R., SILVIS, S., CHANG, S., HAUSER, A. and JACOB, H. (1972). Hyperalimentation hypophosphatemia: a new hematoligic-neurologic syndrome. *Blood*, **40**, 943a.

YAWATA, Y., HEBBEL, R. P., SILVIS, S., HOWE, R. and JACOB, H. (1974). Blood cell abnormalities complicating the hypophosphatemia of hyperalimentation: erythrocyte and platelet ATP deficiency associated with hemolytic anemia and bleeding in hyperalimented dogs. *J. Lab. Clin. Med.* **84**, 643.

Index

A
A-system, 319
A23187, 56, 57, 59, 66, 89, 95, 166, 452
accelerative exchange diffusion, 312
acetamide, 243, 390
acetazolamide, 201, 202
aceturate, 205
acetylcholine, 106
actin, 54
adenyl cyclase, 386
ADH, 241
adrenal steroids, 456
alkylosis, 456
alkyltrimethylammonium compounds, 106
allosteric inhibition, 23
amino acid transport, 301–23, 395–6, 433
   inhibitors, 319
   kinetics, 308–15
   Na-dependence, 307–8
   temperature effects, 309
ammonium chloride lysis, 132
Amphiuma red cells, 96, 97, 130, 140, 142, 177–8, 420
   effect of nucleus, 147
   membrane resistance, 178
amphotericin B, 235, 244
amyl alcohol, 239
anaesthetics, 239
anion distribution, oxygen effects, 119
anion transport, 115–35, 137–40, 147–53, 175–92, 197–218, 389, 443–4
   activation energy, 179, 215
   conductance, 177–80
   exchange, 177–80, 181, 201
   inhibitors, 182, 201–2
   kinetic models, 180–2
   pH effects, 119–33, 181, 216
anisocytosis, 354
ANS, 149, 179, 182–5
APMB, 185
ASC system, 316, 323, 395–6
ATP–ADP exchange, 9
ATP binding, 12
ATPase, 22–3, 346, 353 (*see also* Ca ATPase; sodium pump)

B
beryllium, 22
benzene sulphonate, 205, 208
benzoate, 204
benzol, 239
benzyl alcohol, 109
6-O-benzyl-D-galactose, 281
B-system, 395
black lipid membranes, 160, 169, 233, 235, 241–2
Bohr effect, 121
buffaloes, 363

C
caesium influx, 23
calcium ATPase, 89, 453
calcium binding, 64
calcium buffering, cytoplasmic, 58–62
calcium–calcium exchange, 66, 80, 452
calcium content of red cells, 167, 168
calcium-dependent K-channels, 54, 93–9, 139, 165–6, 349
calcium effect on membrane potential, 165–6
calcium effect on water fluxes, 239
calcium efflux, 73–84, 86–7, 357–8
calcium pump, 54, 166, 349, 356, 452
   inhibitors, 56
   lability, 55
calcium–sodium exchange, 73
calcium transport, 53–90
calcium uptake, 85, 335–6
   ATP depleted, 63
   monovalent cation effects, 71
   temperature dependence, 86
calves, new born, 378
carbachol, 106
carbocyanine dyes, 149
carbon dioxide, 115–16, 175
carbonic acid, 124
carbonic anhydrase, 115, 125, 126, 127, 175, 199
   inhibitors, 214, 215
cardiac glycosides, 3
cat, 138, 228, 258, 427, 457
catalytic centre activity, 11, 12
catecholamines, 392, 416–18
cattle, 46, 228, 363–80, 428, 431
cell water, 221–39, 399
chloride–bicarbonate exchange, 116, 117, 128
chloride conductance, 139, 160–2, 165, 178
   distribution ratio, 140, 146, 397
   hydroxyl exchange, 124, 202
chlormedrin, 277
chloroform, 239

chlorpromazine, 169, 184, 185, 266, 267, 280, 452
cholera toxin, 418
cholesterol, 234–5, 244, 347
choline transport, 99–114
Christiansen's allosteric model, 110
chronic acidosis, 121
citric acid cycle, 388
colchicine, 448
collodion membranes, 176, 197, 198
cyclic AMP, 241, 416–18
cysteine system, 322, 323, 324
cytochalasin, 258, 275, 276, 277, 285

D
DAS, 185
decamethonium, 109
diamide, 320, 328
dicarboxylic acids, 205
dicyclohexylcarbodiimide, 22, 23
DIDS, 187–8, 241
dimethyladipidate, 343
1,3-dimethylurea, 243
dinitrophenol, 204, 392
di-O-C_6, 149
dipyridimole, 148, 182, 189, 214
di-S-C_3, 130, 132, 149, 401, 412
DNFB, 187–8
dog red cells 121, 138, 228, 232, 234, 258, 427–457
2,3-DPG, 121, 122, 388, 430, 442
double membrane effects, 238

E
echinocytes, 182, 184
Eilam's modified tetramer model, 271–3
electro-diffusional leak, 42, 46
electrophoretic mobility, 386
electrostatic effects, 185–6
elliptocytosis, 354
enthalpy of glucose binding, 278–9
erythritol, 265, 389, 432, 445
ethacrynic acid, 215, 343
ethyl alcohol, 239
exchangeable anions, 117, 118
external sodium site of pump, 23–5

F
F(ab), 377
FDNB, 109, 110, 275, 276, 294
filtration coefficient, 228
fish red cells, 390, 420
fixed charge hypothesis, 176
fluorescent probes, 130, 132, 149, 177, 182, 183, 187–9, 401, 412
fluoride, 97, 333, 442,
fluoroglucose derivatives, 274
foetal cells, 436
formamide, 243
formate, 207

freeze-fracture experiments, 222
friction coefficients, 229
fructose, 265, 295
furseimide, 97, 215, 338, 342–3

G
γ-glutamyl cycle, 303, 319
γ-glutamyl transpeptidase, 327
galactose, 264, 265, 274
Gardos effect (see calcium-dependent K channels)
Geck's asymmetric carrier model, 267–70, 272
glucose carrier, 391–2
  diffusion coefficient, 266
  metabolism, 387, 390
glucose-6-P-dehydrogenase deficient cells, 332
glucose oxidase, 282
glutathione, 301, 327–35
  deficiency, 303, 305, 307, 311, 319, 320
  turnover rate, 327
glycerol, 228, 389, 432
glycine transport, 309, 313
glycolysis, 387, 442, 447
glycophorin, 240, 241
goats, 363–80
Goldman equation, 173, 177
Gouy–Chapman equation, 186
gramicidin, 128, 129, 177, 395
ground permeability to K, 42, 46
GSSG, 328–34
  transport, 321, 328–9, 397
  inhibitors, 333
  kinetics, 333

H
haemoglobin, 15, 176, 181, 282, 283, 328, 334, 342, 388, 456
  carbamino groups, 124
  CO_2 binding, 120, 121
  Hammersmith, 354
  osmotic coefficient, 123
  viscosity, 283
haemolysis, in ammonium salts, 199
  time, 226–7
haemolytic anaemia, 354, 456
halide fluxes by flow apparatus, 179
Hamburger shift, 138
Heinz bodies, 456
hemicholinium HC 3, 103, 106, 112
Henderson regime, 141
hereditary spherocytosis, 350–4
hereditary stomatocytosis, 339–49, 457
hexose monophosphate shunt, 387
HK cells, 363, 404
hippurate, 205
Haldane effect, 119
H site, sugar transport, 268
hydrophilic pore, 240
hydroxyl concentration ratio, 116
hydroxyl conductance, 165, 199

INDEX

I
inosine, 50, 63, 332
insulin, 267, 277, 280
internal K inhibition, 24, 366–71
interorgan transport, 322
intracellular pH (DMO method), 147
iodoacetamide, 63, 94, 442

J
Jacobs–Stewart cycle, 131, 132
junction potentials, 141

K
kinetics
  amino acid transport, 308–16
  anion exchange, 179–81
  choline transport, 102–6
  GSSG transport, 333
  HK and LK cells, 365–71
  sodium pump, 27, 29–32, 365–71
  sugar transport, 258–93
"kinks" hypothesis, 242

L
lactate permeability, 215, 216
lamb red cells, 372
L-antigen, 364, 375–6
lattice pore theory, 265–7, 270
lead, 97
leak potential, 144
Lefevre's introverting hemiport model, 270, 272
leucine transport, 395
lipid bilayers, 160, 169, 183, 235, 241–2, 305, 306
liquid ion exchange membranes, 178
lithium, 4, 23, 27, 48, 111, 448
LK cells, 364-82
local anaesthetics, 169, 182
long pore effect, 259
LP system, 395
L site, sugar transport, 268
lung capillaries, 175
lyotropic agents, 443–5
Ly$^+$ system, 318, 319

M
malate, 205
maleic anhydride, 187
mannose, 264, 265, 274
M antigen, 364, 375–6
membrane calcium, 359
membrane capacitance, 153–4
membrane lipids, 228, 354, 375, 430
membrane potential, 130, 137–70
  Amphiuma red cells, 141–7
  avian cells, 410–12
  definition, 133
  human cells, 142–3, 146
  semantics, 173–4
methaemoglobin, 115, 116
3-O-methyl glucose, 391
microcytosis, 354
microelectrode studies, 140–2
microtubules, 385
MNT, 187–8
mobile carrier kinetics, 264–5

N
Naftalin's pore model, 110
narcotics, 446
NEM, 22, 106, 108, 109, 327–8, 320
nitrene labelling, 190
NMR method for water, 224
nonelectrolytes
  H bonding, 244
  lipid solubility, 243
  molar volume, 244
  temperature effects, 245–6
  steric effects, 244
norepinephrine, 400, 407, 409, 410, 414, 417–18
nuclear volume, 147, 384
nucleoside transport, 436
nystatin, 152, 180, 244, 364, 375

O
OH transport, 132
oligomycin, 9, 10, 97
o-phenanthroline, 218
organic anions, 179, 197–18
osmotic coefficient, 228
osmotic flow equation, 226
ouabain, 17–22, 97, 346, 364, 371, 402
oxalate exchange, 212, 216
oxygen transport, 115

P
PAH, 161, 205
passive cation transport, 40–2, 46–50, 338, 339, 342-2 436, 448
Patlack's "gate" model, 110
PCMBS, 56, 106, 152, 179, 187, 236, 241, 247, 248, 249, 277, 280, 320, 364, 403, 433
permeability coefficient, equation, 226
  lipophilic molecules, 242–3
pH, 115–33
  effects on water transport, 239
  effects on Cl transport, 147, 161
phenylalanine transport, 395
phloretin, 148, 169, 182, 183, 184, 186, 190, 218, 247, 248, 249, 251, 252, 269, 275, 279, 282, 284, 433, 446
phloridzin, 148, 169, 214, 218
phosphate fluxes, 179, 181, 251, 435
phosphoglycerate kinase, 442
phytic acid, 387, 388
PMR studies, 285
PNPPase, 15–17, 372
polar pore model, 289
polycythaemia vera, 89
potassium, congeners, 26
  influx, 2, 23, 42, 369, 438
  permeability Ca effects (*see* calcium-dependent K channels)
  exchange, 7, 14, 41, 42, 44–5, 49

potential-sensitive fluorescent dyes, 149–52
pronase, 188–9, 241
propranolol, 418
6-O-propyl-D-glucose, 281
protein band 3, 240, 282, 285
pump II, 39, 48
puppies, 428, 439, 449
pyridoxal phosphate, 179, 187–8
pyruvate kinase, 428
  deficiency, 354, 457
pyruvate kinetics, 216, 218

Q

quinine, 97
quinidine, 97

R

rapid mixing technique, 11, 223
rat red cells, 23, 46, 48
red cell, ATP effects, 58, 63
  bound water, 123, 124
  calcium content, 56, 57, 58–63, 357
  deformability, 141
  Donnan effects, 117
  lifespan, 89, 348
  lipid composition, 55, 88, 90, 347, 350, 433
  shape, 142, 182, 184, 185
  storage, 55
Regan and Tarpley's mobile carrier model, 271–2
resealed ghosts, 96, 97
reticulocytes, 347–8, 372–4, 428, 456–7
  amino acid transport, 316–19
reversible haemolysis, 55
ribose, 265
rubidium influx, 23, 49

S

salicylate, 56, 179, 204
sheep, 138, 157, 159, 258, 302, 303, 305, 336, 363, 380, 436, 449
SH reactive agents, 235–6, 392, 432 (see also PCMBS)
shrinking and swelling, 225–6
sialic acid, 187
simultaneous models, 28
SITS, 187–8, 199, 200, 202, 212, 216
sodium ATPase, 12, 14
sodium-dependent amino acid transport, 393–4
sodium fluxes, 3, 8, 23, 45–50, 409, 441, 442, 438
sodium-potassium, ATPase, 22, 364, 366, 386, 449
  cotransport, 43, 338, 414, 439
  stoichiometry of exchange, 4–5
sodium pump, 1–37, 40–1, 45–6, 97, 241 337–8, 365–80, 405, 408, 428
  antibodies to, 8, 17
  avian red cells, 398–9
  calcium inhibition, 90
  circular carrier model, 27
  coupling ratio, 152, 348

dog red cells, 449
EPR and PRR studies, 30
external affinity, 6
flip-flop model, 28
fluxes ouabain-poisoned, 48–50
half the sites reactivity, 28
independence of sites, 25
involvement with Gardos channel, 98
ion selectivity, 29
kinetic models, 25–7
mechanical models, 27
membrane potential contribution, 152
HK and LK cells, 365
ouabain inhibition, 40
partial reactions, 9–23, 371–4
passive K exchange, 41
phosphorylation, 9
stoichiometry, 29
structure, 28
sodium–sodium exchange, 7, 10, 25, 45, 348, 365, 440, 452
solvent drag effect, 231–2
sorbose, 273, 279, 281, 294–5
sphingomyelin, 306
spleen, erythrostasis theory, 354
stilbene disulphonate derivatives, 188
stomatocytes, 182, 339–49
stop-flow technique, 224
substituted phenols, 169
sugar transport, 191, 257–96, 390–3, 434, 436
  classical kinetics, 258–9
  competitive inhibition, 258
  counterflow, 258–9, 262, 292
  pH dependence, 279–80
  specificity, 273–5
  temperature effects, 277–9
sulphate transport, 178, 179, 188, 198, 215, 235, 407, 435
sulphonamides, 182, 204
surface potential, 185
synaptosomes, 112

T

tannic acid, 239, 248, 249, 389, 448
target cells, 340
tartrate, 205
tetramer model, Lieb and Stein, 28, 110, 267, 272
tetramethylammonium, 101, 106, 109
tetrodotoxin, 239
thalassaemia, 354
thallium, 23
thiourea, 251, 389, 390
thiocyanate, 445
tributyl phosphate membranes, 230
TNC, 56
TNBS, 187–8
two-compartment tracer diffusion, 223–4

U

Uncoupled sodium efflux, 8, 17
unstirred layers, 159–60, 229, 265, 266, 27
urea, 243, 248–52, 389, 390, 432

V

valinomycin, 128, 149, 169, 170, 177, 186, 239
volume regulation, 399
volume regulatory decrease (VRD), 400–7, 419–20
volume regulatory increase (VRI), 407–10, 419–20

W

Water fluxes, temperature dependence, 232
  activation energies, 233
  permeability, 221–53, 396, 431–3

X

xylose efflux, 185

Z

zero-*trans* entry and exit, 268, 280
zeta potential, 119
zinc, 446